An Atlas for the

CLINICAL USE OF THE MMPI

AN ATLAS FOR THE Clinical Use of the MMPI

by

STARKE R. HATHAWAY

and

PAUL E. MEEHL

THE UNIVERSITY OF MINNESOTA PRESS · MINNEAPOLIS

Published by the University of Minnesota Press,
2037 University Avenue Southeast, Minneapolis, MN 55414
Printed in the United States of America.
Sixth printing, 1980

ISBN 0-8166-0070-8

Acknowledgments

No publication of this kind is possible through the activities of two persons alone. We well recognize that what is contained in this *Atlas* represents in only a small part the product of our own efforts. The entire staff of the University of Minnesota Hospitals Psychiatric Unit contributed materially, as did many psychiatric residents and other students in training.

Our greatest debt is to Dr. Burtrum C. Schiele, who was chief of the inpatient services during the whole period covered by the cases included in the *Atlas*. His supervision assured a high level of staff thinking and of responsibility for the patient. As chiefs of the clinical staff and heads of the Department of Psychiatry and Neurology, Dr. J. C. McKinley until his retirement and then Dr. D. W. Hastings made the whole work possible through their encouragement of the research attitude and their active cooperation in the many administrative and advisory details that ensure the collection of complicated research material.

In the actual preparation of this volume we owe greatest recognition to the Graduate School of the University of Minnesota, which generously granted funds for the collection of data, the coding of the MMPI profiles, and innumerable other details that are the core of the contribution. The graduate assistants, clerical workers, and typists who have performed this work have at times seemed to be the only reality it had. Marie Ford and Virginia Hathaway edited, and often reshaped, the first rough copies of the shortened case histories in order to give them acceptable style.

Although all these persons and others bore the brunt of the preparation of the manuscript, its final form is our product, and, humble in recognizing the aid we have received, we accept full responsibility for all imperfections.

STARKE R. HATHAWAY
PAUL E. MEEHL

Table of Contents

MAKING, DESCRIPTION, AND USE OF THE *ATLAS*

The Making of the *Atlas*

This *Atlas* was prepared as a case history handbook for professional users of the Minnesota Multiphasic Personality Inventory. It is not a manual telling how to administer and score the Inventory. Neither is it a compendium of present clinical practices or of experimental and scientific findings relative to the use of the Inventory. It is assumed that the user of the *Atlas* will have had experience with the MMPI and will understand the terminology peculiar to it. If he is not already familiar with the literature on the subject, he should read at least the starred articles in the appended bibliography.

The *Atlas* was compiled to provide a reference book that might serve to recall similar cases from the user's own experience by a kind of "consultative" looking up of cases with MMPI patterns similar to the one being considered. Designed, then, to present a representative cross section of clinical experience with the MMPI, the *Atlas* is chiefly a collection of 968 short case histories (458 from males and 510 from females) with the associated MMPI profiles. We have called the collection an "Atlas" because we are chiefly concerned with presenting to the reader clinical information pertinent to the interpretation of the *form* (the *shape*), of MMPI profiles. To a lesser extent the *intensity* (elevation) of the profiles is also stressed, but the main emphasis is on the form. We have called the collection an "Atlas for Clinical Use" because it is intended primarily for use in the clinical situation. The histories are all of persons who were under clinical (although not necessarily medical) examination.

Source of the Cases

The great majority of the persons whose records are in the *Atlas* were seen as inpatients in the Psychiatric Unit of the University of Minnesota Hospitals from about a year after its opening in 1937 up to 1949. The Psychiatric Unit was established by the state legislature as an integral part of the University Hospitals to serve as a special observational and diagnostic unit for mental cases from the state of Minnesota. In addition to its service and research functions, it provides clinical material utilized in teaching the principles and practices of psychiatry to medical students and others engaging in such study. Most of the patients are not held for more than a month. Only a few, considered necessary for teaching, may stay in the hospital for extended periods, during which they receive intensive psychotherapy or extensive physical and other investigations that may be pertinent to proper diagnostic understanding of their disorders.

The patients come from four general sources. Some are referred by family physicians for evaluation and therapy. Others are more severely disturbed patients sent from civic agencies for observation and evaluation, sometimes preceding their review by a sanity commission for commitment to a state hospital, at other times before returning to a state hospital after having been out for a time. Other persons are referred by courts of the state for evaluation and recommendation before disposition by the court. Still others come from various state institutions—reform schools, prisons, and the like—because they have been found to behave in ways that seem definitely to indicate the need for special study.

In economic and other ways the patients probably represent a good cross section of those among the population of the state who are psychologically ill and get psychiatric help. The great majority of the patients are partially subsidized in their hospitalization by the county or from state funds available to the Psychiatric Unit. Some are private patients, however, and not a few are rather prominent in their communities.

In this connection it should be understood that the case histories in this *Atlas* are deliberately blurred so as to assure the patients of anonymity. Occupational and other details have been changed, so that any seeming resemblance to particular individuals is coincidental.

The staff of the Psychiatric Unit is large compared to the number of inpatients, as is properly the case where teaching and research are important functions. The staff is conventionally complete, including as professional members full-time psychiatrists, psychologists, social workers, neurologists, nurses, and occupational therapists. Most of these staff members are also concerned with the operation of a large outpatient clinic for psychiatry and neurology, where many of the patients described in the *Atlas* received follow-up treatment or were studied before admission.

If it seems to the reader that study of an individual was often too brief or lacking in many elements, that therapy was hardly extensive enough, or that patients having good chances of recovery were sent to a state hospital, it should be remembered that the material presented was drawn from a working unit where there was a real press of patients and the staff had to concentrate its efforts where they could be utilized most effectively. For any patient discharged or transferred, another was always awaiting admission. We can only hope that testing devices such as the MMPI will increase efficiency so that with augmented staffs and public support many more of this type of patient can be studied more efficiently and completely, and above all in greater and greater numbers receive more therapeutic aid.

Drawing the case material of the *Atlas* from a single psychiatric service may well have emphasized regional factors in the clinical trends shown. This undesirable emphasis has been mitigated in some degree, we hope, by the interspersion of one hundred and seventy summaries from other clinicians. We consider it very fortunate that we were able to include a number of cases prepared by each of the following:

C. Knight Aldrich, M.D. (C. K. A.), Assistant Professor of Psychiatry, University of Minnesota, Minneapolis, Minnesota. 12 cases.

Marcella Vig Baldwin, Ph.D. (M. V. B.), 558 South 48th Street, Philadelphia, Pennsylvania. 5 cases.

Elaine Barron, M.A. (E. B.), Langley-Porter Clinic, San Francisco 22, California. 20 cases.

Edward S. Bordin, Ph.D. (E. S. B.), Associate Professor of Psychology, University of Michigan, Ann Arbor, Michigan. 6 cases.

Dora F. Capwell, Ph.D. (D. F. C.), Director, Allegheny Vocational Counseling Center, Pittsburgh 13, Pennsylvania. 10 cases.

William M. Hales, Ph.D. (W. M. H.), Chief Clinical Psychologist, Veterans Administration Hospital, St. Cloud, Minnesota. 10 cases.

A. T. Kazan, M.D. (A. T. K.), 731 Webster Avenue, New Rochelle, New York. 11 cases.

R. C. Koeninger, Ph.D. (R. C. K.), Head, Department of Sociology, Sam Houston State Teachers College, Huntsville, Texas. 22 cases.

Carl W. Swedenburg, M.A. (C. W. S.), Clinical Psychologist, Veterans Administration Hospital, St. Cloud, Minnesota. 20 cases.

Anders Sweetland, Ph.D. (A. S.), Department of Psychology, Florida State University, Tallahassee, Florida. 18 cases.

Martha Vidor, Ph.D. (M. V.), Psychologist, North Wales Hospital for Nervous and Mental Disorders, Denbigh, North Wales, England. 36 cases.

In the *Atlas* these cases are identified by the initials of the contributor placed at the end of the summaries. The Contributors' Index also lists separately the histories from each contributor. The case types among these contributions vary with the source, clinic, or facility, and in some degree represent special kinds of problems. There are cases from among college clients, Veterans Administration hospital patients, adult guidance clients, patients in an English hospital, and a special group of self-mutilators that were seen in a Texas prison population. We are particularly grateful to these contributors and feel that their case summaries add greatly to the representativeness of the whole sample of clinical experience and also agreeably spice the larger mass of local material.

Preparation of the Histories

In a sense the *Atlas* histories from the Psychiatric Unit are twice removed from the people whose stories they present. They are summaries of the longer and more comprehensive case histories that were written routinely by the psychiatrist or psychiatric resident responsible for the patients. While the routine case histories were often in error on points of detail or emphasis, for the most part they did present at least one professional view of the patient.

Fortunately, these case histories were written by many different staff doctors. Individual biases, therefore, cannot have markedly influenced the general trend of clinical patterns. On the other hand, it is obvious that local staff trends in diagnosis or emphasis did affect the whole series. The psychiatric staff was not readily characterizable, however, except possibly by "eclecticism"; no system or special trend in psychiatric practice or thinking has been particularly emphasized for practice or teaching.

The shortening of the original case write-ups is likely to have been in some degree prejudicial to the inclusion of certain classes of facts. The summaries, except those contributed from other clinics, were written by Starke R. Hathaway. The flavor of the original case history was preserved as far as possible, and a definite effort was made to include directly observed facts or those given by the patient and other informants without distortion and where possible in direct quotations. The necessary disguising of factual material that might betray the identity of the patient was done as far as possible in such a way as not to change the significance.

The cases selected for inclusion in the *Atlas* were chosen primarily because of completeness of clinical records, representativeness in frequency of diagnostic categories, and other factors not closely related to the MMPI profiles. And the summaries were written from the longer originals without knowledge of the associated profiles. Nevertheless, since the staff member who wrote the original case history may have known the MMPI scores for the patient, it cannot be said that the summaries are wholly free from contamination by the corresponding MMPI profiles. But because they are objective, relating specific events and observations rather than interpretations from these events and statements, such prejudice should be minimal. Also, nearly 15 per cent of the cases were processed before the special scales had been derived. And no case was excluded on the basis of an MMPI profile that did not "fit" the diagnosis or history.

As we have said, the patient's MMPI profile was not known to the writer at the time he prepared the summary of the case history. A minor exception to this general procedure lay in the attempt, after the main body of the summaries was completed, to find cases where the profile codes fell into rare categories so as to provide a few examples of these to round out the collection. With this method of compiling, we hope the *Atlas* truly represents clinical experience—though some cases may prove to be too atypical or trivial to be really useful.

Arrangement and Description of the Data

Key to the History Headings

The *Atlas* histories are arranged in numerical order according to the codes of the MMPI profiles (see the following section on Codes and Coding). Where there are two or more codes, the master code, under which the case history is located in the *Atlas,* is that of the MMPI administration most closely associated in time with the data on the person's complaints or problem situation. Each history begins with a summary of data like this:

a	b_1 b_2 b_3 b_4	*c*	*d*	*e*	*f g h*
Ps. Paranoid	M:30:S:83	+1	12738′469–	(67)	4:8:14
Schizoid		+93	32781′496–	(59)	1:5:7

In these history headings

a = Diagnostic or descriptive terms
b = Personal data (b_1 = sex; b_2 = age at admission; b_3 = marital status; b_4 = days in hospital)
c = Time of MMPI administration in days before (—) or after (+) admission to hospital
d = Profile code
e = Mf T score (when available)
f = L score
g = F score
h = K score

When there are two or more hospital admissions for one patient the history heading will look like this:

Ps. M-D., Depr.	M:50:M:40	+3	2′31478–96	(61)	9:1:23
Paranoid		+27	89′764–2X	(65)	2:20:8
Ps. M-D., Depr.	M:51:M:28	+1	2′3478–	(53)	7:0:20

In this case the patient entered the hospital twice. In the second admission (a year after the first since the patient was a year older) the diagnosis was psychosis, manic-depressive, depressed (see page xiii). The patient was male, 51 years old, and married; he remained in the hospital for 28 days. The MMPI was administered 1 day after his admission to the hospital. The code of his MMPI profile was 2′3478–; his Mf T score was 53; and his L, F, and K raw scores were 7, 0, and 20.

Each of these groups of data is described in some detail in the sections that follow.

ARRANGEMENT AND DESCRIPTION OF DATA

The Codes and Coding

The codes found in the history headings for each case give some information about both the shape and the intensity of the profile. The coding system is that described by Hathaway except for the omission of the Mf scale (see the discussion of the Mf scale, page ix).

The eight coded clinical scales are indicated with the numbers 1, 2, 3, 4, 6, 7, 8, and 9 in order from left to right in the usual profile arrangement;* that is to say, omitting Mf, which would be 5:

1 = Hs	4 = Pd	8 = Sc
2 = D	6 = Pa	9 = Ma
3 = Hy	7 = Pt	

One may therefore refer to the various scales by number rather than by the letters conventionally used. For a number of reasons it would probably have been better to have used numbers instead of letters from the first. It is recommended that users of this *Atlas* should gradually institute the practice of referring to the scales by number rather than by letter.

THE HIGH-POINT CODE

The writing of a code from an MMPI profile begins by identifying the highest T score value in the profile as found among the eight coded scales. The number assigned to this scale (according to the equivalents given above) is then written as the first number of the code. For example, if Hy, which is scale 3, is the highest point on the profile, one would begin the code by writing down a 3. The scale numbers of other profile points *above* $T = 54$ are written in the same way, in order of decreasing T scores. For example, if Hy is the highest score at $T = 65$, Ma the second highest at $T = 60$, and Pa the third at $T = 58$, then the code for these three points would be 396 in that order.

The dash. If these were the only points on the profile that exceeded T score 54, a dash would follow. This would then make 396–. The dash signifies the band of T scores from $T = 54$ down to $T = 46$ inclusive. Thus, scales in the interval $46 \leqq T \leqq 54$ are not coded. The code, as written up to the dash, is referred to as the "high-point" code. It shows the numbers of all scales, however many they may be, that exceed $T = 54$ on the profile. In some high-point codes all eight of the coded scales will be above 54.

The prime. Within the high-point code, a prime is placed to indicate the point where the $T = 70$ line is crossed. In the example given above, the prime would be placed to the left of all three since all the high points are below 70. Addition of the prime completes the high-point code in this example, making it ′396–. If the Hy had been 70 or above, the prime would have followed the 3, and the high-point code would have been written 3′96–.

*A tenth scale, Si (social introversion) has been developed by Drake and is widely used. When included in the code, this scale is usually designated by zero. It is omitted in this *Atlas,* partly because it is not strictly a clinical scale, but chiefly because in some of the earlier case records it could not be scored since the Si scale overlaps Mf items that were added later. If such an *Atlas* as the present one were prepared for use in interpretation of more nearly normal problem cases, it would appear highly desirable that the Si scale should be coded, and possibly also several other scales such as those developed by Friedman, Gough, Hanvik, and Gough, McClosky, and Meehl.

With the exception of this prime indicating the 70 level, no other code indication is included to show absolute intensity, although relative intensity is of course indicated by the succession of the code numbers. In reading such a high-point code, one merely knows that the scales indicated to the left of the prime exceeded 69 by an indeterminate amount. Similarly, those to the right of the prime lay in the interval $55 \leqq T \leqq 69$.

Underlining. In writing the code, those code numbers that represent T scores equal to one another *or within one T score point of one another* are underlined. A code beginning ′48 would therefore signify that the T scores for Pd and for Sc were either equal or within one point of each other, the 4 being one point higher than the 8 in the latter case. (Conventionally, if the Sc is one point more than the Pd we write 84, instead of the 48 that would be used if the two scores were equal or if Pd exceeded Sc by one point.) The underlining is continued for as many scales as are equal or within one point of one another. It is therefore possible, for example, in the code ′468–, that the 4 and the 8 may be separated by as much as two points; that is, the 4 could be at $T = 65$, the 6 at $T = 64$, and the 8 at $T = 63$. Although it rarely occurs, it is theoretically possible for the beginning coded scale among a string of underlined scales to be more than three T points different from an end code value. In the code 12 738′469–, the scales in each of the pairs 12, 73, and 69 are equal or within one point of each other, *but scales 2 and 7 are not.* Thus, a space within a code indicates a break in the series of scores equal or within one point of one another.

THE LOW-POINT CODE

After writing the high-point code and placing a dash at the end, one next writes the low-point code. The procedure here is similar to the writing of the high-point code except that one first sets down the code number of the scale having the *smallest* T score and follows this successively by the code numbers of scales in ascending order up to, but not including, $T = 46$. In writing the low-point code, no indication of intensity corresponding to the prime of the high-point code is included. Underlining is used as with the high-point code.

A completed code of a profile having some scale values above 54 and some below 46 is therefore made up of a high-point code and a low-point code separated by a dash. When there is no clinical scale T score$>$54, the code *begins* with a dash; when there is no clinical scale T score$<$46, the code *ends* with a dash.

THE MF SCALE

The Mf scale was not included for several reasons. Chief among these was that it is not strictly a clinical diagnostic scale. While it is frequently elevated in clinical cases of male homoeroticism, there is considerable evidence that its T score may be high without such clinical implication. With females the interpretation is still more ambiguous. Some unpublished research data indicate that it is a rather variable score. Finally, a great many of our older records, including the basic norm group, were obtained with an earlier form of the Inventory that did not include some of the Mf items added later. Scoring Mf was therefore impossible on all those cases. Where Mf scores were available on a case, the T score is always given in parentheses following the MMPI code. The Mf Index contains a listing of all Mf scores in a frequency distribution by fives beginning with the score 60 upward and with the score 40 downward. Those interested in interpretation of the Mf deviations as based on these *Atlas* summaries may begin with the index references.

THE L, F, AND K SCORES

Following the code and the Mf score, if any, in parentheses, three numbers separated by colons indicate the L, F, and K raw scores in that order. Raw scores are used because experience subsequent to the publishing of the T tables for L, F, and K has shown that our arbitrary choices of T equivalents for L and F were not good. T scores were set too leniently for L and too rigorously for F. Instead of the published values 10 and 12, the tables should have shown a raw score L of about 7 as T = 70 and a raw score F of about 16 as T = 70. In view of the various factors involved, it has seemed better not to try to change the tables that are now in such wide use but rather to adopt some new alternative. It is not difficult for the clinician to remember the interpretation of these two scales in raw score form, so they are here given in that way. Those codes followed by a capital X are profiles where the raw score L ≧ 10 or the raw score F ≧ 16. For most research work, all such possibly invalid profiles should be omitted. In this *Atlas*, however, many X codes are included because a part of clinical interpretation depends upon proper consideration of such validity scores. The cases included were not considered invalid either because other evidences in the profiles indicated validity or because there was outside evidence of it. No case has been included, however, in which the Cannot Say value exceeded T = 70.

The K score is included with the L and F scores in the same raw score form Since K contributes to the scale levels as expressed by the code, there is not so much argument for its repetition, but some clinicians like to know the actual value. It seems to have its own personality significance and is used in Gough's F-K index.

As with Mf, the L Index, the F Index, and the K Index list the master codes of cases having deviant values on L, F, or K.

The following examples illustrate most of the problems in coding profiles. The code numbers used for the scales are printed below the scales. To repeat, the Mf T score is placed in parentheses following the code. After the Mf the three numbers are the L, F, and K raw score values in that order. The reader should study the examples until he feels sure of understanding how the profile data are translated into the numerical code.

Profile Data													*Code*
?	*L*	*F*	*K*	*Hs* 1	*D* 2	*Hy* 3	*Pd* 4	*Mf*	*Pa* 6	*Pt* 7	*Sc* 8	*Ma* 9	
50	50 (4)	50 (3)	61 (18)	53	49	63	53	42	43	46	63	55	'389–6 (42) 4:3:18
53	53 (5)	70 (12)	40 (7)	62	82	79	60	51	67	84	80	54	7283'614–(51) 5:12:7
50	50 (1)	53 (14)	53 (14)	49	34	51	47	55	65	48	52	59	'69–2 (55) 1:4:14
50	53 (5)	50 (1)	55 (15)	51	48	55	56	57	42	43	46	72	9'43–67 (57) 5:1:15
50	50 (2)	78 (15)	44 (9)	76	92	70	76	63	77	96	94	68	7826143'9–(63) 2:15:9
50	56 (6)	80+ (19)	31 (2)	66	96	75	60	59	59	67	56	50	23'71 468–X (59) 6:19:2
50	70 (10)	53 (4)	66 (21)	67	69	66	65	50	55	68	61	53	'2713486–X (50) 10:4:21
50	53 (5)	50 (3)	61 (18)	49	41	53	53	69	53	50	46	48	–2 (69) 5:3:18
50	50 (0)	53 (4)	53 (14)	45	52	44	48		52	50	46	54	–31 0:4:14

It is remarkable how closely these codes indicate the intensity and shape of the profiles in spite of the fact that the codes are greatly simplified. The reader who wishes to familiarize himself thoroughly with coding should choose several coded profiles and attempt to reproduce the profiles from the codes alone. He should then compare these with the original profiles. The average profile will be found to be reproducible rather adequately from its code. Only the extreme deviations will be badly represented.

The authors recognize that this coding does not convey all the information about profiles. This *Atlas* is not presented as a research tool or source. We recommend highly the much more complete coding suggested by Welsh for research and possibly even for routine filing. It is our feeling that in attempting to convey clinical experience with an instrument as complex as this, one must make a compromise between giving all the profile data, which would become too confusing for the study of patterns, and giving too little, so that the complexities would not be expressed well enough to convey most of the useful meaning. The present coding was adopted in the hope that it is a fair compromise. The codes are complex enough so that few exact duplicates occur among the cases presented here. And even in our very extensive clinical files there are not many duplicates. From this standpoint the information conveyed in the codes appears to be highly individual and could, perhaps, be considered still too complex.

Diagnostic Terms

In addition to a code, each case history (with the exception of a few of the contributed summaries) is accompanied by one or more diagnostic or descriptive terms. The first of these listed for each history is the one most emphasized as characteristic by the psychiatric staff or other contributor. Usually this is in the form of a psychiatric diagnosis. Below this main diagnosis there may be several others that are always less certain and are included merely to show the complexity and breadth of the case. In addition to the more formal diagnoses some adjectives are used. There was no very rational basis on which the adjectives were selected, and no doubt others may seem to have been better choices. The ones used were adopted chiefly because they were adjectives frequently used in the diagnostic summary that accompanied the longer case histories.

It is not our intent to emphasize the diagnostic categories; these are frequently unsatisfactory, and they vary as applied to patients seen over a period of time. On the other hand, it seemed desirable to give indications as to the class of diagnoses, if not the specific ones.

Following is the list of the diagnostic and descriptive terms in order as they occur in the Diagnosis Index. After each one a note indicates the kind of patient to whom this term was usually applied. The letter B. is an abbreviation for behavior problem, P. for psychoneurosis, and Ps. for psychosis.

Alcoholism. This appears here occasionally as a primary diagnosis. In those cases it indicates a person in whom alcoholism seemed to be the main difficulty and the patient was without psychosis. If there was much asocial or antisocial behavior mixed with the alcoholism, or if there was variable emotionality, the patient was usually referred to as some type of psychopathic personality. Mostly the word *alcoholism* is used secondarily and is descriptive of a condition not felt to be primary for the patient. Alcoholism is similar to drug addiction but is treated separately in recognition of its more common occurrence and special social significance.

B. Pri., Child. Primary behavior problem of childhood. This term was applied to patients, mostly of age 16 or less, who were without psychosis but exhibited what was felt to be a deep-seated personality disorder.

B. Psth., Asocial. Psychopathic personality, asocial, amoral type. This included persons similar to those who have been usually described under that heading in conventional literature. In the terminology peculiar to the MMPI this class would be called "psychopathic deviate." They were usually free from psychosis and experienced shallow affect. Some had transient psychotic episodes.

B. Psth., Mixed. Psychopathic personality, mixed type. This included the conventionally described psychopaths who showed behavior disorders similar to more than one of the specific subtypes.

B. Psth., Path. Emot. Psychopathic personality, pathologic emotionality. This term was applied to those patients conventionally described as having uncontrollable tempers or as being unpredictable in mood and behavior without obvious neurosis or psychosis.

B. Psth., Path. Sexuality. Psychopathic personality, pathologic sexuality. This diagnostic term refers in the greater part to males with a repeated history of homosexuality or other sexual activities abhorred by society. In general the staff was reluctant to use this term unless the behavior showed repeated occurrences with the traditionally emphasized failure to change following punishment or social disapproval.

B. Simple Adult Maladj. Simple adult maladjustment. This description was used infrequently by the psychiatric staff and refers to those adult cases, roughly comparable to the primary behavior disorders of childhood, in whom there was no psychosis and neurotic components were obscure but who did not seem to have such deep character disorders as did the psychopathic personality cases.

Deteriorated. This term was applied to those cases in which there was good neurological evidence of organic brain damage from whatever cause.

Drug Add. Drug addiction. These descriptive words were applied to all patients taking some drug to a detrimental degree, whether the drug was one of the addiction-prone drugs or not. Thus the "non-habit forming" barbiturates were included among the drugs.

Epilepsy. This diagnosis has its usual meaning.

Mental Deficiency. This term was very loosely applied to all persons whose I.Q.'s were below 80. The reader should not think of the term as certainly diagnostic.

Mutilative. This adjective was chiefly applied to the special block of cases from Texas prisons that was mentioned in the section on Making of the Atlas. The term was also extended to cover a few Psychiatric Unit cases that persistently or episodically injured themselves.

P. Anxiety State. This was applied to cases fitting the conventional diagnostic category.

P. Hypo. Psychoneurosis, hypochondriasis. This diagnosis was used as the near equivalent of the older term *neurasthenia.* It was applied to patients who had multiple complaints, usually of a vague and indefinite character. The staff did not use the term *hypochondriasis* for that special group of patients that centered their physical complaint about a single tissue, limb, or organ. For the most part this latter type was classed as "psychoneurosis, hysteria."

P. Hys. Psychoneurosis, hysteria. This term was used for cases meeting conventional symptomatic requirements for the category. These patients frequently had conversion symptoms or they may have exhibited seizures or other disturbances of motor function. A certain number of them had disturbances of sensation; mostly this was difficulty in vision or paresthetic sensations.

P. Mixed. Psychoneurosis, mixed. This was applied to cases where several different psychoneurotic patterns appeared in the same patient.

P. Psychas. Psychoneurosis, psychasthenia. This category included chiefly the phobic and obsessive patients, although some cases so diagnosed were characterized by indecisiveness and anxious doubt.

P. React. Depr. Psychoneurosis, reactive depression. This characterizes the patients in whom depression seemed the outstanding symptom and the cases in which the life situation of the patient was felt to be an important etiological factor. Obvious reactive depressions occurred with the death of friends or family, with economic setbacks, with frustration of basic or habitual tendencies to action, and the like.

Paranoid. As an adjective this term was applied to a number of patients who, while not primarily paranoid, nevertheless showed evidences of paranoid thinking or ideation.

Ps. Invol. Melan. Psychosis, involutional melancholia. This term was used in the traditional meaning.

Ps. M-D., Depr. Psychosis, manic-depressive, depressed. The term was used in the traditional meaning. It signifies that the staff felt the patient to be more deeply disturbed than is usually the case for the reactive depression; more often than not the patient had had previous episodes of illness, either manic or depressive or both.

Ps. M-D., Manic. Psychosis, manic-depressive, manic. This characterizes overactive persons fitting the usual description. Both these and the depressed patients often changed before they actually took the MMPI, so that the record failed to agree with the presenting symptoms.

Ps. M-D., Mixed. Psychosis, manic-depressive, mixed. This term was used for agitated persons in whom both depression and overactivity with flight of ideas were noticeable. It was also used for patients where alternation between depression and hypomania occurred rapidly so that it was difficult to refer to the illness as either manic or depressed in character.

Ps. Paranoid. Psychosis, paranoid. This diagnosis was applied in a general way to include all paranoid psychoses except schizophrenia. A few of the cases were true paranoia; some were paranoid condition; and one or two were involutional melancholia, paranoid type.

Ps. Postpartum. Psychosis, postpartum. The term was used in the conventional sense.

Ps. Psth. Psychosis with psychopathic personality. This term was applied to patients where a psychopathic personality seemed accompanied by episodes of psychosis during one of which the patient was admitted.

Ps. Senile. Psychosis, senile. This category included senile and presenile cases, most of whom were also deteriorated.

Ps. Sz., Cat. Psychosis, schizophrenia, catatonic. The patients so classed were conventional types.

Ps. Sz., Hebe. Psychosis, schizophrenia, hebephrenic. These patients were conventional examples of this class.

Ps. Sz., Mixed. Psychosis, schizophrenia, mixed. Here the patients were schizophrenic but showed mixed classificatory symptoms.

Ps. Sz., Paranoid. Psychosis, schizophrenia, paranoid. This diagnosis was applied to cases with prominent paranoid symptoms, usually ideas of reference or schizoid hallucinations, but in whom the paranoid process was considered secondary to schizophrenia.

Ps. Sz., Simple. Psychosis, schizophrenia, simple. A strong determining factor in these cases was a relatively long history of an inadequate personality.

Ps. Toxic. Psychosis, toxic. This diagnosis was somewhat loosely applied to confusional states and all other psychotic conditions felt to derive from a chemical agent. Some of these were drug addiction cases, some were alcoholism, and still others were cases of lead or other toxic encephalopathies.

Schizoid. This, as an adjective, was applied in cases where schizophrenia did not seem to be justified as a diagnosis but where some of the observed behavior or symptoms seemed similar to the schizophrenic pattern.

Suicidal. For the most part this refers to patients who had made attempts at suicide or who seemed in their discourse to be real suicidal risks.

Twin. The term includes the few case histories available for one or both twins.

Personal Data

For each case history, lying between the diagnostic terms at the left of the page and the MMPI code at the right, symbols and numbers are given as follows: First, an M or F for male or female. After this a number indicates the age of the patient at the time of admission. Next follows a letter showing the marital status: M, married; S, single; D, divorced; and W, widowed. Finally, when, as is usually the case, the patient has been in the hospital, a number shows the days spent in admission.

For example, F:24:M:25 means that the case history is that of a female, 24 years old at the time of admission, married, and in the hospital 25 days. If the series had been M:50:D:40 it would indicate a male, 50 years old, who was divorced and who stayed 40 days in the hospital.

Time of MMPI Administration

A number, with plus or minus sign, is placed in front of each MMPI code to indicate the relation of the MMPI administration time to the date of the patient's admission to the hospital or to the date of the first interview. A +2 would mean that the patient was given the MMPI two days after admission to the hospital. If, as sometimes happens, the patient took the Inventory before admission, one might find the time indicated by —12; this would mean that the Inventory predated admission to the hospital by 12 days. A zero means that the MMPI was administered on the day of admission. In a few cases, where the time of administration could not be determined, there is a question mark to the left of the code.

ARRANGEMENT AND DESCRIPTION OF DATA

Where a number of MMPI profiles were available on a patient, they are arranged in order as they occurred in relation to the admission date. The one closest in time to admission is always considered the primary profile, and its code is the master code under which the history is located in the *Atlas*. Presumably this will usually be most closely related to the personality as described in the admission notes. Whenever one studies cases in this *Atlas*, he should notice the relation of the time of administration of each MMPI to the admission date for the patient as shown by these numbers. Unfortunately, however, some of the indicated administration times are probably wrong. They were determined by reading the charts; and some entries by nurses and clerks on the time of administration may have been put off and merely entered as rough estimates when the patient's chart was assembled for filing after his discharge.

It might have been desirable, from certain considerations, to include only cases tested within plus or minus two days relative to admission time; however, we felt there was value in including cases in which the data were from a test given considerably before or after the illness. There seemed likely to be a special value in including patients on whom several different codes were available. These would afford the reader an opportunity to see what happened as the patient changed in pattern from illness to better or worse or from one type of disorder to another. Often changing validity scores are of interest since they indicate greater or less defensiveness on the part of the patient.

Where a patient was admitted more than once, diagnostic and other data are repeated for each admission in order as they occurred. These separate admissions are indicated by the repetition of the orientational and diagnostic data, and are separated by extra space. MMPI codes for each admission are related in time to that particular admission. The time between the admissions themselves is usually indicated either by the change in age of the patient, or in the body of the case history.

The Case Summaries

The case histories usually fall into three parts. The first describes the patient at the time he enters the hospital or first comes to the attention of the therapist. The complaints that led to hospitalization (or the interviews) are listed, and a brief account of the patient's recent behavior is given whenever relevant.

The second part includes the pertinent historical information on the patient: past health, intelligence, general personality. His education and work history are often given here, as well as his family or marital history, when these seem significant for the present problem.

Finally there is a description of the patient as he appeared to the therapist or to the staff of the hospital. After a summary of the patient's attitude, his behavior on the ward or during interviews, his response to treatment, and the like, the history usually concludes with a prognosis. If follow-up information is available, it may be mentioned briefly to indicate more certainly the course of the patient in the future.

The emphasis in these histories is on *description*, on giving a factual, objective picture of the patient as the professional worker responsible for him saw it. Thus, except in one or two instances, there is no attempt to relate the history and the MMPI profile, or to explain discrepancies between them.

The Use of the *Atlas* and Its Indexes

It should be understood, of course, that these cases are not necessarily representative of all the patterns seen in other clinics. It is particularly likely that many of the profiles observed in a nonmedical setting would be different. Users of the *Atlas* should be constantly aware that its cases and interpretative data are directed at, and mostly representative of, experience in a hospital setting. When one prepares to interpret an MMPI profile, he should first know if the person represented is in social trouble because of his behavior, is considered maladjusted, or considers himself maladjusted. Interpretative suggestions should change greatly according to such facts about the person. All the individuals presented in this *Atlas* were either in trouble with society or considered themselves to be in need of some sort of help (although not necessarily psychiatric). These people took the MMPI in an atmosphere of professional protection and many of them had come voluntarily. Although some of them remained highly on the defensive and no doubt frequently responded to the items in as diverse ways as would people not in such an atmosphere, there was nevertheless a greater likelihood of candid cooperation than is present in school testing programs or in the testing done as part of an industrial personnel program. We therefore feel that a separate *Atlas* would be required for *unqualified* use with nonclinical clients.

But we also feel that experience with clinical interpretation should be a part of the training of one who expects to use the MMPI in nonclinical settings and that all users of the MMPI should study this *Atlas* extensively. Some users may protest that they rarely see "the kind of person" presented in this *Atlas,* but this statement is patently false. Well over one in twenty persons will spend some time in a mental hospital during their lives; an undetermined but much greater per cent will be psychosomatically ill or will be chronically unhappy or handicapped by other psychological maladjustments. The patients in this *Atlas* happened to be a little worse or, more often, a little luckier in having someone recognize their illness. They were often not psychotic as the lay person would see it. It is in part the general refusal to recognize minimal psychological illness that permits so many people with less severe maladjustments to go untreated. No counselor in an industrial or school program fails to see a fair percentage of persons who are as ill, or nearly so, as many of the people in this *Atlas*. A counselor may not be aware of the more severe maladjustments among his clients, or he may choose to disregard them. The former is inexcusable; the latter may be a deliberate decision in the role he plays as part of an agency or as a professional practitioner.

USE OF THE *ATLAS*

The case histories in this *Atlas* are the adult developments that counseling should help to avoid or should at least recognize early so as to institute routine treatment. No counselor who feels himself at all responsible in his assessment of his clients or who is aware of his usefulness in society can afford not to be familiar with the end products of his failures or the inevitable outcomes of what he sees in early form.

We are not here attempting to present interpretative methods or rules or findings of a scientific nature relative to the use of the MMPI. Rather, as we indicated in the section of Case Summaries, we are trying to convey an honest picture of the persons whose case histories are included, giving in simple exposition their symptoms, the way they acted, and how others, or they themselves, described them as they appeared before the illness.

Thus, this *Atlas* represents a new way of showing the validity and defining the scales of the Inventory. Since the selection of the cases was only slightly determined by the MMPI profiles, the relationships between the profile shapes and the problems of the people described are evidences of the validity of the Inventory as a characterizer of personality. Instead of means and other cross-sectional data as produced by statistical processing, the untabulated findings are given here. It is left to the reader to draw from the material such relationships and generalizations as he finds useful or regards valid.

Suppose we had attempted to derive generalized interpretations and to write long descriptions of the kinds of persons we thought we had seen with each shape of profile, or with each special type of deviation. We might have missed many points, emphasized wrong ones, and in general communicated a mixture of truth with our own possibly false summaries of a kind of experience that could hardly be adequately organized or tabulated, let alone statistically validated.

The user of this *Atlas* may also learn directly the clinical characteristics of the separate scales. Here there is no distortion from another person's generalizations about what a scale measures. There is less semantic warping than occurs when one person's short description of what a scale measures must be translated into clinical applications by another. Each is here provided with the material to fashion his own description of scales and of profile patterns. Possibly this method will not contribute to the much needed improvement of the current psychiatric classificatory system, but we feel that it is superior to the latter as a basis for practical use of the MMPI. Undoubtedly, individual workers will develop their own procedures for using the *Atlas*, and the following suggestions are made merely to indicate the range of possibilities.

Histories with Similar Codes

The simplest use of the *Atlas* consists in the reading of all case histories having similar codes, i.e., appearing together in the *Atlas*. To learn clinical interpretation in this way, one simply reads, for example, all the cases with codes beginning with a 4. One might, to limit the amount of reading he did, study only those beginning with a 4 where the 4 is to the left of the prime, or, perhaps with somewhat less profit, he could read those fewer cases where the code begins ′4. This same type of study could be done with the histories having given low-point codes except that these would have to be found by first referring to the Low-Point Index, where all such low-point codes are listed. More often, and for the most frequently occurring codes, one would choose to read the case histories for all codes having a selected pair of high points, for example the 49 (read as "four, nine," *not* as "forty-nine"). It should be remembered in looking up such pairs of code numbers that codes with an underlined 49 are practically equivalent to those with an underlined 94. It is appropriate, therefore, to read the case histories for underlined numbers in both orders.

In the High-Point Index all codes having the first two figures underlined are presented in the two possible permutations. For example, if a code begins with 49 underlined (e.g., 49′6–2) and if that is the code under which the case history is presented, the High-Point Index will show the code as 49 . . . and will also list it as a 94 . . . among the nines. The latter listing will be followed, on a separate line, indented, by the basic form 49 . . . (e.g., 94′6–2 over 49′6–2) so that the reader may immediately find the case history under the master code beginning 49 in the body of the *Atlas*.

Where the first three or four numbers of the code are all underlined, the High-Point Index shows all combinations and permutations of these numbers taken two at a time, as illustrated in the accompanying Example A. Each of the alternative entries is, of course, followed by the master code in order to locate the corresponding summary in the *Atlas*. When three numbers are underlined, there will be six index entries; if four numbers are underlined, there will be twelve entries.

In a similar way, if the second number of the code is underlined along with one or more of the succeeding high points, the index will also show all of the forms where the first code number appears with each of the succeeding underlined code numbers in turn. For example, a code like 4′3726–9 will be presented in the *Atlas* case history section at that place but will appear in the index under four entries, as shown in Example B.

Example A	*Example B*
312′784–9	4′3726–9

321′784–9
  312′784–9
	4′7326–9
	  4′3726–9

213′784–9
  312′784–9
	4′2376–9
	  4′3726–9

231′784–9
  312′784–9
	4′6372–9
	  4′3726–9

123′784–9 312′784–9	
132′784–9 312′784–9	

If the reader embarks upon the task of familiarizing himself with the similarities among case histories that occur under various code combinations, he should also pay particular attention to those case histories that do not seem to fit in with others. These are sometimes called "misses," with reference to the fact that the case does not seem to have been properly characterized by the profile. In many of these instances the clinician will at least be able to form rational hypotheses that will explain them. Frequently they are explicable by reference to deviant validity scores or perhaps by the failure of the clinical write-up to emphasize points that might have been brought out to tie the case in with others having similar codes. In other instances the patients might have been tested after they had shifted rather radically in personality from the picture that was seen as a basis for the case history. This latter occurrence was all too frequent. As an example of this, the staff of the Psychiatric Unit was always faced with a problem when a patient entered the hospital as a manic, overactive individual and within a relatively short time shifted to depression. It was impossible to know for sure the phase in which the patient answered the items of the MMPI, and frequently the write-up of the case would also tend to disregard one or the other aspect of the clinical picture.

In the clinical use of an instrument such as the MMPI there is frequently as much useful information to be gained through proper consideration of the "misses" as there is in proper interpretation of the "hits." For example, if a patient seems clinically not depressed, yet obtains a high 2 score, one knows that he is, within the limits of the testing, responding to the items in the ways that depressed persons tend to respond. One is therefore challenged to explain the fact and may discover significant trends he would otherwise overlook.

Similarly, when a patient is admitted to the psychiatric hospital with a history of paranoid activities or with other evidence of the presence of paranoid ideas and yet obtains no deviant scores on the MMPI profile, one can, with rather high probability, assume the operation of "cover up" behavior. This in turn indicates that the patient is relatively under control and not disposed to view himself candidly. In this *Atlas* it will be observed that many paranoid individuals who are well oriented and intact in sensorium and intellect obtain fairly normal MMPI codes. A patient admitted to a psychiatric hospital because of certain complaints (usually by others) about his behavior or psychological state who obtains a normal appearing code is very likely to be basically paranoid but with enough self-control and contact with the environment to be able to hide the fact. It is well known that a clinical staff interviewing a paranoid patient without the benefit of an independent history of the complaints against the patient is often unable to discover anything deviant in his behavior or discourse.

Probably the main value of the *Atlas* will be its use as a source where one may find case histories of persons having codes similar to that of a patient. As an example of this procedure, let us assume that we have a woman's profile with the code 4′6379–12. From what has been said above, it should be immediately recognized that this code is practically the equivalent of 4′3679–12, and similarly, it is like each of these two codes with a low-point code written –21. It is also rather like any code beginning with 64 or 34, especially if one or more of the other three high-point code numbers follows. Sometimes the clinician may feel that a code such as 4 . . . –1 . . . is still more similar. That viewpoint would chiefly emphasize the combination of the highest point on the profile with the lowest.

The authors know of no a priori rules that will determine which codes are most "like" others. The accompanying Example C shows some of the *Atlas* codes from the High-Point and Low-Point indexes that are, in various ways, like the given code. These codes have the prime in a somewhat similar position

Example C

Given code: 4′6379–12 F

Similar Codes from High-Point Index

4′63– F

′463–2 F

4′6318– F

4′6328– F

4′6372–9 F
4′3726–9

′4638– F

46′3819– F

4′638 2179– F

46′3897– F
46′829 37

′46392–718 M
462378′91–

′46398– M
7289′6–

′43 619 278–X F
′34 619 278–X

′436 218– F
′7243–

4′36271–9 F
3′46271–9

′43 69–2 F
′34 69–2

Similar Codes from Low-Point Index

′49–1267 M

′49876–21 M

and at least three deviant score similarities. Eleven codes are listed beginning with 463 and four beginning 436. Thirteen of these are females. Only two codes are listed in the Low-Point Index as having –12 or –21 with 4 as the first scale of the high code. If the given case had deviant scores on L, F, K, or Mf, these points could be cross-checked by reference to the corresponding indexes. The user of the *Atlas* will simply have to decide for himself how rigorously he will define "similar" as applied to codes. If the code one seeks to match is a rare one, then frequently only one or two cases can be found that are at all similar and even then considerable latitude may need to be allowed. But a little practice with the looking up of profiles, particularly if one checks all the variations, will usually lead to a goodly number of cases from which interpretative ideas may be drawn.

We feel that it would be undesirable to suggest outlines or rules to be followed in applying ideas gained from the *Atlas* histories to specific persons whose codes seem to match. We cannot readily determine the validity of such ideas; the clinician must be left to work out his own concepts of validity. It is obvious that if a given code, as represented in a number of variations discoverable in the *Atlas,* should lead to several case histories having backgrounds, symptoms, or outcomes similar among themselves, then at least there would be evidence enough to justify careful investigation of the client to identify either the similarities to the commonly found type or to indicate why the similarities do not appear.

Code Frequencies and the Diagnostic Patterns

One of the most interesting points about the code of a patient is its relative frequency. Some codes are very common, at least in their main deviant characteristics, while others are nearly unique. Presumably an uncommon code denotes a case having unusual features.

Figures 1 and 2 show, in graphic form, the relative frequencies of master code characteristics found in a sample of general inpatients at the University of Minnesota Hospitals Psychiatric Unit over about ten years of experience. Figures 3 and 4 show, in similar form, the frequencies as observed among the original sample of Minnesota "normals" obtained during the earliest stages of MMPI development. Figures 5 and 6 show the observed frequencies among University of Wisconsin students.* Finally, Figures 7 and 8 show the distributions for a nearly total population sample of public school ninth-grade children in Minneapolis.† Tables I through VIII show another aspect of code frequency. Here the highest and lowest points are emphasized. One may check the observed frequency of any combination of highest and lowest scale values.

We have assumed, since the earliest publications of MMPI data, that the clinician would consider the diagnostic categories implied in the names of the various scales as minor in the derivation and use of the Inventory. Although the separate scales were based upon common psychiatric categories, we have emphasized that particular patients usually show multiple syndromes. For example, most schizophrenic patients are depressed to an extent that makes the D score as high or higher than the Sc score. What is presumably useful for diagnostic and descriptive purposes lies in the *profile* interpretation as well as in the elevation of specific scales. Although we expect to deal with the subject more fully in other publications, the Diagnosis Index gives an idea of the frequency of various code patterns as related to diagnosis from our experience. The relative frequency of the patterns in this index have to be considered by comparing the frequencies with those presented in Figures 1 and 2, and, more readily, by a study of Tables IX to XXIII. As an example from Table XXIII, the patterns occurring under the term *Suicidal* are deficient in codes beginning with 13. Codes with 13 make up 6.6 per cent of all the clinic cases but only 2.8 per cent of the codes of suicidal persons as we have seen them. Though this general approach can only be hinted at here, we feel it to be of supreme significance and hope that readers may be stimulated to further research along these lines.

*Data contributed by L. E. Drake from a relatively unselected sample of University of Wisconsin students.

†Data obtained by E. Monachesi and S. R. Hathaway as part of another project subsidized by research funds from the University of Minnesota Graduate School.

For Figures 1 to 8 the N used to calculate the percentage values was the number of codes that were not "X" codes. The codes with underlined scales in the first two places (12...,–) are evenly distributed in the two permutations (12... and 21...). Codes with the second and third scales underlined (123...–) are divided between the two combinations (12 and 13). Codes with the second and two or more following scales underlined are classified without regard to the underlining (1234...– would be called a 12). Codes having the first three or more scales underlined are listed as indeterminate (?). Codes with no "high point" are indicated by a dash (–).

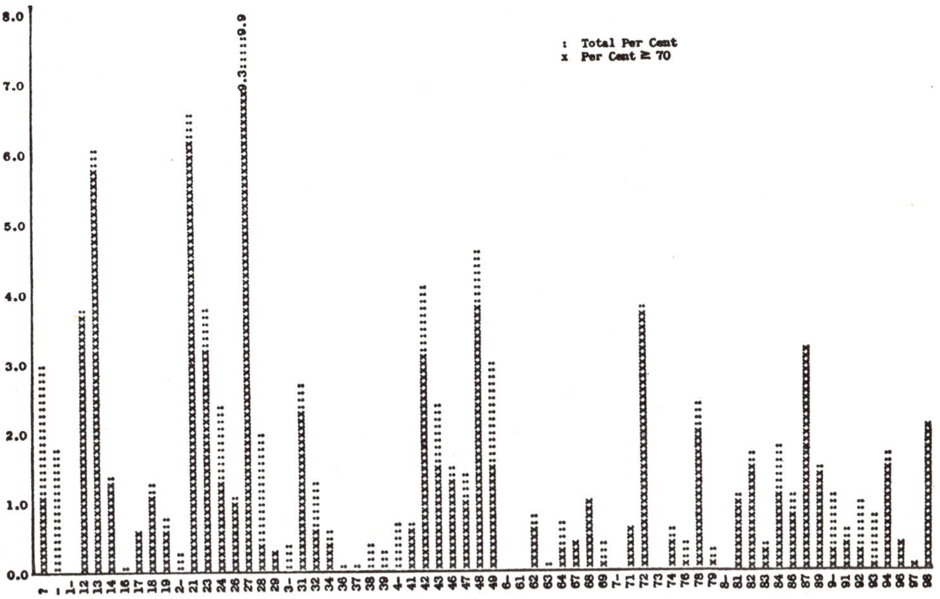

Figure 1. Relative frequencies of various high-point codes from a sample of 710 male adult Psychiatric Unit inpatients

Figure 2. Relative frequencies of various high-point codes from a sample of 1053 female adult Psychiatric Unit inpatients

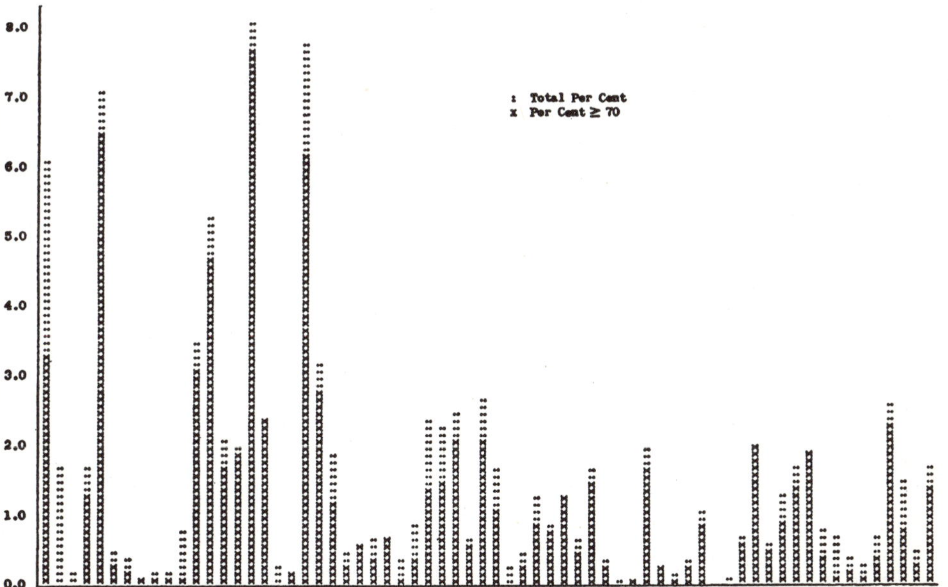

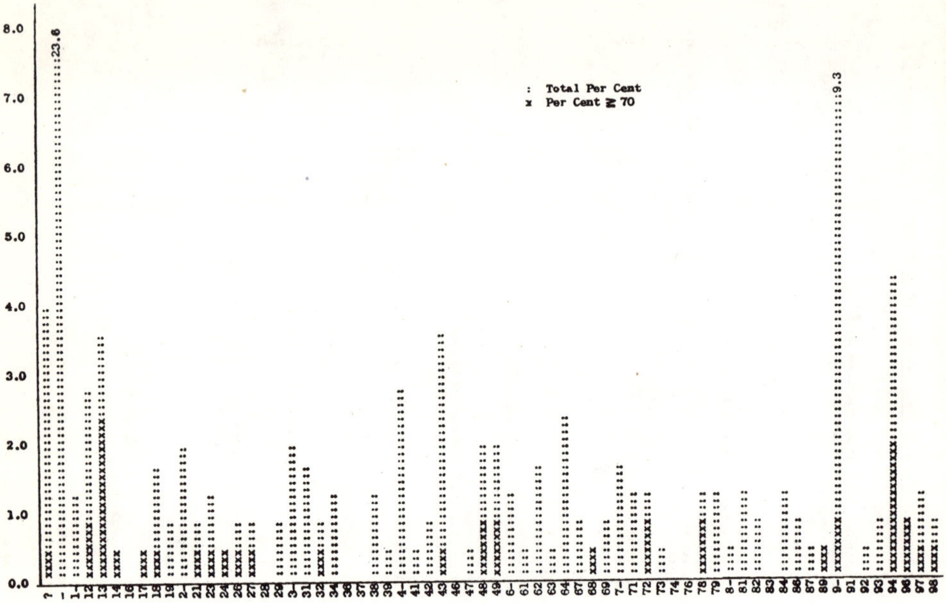

Figure 3. Relative frequencies of various high-point codes from a sample of 258 male adult "normals" in Minnesota

Figure 4. Relative frequencies of various high-point codes from a sample of 360 female adult "normals" in Minnesota

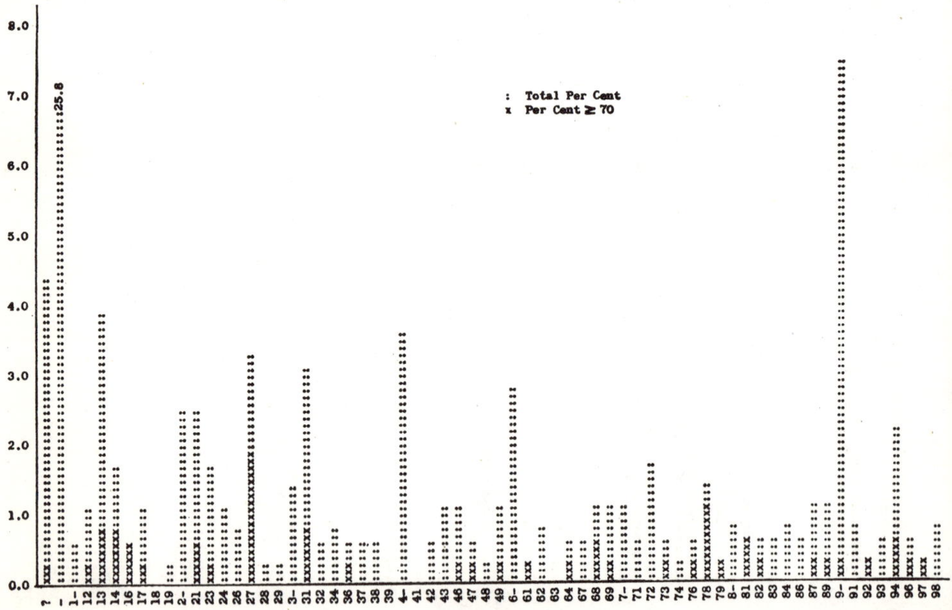

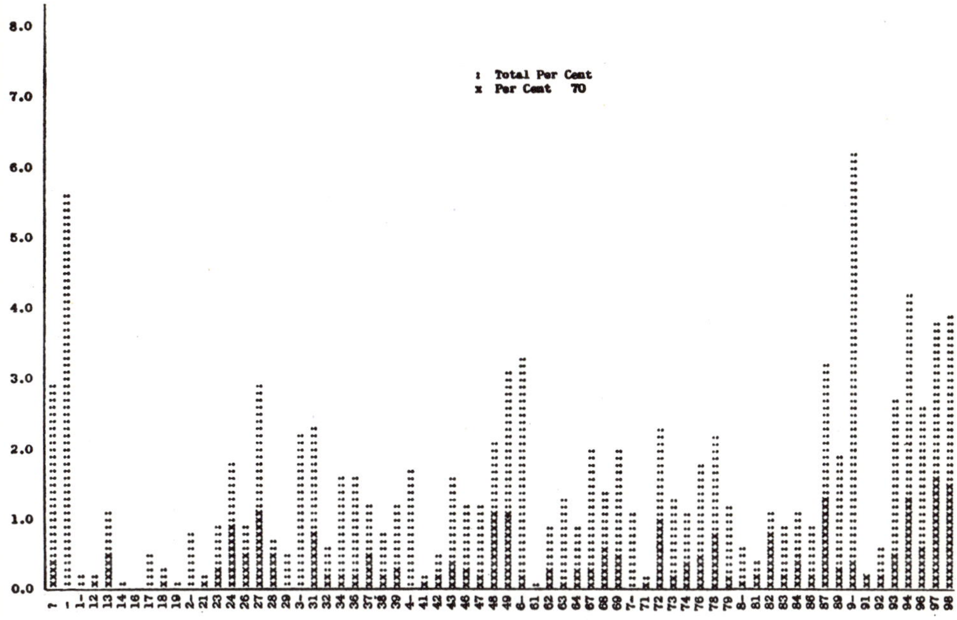

Figure 5. Relative frequencies of various high-point codes from a sample of 2805 University of Wisconsin male students

Figure 6. Relative frequencies of various high-point codes from a sample of 1367 University of Wisconsin female students

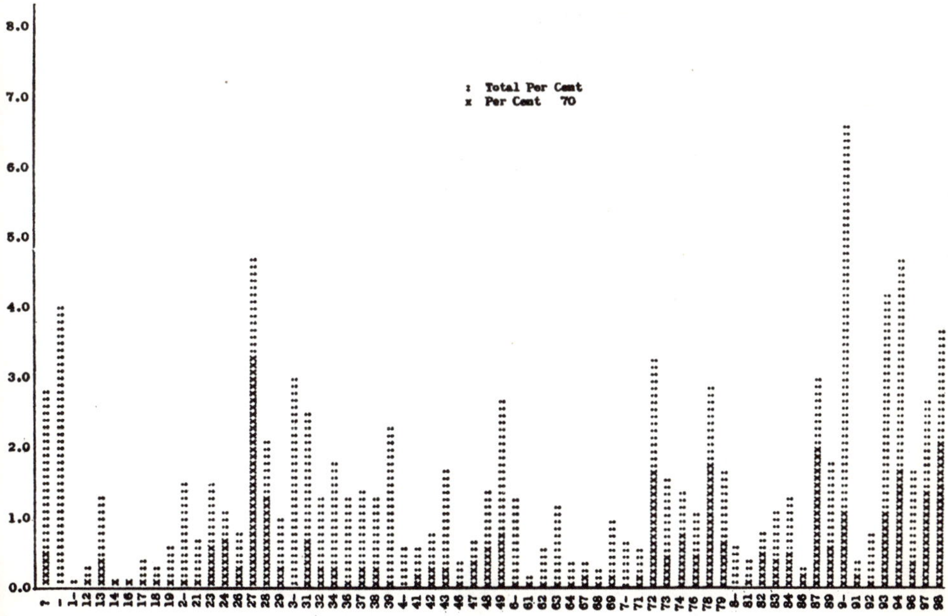

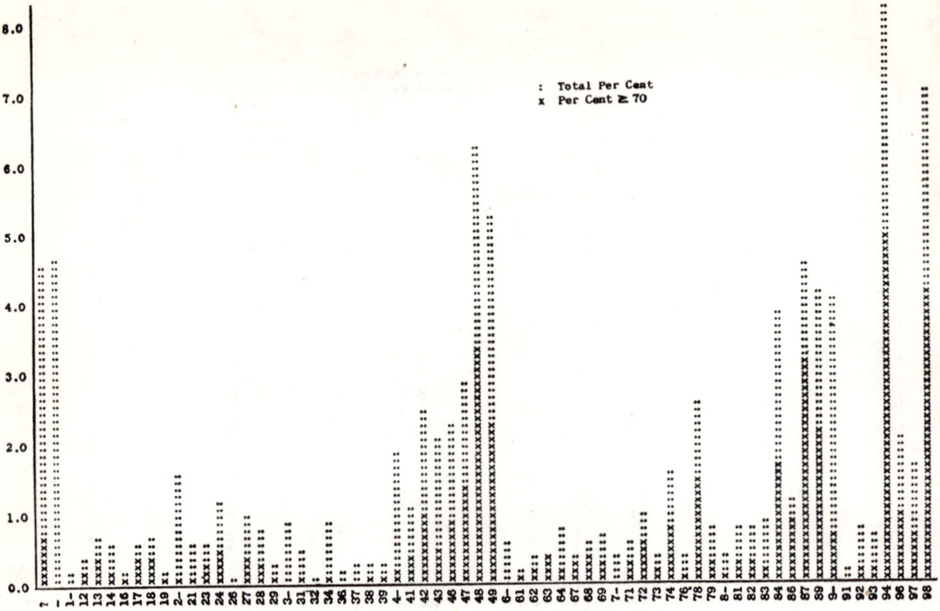

Figure 7. Relative frequencies of various high-point codes from a sample of 1816 ninth-grade schoolboys in Minneapolis

Figure 8. Relative frequencies of various high-point codes from a sample of 1937 ninth-grade schoolgirls in Minneapolis

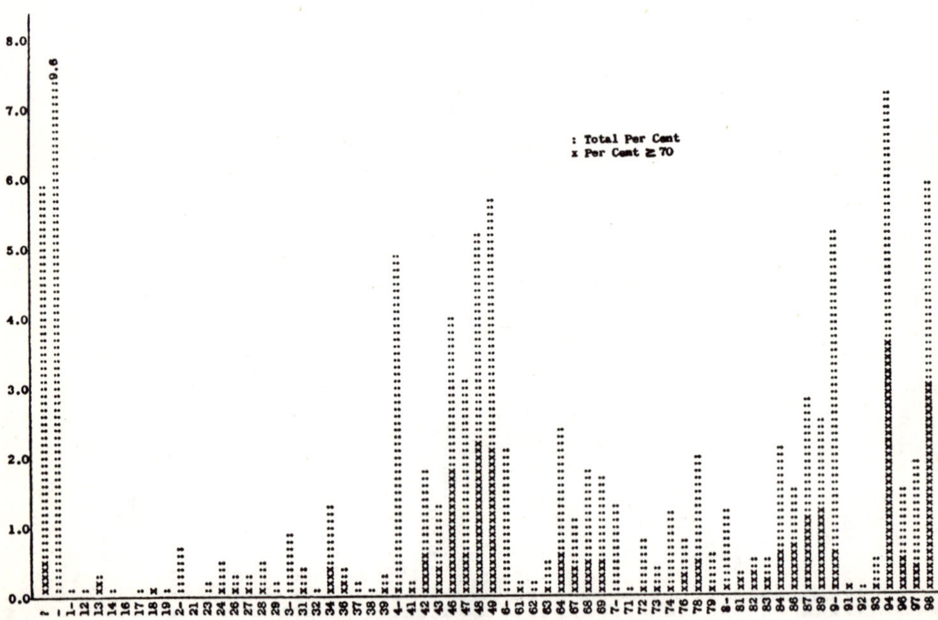

Table I. Relative frequencies of various combinations of scales as "highest" and "lowest" in the codes of a sample of 710 male psychiatric inpatients from the Psychiatric Unit

	High Point									
Low Point	–	1	2	3	4	6	7	8	9	Total
–	.0	8.3	12.4	3.4	10.5	1.1	5.1	7.5	2.1	50.4
1	.4		1.1	.0	2.1	.7	.6	.7	.8	6.4
2	.3	.1		.0	1.4	.1	.4	.4	1.5	4.2
3	.1	.0	.1		.4	.3	.0	.3	1.4	2.6
4	.3	.6	.7	.3		.1	.4	.1	.3	2.8
6	.1	2.0	1.1	.6	1.1		.1	.4	1.3	6.7
7	.0	.3	.4	.3	.1	.3		.3	.6	2.3
8	.3	.3	1.4	.0	.0	.0	.1		.1	2.2
9	.3	3.4	9.8	2.1	2.4	1.3	1.7	1.1		22.1
Total	1.8	15.0	27.0	6.7	18.0	3.9	8.4	10.8	8.1	99.7

Table II. Relative frequencies of various combinations of scales as "highest" and "lowest" in the codes of a sample of 1053 female psychiatric inpatients from the Psychiatric Unit

	High Point									
Low Point	–	1	2	3	4	6	7	8	9	Total
–	.1	6.1	13.6	10.0	9.1	5.2	2.6	8.6	2.9	58.2
1	.1		.1	.1	.9	.6	.1	.3	1.0	3.2
2	.3	.1		.6	.4	.3	.0	.2	2.1	4.0
3	.0	.2	.2		.0	.5	.0	.3	.8	2.0
4	.4	.9	.7	1.0		.0	.3	.1	.2	3.6
6	.1	.9	.9	1.1	1.3		.2	.1	.7	5.3
7	.1	.4	.1	.1	.5	.3		.2	.8	2.5
8	.2	.2	.2	.5	.1	.0	.0		.1	1.3
9	.3	2.8	9.2	4.5	1.4	1.0	1.4	.3		20.9
Total	1.6	11.6	25.0	17.9	13.7	7.9	4.6	10.1	8.6	101.0

Table III. Relative frequencies of various combinations of scales as "highest" and "lowest" in the codes of a sample of 256 male adult "normals" in Minnesota

	High Point									
Low Point	–	1	2	3	4	6	7	8	9	Total
–	.0	3.9	.8	.8	3.1	.8	1.2	.8	.8	11.4
1	3.9		.8	.0	.8	2.3	.4	.8	4.7	13.7
2	3.9	1.2		1.2	1.2	.8	1.2	1.2	5.8	17.3
3	1.9	.0	.8		.8	2.7	1.2	.8	1.6	9.8
4	3.5	.4	1.9	.4		.8	.4	.4	.8	8.6
6	3.5	2.3	.0	1.2	2.3		.4	.4	1.9	12.0
7	1.9	1.2	.8	.0	.4	.0		.0	1.9	6.2
8	4.3	.8	.4	.0	.4	.4	.0		.8	7.1
9	.8	3.1	2.7	3.5	2.3	.8	1.9	.4		15.5
Total	23.7	12.9	8.2	7.1	11.3	8.6	6.7	4.8	18.3	101.6

Table IV. **Relative frequencies of various combinations of scales as "highest" and "lowest" in the codes of a sample of 360 female adult "normals" in Minnesota**

	High Point									
Low Point	–	1	2	3	4	6	7	8	9	Total
–	.3	3.3	2.2	2.2	.8	1.4	1.7	3.9	.0	15.8
1	3.6		.6	.0	2.5	1.1	.8	.3	3.3	12.2
2	2.8	1.1		.8	1.1	1.1	.3	.6	3.9	11.7
3	2.5	.0	.8		.6	.8	.8	1.1	.6	3.9
4	6.1	2.5	1.4	.3		.8	1.1	.3	.8	14.4
6	1.9	.8	1.9	1.1	1.1		.0	.0	1.7	10.7
7	1.9	.6	.6	.3	.8	.3		.0	2.2	6.7
8	1.1	.6	.6	.6	.0	.6	.3		.3	4.1
9	5.6	3.3	5.8	1.9	1.4	1.1	1.1	.3		20.5
Total	25.8	12.2	13.9	7.2	8.3	7.2	6.1	6.5	12.8	100.0

Table V. **Relative frequencies of various combinations of scales as "highest" and "lowest" in the codes of a sample of 2805 University of Wisconsin male students**

	High Point									
Low Point	–	1	2	3	4	6	7	8	9	Total
–	.2	1.4	5.5	6.2	3.7	1.4	6.5	4.8	6.3	36.0
1	.8		2.1	.3	.9	.8	1.8	1.0	3.6	11.3
2	1.0	.2		2.5	1.3	.9	.5	.7	7.5	14.6
3	.0	.0	.3		.0	.1	.4	.3	.4	1.5
4	1.0	.4	1.0	.8		.6	1.1	.1	1.7	6.7
6	.8	.3	1.7	.9	1.2		1.3	1.1	3.5	10.8
7	.9	.0	.3	1.0	.4	.2		.3	1.8	4.9
8	.4	.1	.3	.6	.2	.2	.2		.8	2.8
9	1.2	.6	2.7	3.1	.8	.9	1.6	.7		11.6
Total	6.3	3.0	13.9	15.4	8.5	5.1	13.4	9.0	25.6	100.2

Table VI. Relative frequencies of various combinations of scales as "highest" and "lowest" in the codes of a sample of 1367 University of Wisconsin female students

	High Point									
Low Point	–	1	2	3	4	6	7	8	9	Total
–	.4	1.2	3.5	3.8	4.7	3.4	5.0	4.4	6.7	33.1
1	1.4		1.2	.2	1.7	2.3	1.8	1.3	5.2	15.1
2	1.7	.4		2.6	2.2	1.7	.6	1.3	6.3	16.8
3	.4	.0	.4		.1	.7	.9	.7	1.2	4.4
4	2.3	.2	.4	.6		1.2	.9	.4	1.1	7.1
6	1.1	.1	1.1	.7	.8		.7	.6	2.2	7.3
7	.9	.1	.0	.8	.4	.7		.1	.7	3.7
8	.6	.1	.3	.4	.0	.1	.1		.1	1.7
9	2.1	.2	1.1	2.1	1.2	1.8	1.4	.7		10.6
Total	10.9	2.3	8.0	11.2	11.1	11.9	11.4	9.5	23.5	99.8

Table VII. **Relative frequencies of various combinations of scales as "highest" and "lowest" in the codes of a sample of 1816 ninth-grade schoolboys in Minneapolis**

Low Point	High Point									
	–	1	2	3	4	6	7	8	9	Total
–	.1	2.0	2.1	1.7	11.1	1.8	3.4	7.6	5.1	34.9
1	.3		.6	.0	1.6	.8	.9	1.8	4.0	10.0
2	1.3	.4		1.0	4.4	.8	.5	2.5	8.3	19.2
3	.4	.0	.6		1.5	.2	1.0	1.8	3.7	9.2
4	.3	.1	.5	.1		.1	.3	.7	.6	2.7
6	.7	.4	1.1	.3	3.6		1.0	1.5	2.5	11.1
7	.6	.1	.2	.1	.7	.2		.2	1.3	3.4
8	.4	.1	.3	.0	.2	.0	.1		.2	1.3
9	.6	.9	1.6	.9	2.2	.4	.9	.7		8.2
Total	4.7	4.0	7.0	4.1	25.3	4.3	8.1	16.8	25.7	100.0

Table VIII. **Relative frequencies of various combinations of scales as "highest" and "lowest" in the codes of a sample of 1937 ninth-grade schoolgirls in Minneapolis**

Low Point	High Point									
	–	1	2	3	4	6	7	8	9	Total
–	.1	.3	.4	1.4	8.6	2.4	1.7	4.1	3.5	22.5
1	2.3		.5	.3	5.0	1.9	1.6	2.0	5.3	18.9
2	1.6	.2		1.7	6.3	2.6	1.3	2.1	7.6	23.4
3	.9	.0	.3		2.1	1.0	.9	1.8	2.6	9.6
4	1.0	.1	.1	.1		.4	.2	.2	.1	2.2
6	.9	.2	.3	.4	2.5		1.0	.7	2.2	8.2
7	.5	.1	.1	.3	1.2	.3		.0	.4	2.9
8	.1	.0	.1	.1	.1	.2	.1		.1	.8
9	2.3	.4	1.1	1.1	3.4	1.7	1.1	1.0		12.1
Total	9.7	1.3	2.9	5.4	29.2	10.5	7.9	11.9	21.8	100.6

In Tables IX to XXIII the Normal Population indicates the percentage occurrences of the given codes as shown in samples from the normal population (Figures 3 and 4, averaged) and the percentage occurrences in a general clinical sample (Figures 1 and 2, averaged). All codes were included in the abbreviated tables when any one of the three columns of the complete code frequency table showed a percentage of 4 or larger. Codes with no "high point" are indicated by a dash (–).

Table IX. Alcoholics: an abbreviated table contrasting the observed frequencies of certain common codes, in percentages, among normal and general clinical samples with the frequencies obtained from the 74 alcoholics in this *Atlas*

Code	In Normal Population	In Clinical Samples	Among Alcoholics in *Atlas*
–	24.7	1.8	1.3
13	3.7	6.6	2.7
21	1.7	5.0	2.0
23	1.4	4.5	3.4
27	2.0	9.0	4.7
31	2.3	5.3	1.3
46	.6	2.0	4.7
49	1.5	2.3	6.1
72	1.4	2.9	4.0
9–	8.4	.9	.0
98	.8	1.9	6.7

Table X. Psychopathic Personality, Asocial, Amoral: an abbreviated table contrasting the observed frequency of certain common codes, in percentage, among the normal and clinical general samples with the frequencies obtained from the 94 psychopathic personalities of the asocial type in the *Atlas*

Code	In Normal Population	In Clinical Samples	Among Psychopathic Personalities, Asocial Type, in *Atlas*
–	24.7	1.8	.0
13	3.7	6.6	.0
21	1.7	5.0	.5
23	1.4	4.5	1.1
27	2.0	9.0	.0
31	2.3	5.3	1.1
42	.7	3.3	7.4
46	.6	2.0	6.4
48	1.1	3.6	16.5
49	1.5	2.3	12.8
89	.7	1.2	4.3
9–	8.4	.9	1.1
98	.8	1.9	4.3

Table XI. Psychopathic Personality, Mixed: an abbreviated table contrasting the observed frequency of certain common codes, in percentage, among the normal and clinical general samples with the frequencies obtained from the 86 patients in the *Atlas* diagnosed as having psychopathic personalities of the mixed and pathological emotionality types

Code	In Normal Population	In Clinical Samples	Among Psychopathic Personalities, Mixed Type, in *Atlas*
–	24.7	1.8	.0
13	3.7	6.6	7.6
21	1.7	5.0	.7
23	1.4	4.5	2.3
27	2.0	9.0	6.4
31	2.3	5.3	3.5
42	.7	3.3	6.4
43	2.3	2.3	4.6
46	.6	2.0	10.2
48	1.1	3.6	10.2
84	1.0	1.5	4.1
87	.8	2.5	5.8
9–	8.4	.9	.0

Table XII. Organic types: an abbreviated table contrasting the observed frequency of certain common codes, in percentage, among the normal and clinical general samples with the frequencies obtained from 52 patients in the *Atlas* with organic brain damage

Code	In Normal Population	In Clinical Samples	Among Patients in *Atlas* with Brain Damage
–	24.7	1.8	.0
13	3.7	6.6	4.8
21	1.7	5.0	9.6
23	1.4	4.5	5.7
27	2.0	9.0	6.7
31	2.3	5.3	2.9
42	.7	3.3	7.7
48	1.1	3.6	4.8
9–	8.4	.9	3.8
92	.4	.6	8.6
98	.8	1.9	3.8

Table XIII. Psychoneurosis, Hypochondriasis: an abbreviated table contrasting the observed frequency of certain common codes, in percentage, among the normal and clinical general samples with the frequencies obtained from the 106 patients in the *Atlas* diagnosed as having psychoneurosis, hypochondriasis

Code	Among Normal Population	In Clinical Samples	Among Patients in *Atlas* with Psychoneurosis, Hypochondriasis
–	24.7	1.8	.0
12	1.9	2.7	10.9
13	3.7	6.6	18.4
21	1.7	5.0	18.0
27	2.0	9.0	4.7
31	2.3	5.3	18.4
9–	8.4	.9	.0

Table XIV. Psychoneurosis, Hysteria: an abbreviated table contrasting the observed frequency of certain common codes, in percentage, among the normal and clinical general samples with the frequencies obtained from the 85 hysteria patients in the *Atlas*

Code	In Normal Population	In Clinical Samples	Among Hysteria Patients in *Atlas*
–	24.7	1.8	4.7
13	3.7	6.6	8.8
21	1.7	5.0	4.7
23	1.4	4.5	3.5
27	2.0	9.0	3.5
31	2.3	5.3	21.7
87	.8	2.5	4.1
9–	8.4	.9	1.2

Table XV. Psychoneurosis, Mixed: an abbreviated table contrasting the observed frequency of certain common codes, in percentage, among the normal and clinical general samples with the frequencies obtained from the 133 mixed-psychoneurotic patients in the *Atlas*

Code	In Normal Population	In Clinical Samples	Among Mixed-Psychoneurotic Patients in *Atlas*
–	24.7	1.8	.0
13	3.7	6.6	7.6
21	1.7	5.0	8.0
23	1.4	4.5	9.2
28	.2	2.2	5.7
31	2.3	5.3	9.2
32	.7	2.3	5.7
82	.7	1.8	5.0
87	.8	2.5	4.6
9–	8.4	.9	.0

Table XVI. **Psychoneurotic, Psychasthenic: an abbreviated table contrasting the observed frequency of certain common codes, in percentage, among the normal and clinical general samples with the frequencies obtained from the 91 psychasthenic patients in the *Atlas***

Code	In Normal Population	In Clinical Samples	Among Psychasthenic Patients in *Atlas*
–	24.7	1.8	1.1
13	3.7	6.6	.5
21	1.7	5.0	5.4
23	1.4	4.5	6.5
27	2.0	9.0	23.5
31	2.3	5.3	1.1
72	1.4	2.9	16.3
78	1.3	1.7	9.8
87	.8	2.5	9.2
9–	8.4	.9	.0

Table XVII. Reactive Depression: an abbreviated table contrasting the observed frequency of certain common codes, in percentage, among the normal and clinical general samples with the frequencies obtained from the 110 reactive depressives in the *Atlas*

Code	In Normal Population	In Clinical Samples	Among Reactive Depressives in *Atlas*
–	24.7	1.8	.0
13	3.7	6.6	1.8
21	1.7	5.0	3.6
23	1.4	4.5	12.3
27	2.0	9.0	22.0
28	.2	2.2	5.5
31	2.3	5.3	5.5
48	1.1	3.6	.0
72	1.4	2.9	8.6
9–	8.4	.9	.0

Table XVIII. Paranoid: an abbreviated table contrasting the observed frequency of certain common codes, in percentage, among the normal and clinical general samples with the frequencies obtained from 128 paranoid patients in the *Atlas*

Code	In Normal Population	In Clinical Samples	Among Paranoid Patients in *Atlas*
–	24.7	1.8	2.3
13	3.7	6.6	3.9
21	1.7	5.0	3.9
23	1.4	4.5	7.4
26	.8	1.6	4.3
27	2.0	9.0	3.9
31	2.3	5.3	1.6
43	2.3	2.3	4.3
46	.6	2.0	4.3
48	1.1	3.6	5.5
68	.8	1.3	4.3
9–	8.4	.9	.0
94	3.2	2.2	5.5

Table XIX. Psychotic Depression: an abbreviated table contrasting the observed frequency of certain common codes, in percentage, among the normal and clinical general samples with the frequencies obtained from 121 persons in the *Atlas* diagnosed as being manic-depressive, with depressed and involutional melancholia

Code	In Normal Population	In Clinical Samples	Among Patients in *Atlas* with Psychotic Depression
–	24.7	1.8	.8
13	3.7	6.6	2.1
21	1.7	5.0	5.0
23	1.4	4.5	7.0
27	2.0	9.0	26.0
28	.2	2.2	6.6
31	2.3	5.3	.8
72	1.4	2.9	7.4
82	.7	1.8	7.4
9–	8.4	.9	.8

Table XX. Hypomania: an abbreviated table contrasting the observed frequency of certain common codes, in percentage, among normal and clinical general samples with the frequencies obtained from the 47 manic-depressives, manic type, of the *Atlas*

Code	In Normal Population	In Clinical Samples	Among Patients in *Atlas* with Hypomania
–	24.7	1.8	2.1
13	3.7	6.6	1.1
21	1.7	5.0	.0
23	1.4	4.5	1.1
27	2.0	9.0	.0
31	2.3	5.3	2.1
48	1.1	3.6	4.3
49	1.5	2.3	4.3
68	.8	1.3	6.4
9–	8.4	.9	2.1
94	3.2	2.2	30.0
96	.7	.9	5.3
98	.8	1.9	16.0

Table XXI. Psychosis, Schizophrenia: an abbreviated table contrasting the observed frequency of certain common codes, in percentage, among normal and clinical general samples with the frequencies obtained from the 161 schizophrenics of all types of the *Atlas*

Code	In Normal Population	In Clinical Samples	Among Schizophrenics in *Atlas*
–	24.7	1.8	1.2
13	3.7	6.6	1.2
21	1.7	5.0	3.7
23	1.4	4.5	2.5
27	2.0	9.0	5.3
31	2.3	5.3	.8
48	1.1	3.6	4.0
68	.8	1.3	5.0
82	.7	1.8	4.3
86	.7	1.4	7.2
9–	8.4	.9	1.2

Table XXII. Schizoid: an abbreviated table contrasting the observed frequency of certain common codes, in percentage, among normal and clinical general samples with the frequencies obtained from the 78 persons in the *Atlas* diagnosed as being schizoid

Code	In Normal Population	In Clinical Samples	Among Schizoid Patients in *Atlas*
–	24.7	1.8	.0
13	3.7	6.6	2.6
21	1.7	5.0	1.9
23	1.4	4.5	1.3
27	2.0	9.0	13.4
31	2.3	5.3	3.2
48	1.1	3.6	6.4
72	1.4	2.9	5.8
82	.7	1.8	4.5
86	.7	1.4	3.9
87	.8	2.5	8.3
9–	8.4	.9	.0
94	3.2	2.2	4.5

Table XXIII. Suicidal: an abbreviated table contrasting the observed frequency of certain common codes, in percentage, among normal and clinical general samples with the frequencies obtained from the 107 persons of the *Atlas* with suicidal tendencies

Code	In Normal Population	In Clinical Samples	Among Patients in *Atlas* with Suicidal Tendencies
–	24.7	1.8	.9
13	3.7	6.6	2.8
21	1.7	5.0	3.3
23	1.4	4.5	5.6
27	2.0	9.0	15.4
28	.2	2.2	6.5
31	2.3	5.3	4.2
32	.7	1.8	6.1
37	.8	2.5	6.1
9–	8.4	.9	.9

Bibliography

This list includes most papers which make more than a passing reference to the MMPI (through November 1950). It covers psychological, medical, and sociological literature. Starred entries are considered basic reading for clinicians expecting to use the Inventory.

Aaronson, B. S., and G. S. Welsh. "The MMPI as diagnostic differentiator: A reply to Rubin." *J. consult. Psychol.*, 14:324–25 (1950).

Abramson, H. A. "The effect of alcohol on the Personality Inventory (Minnesota); preliminary report." *Psychosom. Med.*, 7:184–85 (1945).

———. "The effect of alcohol on the Personality Inventory." *Ann. N.Y. Acad. Sci.*, 46:535–57 (1946).

———. "The Minnesota Personality Test in relation to selection of specialized military personnel." *Psychosom. Med.*, 7:178–84 (1945).

——— and others. "Non-projective personality tests." *Ann. N.Y. Acad. Sci.*, 46:531–678 (1946).

Adjutant General's Office, Personnel Research Section. "Analysis of item responses of WAC's and WAC applicants on the MMPI and Cornell Selectee Index." PRS No. 726, 1944. Pp. 22.

———. "Measurement of personal characteristics of War Department personnel." PRS No. 669, 1944. Pp. 13.

———, Personnel Research and Procurement Branch. "Research on personality testing." *Bull. milit. clin. Psychol.*, 1:33–41 (1946).

Albee, G. W. "Psychological concomitants of pulmonary tuberculosis." *Amer. Rev. Tuberculosis*, 58:650–61 (1948).

Altus, W. D. "The adjustment of army illiterates." *Psychol. Bull.*, 42:461–76 (1945).

———. "A college achiever and non-achiever scale for the MMPI." *J. appl. Psychol.*, 32:385–97 (1948).

———. "Some correlates of the group Rorschach and the schizophrenia scale of the group MMPI among two groups of 'normal' college students." *J. consult. Psychol.*, 12:375–78 (1948). Also abstracted in *Amer. Psychologist*, 3:349 (1948).

——— and H. M. Bell. "An analysis of four orally administered measures of adjustment." *Educ. psychol. Measmt.*, 7:101–15 (1947).

———. "The validity of certain measures of maladjustment in an army special training center." *Psychol. Bull.*, 42:98–108 (1945).

Anderson, A. L. "Personality changes following pre-frontal lobotomy." *J. consult. Psychol.*, 13:105–7 (1949).

Arthur, G. "An experience in examining an Indian twelfth-grade group with the MMPI." *Ment. Hyg.*, 28:243–50 (1944).

Baker, G., and J. G. Peatman. "Tests used in Veterans Administration guidance units." *Amer. Psychologist*, 2:99–102 (1947).

Bard, P. "A note on MMPI (Pd) scores of state training school boys." *Minn. Counselor*, 4(No. 2):21 (1950).

Barnabus, B. "Twelve tests that have been proved practical in commercial application." *Trans. Kans. Acad. Sci.*, 50:204–7 (1947).

Benton, A. L. "The MMPI in clinical practice." *J. nerv. ment. Dis.*, 102:416–20 (1945).

———. In Buros's *The third mental measurements yearbook*. New Brunswick, N.J.: Rutgers University Press, 1949. Pp. 104–7.

——— and K. A. Probst. "A comparison of psychiatric ratings with MMPI scores." *J. abnorm. soc. Psychol.*, 41:75–78 (1946).

Berdie, R. F. "Range of interests and psychopathologies." *J. clin. Psychol.*, 2:161–66 (1946).

Berkshire, J. R., S. F. T. Bugental, and F. P. Cassens. "Test preferences in guidance centers." *Occupations*, 26:337–43 (1948).

Bier, W. C. (S.J.). "A comparative study of a seminary group and four other groups on the MMPI." *Stud. Psychol. Psychiat.*, 7:1–107 (1948).

BIBLIOGRAPHY

Birnberg, V. K. "The relationship between food aversions and the MMPI for college women." Unpublished M.A. thesis, University of Minnesota, 1945.

Blake, R. R., and G. P. Wilson. "Perceptual Selectivity in Rorschach Determinants as a Function of Depressive Tendencies." *J. abnorm. soc. Psychol.*, 45:459–72 (1950).

Blum, L. P. "A comparative study of students preparing for five selected professions including teaching." *J. exp. Educ.*, 16:31–65 (1947).

Bolander, W. G. "A study of the MMPI as an indicator in the prediction of college success." Unpublished M.A. thesis, University of Oregon, 1947.

Bortin, A. W., and I. Brill. "Psychiatric studies based on new personality test." *Milit. Surg.*, 96:497–503 (1945).

Brower, D. "The relation between intelligence and MMPI scores." *J. soc. Psychol.*, 25:243–45 (1947).

———. "The relations between MMPI scores and cardio-vascular measures before and after experimentally induced visuo-motor conflict." *J. soc. Psychol.*, 26:55–60 (1947).

———. "The relations of visuo-motor conflict to personality traits and cardio-vascular activity." *J. gen. Psychol.*, 38:69–99 (1948).

Brown, D. G., and W. L. Lowe. "A study of religious beliefs and personality differences in college students." Unpublished M.A. thesis, University of Denver, 1948.

Brown, H. S. "An investigation of the validity of the MMPI for a college population, and the relationship of certain personality traits to achievement." Unpublished Ph.D. thesis, University of Minnesota, 1947.

———. "Similarities and differences in college populations on the Multiphasic." *J. appl. Psychol.*, 32:541–49 (1948).

*Brown, M. A. "Alcoholic profiles on the Minnesota Multiphasic." *J. clin. Psychol.*, 6:266–69 (1950).

Brozek, J. "Psychology of human starvation and nutritional rehabilitation." *Sci. Mon.*, 70:270–74 (1950).

——— and N. K. Erickson. "Item analysis of the psychoneurotic scales on the MMPI in experimental semistarvation." *J. consult. Psychol.*, 12:403–11 (1948).

———, H. Guetzkow, and A. Keys. "A study of personality of normal young men maintained on restricted intakes of vitamins of the B complex." *Psychosom. Med.*, 8:98–109 (1946).

——— and B. C. Schiele. "Clinical significance of the Minnesota Multiphasic F scale evaluated in experimental neurosis." *Amer. J. Psychiat.*, 105:259–66 (1948).

Burton, A. "The use of the masculinity-femininity of the MMPI as an aid in the diagnosis of sexual inversion." *J. Psychol.*, 24:161–64 (1947).

———. "The use of psychometric and projective tests in clinical psychology." *J. Psychol.*, 28:451–56 (1949).

——— and C. J. Bright. "Adaptation of the MMPI for group administration and rapid scoring." *J. consult. Psychol.*, 10:99–103 (1946).

Canning, W., G. Harlow, and C. Regelin. "A study of two personality questionnaires." *J. consult. Psychol.*, 14:414–15 (1950).

Capwell, D. F. "Personality patterns of adolescent girls: I. Girls who show improvement in I.Q." *J. appl. Psychol.*, 29:212–28 (1945).

*———. "Personality patterns of adolescent girls: II. Delinquents and non-delinquents." *J. appl. Psychol.*, 29:289–97 (1945).

Carp, A. "MMPI performance and insulin shock therapy." *J. abnorm. soc. Psychol.*, 45:721–26 (1950).

Cauffiel, P. W. "A comparison of the P-S experience blank with the MMPI." Unpublished M.A. thesis, Pennsylvania State College, 1950.

Chyatte, C. "Personality traits of professional actors." *Occupations*, 27:245–50 (1949).

Cillis, O. E. de, and W. D. Orbison. "A comparison of the Terman-Miles M-F test and the Mf scale of the MMPI." *J. appl. Psychol.*, 34:338–42 (1950).

Clark, J. H. "Additional applications of the Altus thirty-six point adjustment test as a screening instrument." *J. gen. Psychol.*, 40:261–65 (1949).

———. "The adjustment of army AWOL's." *J. abnorm. soc. Psychol.*, 44:394–401 (1949).

———. "Application of the MMPI in differentiating AWOL recidivists from non-recidivists." *J. Psychol.*, 26:229–34 (1948).

———. "Clinical use of the Altus thirty-six point adjustment test in screening army AWOL's." *J. consult. Psychol.*, 12:276–79 (1948). Also abstracted in *Amer. Psychologist*, 2:411 (1947).

———."Intertest variability on the California Test of Mental Maturity in relation to the MMPI." *J. consult. Psychol.*, 14:32–34 (1950).

———. "Some MMPI correlates of color responses in the group Rorschach." *J. consult. Psychol.*, 12:384–86 (1948). Also abstracted in *Amer. Psychologist*, 3:349 (1948).

BIBLIOGRAPHY

Cofer, C. N., J. Chance, and A. J. Judson. "A study of malingering on the MMPI." *J. Psychol.,* 27:491–99 (1949).

———, A. J. Judson, and D. V. Weick. "On the significance of the psychogalvanic response as an indicator of reaction to personality test items." *J. Psychol.,* 27:347–54 (1949). Also abstracted in *Amer. Psychologist,* 3:303 (1948).

Cook, E. B., and R. J. Wherry. "A factor analysis of MMPI and aptitude test data." *J. appl. Psychol.,* 34:260–65 (1950).

Corsini, R. J. "A time and motion study of hand scoring the individual MMPI." *J. consult. Psychol.,* 13:62–63 (1949).

Cottle, W. C. "Consideration of correlation coefficients of the card versus booklet forms of the MMPI as reliability coefficients." *J. appl. Psychol.,* 34:255–59 (1950).

———. "A factorial study of the Multiphasic, Strong, Kuder, and Bell inventories using a population of adult males." *Psychometrika,* 15:25–47 (1950).

———. "Relationships among selected personality and interest inventories." *Occupations,* 28:306–10 (1950). Also abstracted in *Amer. Psychologist,* 4:292–93 (1949).

——— and J. O. Powell. "Relationship of mean scores on the Strong, Kuder, and Bell inventories with the MMPI Mf scale as a criterion." *Trans. Kans. Acad. Sci.,* 52:396–98 (1949).

Crook, G. H. "The measurement of personal characteristics: Are available tests of personality of use in the army?" Adjutant General's Office, Personnel Research Section, Report No. 669, 1944. Pp. 5.

Cross, O. H. "Adaptation of the MMPI for use with the blind." Unpublished M.A. thesis, University of Minnesota, 1945.

———. "Braille edition of the MMPI for use with the blind." *J. appl. Psychol.,* 31:189–98 (1947).

Daly, J. M. "Relationship of MMPI and Kuder Preference Record scores." Unpublished M.A. thesis, Catholic University, 1948.

Daniels, E. E., and W. A. Hunter. "MMPI personality patterns for various occupations." *J. appl. Psychol.,* 33:559–65 (1949).

Darley, J. G., and D. G. Marquis. "Veterans' guidance centers: A survey of their problems and activities." *J. clin. Psychol.,* 2:109–16 (1946).

Davis, C. E. "The MMPI: A new method of scoring and analysis." *J. clin. Psychol.,* 3:298–301 (1947).

Drake, L. E. "A method for machine scoring the card form of the MMPI." *J. educ. Res.,* 41:139–41 (1947).

———. "A social I.E. scale for the MMPI." *J. appl. Psychol.,* 30:51–54 (1946).

——— and W. B. Thiede. "Further validation of the social I.E. scale for the MMPI." *J. educ. Res.,* 41:551–56 (1948).

Ellis, A. "Personality questionnaires." *Rev. educ. Res.,* 17:53–63 (1947).

———. "The validity of personality questionnaires." *Psychol. Bull.,* 43:385–440 (1946).

——— and H. S. Conrad. "The validity of personality inventories in military practice." *Psychol. Bull.,* 45:385–426 (1948).

Eysenck, H. J. In Buros's *Third mental measurements yearbook.* New Brunswick, N.J.: Rutgers University Press, 1949. Pp. 107–8.

Falls, R. P., and R. R. Blake. "A quantitative analysis of the Picture-Frustration study." *J. Personality,* 16:320–25 (1948).

Farberow, N. L. "Personality patterns of suicidal mental hospital patients." *Genet. Psychol. Monogr.,* 42:3–80 (1950).

Feldman, M. J. "A prognosis scale for shock therapy." *Amer. Psychologist,* 3:348 (1948). Abstract.

Ferguson, R. G. "A useful adjunct to the Minnesota Personality Inventory scoring and analysis." *J. clin. Psychol.,* 2:248–53 (1946).

Foster, K. "A study of WPA white collar workers with respect to job satisfaction and personality characteristics." Unpublished M.S. thesis, University of Minnesota, 1941.

Friedman, S. H. "Psychometric effects of frontal and parietal lobe brain damage." Unpublished Ph.D. thesis, University of Minnesota, 1950.

Fry, F. D. "A study of the personality traits of college students and of state prison inmates as measured by the MMPI." *J. Psychol.,* 28:439–49 (1949).

Gilliland, A. R. "A comparison of two personality tests." *Amer. Psychologist,* 4:258 (1949). Abstract.

Gjerde, C. M. "Parent-child resemblances in vocational interests and personality traits." Unpublished Ph.D. thesis, University of Minnesota, 1949.

Goffard, S. J. "Some diagnostic correlates of sociometric status." Unpublished Ph.D. thesis, University of Minnesota, 1949.

*Gough, H. G. "Diagnostic patterns on the MMPI." *J. clin. Psychol.,* 2:23–37 (1946).

BIBLIOGRAPHY

———. "The F-K dissimulation index for the MMPI." *J. consult. Psychol.*, 14:408–13 (1950).

———. "Factors relating to the academic achievement of high school students." *J. educ. Psychol.*, 40:65–78 (1949).

———. "A new dimension of status: I. Development of a personality scale." *Amer. sociol. Rev.*, 13:401–9 (1948).

———. "A new dimension of status: II. Relationship of the St scale to other variables." *Amer. sociol. Rev.*, 13:534–37 (1948).

———. "A new dimension of status: III. Discrepancies between the St scale and 'objective status'." *Amer. sociol. Rev.*, 14:275–81 (1949).

———. "A note on the security-insecurity test." *J. soc. Psychol.*, 28:257–61 (1948).

———. "Personality correlates of social and ethnic attitudes among high school students." Unpublished Ph.D. thesis, University of Minnesota, 1949.

———. "Personality correlates of socio-economic status." *Amer. Psychologist*, 3:360 (1948). Abstract.

———. "A research note on the MMPI social I.E. scale." *J. educ. Res.*, 43:138–41 (1949).

———. "Simulated patterns on the MMPI." *J. abnorm. soc. Psychol.*, 42:215–25 (1947).

———, H. McClosky, and P. E. Meehl. "A scale for measuring social responsibility." *J. abnorm. soc. Psychol.*, in press.

———. "A scale for measuring dominance." *J. abnorm. soc. Psychol.*, in press.

Grant, H. "A rapid personality evaluation based on the MMPI and the Cornell Selectee Index." *Amer. J. Psychiat.*, 103:33–41 (1946).

Guetzkow, H., and others. "Recovery after 12 weeks of controlled nutritional rehabilitation following experimental semi-starvation in man: Part III. Personality." *Amer. Psychologist*, 2:330–31 (1947). Abstract.

Gulde, C. J., and H. L. Roy. "A note on the scoring of the MMPI." *J. consult. Psychol.*, 11:221–22 (1947).

*Guthrie, G. M. "Six MMPI diagnostic profile patterns." *J. Psychol.*, 30:317–23 (1950).

———. "A study of the personality characteristics associated with the disorders encountered by an internist." Unpublished Ph.D. thesis, University of Minnesota, 1949.

Hales, W. M., and W. Simon. "MMPI patterns before and after insulin shock therapy." *Amer. J. Psychiat.*, 105:254–58 (1948).

Hampton, P. J. "The MMPI as a psychometric tool for diagnosing personality disorders among college students." *J. soc. Psychol.*, 26:99–108 (1947).

Hanvik, L. J. "Some psychological dimensions of low back pain." Unpublished Ph.D. thesis, University of Minnesota, 1949.

Harmon, L. R., and D. N. Wiener. "Use of the MMPI in vocational advisement." *J. appl. Psychol.*, 29:132–41 (1945).

Harris, R. E. "Measured personality characteristics of convulsive therapy patients: A study of diagnostic and prognostic criteria." *Psychol. Bull.*, 42:535 (1945). Abstract.

———, K. M. Bowman, and A. Simon. "Studies in electronarcosis therapy: III. Psychological test findings." *J. nerv. ment. Dis.*, 107:371–76 (1948).

*——— and C. Christiansen. "Prediction of response to brief psychotherapy." *J. Psychol.*, 21:269–84 (1946).

——— and V. M. Ives. "A study of the personality of alcoholics." *Amer. Psychologist*, 2:405 (1947). Abstract.

Hathaway, S. R. "A coding system for MMPI profiles." *J. consult. Psychol.*, 11:334–37 (1947).

———. "Multiphasic Personality Inventory." *Modern Hospital*, 66:65–67 (1946).

———. *Supplementary manual for the MMPI.* Part I, "The K scale and its use." Part II, "The booklet form of the MMPI." New York: Psychological Corporation, 1946.

*——— and J. C. McKinley. *Manual for the MMPI.* New York: Psychological Corporation, 1945.

———. "The measurement of symptomatic depression with the Minnesota Multiphasic Personality Schedule." *Psychol. Bull.*, 37:425 (1940). Abstract.

———. *The Minnesota Multiphasic Personality Schedule.* Minneapolis: University of Minnesota Press, 1942.

———. "A multiphasic personality schedule (Minnesota): I. Construction of the schedule." *J. Psychol.*, 10:249–54 (1940).

———. "A multiphasic personality schedule (Minnesota): III. The measurement of symptomatic depression." *J. Psychol.*, 14:73–84 (1942).

Hawkes, G. R. "Use of the MMPI in screening college students for counseling purposes." *J. educ. Psychol.*, 41:116–21 (1950).

Henderson, C. R., and others. "Changes in personality appraisal associated with a restricted intake of B vitamins and protein." *Amer. J. med. Sci.*, 213:488–93 (1947).

BIBLIOGRAPHY

Heston, J. C. "A comparison of four masculinity-femininity scales." *Educ. psychol. Measmt.,* 8:375–88 (1948).

Hewitt, C. C. "A personality study of alcohol addiction." *Quart. J. Stud. Alcohol,* 4:368–86 (1943).

Hibbeler, H. L. "Personality patterns of white adults with primary glaucoma." *Amer. J. Ophthal.,* 30:181–86 (1947).

Holzberg, J. D., and S. Alessi. "Reliability of the shortened MMPI." *J. consult. Psychol.,* 13:288–92 (1949).

Houk, T. W. "MMPI in diagnosis of psychoneuroses." *Northwest Med.,* 45:248–52 (1946).

——— and Y. Robertson. "Diagnosis of hypoglycemia-neurosis with the MMPI." *Northwest Med.,* 45:923 (1946).

Hovey, H. B. "Detection of circumvention in the MMPI." *J. clin. Psychol.,* 4:97 (1948).

*———. "Somatization and other neurotic reactions and MMPI profiles." *J. clin. Psychol.,* 5:153–56 (1949).

Hunt, E. L., and G. F. J. Lehner. "Relationships of the Hildreth feeling and attitude scales to the MMPI." *J. clin. Psychol.,* 4:412–14 (1948). Also abstracted in *Amer. Psychologist,* 2:417 (1947).

Hunt, H. F. "The effect of deliberate deception on MMPI performance." *J. consult. Psychol.,* 12:396–402 (1948). Also abstracted in *Amer. Psychologist,* 3:349 (1948).

——— and others. "A study of the differential diagnostic efficiency of the MMPI." *J. consult. Psychol.,* 12:331–36 (1948). Also abstracted in *Amer. Psychologist,* 2:417 (1947).

———. "A study of the effect of the K correction on the differential diagnostic efficiency of the MMPI." *Amer. Psychologist,* 2:273–74 (1947). Abstract.

Hunt, W. A., and I. Stevenson. "Psychological testing in military clinical psychology: II. Personality testing." *Psychol. Rev.,* 53:107–15 (1946).

Jeffery, M. E. "Some factors influencing answers on the Multiphasic K scale." Unpublished Ph.D thesis, University of Minnesota, 1946.

Jennings, L. S. "MMPI: Differentiation of psychologically good and poor combat risks among flying personnel." *J. Aviat. Med.,* 19:222–26, 237 (1948).

Jensen, M. B., and J. B. Rotter. "The value of thirteen psychological tests in officer candidate screening." *J. appl. Psychol.,* 31:312–22 (1947).

Johnson, R. H., and G. L. Bond. "Reading ease of commonly used tests." *J. appl. Psychol.,* 34:319–24 (1950).

Johnson, R. L. E. "The relation of religious attitudes and selected personality characteristics." Unpublished M.A. thesis, University of Minnesota, 1948.

Kahn, H., and E. Singer. "An investigation of the factors related to success or failure of school of commerce students." *J. educ. Psychol.,* 40:107–17 (1949).

Kalhorn, J. "Personality and parent behavior." *Amer. Psychologist,* 2:425 (1947). Abstract.

Kamman, G. R. "Psychosomatic diagnosis." *J. Lancet,* 67:102–7 (1947).

Kazan, A. T., and I. M. Sheinberg. "Clinical note on the significance of the validity score (F) in the MMPI." *Amer. J. Psychiat.,* 102:181–83 (1945).

Kelly, E. L., and D. W. Fiske. *The selection of clinical psychologists. Progress report and preliminary findings.* Ann Arbor: Edwards Letter Shop, 1948.

Keys, A., and others. *Biology of Human Starvation.* Vol. II. Minneapolis: University of Minnesota Press, 1950.

———. "Later stages of rehabilitation following experimental starvation in man." Laboratory of Physiological Hygiene Report, University of Minnesota, 1946.

———. "Rehabilitation following experimental starvation in man." Laboratory of Physiological Hygiene Report, University of Minnesota, 1946.

Kinsala, J. E., and E. L. Phillips. "Personality characteristics of veterans with no primary interest on the Strong Vocational Interest Test." *Minn. Counselor,* 4(No. 1):13–17 (1949).

Koskaff, Y. D., and E. Wheeler. "Psychometric evaluation of non-institutionalized epileptic patients with varying degrees of cerebral dysrhythmia." *Trans. Amer. Neurol. Assoc.,* 1946 (71st meeting), p. 173. Abstract.

Krise, E. M. "A common error in scoring the MMPI." *J. clin. Psychol.,* 2:180–81 (1949).

———. "A short method of scoring the MMPI." *J. clin. Psychol.,* 3:386–92 (1947).

Lagerstedt, B. "Investigation of personality and attitudinal changes in three SPAN groups." Unpublished M.A. thesis, University of Minnesota, 1950.

La Tourelle, C. W. "A study of the relationship of the subtest deviations on the Wechsler-Bellevue intelligence scale and scores of the MMPI." Unpublished M.A. thesis, University of Southern California, 1946.

Leton, D. "A study of the relationship between the Kuder Preference Record and the MMPI." *Minn. Counselor,* 4(No. 1):18–22 (1949).

BIBLIOGRAPHY

Leverenz, C. W. "MMPI: An evaluation of its usefulness in the psychiatric service of a station hospital." *War Med.*, 4:618–29 (1943).

Lewis, J. A. "Kuder Preference Record and MMPI scores for two occupational groups." *J. consult. Psychol.*, 11:194–201 (1947).

———. "Occupational interests and personality tendencies." Unpublished M.A. thesis, University of Minnesota, 1946.

Lively, M. L. "An investigation of some clinical aspects of the Heidbreder introversion-extroversion variable." Unpublished M.A. thesis, University of Minnesota, 1943.

Loth, N. N. "Correlations between the Guilford-Martin inventory of factors STDCR and the MMPI at the college level." Unpublished M.A. thesis, University of Minnesota, 1945.

Lough, O. M. "Teachers college students and the MMPI." *J. appl. Psychol.*, 30:241–47 (1946).

———. "Women students in liberal arts, nursing, and teacher training curricula and the MMPI." *J. appl. Psychol.*, 31:437–45 (1947).

Louttit, C. M., and C. G. Browne. "The use of psychometric instruments in psychological clinics." *J. consult. Psychol.*, 11:49–54 (1947).

Mann, W. A. "Validation of the Cornell Index for freshmen at Michigan State College." Unpublished Ph.D. thesis, Michigan State College, 1949.

Manson, M. P. "A psychometric analysis of psychopathic characteristics of alcoholics." *J. consult. Psychol.*, 13:111–18 (1949).

——— and H. M. Grayson. "Keysort method of scoring the MMPI." *J. appl. Psychol.*, 30:509–16 (1946).

McKinley, J. C., and S. R. Hathaway. "The identification and measurement of the psychoneuroses in medical practice." *J. Amer. med. Assoc.*, 122:161–67 (1943).

———. "A multiphasic personality schedule (Minnesota): II. A differential study of hypochondriasis." *J. Psychol.*, 10:255–68 (1940).

———. "A multiphasic personality schedule (Minnesota): IV. Psychasthenia." *J. appl. Psychol.*, 26:614–24 (1942).

———. "The MMPI: V. Hysteria, hypomania and psychopathic deviate." *J. appl. Psychol.*, 28:153–74 (1944).

*——— and P. E. Meehl. "The MMPI: VI. The K scale." *J. consult. Psychol.*, 12:20–31 (1948).

Meehl, P. E. "Configural scoring." *J. consult. Psychol.*, 14:165–71 (1950).

*———. "The dynamics of 'structured' personality tests." *J. clin. Psychol.*, 1:296–303 (1945).

———. "An investigation of a general normality or control factor in personality testing." *Psychol. Monogr.*, 59, No. 4 (1945). Pp. vi, 62.

*———. "Profile analysis of the MMPI in differential diagnosis." *J. appl. Psychol.*, 30:517–24 (1946).

*——— and S. R. Hathaway. "The K factor as a suppressor variable in the MMPI." *J. appl. Psychol.*, 30:525–64 (1946).

Michael, J. C., and C. Bühler. "Experiences with personality testing in a neuropsychiatric department of a public general hospital." *Dis. nerv. Syst.*, 6:205–11 (1945).

Miller, D. R. "Levels of aspiration of hysterics and neurasthenics." *Amer. Psychologist*, 2:406 (1947). Abstract.

Mitchell, M. B., and H. F. Rothe. "Validity of an emotional key or a short industrial personality questionnaire." *J. appl. Psychol.*, 34:329–32 (1950).

*Modlin, H. C. "A study of the MMPI in clinical practice with notes on the Cornell Index." *Amer. J. Psychiat.*, 103:758–69 (1947).

Monachesi, E. D. "Personality Characteristics and socio-economic status of delinquents and non-delinquents." *J. crim. Law Criminol.*, 40:570–83 (1950).

———. "Some personality characteristics of delinquents and non-delinquents." *J. crim. Law Criminol.*, 38:487–500 (1948).

Morris, W. W. "A preliminary evaluation of the MMPI." *J. clin. Psychol.*, 3:370–74 (1947). Also abstracted in *Amer. Psychologist*, 1:264 (1946).

Morton, M. A. "The army adaptation of the MMPI." *Amer. Psychologist*, 3:271–72 (1948). Abstract.

Mullen, F. A. "The MMPI: An extension of the Davis scoring method." *J. clin. Psychol.*, 4:86–88 (1948).

O'Gorman, W. D., and E. C. Kunkle. "Study of the relation between MMPI scores and 'pilot error' in aircraft accidents." *J. Aviat. Med.*, 18:31–38 (1947).

Owens, W. A., and W. C. Johnson. "Some measured personality traits of collegiate underachievers." *J. educ. Psychol.*, 40:41–46 (1949). Also abstracted in *Amer. Psychologist*, 3:363 (1948).

Pacella, B. L., Z. Piotrowski, and N. D. C. Lewis. "The effects of electric convulsive therapy on certain personality traits in psychiatric patients." *Amer. J. Psychiat.*, 104:83–91 (1947).

BIBLIOGRAPHY

Page, R. B. "Application of the MMPI to tuberculosis patients." Unpublished Ph.D. thesis, University of Minnesota, 1947.

Pearson, J. S. "Prediction of the response of schizophrenic patients to electroconvulsive therapy." *J. clin. Psychol.*, 6:285–87 (1950).

Penrose, L. S. In Buros's *Third mental measurements yearbook.* New Brunswick, N.J.: Rutgers University Press, 1949. Pp. 108–9.

Perlman, M. "Social class membership and test-taking attitude." Unpublished M.A. thesis, University of Chicago, 1950.

Phillips, E. L., and D. N. Wiener. "Relationships between selected disability and disease groups and the MMPI." *Amer. Psychologist,* 2:274 (1947). Abstract.

Portenier, L. G. "Personality tests in a university guidance program." *J. educ. Psychol.,* 39:479–87 (1948).

Rashkis, H. A., and D. A. Shaskan. "The effects of group psychotherapy on personality inventory scores." *Amer. J. Orthopsychiat.,* 16:345–49 (1946).

Richards, T. W. *Modern clinical psychology.* New York: McGraw-Hill, 1946.

Rose, A. A. "A study of homesickness in college freshmen." *J. soc. Psychol.,* 26:185–202 (1947).

Rosen, H. "Correlations between the Schellenberg free association test and the MMPI." Unpublished M.A. thesis, University of Minnesota, 1944.

Rosenzweig, S. "The dynamics of an amnesic personality." *J. Personality,* 15:121–42 (1946).

Rotter, J. B. In Buros's *Third mental measurements yearbook.* New Brunswick, N.J.: Rutgers University Press, 1949. Pp. 109–10.

Rubin, H. "The MMPI as a diagnostic aid in a veterans hospital." *J. consult. Psychol.,* 12:251–54 (1948).

———. "A note on 'Reply to Rubin'." *J. consult. Psychol.,* 14:327–28 (1950).

Ruesch, J. "Personality structure, lactic acid production and work performance in psychiatric patients." *J. Psychol.,* 20:381–90 (1945).

———. "Psychophysiological relations in cases with head injuries." *Psychosom. Med.,* 7:158–68 (1945).

——— and K. Bowman. "Prolonged post-traumatic syndromes following head injury." *Amer. J. Psychiat.,* 102:145–63 (1945).

———, R. E. Harris, and K. M. Bowman. *Pre- and post-traumatic personality in head injuries.* Assoc. Res. Nerv. Ment. Dis. Monogr. 24. Baltimore: Williams & Wilkins Co., 1945.

*——— and others. *Chronic disease and psychological invalidism: A psychosomatic study.* Amer. Soc. Res. Psychosom. Problems. New York: Hoeber, 1946.

———. *Duodenal ulcer: A socio-psychological study of naval personnel and civilians.* Berkeley: University of California Press, 1948.

———. "Psychological invalidism in thyroidectomized patients." *Psychosom. Med.,* 9:77–91 (1947).

Schiele, B. C., A. B. Baker, and S. R. Hathaway. "The MMPI." *J. Lancet,* 63:292–97 (1943).

——— and J. Brozek. "'Experimental neurosis' resulting from semistarvation in man." *Psychosom. Med.,* 10:31–50 (1948).

Schmidt, H. O. "Notes on the MMPI: The K factor." *J. consult. Psychol.,* 12:337–42 (1948).

*———. "Test profiles as a diagnostic aid: The MMPI." *J. appl. Psychol.,* 29:115–31 (1945).

Schneck, J. M. "Clinical evaluation of the F scale on the MMPI." *Amer. J. Psychiat.,* 104:440–42 (1948).

*———. "The double-spike pattern on the MMPI." *Am. J. Psychiat.,* 104:443–45 (1948).

Schneider, R. A., J. S. Gray, and C. U. Culmer. "Psychological evaluation of surgical patients." *Bull. University of Minnesota Hospital and Minnesota Medical Foundation,* 20:201–11 (1948).

Schofield, W. "Changes in responses to the MMPI following certain therapies." *Psychol. Monogr.,* 64, No. 5 (1950).

Shacter, H. "Personality profiles of psychoneurotics before and after treatment." *Amer. Psychologist,* 2:420 (1947). Abstract.

Sherman, A. W. "Personality factors in the psychological weaning of college women." *Amer. Psychologist,* 2:423 (1947). Abstract.

Shneidman, E. S. "Prospectus of the Make-A-Picture Story (MAPS) projective personality test." *Amer. Psychologist,* 2:407 (1947). Abstract.

———. "A short method of scoring the MMPI." *J. consult. Psychol.,* 10:143–45 (1946).

Simon, W. "Attempted suicide among veterans." *J. nerv. ment. Dis.,* in press.

——— and W. M. Hales. "Notes on a suicide key in the MMPI." *Amer. J. Psychiat.,* 106:222–23 (1949).

Sisk, H. L. "A reply to Winfield's study of the multiple choice Rorschach." *J. appl. Psychol.,* 31:446–48 (1947).

BIBLIOGRAPHY

Snoke, M., and N. Ziesmer. "Relationship between subtle-obvious keys and K scale of the MMPI." V.A. Voc. Rehab. and Educ. Div., Inform. Memo., 1946, No. 6, p. 7.

Staudt, V. M. "The relationship of certain personality traits to errors and correct responses in several types of tasks among college women under varying test conditions." *J. Psychol.*, 27:465–78 (1949). Also abstracted in *Amer. Psychologist*, 3:273 (1948).

Strangio, V. "A psychiatric test for general practice: Part I. The personality in terms of the psychiatric components." *J. Osteopathy*, 57:20–23 (1950).

———. "A psychiatric test for general practice: Part II. Clinical applications." *J. Osteopathy*, 57:16–19 (1950).

Sweetland, A. "Hypnotic neurosis: Hypochondriasis and depression." *J. gen. Psychol.*, 39:91–105 (1948).

Thompson, G. M. "MMPI correlates of certain movement responses in the group Rorschachs of two college samples." *J. consult. Psychol.*, 12:379–83 (1948). Also abstracted in *Amer. Psychologist*, 3:348 (1948).

Triggs, F. O. "A study of the relationship of measured interests to measured mechanical aptitude, personality, and vocabulary." *Amer. Psychologist*, 2:296–97 (1947). Abstract.

Van Vorst, R. B. "An evaluation of test performances of a group of psychopathic delinquents." *Psychol. Bull.*, 50:583 (1943). Abstract.

Verniaud, W. M. "Occupational differences in the MMPI." *J. appl. Psychol.*, 30:604–13 (1946).

Veterans Administration Guidance Center, St. Cloud. "A study of the Bell Adjustment Inventory and deviant scores on the MMPI." *Minn. Counselor*, 3 (No. 1):1–7 (1948).

Vig, M. J. "A clinical investigation into the psychological aspects of multiple sclerosis." Unpublished Ph.D. thesis, University of Minnesota, 1947.

Walch, A. E., and R. A. Schneider. "The MMPI: An evaluation of its use in private practice." *Minn. Med.*, 30:753–58 (1947).

Waters, R. O. V., and E. V. Semrad. "Use of the MMPI in assessing the Pd factor in psychopathic personalities." *Dis. nerv. Syst.*, 10:267–72 (1949).

Wauck, L. A. "Schizophrenia and the MMPI." *J. clin. Psychol.*, 6:279–84 (1950).

Welsh, G. S. "An anxiety index and an internalization ratio for the MMPI." *J. consult. Psychol.*, in press.

*———. "An extension of Hathaway's MMPI profile coding system." *J. consult. Psychol.*, 12:343–44 (1948).

———. "A projective figure-preference test for diagnosis of psychopathology: I. A preliminary investigation." Unpublished Ph.D. thesis, University of Minnesota, 1949.

Wesley, E. "Correlations between the Guilford-Martin personality factors O, Ag, Co and the MMPI at the college level." Unpublished M.A. thesis, University of Minnesota, 1945.

Wesley, S. M., B. Stewart, and D. Corey. "A study of the intra-individual relationships between interest and ability." *Amer. Psychologist*, 2:411 (1947). Abstract.

Wiener, D. N. "Advisement factors in successful and unsuccessful rehabilitation trainees." V.A. Voc. Rehab. and Educ. Div., Inform. Memo., 1946, No. 6, pp. 1–4.

———. "A control factor in social adjustment." *J. abnorm. soc. Psychol.*, in press.

———. "Differences between the individual and group forms of the MMPI." *J. consult. Psychol.*, 11:104–6 (1947).

———. "MMPI K-correction results for non-institutionalized neuropsychiatric cases." *Minn. Counselor*, 3:12–13 (1948).

———. "Personality characteristics of selected disability groups." *J. clin. Psychol.*, 4:285–90 (1948).

———. "Personality characteristics of selected disability groups." *Genet. Psychol. Monogr.*, in press.

———. "Selecting salesmen with subtle-obvious keys for the MMPI." *Amer. Psychologist*, 3:364 (1948).

———. "The subtle-obvious factor in vocational and educational success." *Amer. Psychologist*, 3:299 (1948). Abstract.

———. "Subtle and obvious keys for the MMPI." *J. consult. Psychol.*, 12:164–70 (1948). Also abstracted in *Amer. Psychologist*, 2:296 (1947).

——— and L. R. Harmon. "Subtle and obvious keys for the MMPI: Their development." Advisement Bull., Minneapolis Regional V.A. Office, No. 16, 1946.

——— and E. L. Phillips. "A study of progress in psychotherapy." *J. clin. Psychol.*, 4:201–6 (1948).

——— and W. Simon. "Personality characteristics of embalmer trainees." *J. appl. Psychol.*, in press.

Winfield, M. C. "The use of the Harrower-Erickson multiple choice Rorschach test with a selected group of women in military service." *J. appl. Psychol.*, 30:481–87 (1946).

CASE HISTORIES

Ps. Psth.	M:30:M:7	−1	-34(57)	4:6:8
Ps. Paranoid		−1	9'86274-3(69)	5:8:10
Alcoholism				

This patient had a long history of personality difficulties dating back to childhood. Always restless, he was an extremist, had a bad temper, and had had difficulty sticking to any line of action. There was a history of heavy periodic drinking, promiscuity with women, window peeping, homosexual interests, and other unusual sexual practices. He had been in a state hospital for nearly a year and a half, being released about three years before this present admission, but since then he had again become unmanageable, chiefly because of exaggerated ideas of personal importance.

The past history was not particularly contributory. He had contracted gonorrhea three or four times, the last time about five years before admission. It was difficult to get details of his earlier life, but apparently he had graduated from high school and spent some time at a university, although he had no college degree and his grade and work records were extremely poor at all times. He had never held any position for longer than a few weeks, usually quitting because he felt he was capable of doing something much better.

In the hospital he showed impulsive behavior, marked irritability, and poor judgment. He described a number of fantastic delusions, among them that he had supplied the master plan governing the Allied war strategy in Europe, and that he had positive proof he was to be the next president of the United States. On admission he was pleasant and social, but he soon became insolent, demanding, noisy, and threatening. He felt that he should be given all the privileges of the staff; and when he was not accorded them, he became sarcastic, threatening the staff, members of his family, and prominent citizens in his town. Because he was not allowed an unlimited supply of cigarettes, he went on a hunger strike for four days. When he was finally told that if he did not try to cooperate he could not remain in the psychopathic unit but would have to return to the state hospital, he elected the latter and was discharged for transfer there.

The two MMPI profiles for this patient illustrate the variability that may appear in a short time. During the first test he had no real intention of cooperating at all with the staff; and the profile was manifestly not a true picture of him. He was given a terse and realistic summary of his situation and told to choose cooperation or direct state hospital commitment. When he chose, at least at first, to undergo study, he was asked to repeat the test.

P. Hys.	F:19:S:36	+2	-41<u>89</u>	6:2:11

Dyspnea, present ever since she could remember but recently much worse, brought this young woman into the hospital. The condition—an irresistible desire to take a deep breath or sigh every few minutes—was worse at night, especially during insomnia, and also when she became nervous or was in the presence of strangers. During the last three years she had suffered from pain in the chest at the height of breath inspiration and this symptom had been growing worse. She was subject also to crying spells, and she complained of hearing "keys in locks," an illusory or possibly hallucinatory experience.

The patient's general health had been good and there appeared to have been no abnormalities of physical or psychological development. Her intelligence was in the average range. She finished the eighth grade, failing only one subject throughout her schooling. She had a persistent ambition to become a traveling preacher, but for the most part she had done housework. Outside work and sports appealed to her, especially those with boys, such as skating and skiing. Friendly, cheerful, even-tempered, kind, and thoughtful, she was also, according to her mother, secretive and stubborn. She insisted upon wearing long, plain, homemade dresses, black cotton stockings, and black shoes. She used no make-up and braided her hair tightly. She objected, although passively, to slacks, smoking, drinking, and the radio. Girl friends were numerous, but there was no one she called "special." A boy friend, eleven years her senior, was described as "shiftless," and the family had insisted that she give him up. She said at the time of admission that she now "agreed with the family about him."

In the hospital her predominant mental trends were religious, but vaguely described. Apparently she had no affiliation with an organization, but she said that her family held meetings and believed in "just following the teachings of the Bible." She always appeared happy and smiling and could not see "any possible connection" between her difficulty and psychological factors. Excessively agreeable and pleasant, she showed no tensions, cooperated, and readily formed friends among the other patients. Under the influence of sodium amytal she stated that it was "a sin to have two things on my mind at once." She also talked of inability to forget about her previous boy friend and a desire to "preach the gospel." She later repudiated any interest in marriage. The gasping respiration and other symptoms ceased when diaphragmatic breathing was suggested as a substitute. Although the presenting symptoms disappeared, the therapy was recognized as being exceedingly superficial and she was discharged to be followed in outpatient contact.

P. Psychas. F:46:M:28 +15 –467823 (68) 5:2:10
P. Hys.

This woman became obsessed with the idea that she had done injury to her mouth thirty years ago, and she now felt there was something wrong with her jaw. She was depressed and complained of various pains. Owing to some trouble with her gums, ears, throat, etc., she thought she was going blind. She was admitted to the hospital as a voluntary patient.

Little was known about her early history. Her father was aggressive, self-assertive, and domineering with his family. She married at the age of 30.

The diagnosis was obsessional neurosis, and she underwent a course of electric convulsion therapy. She improved and her symptoms, though still present, became weaker. There seemed to be hysterical features as well. According to a recent report, improvement was maintained fairly well. M. V.

Ps. Invol. Melan. M:55:M:32 +19 –47 13 (51) 2:6:10
Paranoid

The illness really began about two years before admission when the patient became nervous and developed paranoid ideas concerning his wife and neighbors. The symptoms disappeared after he had taken a six weeks' vacation. Some months later he had another attack with the same symptoms and, in addition, a fear of being with people. He recovered from this also after a couple of months and went through still another similar episode before the one during which he was admitted. This last was his worst upset.

He had attended agricultural college for two years, then married and bought himself a farm. He lost the farm and went deeply into debt. In the next years, however, he completed paying for his father's farm, which he operated. He was a quiet and withdrawn person, always a hard worker who kept things to himself. He had always been suspicious and jealous. His family had learned to humor him. He was described as rigid, very honest, and ambitious.

In the hospital he talked little. His mental content appeared to be delusional with paranoid ideas involving a number of persons, not centering on any one. The delusions were poorly systematized. He was well oriented and his intellect appeared unimpaired. He kept to himself and seemed depressed. With six electroshock treatments his paranoid delusions disappeared, but he became confused and restless, complained bitterly of lonesomeness, and again and again pleaded to be discharged and allowed to go back to his family. At the time of discharge he seemed to have a fairly complete remission of the symptoms.

P. Hys. F:25:M:47 +10 –72 (70) 6:1:17
Suicidal

Soon after her marriage this young woman began wandering away from home for periods up to 24 hours. She had no recollection of them afterward. She also attempted suicide several times, by drowning and taking overdoses of phenobarbitone. Shortly after the most recent of these attempts on her life, she was admitted to the hospital as a voluntary patient.

Little was known about her early history. She was the youngest of three children and received an elementary education. She worked in a factory on leaving school.

The diagnosis was anxiety hysteria, and her condition improved after one electroshock. M. V.

P. Hys. F:18:S:50 +30 –796 5:6:10
Mental Deficiency

This girl was admitted because of rapid abdominal breathing and complaints of choked feelings in her neck and chest. These difficulties began three weeks before admission and were associated with insomnia, confusion, and increased irritability.

-9164387

At first present only at night, the symptoms gradually began to be continuous. When she began to be troubled also with tinnitus, diarrhea, and polyuria, she was admitted to the psychiatric unit.

There had been a similar illness four years earlier, of one week's duration. Otherwise the previous physical history was noncontributory. In the second year of high school at the time of admission, the patient had always found schoolwork difficult and had failed the seventh grade. However, her teachers had been lenient and had often given her passing grades when she had not earned them. Always a sensitive, nervous, shy, bashful person, she learned slowly and had a marked dislike for housework. She had never shown interest in sex and seldom even expressed the desire for companionship. She rarely exhibited joy or sorrow. Reciting in front of the class always upset her, and the present illness began one day before she was to present a book report in class.

Except for the rapid breathing and the accompanying to and fro motion of the pelvis, the physical findings were negative. Her tested I.Q. was 57. The patient felt that her illness was due to "heart trouble and nervousness." She appeared happy and contented, and she was neat and cooperative on the ward. The excessive breathing motions appeared most obvious whenever anyone was watching her. During the first weeks of hospitalization no change occurred. She was then told that the muscles of her abdomen needed to be strengthened, and she was given, along with this suggestion, faradic stimulation to the abdominal region. This stimulation was applied several times a day with the suggestion that "it would help." The movements quickly decreased in amplitude, and by the fourth day of treatment, she was free of symptoms. The recommendation was made that she leave school and, if possible, be placed in a training school for subnormal students. At the time of discharge she had apparently recovered from the present illness.

Ps. Sz., Paranoid M:32:M:95 +82 -9164387 (51) 9:4:12

This man was invalided out of the army with gunshot wounds in the chest and associated nervous symptoms, including psychosis. He developed delusions, signaled from his window, and talked about Germans and fifth columnists around him. He spent six months in a mental hospital but returned home because his wife was expecting a baby. He then became obsessed with such bizarre ideas as that his wife was a German in disguise. He entered the hospital as a voluntary patient.

He was the fifth of nine children, two of whom had died in childhood. He attended a technical college and was a good draughtsman. As a child he was well liked and sociable but had periods of absent-mindedness. He did not appear to be interested in girls until he met his wife. He worked for a firm as a process artist, and his work was highly appreciated by his employers.

The diagnosis was schizophrenia, and he underwent a course of electric convulsion and deep insulin therapy. His condition improved. M. V.

Ps. Paranoid F:29:M:11 +1 –97X 11:5:17
Ps. Sz., Paranoid

For about eighteen months the patient had had the idea that people thought she was peculiar, and she believed that they controlled her mind. There were intervals during which these ideas were not verbalized, but according to the family they had always been present. Many of her delusions were built around a physician who she feared would separate her from her husband, paralyze her bowels, and give her a brain tumor. All this was to be done by spiritual means because she would not "yield to the doctor's demands." She was unresponsive to direct questioning, and frequently she sat smiling and laughing to herself. She had the notion that she had been pregnant five times in spite of the fact that her husband said she had at no time missed a menstrual period.

An eighth-grade graduate, she had dropped out of school to take care of her mother. She had always enjoyed outdoor life, and she was active on her husband's farm. Although they were apparently compatible, her husband was a poor provider, and at the time of her admission they lived on relief in a three-room shack. There were no children. A plodding, shy, retiring person, she had low average intelligence. She had always been sensitive and overly quick to take offense.

In the hospital she was inconspicuous in manner. Occasionally she was depressed, but for the most part she appeared more apathetic. Although her attitude was cooperative, she consistently denied all her paranoid trends. When asked specifically about a given pain, she said, "I just took cold in my feet." She was so fearful that she would not be allowed to return home that one had the impression she deliberately concealed the nature of her thoughts. So successfully did she hide her symptoms that manifestations of apathy and reticence were all that could be identified as abnormal, and since it did not seem possible to treat her she was discharged to try living at home again.

Ps. Psth. M:31:M:28 +16 1'2-<u>96</u>(32) 8:6:18
Paranoid
Alcoholism

The patient's admission complaints were paranoid ideas, irresponsibility, and sinusitis and asthma, with which he had been troubled for many years and which he said were the reason for his inability to work and support his family. Because of his irresponsibility and drunkenness, his family had been sent to a county poor farm, but he claimed that his father, toward whom he had become antagonistic, had taken his wife and children away from him. While intoxicated he made an attempt to take his family forcibly out of the poor farm, and as a result he was arrested and jailed, and later was sent to the hospital for treatment of the sinusitis and for psychiatric study.

A long history of asthma and intermittent draining of his ears from the sinusitis apparently had made it impossible for him to remain employed for any length of time. Since he was never able to get along with people and had always had an irresponsible attitude in regard to his family, the mental symptoms had evidently been present for many years. He had completed the third grade at the age of 14, presumably having been retarded by his hearing difficulty. Because of his inability to hold a job, he did much begging from welfare organizations and his family, as well as his father's, was known to many agencies.

The physical examination on admission showed definite hearing loss and a disturbance of position sense. It appeared that there might be some cerebral damage. He was restless, irritable, impulsive, uncooperative, and talked antagonistically about his father and the welfare agencies, threatening to sue the latter, the state, and the hospital for the way they treated him. He had a tendency to falsify and exaggerate, and he was anxious to impress others with his strength, telling of his temper and of fights he had been in. He was well oriented, his I.Q. was found to be about 85, and he had no queer mannerisms, but he was reluctant to participate in social activities. He was discharged back to the county authorities with the recommendation that he be committed to a state hospital.

P. Hypo. F:39:M:29 +5 12'3467–98 8:1:16

Two years before the patient came to the hospital she had "flu," became weak and bedridden, and began to complain of abdominal pain, nausea, constipation, and anorexia. Later other symptoms appeared, such as headaches, precordial pain, dyspnea, choking spells, and paresthesias. Greatly concerned, the patient decided she had an organic disease, perhaps an infection, and consulted a physician who treated her for a presumed focal infection. In spite of the treatment she remained practically bedridden and the symptoms persisted.

Thirteen years earlier, the patient had suffered a "nervous breakdown" following the death of a young son. The symptoms at that time appear to have been similar. She recovered in a year's time without hospitalization. Otherwise the past history was not contributory. The patient grew up on a farm near a small town. An eighth-grade graduate, she did housework until marriage. Energetic, outgoing, and hard working as a young person, she later became worrisome, less cheerful, and seclusive. There was a degree of sexual incompatibility with the husband. Otherwise they got along rather well. After she developed leucorrhea the husband refused sexual relations altogether, and this was correlated, to some extent, with the patient's symptomatology. Apparently she liked their four children and was a good mother.

The patient was a small, sickly appearing woman, lacking in energy and vitality. A purulent vaginal discharge was present. Her dominating concern was ill health; her complaints were numerous and there were obvious manifestations of anxiety. Mentally she seemed to be intact, with the exception of the delusional pattern. She was variable in mood and cried at times. Fairly willing to accept psychological elements as factors in her disorder, she was nevertheless convinced that a physical illness was present. She was hesitant about revealing much concerning her private life and was, of course, difficult to approach psychotherapeutically. On the ward she usually moped, asked frequently for attention, and showed only mild interest in what went on around her. During her stay she had ups and downs but on the whole improved. Considerable effort was directed toward improving the patient's physical condition since this was felt to be correlated with her problem. At discharge social service follow-up plans were outlined carefully, and work, on an outpatient basis, was to be continued.

Ps. Paranoid	M:46:M:73	+1	1234′678–9 (63)	4:13:17
P. Hypo.		+60	1342786′– (59)	4:9:19

The patient was admitted complaining of attacks of severe dyspnea, palpitation, anginal pain, and weakness. About two years before he had experienced these same symptoms accompanied by other vague somatic complaints. Concerned about the possibility of cancer, he had gone to a clinic, where his ailment was diagnosed as diverticulosis and cholelithiasis. He lost one job because of this illness, took another, but left that after experiencing a "cardiac attack." After this the patient began to visit numerous physicians and was told by all but one that nothing serious was wrong with his heart. However, he clung tenaciously to the belief that his cardiac condition was serious, took every medicine prescribed, spent months in hospitals, and throughout the two years expected his wife to work and support him. At home he became intolerable, openly accusing his wife of infidelity and threatening her during temper outbursts. He became increasingly suspicious not only of his wife but of other people and demanded more and more of his wife's attention because of his "cardiac condition."

The patient had always been in poor health, and he listed many complaints about his past physical condition. He had once won a lawsuit from a railway company on the basis of an injury which he felt he had sustained while working and which, according to him, had been treated incorrectly. At one time he contracted gonorrhea and at the age of 17 was addicted to morphine. When that habit was broken he turned to alcohol, later to phenobarbital. About average in learning ability, he had gone only through the eighth grade in school, then worked at occupations ranging from male nurse to W.P.A. foreman. A roamer, he was never satisfied. Adventure and true story magazines and medical textbooks interested him. He had few friends and continually found fault with those he had. He was acutely jealous of his wife, he was never cheerful, and he was persistent to a fault.

The medical findings were relatively negative. He was exceedingly hypochondriacal on admission, felt he would die from the cardiac condition, and wrote to his wife stating that fact. His sporadic attacks of dyspnea were most marked when someone was taking his pulse. As he was observed in the hospital, the paranoid trends became progressively more and more apparent. There were retrospective falsifications, suspicion of his wife's ulterior motives, ideas of persecution by his brother-in-law, and other ideas. These he wove into a grand delusional pattern centering on the fact that he had once contracted gonorrhea. Self-sympathetic, he had little or no insight, and he became increasingly suspicious of being "framed" by the psychiatric staff. He fluctuated between anxiety that he would be committed and attempts at composure. At times the only way he could be controlled was by the threat of commitment. When this happened he moved about the ward carefully, attempting to appear normal although not "overdoing." His wife finally took him home against the staff's advice that he be committed immediately.

Ps. M-D., Manic F:49:M:63 +7 123'4687–X 10:2:25

The patient was admitted because of marked overactivity, insomnia, and bizarre behavior which had been increasingly noticeable over a period of six months. About a month before admission the condition had become extreme. Unusual behavior included buying an icebox that she could not afford, striking her sister-in-law because the latter interfered with her home life, and volunteering to give a speech at the local high school, a task for which she was incompetent. She was afraid to be left alone because she felt she might commit suicide.

She had been nervous as a girl, and there had been an episode five years before admission when the doctor diagnosed the cause of her symptoms as a brain tumor. There had been no operation, and further details could not be ascertained. She was a practical nurse and had been married twice, divorced once. An open, pleasant, and unselfish person, she was interested in people about her almost to the point of being domineering. She had always worked very hard, enjoying few luxuries. Her mother had committed suicide by jumping into a well.

Her intelligence was average. She was conventional and perhaps overtalkative, and at times her conversation was irrelevant. For the first few days after admission she was disoriented, but when she became clear mentally she took an interest in her surroundings and seemed almost completely normal from that time on. She was almost overly interested in working around the ward, and it was difficult to make a diagnosis of her condition. There was a fair possibility that her entire pattern of reaction could be traced to the fact that her husband worked on the sister-in-law's farm to the point of neglecting his wife and family, to the patient's great irritation.

P. Mixed F:54:M:59 +9 123'476–(59) 6:5:19

The patient was admitted with constant acute abdominal and lumbar pains, the onset of which occurred about three months before admission when she became emotionally disturbed about her daughter's divorce and about finding a bottle of liquor in her husband's pharmacy. She began to swear frequently and raved and found fault incessantly. The pains became worse, interfering with her taking food, and she lost thirty pounds. Hospitalization at a clinic disclosed no organic basis for the symptoms. She grew so irritable and depressed that her daughter had to feed her. Taken to a hospital, she was upset and excited and fell out of bed several times; when she heard someone mention shock therapy she refused all forms of treatment. Sedative drugs precipitated a more severe attack. Her memory was cloudy and she had severe crying spells with continuous moaning. She refused further treatment and had to be taken home, where she stayed until the present admission.

There was little that was pertinent in her previous history. After completing the second year of high school she had entered a conservatory to study piano, and she had taught piano for two years after her marriage, which occurred at age 20. Not a very social person, she was self-reliant, her attention being focused largely on her home and on saving money. She was of average intelligence and apparently was quite capable as an assistant in the operation of her husband's pharmacy. According to her daughter, she was always "grasping for money." Her interest was centered on her only son, and she was intolerant of the rest of the family. Hypercritical and vain, she based her attitude toward others on whether the relationship would be a profitable one. Otherwise, "she would pick people apart." She had hypochondriacal trends and numerous long-standing fears. Although she was emotionally unstable and always irritable, she was immaculate in her dress, and her taste in clothes was exceptionally good. While her husband was a fairly stable person, he had a "mean disposition," occasionally beating the children.

On admission the patient was mainly concerned with her pain, and although the laboratory findings and physical examinations were essentially negative, she complained incessantly. She referred frequently to finding the liquor bottle in her husband's store, an incident that worried her because of what might have happened to him since he had no license. Although she complained of black spots in front of her eyes, there were no clear-cut hallucinations or delusions. She appeared to be intact mentally and of average intelligence, and she changed very little in the early part of her hospitalization. Although she was pleasant and agreeable on approach, she was so concerned about her symptoms that she would discuss nothing else. While she disliked being alone, she craved company only to obtain sympathy, and she made little effort to mix with others or to enter into ward activities. After several weeks in which she continually found fault with the food, with other patients, and with the personnel, she became more cooperative and began to get some insight into her problems. There was definite improvement when she was discharged, but it was suggested that she continue in the outpatient clinic. Six months later she was readmitted to the medical department with what appeared to be carcinoma of the pancreas. It was impossible to say how much of her original problem was neurotic, how much somatic. It was certain, however, that both factors contributed to the picture in the hospital.

P. Hypo. M:45:M:30 +2 1234876′–9 8:13:20
Suicidal

During about four months the patient had been seeking help from a county welfare board, saying that he was unable to work because of rheumatism, gas pains, and nervous spells. He worried about his financial status and wondered what would happen to his family. He alarmed his wife by threatening suicide and finally she appeared before the welfare board asking that her husband be committed as a mental case. He had a multiplicity of somatic complaints. Symptoms had really been present for twenty years.

He discontinued school at age 16, when he was in the fifth grade. He had never been free from worry over money matters and had always had difficulty planning for his family. He was generally friendly toward others and enjoyed being in the limelight at parties. Usually he got his own way about things, exhibiting a quick temper but being on the whole a cheerful person. At one time he had been in jail for six months for moonshining. He came from a family of 22 children, and he and his wife had, at the time of his admission, 23 children living; 4 had died in infancy. The patient's I.Q. was about 90 and that of his wife about 70.

In the hospital he was mainly concerned with his physical complaints and the problems of his home security. He did not place any emphasis on suicidal thoughts and there were no gross disturbances of intellect or sensorium. He agreed that the hospital might help him but thought that the psychiatric ward was certainly no place for him. He was alert, was interested in the examinations, and fell fairly well into ward routines. He gradually improved during the hospitalization and some of his complaints disappeared. At one time he said that his wife had told him he was a failure and she would be better off without him. He was discharged to a boardinghouse where he was to remain until his county social welfare board could thoroughly investigate the home situation and try to arrange matters so that the patient could carry less burden.

Ps. Invol. Melan.	M:65:M:37	+1	123'497–(49)	7:5:16
P. Hypo.		–28	12379'846–(53)	8:8:19
		+61	'129374–(47)	9:4:16

This man had felt perfectly well until about three years before admission, when he began to notice a ringing in the left ear. This made him nervous but not enough to quit his job as a salesman in a department store. His work was, however, trying to him. One day at work a month later he suddenly felt a severe pain in the epigastrium. From then on he experienced continual crawling sensations in his stomach. Eventually he stopped working. Irritability rose to a pitch, and periods of confusion occurred so frequently that the family dared not let him leave the house alone. Insomnia developed and also spells of weeping, usually not preceded by sad situations. After three electroshock treatments at a private hospital he felt somewhat better. However, he was far from well and began to take barbiturates to sleep.

On admission he said a similar episode had occurred three months after his marriage at age 32. This first illness he called not so severe, and since that time there had been no difficulty. Just before the present hospitalization he underwent an operation to "cut the nerve that was making the buzzing." This procedure did not, however, stop the sound. The patient was raised in strict but apparently happy surroundings. His school record was good, but he withdrew at an early age, held a number of jobs, and finally became a shoe salesman. He liked this work but it often led to predicaments which made him nervous. His entire work history was a sequence of changing from one job to another following outbursts of indignation during which he would quit or be fired. He liked to mingle with people and enjoyed conversation.

In the hospital the patient appeared as an extremely emotional man, with an anxious and depressed countenance. He was verbose, repeated himself frequently, and became very excited if he suspected he was not believed. There was no good evidence for arteriosclerosis. His stream of thought was normal and his mentality appeared intact. Although he appeared to have fair insight he did not view his problems in correct perspective. Electroshock therapy was instituted. After eleven treatments there was noticeable improvement. Occasional irrationality and confusion remained, however. He was discharged to his home in the hope that he might continue to improve, and it was recommended that he continue in the outpatient clinic.

Ps. Sz., Paranoid   F:47:S:110   +24   123′6874–9   8:9:25

The primary problems for this patient were withdrawal, bizarre feelings of influence, depression, and impaired judgment, all dating back to the onset of the menopause five years earlier. At that time she began to be depressed and retarded, slept much of the day, and was sleepless at night. Gradually delusions of persecution and ideas of reference developed more clearly, and depression became even more profound when the patient lost a large amount of money in a bank failure. She began to make foolish purchases and often called strangers, asking them to deposit money in the bank for her. A month before admission she became irritable, depressed, and paranoid, insisted on clean sheets for her bed every night, refused to eat, and lost much weight. At age 34 she had had a similar attack and during that episode (which lasted about a year) she had also complained of uncleanliness about the home, was depressed, and cried a great deal.

After three years in high school the patient spent one year in normal school. Before her illness she was employed as a clerk in a store, where she received a fairly adequate salary. Although always more or less shy in the presence of men, she had not been thought of as outstandingly maladjusted in any way. She had a strong interest in gardening, always exhibited good judgment, and was thoughtful of others.

In the hospital the patient insisted that she had been "sent here" because of the family's concern over her loss of weight. This weight reduction she attributed to a "shedding of iron," which she believed took place only when she was outside. She attributed her ill health to some "spoiled spinach and milk" she had eaten, and she was firmly convinced that someone had "seen to it that the food was spoiled." Orientation was good and her memory and mental processes seemed sound. Tense, preoccupied, and apprehensive, she nevertheless admitted no depression or anxiety. Her answers to questions were relevant and coherent, although brief, evasive, and disinterested. Markedly restless, she paced the floor, refused food several times, and four days after admission swallowed a large piece of soap. As time went on her behavior definitely improved and the somatic delusions became less prominent. She remained, however, grossly defective in insight and continually demanded to be discharged. It was finally decided that there might be a mild thyrotoxicosis, and she was given appropriate medication. Under this treatment, she became better and added a little weight. Gains were chiefly in the physical condition, however, and at the time of discharge she was still grossly delusional, had defective insight, and retained some of the paranoid ideas. She returned to her home pending commitment to a state hospital.

P. Hypo. M:46:M:29 0 123'7–94 2:4:8

Although he had been restless and irritable for many years this man's difficulties had become more pronounced in the last five years. Increasingly troubled by gastric distress, associated with impaired appetite, he also showed marked weakness and weight loss. After surgery in which a renal calculus was removed he had fair health for several months and then the symptoms reappeared. Told he had a prostatic infection, he underwent treatment. Since he felt unable to continue work he sold his farm. His recovery from the prostatitis was slow and he was given more extensive treatment. It was noted that the psychological complaints were not well correlated with the somatic findings, and he was referred to the psychiatry outpatient clinic, where he was diagnosed as psychoneurotic. There were transitory attacks in which he was unable to speak. Gradually he became worse, worried excessively, and finally was urged by his wife to come into the hospital, chiefly because of his depression. There were earlier illnesses in his life, among them otitis from mumps when he was 18, otitis media, an operation for varicocele, and the like. He had contracted a gonorrheal infection at age 20.

Finishing the eighth grade at 14, the patient ran away from home three years later to join the navy. Spending four years in the navy at that time, he later enlisted for an additional two years. After working for a while as a laborer he took up farming. As long as his wife had known him he had been irritable and restless. Interested in baseball, prize fighting, football, and travel, he showed almost no interest in his home. His wife, who was 18 years younger, found it difficult to accept his illness, especially since she herself had not been in good health. There were two children. For the past year the family had been on relief.

In the hospital the patient showed a marked degree of somatic concern and talked at length about his numerous difficulties, with special reference to his gastrointestinal and urinary systems. Despite his belief that much of his difficulty was due to residual kidney disease, he did recognize that his symptoms were more prominent when he was emotionally upset. He showed interest in the examination and was, at least on the surface, quite cooperative. There was gradual but progressive improvement up to the time of discharge. On the other hand his inability to accept searching or analytic psychotherapeutical approaches made it impossible to change him much.

P. Hys. M:24:S:49 +31 12378′46–(49) 6:8:18

At the age of 23 this young man developed abdominal pains with vomiting and underwent an operation. The pains continued and he attributed them to venereal disease "brought on by masturbation." It appeared that he had experienced impotency before the abdominal pains started. He was coughing and thought he had tuberculosis. He became very depressed and feared losing his mind. He entered the hospital as a voluntary patient.

The younger of two children of working-class parents, he was a nervous child, not interested in sports or reading. He left school at 14 and worked as a quarry laborer until he joined the navy, in which he served as an able-bodied seaman, refusing to become a leading seaman because he would then have lost his friends. He resumed employment on demobilization but could not settle down. For two years he had courted a girl whom he wished to marry.

He was diagnosed as having anxiety hysteria and underwent a course of modified insulin therapy and two shocks of electric convulsion therapy. His condition improved. M. V.

Ps. M-D., Depr. M:50:M:15 +11 12378′496–X 10:7:17

The presenting complaints were insomnia, depression, and inability to continue a daily routine. This pattern had apparently started nine months earlier, when one night the patient had gone to bed complaining of severe pain in his abdomen. He stayed in bed six weeks, and gradually the pain eased. However, he felt that he had not regained his strength. He lost all interest in activities and spent entire days in bed, even when the pain was not severe. Growing more and more depressed, he said that no one cared for him any more and that his condition was hopeless. When he entered the hospital he told his wife that he expected to die a natural death within the next few months. There were occasional periods of extreme agitation when he would walk the room, wringing his hands and weeping.

About twenty years before, the patient had suffered a similar attack from which he recovered over a period of two years. Otherwise the past history was not contributory. He had always been active, energetic, and hard working. His

12'3786–

wife said that he worked "too hard," usually under considerable tension, and spent more energy than was necessary. He paid little attention to recreation but was known as a sociable and generous man. Insignificant failures affected him to an unusual degree.

In the hospital the patient showed some hypochondriacal tendencies. He complained of headaches and other difficulties. Well oriented and intact in sensorium and intellect, he showed considerable psychomotor retardation and was emotionally depressed. At times he complained of a feeling of impending disaster. He realized he was mentally ill and suffering from depression. His answers to questions were adequate but accompanied by great deliberation. He was neat and careful in his personal appearance, and although he spoke as though he felt downhearted, his facial expression was cheerful and he smiled frequently. In the hospital he did not improve and therapy seemed to help little. Arrangements were made for him to be cared for by a sister who planned to keep him until he was much better.

P. Hypo. M:56:M:18 +1 12'3786–(53) 6:0:17

The admission complaints centered around gastrointestinal difficulties characterized by "gas pains" and constipation, both present for more than thirty years. There was no apparent initiating event and the attacks had only recently become more severe and numerous. At first laxatives brought belief, but later they became ineffective. The patient consulted a number of physicians and was treated but without result. Physical studies proved noncontributory, and finally he was admitted to the psychiatric ward for study.

Although his general health had always been poor, there were no outstanding events in his past medical history. He left school at the end of the fifth grade, according to his wife, because he was afraid of being beaten up by his classmates. From early childhood he was considered cowardly and timid. His income was small but steady. Described as a reserved, shy, secretive person with few interests, he associated little with others. Although his wife was a different type, outgoing and well adjusted, they appeared compatible. There were no children.

When admitted to the ward he was again studied extensively for physical disease but there were no contributory findings. Psychologically he was dull and apathetic but composed. This mood was constant regardless of what was discussed or what happened around him. He appeared intelligent. Preoccupied with his somatic difficulties, he accepted hospital routine but mixed little with other patients and did not enter into games and ward activities. Much of the time he walked back and forth, with a blank, mournful expression. He resented any implication that his trouble was not organic and was so inaccessible to psychological treatment that there was little improvement. The long duration of the illness indicated that the pattern was fixed and there was little hope that this patient would change much in the future.

P. Hypo. M:49:M:36 +2 12′38467–9 7:4:22
—26 2′134687–9 3:8:13

Ten months before admission this man developed a cold which gave him a great deal of trouble. This was followed by low back pain of a dull, aching character which persisted. During the past two months it had developed into a tingling sensation and was accompanied by leg weakness, dizzy sensations, and difficulty in concentration. There were also tingling sensations over the base of the penis. The patient had been bothered by constipation for years and this became more severe. Considerable medical study revealed no pertinent findings.

Except for a gonorrheal infection at the age of 19 there were no significant medical data in the past history. Throughout his boyhood the patient was "spoiled," it was said, by his mother. She died when he was 14 years old, however. Of his father he said, "He got rid of me as quick as he could." He then lived with his grandmother. After graduating from high school he spent some time in the army, and then he became a skilled workman. His intelligence was average. Always able to find a job and make a living, he apparently changed jobs often. He preferred outdoor life. Aloof and overly serious, he was thought to be rigid in setting standards for himself. He summed up his personality thus: "I was born old." His wife and he appeared relatively well adjusted even though she often had to work to help support them because of his irregularity. There were no children.

When the patient was admitted to the ward his ideas revolved about his physical complaints. He felt he had a weakness in the sexual organs that had been present for years. He believed his nerves were "too sensitive," and he "couldn't stand" to see books on "love or sex" since his wife had left him to spend several weeks in the South. He seemed tense and somewhat nervous; he was not obviously depressed but appeared to be anxious. A "nervous condition" was the trouble, he thought, and it was "up to the doctors" to find out the cause. Whenever he could find a listener, he talked constantly about his problems. At all times he was cooperative, but in spite of this there was present a degree of intellectual separation or abstraction that prevented very effective psychotherapeutic contact. At discharge he was little improved.

P. Hypo. M:49:M:44 +8 123′847– 9:2:21

This man complained of nervousness that had extended over the last six years, stomach trouble, an "ulcer" for ten years, and skin lesions of recent origin. All these symptoms the patient dated from a "heat stroke" he had suffered eight years earlier. However, for longer than that he had associated vague intestinal aches and pains with certain foods. Gradually he became increasingly sensitive to heat, as evidenced by several attacks of "heat prostration" followed by abdominal muscle cramps which forced him to quit work for a few days at a time. Finally, these persisted so that he was forced to quit farm work entirely. A cholecystectomy was performed without relief of the symptoms, and then he began to develop prostration attacks from cold as well as heat.

The patient had lived most of his life on a farm near a small town. In the seventh grade he left school to work on his father's place. Of a pleasant and likable disposition, he was, however, considered to be lazy and indifferent and, in fact, was known to be an occasional malingerer. Until the present illness he had managed his marital and financial affairs fairly well. Whenever he was ill, he required considerable sympathy; otherwise he was cheerful.

When admitted to the ward the patient was apathetic and indifferent toward things in general. Showing only slight concern about his condition, he conveyed an impression of self-satisfaction. He was well oriented and apparently adequate in general intellectual reactions, although he was of dull normal intelligence. At times he had crying spells and exhibited ambivalence. There was some depression. Intensely preoccupied with his somatic complaints, he spoke only when urged and tended to be physically inactive. He changed little and himself summed up the experience with the words, "Improvement not anything to talk about." Seemingly satisfied with his lot, he went home—probably later to seek some other medical attention.

P. Mixed F:54:M:43 +1 123′864–9X (53) 11:6:18
Mental Deficiency

For fifteen years the patient had complained of periods of nervousness which had gradually become more severe. She had an increasing tendency to worry about money, about the illness of her husband, and about her epileptic son. She had always been very dependent on her mother, who had suddenly died recently. After this the symptoms had become worse. About five months before admission she fell to the floor while working in the kitchen. She was put to bed for ten days, agitated and apparently hallucinatory. She showed no improvement and was moved to a hospital, where her disorientation immediately disappeared. She remained in the hospital for two weeks and then left. But shortly thereafter she developed numerous somatic complaints and returned for the present admission.

Apparently she had always been given to hypochondriacal complaints, and there had been one period fifteen years before when she had suffered from a definite "nervous breakdown." The nature of this she could not describe. She had otherwise been able to get along in a borderline way. She was described as a pleasant, outgoing, "harmless" person who had enjoyed people until the onset of the present illness but who had been gradually withdrawing. She had always been dependent on others. Her I.Q. was 70.

Her chief mental content centered about the worries over her finances, her husband's health, and her epileptic son. There were also mild hypochondriacal trends. She had a kind of insight into her condition, but still the staff felt that she showed a *belle indifférence*. At times when she had pains she would appear concerned, but the apparent affect did not fit her complaints. She was eager to please and an active worker. She had an ingratiating manner. She was given several electroshock treatments and showed substantial improvement. There was some psychometric evidence for mental deterioration and the possibility of an early senile deterioration was considered. She was discharged with a fairly good prognosis.

P. Hypo. M:27:S:24 +3 12386<u>'7</u>-(59) 7:6:9
+20 '93-<u>4126</u>(43) 6:1:18

Approximately six months before admission the patient suddenly began having upper abdominal "gas pains" which seemed to press against his heart. In addition to these attacks, which usually came at night, there was nausea, a hacking cough, numbness and tingling in his extremities, tinnitus, and a tired feeling which made him unable to work. Neither treatments of his own nor those suggested by a local physician relieved the symptoms. Although hard work apparently made the pain more severe, rest did not seem to help him in any way.

There were a number of episodic illnesses in his past history, including a tonsillectomy and an appendectomy. At one time he was hospitalized four months for tachycardia and associated nervousness.

The patient attended a country school until he was 16; he did fairly well, but his numerous illnesses prevented him from continuing his education, and from that time on he did farm work. He enjoyed track and baseball, apparently got along well with people, and was fairly adequate socially. He had always lived with his parents, who more or less told him what to do. Although he wanted to be an electrician or a mechanic, his family made it plain to him that they thought he should stay on the farm. His only spending money came from such work as he could do for his neighbors. He had had several girl friends and had had intercourse a number of times. His illness kept him from marrying.

When he was admitted to the hospital his mental content and general mental abilities appeared normal. He expressed a desire to get rid of his "gas pains" (which became better almost immediately on admission). There were no obvious disturbances of mentation. He was low normal in intelligence. His emotional tone was good. He was cheerful, friendly, cooperative, and easy to talk to, although he had poor insight into the possible psychological background of his problems. He got along very well, made friends, and entered into ward routine. It was felt that he might be better adjusted if he could in part break away from his family ties and take some such job as filling station attendant, since he disliked farm work. At the time of discharge he was markedly improved, but of course he was still a very inadequate person.

P. Hypo. F:39:M:2 —14 1'238<u>674</u>-9 3:5:10

For five years the patient had noted a burning pain in the lower area of her back. It was worse when she sat, but there was some relief when she walked. She was bothered also by nausea and became unable to eat well. Later she developed lower abdominal pain, burning, painful micturation, tachycardia, and "pus" in the menstrual flow. The patient dated the symptoms from an appendectomy and "ovarian operation," both performed twelve years earlier. In addition to these complaints she was deeply concerned about her nervousness and weakness.

At 18 the patient developed a scaly body rash which was called eczema. Menstruation was irregular until the unilateral ovariectomy which was resorted to when the patient was emotionally upset over the death of three members of her family, and after that she menstruated regularly. At about the same time evidences of syphilitic infection were discovered and she was given treatment for that disease, although not a complete course of therapy.

The patient's school life ended at the eighth grade. She had no special learning difficulties. She traveled about, doing odd jobs as housemaid, waitress, and the like. The wages she earned were low but she was self-supporting. At 18 she became sexually promiscuous and continued so until marriage, then became a steady helpmate and contented housewife. She was thought of as average in intelligence and of sound judgment. Without hobbies or outside interests, she seemed satisfied to remain at home. Friends and her husband described her as kind, thoughtful, self-reliant, and usually cheerful. Since the onset of the present illness she had exaggerated her symptoms and showed depression and worry. Both the patient and her husband had wanted children but were unable to have them.

On admission there was a doubtful positive Wassermann and some slightly positive findings in the neurological examination, indicating the possibility of an active luetic infection. Although she was hospitalized only briefly for spinal puncture and neurological study, her mental state within that time was also carefully studied. She was found to be preoccupied with her somatic delusions. Her facial expression when discussing her problem was worried and anxious; otherwise she seemed well composed. On one occasion she said, "My small intestine turns around and hums like a motor." This was felt to be not so much significant of unusual thinking as representative of the kind of statement she was likely to make. Extremely sensitive to any implication that she might have a functional illness, the patient and her husband both showed strong and united resistance to the psychological investigation. In summary, there was little doubt that this woman had a severe psychological disorder, whatever else may have been present or developing. It was agreed by the staff that if adequate treatment were acceptable to this patient she would probably recover but that under the circumstances there was little likelihood of improvement.

B. Psth., Asocial M:33:D 124'379–(55) 6:3:12
Suicidal
Mutilative

This prison inmate mutilated himself by cutting off the end of the little finger of his left hand. According to his story, a group of fellow prisoners had drawn numbers to see who would mutilate himself in order to attract attention to the pressing need for improved conditions.

This man's mother had died when he was 3 and he had been left to the care of his father, who made a living as a transient sawmill laborer. School records indicated that he completed the eighth grade. He was married once and divorced. Army papers showed that he was dishonorably discharged. Committed to the state hospital for attempting to commit suicide on two different occasions, he was diagnosed as "a psychotic with pulmonary T.B." The subject's F.B.I. record dated back to his first arrest at the age of 23; it included eight arrests for forgery, robbery with firearms, and assault with intent to murder. He had served two jail sentences and two previous prison sentences. During both previous terms he had acted as a trusty. The subject's present sentence is for 22 years for assault with intent to murder and robbery with firearms. While being arrested he was shot in the shoulder.

Since coming a third time to the penitentiary the subject has regressed, although during previous terms he maintained good behavior and was discharged on good time. Physically not well, he is not able to do the usual day's work for an inmate. As to rehabilitative prospects, the prognosis is considered poor.

R. C. K.

P. Hypo. F:55:M:33 ? 126′378–4 0:4:11

For about a year the patient had complained of general fatigue and weakness, which in combination with vague pains in the abdomen, headaches, dizziness, and difficulty in breathing frequently made it necessary for her to go to bed. Seven months before admission her local physician told her she had colitis. Medication gave her no relief, and after a change of physicians and a three-week stay in her home-town hospital she still was unable to take responsibility for household affairs. Until the time of admission she had been a semi-invalid in her home, having spells of dizziness.

About three years before admission she had gone through a nervous episode which had seemed to be cured with one treatment for hyperacidity and a couple of weeks of rest. Otherwise she had been free from illness.

Her education stopped at the sixth grade because she had to assume responsibility in her home. No unusual childhood problems were apparent. A person of good judgment, she had managed the household affairs, paying bills, keeping receipts, and balancing the family budget. The children always went to her for counsel and advice. Although she had kept aloof from most people and had had few warm friendships, she was gentle and kindly toward her children. Her chief hobbies were gardening and flowers. Her husband was of a different religious faith, but the family seemed to be relatively harmonious in spite of the fact that the husband, a heavy drinker, was quarrelsome and abusive when intoxicated. At the time of admission he was incapacitated with arthritis, and the family had been on relief for some time.

On admission the patient was mainly concerned with her somatic complaints, especially gastrointestinal pains. Well oriented and apparently psychologically intact, she answered questions adequately and normally. She knew little about current affairs, and her understanding of her illness was defective. Changeable in emotional tone, she varied between cheerfulness and irritability, but as she gradually adjusted herself to hospital routine, she became more cooperative and stable. When finally discharged after receiving social service aid on her home problems, she seemed to be considerably better.

P. Hypo. M:45:M:17 +1 12'639–84 (67) 6:3:10
+2 yrs. 1273'864–(61) 6:2:22

About twenty years before admission the patient had developed epigastric distress, had become nervous, and was said to have a duodenal ulcer, which healed in three months under conservative treatment. Since then there had been a history of multiple complaints with a blending of one symptom into another. He had had five or six attacks of cholecystitis, and a cholecystectomy was performed. Severe constipation which gradually became more acute appeared about that time, and although a rectal prolapse was repaired it had no beneficial effect on the complaint.

About two years before admission the patient had had a nervous breakdown from which he recovered in five months, but his somatic complaints continued until the time of admission. There were a number of other surgical interventions extending back to the time when the patient was about 20 years old. As a child he apparently had good health.

An immigrant, the man had finished the eighth grade in Sweden and had come to this country when he was about 21 years old. He was a skilled worker. Described as a friendly, kind, and sensitive person, he was high-strung, energetic, and frequently upset. He was so overly concerned about his health that he became hostile when he was told he was not as sick as he imagined himself to be. He was apparently quite capable in managing his life financially, and there seemed to be a good relationship between him and his wife.

In the hospital he was cooperative and well oriented, but he was primarily concerned with his many complaints, chiefly insomnia, constipation, and fleeting leg pains. Although he recognized that "nervousness" was a part of his illness, he did not like the idea that it could be an important part. Efforts were made to build him up by careful physical treatment during his short stay in the hospital, and he showed steady improvement. Psychotherapy was directed toward reassurance and development of some insight. At the time of discharge it was thought that he would probably be able to make a borderline adjustment. Later he was seen in the outpatient clinic. The symptomatic problem was much the same as at the time of admission.

Ps. Paranoid M:30:S:83 +1 12738'469–(67) 4:8:14
Schizoid +93 32781'496–(59) 1:5:7

For twelve years before admission the patient had been bothered by frequent headaches and feelings of pressure on his head, but it was not until about five years before that he had begun to experience such a variety of symptoms that he suffered a "nervous breakdown" which caused him to be rejected by the army. Despite this he was able to work as a skilled technician until three years before admission. At that time he began to have delusions that the federal radio commission was arranging his marriage to a girl with whom he was only slightly acquainted. When he began writing peculiar letters to his parents about these delusions, they finally persuaded him to come home. He went to a private hospital for five weeks where he was given twelve electroshock treatments. Although he was somewhat improved he had to stop work again for a six months' rest because of extreme nervousness. He again started work but the nervousness, daydreaming, paranoid ideas, and hypochondriasis necessitated hospital admission to the psychiatric ward.

There was a history of measles with possibly a measles encephalitis. Although the patient did well in grade school and was known as a "teacher's pet," his high school grades were not good, possibly because he was too interested in radios. Described as shy, retiring, and moody, he never held any one job very long. Since his first difficulty he had been ill at ease in crowds. His usual daydreams included his girl friends and his high school days. There were frequent periods of depression. On the other hand the patient was friendly, and cooperative.

When admitted to the hospital his most marked mental abnormalities were his delusions about his girl friends. The symptoms were all present in varying degrees, but he was easy to manage, interested, and cooperative. His I.Q. was about 120. Although a series of insulin shock treatments made him feel much better and seemed to increase his self-confidence, he remained withdrawn, easily embarrassed, and somewhat defensive. It seemed likely that the basic psychology of the illness was untouched.

P. Mixed Alcoholism M:45:M:17 +1 '127 386–9 (51) 3:4:17

From the time the patient was 15 years of age, he had had intermittent periods of excessive drinking which had gradually become more frequent and more severe, and he was admitted to the hospital on the recommendation of Alcoholics Anonymous because of his desire to be cured of the habit. Three years before admission his wife had insisted that he take "the cure," and the treatment had been effective for eighteen months. Thinking he was cured, he took one drink, and it started him off on another spree.

With the exception of the alcoholic history, his general health in the past had been good. Until shortly before hospitalization the man had taken phenobarbital to help counteract his craving for liquor, but when its use ceased to give him satisfaction he reverted to alcoholism.

Although the patient was above average in intelligence, he had not worked except when he was forced to, and if his wife had not worked the family would have been on relief. When sober he had been a good father and husband, but he gave the impression of always having had his own way, and in spite of innumerable opportunities to get better jobs he had chosen to stay on the farm where he had an adequate income without having to do very much work. For seventeen years, until his father had died, the patient, his wife, and three children had lived with his parents on their farm, and difficulties between his wife and his parents had put the patient under emotional stress from which he escaped by means of liquor. After he and his family left the farm there were periods in which his drinking bouts decreased in number, but there were recurrences at times of increased stress and strain.

On admission the patient was well composed. Although he cooperated fully in giving the history of his life, there were vague spots which did not seem in keeping with his presumed ability to remember, and he seemed to be on his guard in the manner in which he gave his answers. He seemed to recognize the seriousness of his problems, but in spite of what appeared to be an earnest desire to be cured, he was reluctant to talk about details, and it developed that the idea of his entering the hospital had been more his wife's idea than his. Throughout his stay he was very cooperative, but he was not really open to psychotherapeutic approach. There was a tremor of the hands, face, and head, and he was treated with a high caloric diet and vitamins. Childhood associations and family relations probably laid the groundwork for the patient's problem, and the emotional stresses in his life had not been conducive to a smooth personality make-up. In spite of a good many assets and his repeated efforts to get help, he seemed markedly immature. The prognosis on discharge did not seem to be particularly good since little basic change had been effected. He was felt to be chiefly a neurotic type of drinker.

P. Mixed F:27:M:25 +1 '12 783–9 (55) 5:4:24

For three and a half years, until seven weeks before admission, the patient had been in a sanitarium for tubercular patients. Ten days after going home, she began to have symptoms of nervousness, apprehension, anorexia, depression, vomiting, dizziness, diarrhea, and nausea, which usually persisted until early afternoon if she was alone, but which disappeared at once if she was with someone.

Until the onset of tuberculosis her past health had been good. In the sanitarium she underwent a two-stage thoracoplasty, and the tuberculosis showed steady improvement after the operation.

A high school graduate with excellent grades, the patient had hoped to become a private secretary. When she failed to find this kind of work after graduation, she finally took a job as cashier in a store, where she did very well. Four years later she met her husband, and her marriage at age 20 was forced by a three months' premarital pregnancy. The patient had always been strongly attached to her stepmother, the attachment increasing when her father became a chronic alcoholic. Described as thoughtful and sensitive, the young woman was rather friendly but of an independent nature. Except for the unhappiness caused by her father's drunkenness, her family life was happy and her marriage also appeared to be successful. She wanted her only child, but during her stay in the sanitarium the baby had to go to the father's parents, and neither parent had taken care of it since. The husband was described as a happy-go-lucky person and this was a source of some conflict since the patient was ambitious, was more intelligent than he, and wanted intellectual advancement.

In the hospital the patient's primary concern was to rid herself of her nervous symptoms. Although she was apprehensive about the outcome of her problem and cried when she talked about her child, or the loss of her only girl friend, she did not show her symptoms while in the psychiatric hospital until she was "told something about myself by one of the doctors that I didn't know before." This brought on the symptoms in a sudden attack that lasted for only one day. Several times she complained of being bored. She wanted to go home, and she was continually thinking of ways in which to occupy herself there so that she would not become sick again. While it was possible that her husband's tendency toward alcoholism had contributed to the development of her symptoms, no very good understanding of them was elicited during her hospitalization.

P. Mixed M:17:S:42 +19 12873'946– 3:6:19
Schizoid +186 8341'7926– 1:4:19

The patient dated the present illness from a rheumatic fever attack about a year before which had kept him out of school for two weeks. Although there had been no pain, his joints had been swollen and red, with the wrists especially affected, and in addition there had been loss of appetite and fever which made him drink great quantities of water. An attending physician, who said something about heart trouble, had remarked that the patient would have joint pain for some time. A few months later the boy developed palpitation and weakness while playing ball, with such a severe throbbing in his chest that he was unable to stand. There was also a roaring in his head. Of the two physicians who examined him for headache and pain in the stomach, one told him there was nothing wrong with his heart, and the other said that if he did have a rheumatic heart it was not very acute. After a couple of days in bed he returned to school and finished out the year. On another occasion he had a similar spell when he was left alone at home. The idea of everyone's going away gave him an empty feeling, his heart started to pound, and there was a throbbing pain in his chest. He was in bed for two weeks. For that entire summer he stayed around home most of the time, and when he tried going to a party he became so nauseated that he had to go home. When he finally went to a hospital for three weeks, there was temporary improvement, but with a relapse of symptoms he was sent to the psychiatric unit.

A purulent discharge of his right ear, which had started when he was four years old, was so unpleasant that when he was in the fourth grade students in the class had held their noses. This embarrassment made him cry frequently, and even after he was in high school he was always conscious of this draining ear. Ever since the fourth grade he had had sick headaches that caused him to vomit. His father and sister said that he had been unduly concerned about his health at all times. School was easy for him, and he had been very active in sports until the onset of the present symptoms. Although he was shy among strangers and had no hobby, on the whole he was a normal boy.

The heart examination on admission was negative. There was a small perforation in the left ear drum, and in the right ear there was a foul purulent exudate in the canal. This was diagnosed chronic mastoiditis, and an operation was performed for it while he was in the hospital.

Psychologically, the patient said his reasons for being in the hospital were weakness and sore ears. Although he expressed concern about recovery from these conditions and was anxious to get back to school, most of his conversation centered about his bodily functions; he described such symptoms as throbbing pains in his neck, arms, legs, and chest. When lying down he felt as though he were sinking. He talked slowly and with hesitation and had nervous mannerisms. On one occasion he said he did not want to go home because his mother and father quarreled too much. His intelligence was in the average range, and he made a fair ward adjustment. With time his complaints became less evident. The psychological examiner noted that in the early stages, during the administration of the Wechsler-Bellevue test, the patient occasionally became tense and his mind went blank to the point where he was unable to do the simplest tasks. Social service made a study of home conditions, and after some plans had been made for effecting a better adjustment between the parents, the boy was discharged to live with his sister for a while before going home.

P. Hypo.	F:35:M:14	+6	1'32-4968 (57)	5:3:11
		−330	27138'-(49)	4:5:7
P. Hypo.	F:35:M:25	+2	21'37-4689 (55)	6:3:11
		+25	12'37-9 (51)	5:4:13

This patient's complaints included headaches associated with nausea and vomiting, irregular fever (present for two years), arthritis, and diabetes. In an illness two years before admission, when she had high fever, blurring of vision, sore throat, nausea, and vomiting, she was treated with a sulfa compound to which she reacted with cyanosis and unconsciousness. Following this she spent considerable time in hospitals and was treated for various difficulties, including diabetes, for which there was no good clinical evidence. Her own belief was that her troubles had arisen from the bilateral removal of her ovaries.

The patient's health had never been good and her history showed numerous episodes of unconsciousness and fainting following accidents. Of better than average learning ability she had finished the ninth grade in school. Next she had worked as a waitress, and she had continued in that job after marriage. Always meticulous about housekeeping and clothes, she was described as a constant "driver." Although overtly friendly and pleasant, and always smiling, she was actually sensitive and tended to keep things to herself. She never obviously sought sympathy. She gave numerous rationalizations for the fact that her husband frequently went out at night.

Four months before the present admission (second set of MMPI scores) she had been hospitalized for fourteen days. During that hospitalization she was much disturbed over the locked doors and maintained firmly that her problems all related to the ovarian operation. She did not mix well with other patients and was anxious to leave the hospital. At the time it appeared that she had developed the symptoms partly to retain the love and sympathy of her husband.

On the present admission her face was drawn and haggard and her general appearance was that of nervousness and suffering. In the interim between admissions the symptoms had become progressively worse. She was given thirteen insulin shock treatments with four comas. She showed significant improvement except that her appetite remained poor. Her mental outlook became healthier, and she said that for the first time she could freely discuss the problem which she felt regarding her sister's death. This loss, which had occurred nine years earlier, appeared to have been at least one of the important factors in the illness. At discharge she was advised to continue contact with the outpatient department.

P. React. Depr.	M:60:M:17	+2	13′2–9 (71)	5:2:16
		—22 mos.	2317′486–	6:4:18

On admission the patient's complaints were depression and epigastric pain. About three years before admission the patient began to complain of pain which occurred at nine- or ten-day intervals. The pains, which seemed to be precipitated by excitement or worry, had existed in mild degree for years, and the patient had developed the habit of taking large amounts of Bromo-Seltzer. About a year before admission he became confused and showed partial loss of memory and dizziness. Since then his thinking and memory had improved, but he had become hyperexcitable. Numbness in his left leg made it difficult for him to walk. The death of his son depressed him still more and he began to lose weight. With a long history of outpatient experience for physical problems, the patient had been repeatedly referred to the psychiatric outpatient clinic.

A high school graduate with some college experience, the patient, while always active and a good worker, never stayed long in any particular work, engaging in such varied occupations as miner, wrestling teacher, and insurance salesman. He liked sports. Although his wife thought him stubborn and egotistical he had many friends and was capable in handling himself and his responsibilities. The present wife, his second, was younger than he and there appeared to be considerable incompatibility. His first wife had died, and also two of the children born during that marriage.

The physical examination indicated no demonstrable vascular pathology beyond what was normal for his age, and there was no definite evidence of any physical involvement. Although he was obviously depressed he talked freely, showing much concern over his bodily complaints and his relationship with his family. Aside from the fact that he felt old and wondered why he did not fit in with his younger family, his mental state showed little abnormality, and in most ways he appeared normal and intact. After the first night in the hospital he said that he had slept for the first time in years. While he tolerated the hospital regime well, he did not take much part in activities. Most of the time he sat in the lounge, passively watching what went on. Easy to make a contact with, he liked to talk about himself and his experiences, and he said that he liked the rest he was getting. There was little progress in his adjustment to the problems of his family, although at the time of discharge he was much better in terms of the admission symptoms.

P. Hys.	M:35:M:36	+1	132'4–6 (41)	5:5:13
P. Mixed	M:35:M:93	+49	139'26–4 (51)	8:7:10

This patient was admitted with a history of assaultive behavior and seizures of a peculiar nature that lasted about twelve hours. The attack that brought the patient in was the sixth of a similar nature extending over about a year. There had been an earlier admission to the hospital (first MMPI) for the same problem about four months before. Between admissions, except for headache and some other general complaints, he had been relatively well. The day before admission he fainted, was placed on a couch, regained consciousness, got up, went to the kitchen, fell again, and bruised the back of his head. He then went out into the yard and fought with his brother and with the physician who was called. He was completely disoriented and unmanageable and had to be subdued by force.

Before age 20 the patient had very good health but following that age he experienced an uninterrupted series of severe illnesses, injuries, and multiple somatic complaints. There were long hospitalizations for some of these problems. Among the symptoms were episodes of hiccups. Between severe attacks the patient was serious, temperate, and took an inordinate pride in his ability to work harder than any of his associates. He made a sincere effort to pay his debts and really managed exceptionally well considering his extensive medical bills and the time loss due to illness. His habits were good, and he was friendly and cooperative. He was apparently happily married and interested in his family. He was, however, always quick to see a physician for trivial matters of health.

As indicated, the patient was disturbed and incoherent on admission. He moaned and complained of the pain in his head and was inaccessible except to say "yes" or "no" in answer to questions about his pain. There were no neurological findings consistent with these symptoms and two days after admission he was oriented, composed, and cooperative. Concerned with his headache and bodily pain, he was desirous of attention and denied any recollection of his assaultive episode. He expressed deep sorrow that he was afflicted with the attacks and stated many times that he didn't "want to hurt anyone." He was of average intelligence.

Diagnosis was unusually difficult. It was impossible to be sure that there were no organic factors in the case. On the other hand it was certain that there were psychological factors. Considering his personality as seen in the hospital and the fact that he developed symptoms when psychological pressures were heavy, he was judged to be a case of hysteria. He was relatively inaccessible to psychotherapeutic effort since he was convinced that his problem was organic in nature and since his underlying ambition and self-discipline patterns were exceedingly rigid.

P. Hys. M:40:M:33 +11 132′4–9(47) 5:0:18

The presenting complaints of this man were generalized weakness over the past year, a clamping pain in the chest, and headaches for the last three months. The pain was sharp and well localized, lasting usually five minutes. He believed it to be due to a heart condition and at one time had been advised that he had a heart disorder. Later studies, however, did not bear this out. The headaches would wake him from sleep and were not relieved by aspirin. He became unable to work. Just before admission to the hospital he overheard someone say there was nothing wrong with him and shortly thereafter became disoriented.

Although the patient reported that he had done well in school, other informants denied this, claiming he had been uninterested and a poor student. Family and friends characterized his social life as being at a "low level." He was always cutting up and chasing around with people of low quality, they reported. He had gone from job to job. He had contracted gonorrhea at 17 and syphilis at 25. Both of these were adequately treated. He was described as stubborn, easily provoked, restless, and without ability to plan ahead. He was of average intelligence.

In the hospital the patient's thoughts were almost exclusively concerned with his physical condition. He expressed eagerness to be relieved of these symptoms but there seemed to be little depth to his wishes. He malingered and refused to accept any responsibility for treatment, leaving it all "to the doctor," and so psychotherapeutic efforts were ineffective. Staff members agreed that he was not particularly uncomfortable in spite of the complaints he described in direct conversation. He was discharged without having made significant progress, but it appeared that he might make an average adjustment within the limits defined by his past history.

P. Mixed M:32:M:15 +2 132′478– 7:5:17

The illness began six years before admission when the patient became tense and rather inefficient in his work, which demanded dexterity and speed. From that time on he complained of pain in his arms and legs, headaches, shaking spells, and gradual fatigue from any labor. He was examined at a clinic but nothing significant was found, and he was advised to enter a state hospital on a voluntary basis. He refused, returned to work immediately, developed "chills and fever," and was admitted for study again without significant physical findings. His fellow workmen noted that he was forced to miss days of work now and then and that he complained continuously of aches and pains. Three months before admission he had been transferred to a lighter job, but he soon gave it up because of fatigability and nervous tension.

The patient was well liked by his fellow employees but his complaints of bodily aches and pains wearied them. He had never had good health; one of his difficulties was gonorrhea of ten years' standing. One of the numerous physicians he visited diagnosed his problem as diabetes. He described himself as high-strung and readily excited but never irritable or stubborn. He liked competitive sports and spent a good deal of his spare time raising rabbits and tinkering about the house which he had built himself. He had held a job in a meat-packing plant for a number of years. After failing two grades, he had left school in the fifth grade. His intelligence was low normal.

When admitted to the hospital the patient stated that if he could be assured there was "nothing wrong with his teeth" he would feel much more comfortable. Actually, however, there were many other complaints. The ward routine annoyed him and he was unable to relax. He wished to return to work soon but said that he would follow the advice of the staff. His concern over his illness was a rather passive one; he appeared somewhat unhappy but not deeply depressed. He asked if he should mix with the other patients and in other ways showed a passive dependence. As time went on he entered enthusiastically into cooperative games and by the time of discharge was apparently in fairly good condition. It was recommended that he take a job involving relatively light work.

P. Mixed	M:31:M:9	+1	132'478–(45)	7:4:22
		+3	132'7486–(53)	7:3:26

The patient came in with complaints relating to continuous pain beneath the lower edge of his ribs, and he spoke also of "nervousness." His description of the location and characteristics of the pain was vague. He was certain that he had been nervous all his life but felt it had of late become more serious. His vision was reduced, he reported, and sometimes he "saw double." An ulcer had been diagnosed ten years before admission and had been adequately controlled by diet. He carried a scar from a right frontal sinus operation, but no pathology had been found when the sinus was opened.

A man of average intelligence, the patient was a somewhat below average worker. Schoolwork never interested him and his jobs were not profitable. Eventually he went on relief. Described as pleasant and easy to talk to, he gave one the impression that he was quite normal and self-reliant, although he did not feel himself to be so. He had been married six years before and had two children. The marriage was fairly satisfactory although the patient stated he would not marry his wife again if given the choice. He accused her of infidelity, and was himself untrue to her.

In the hospital the patient appeared irresponsible and facetious. He engaged freely in ward activities, conversations, and games. He said, "I am beyond the state of worrying about my condition or anything else, for that matter. I used to worry a lot, but I found that it doesn't pay." He showed little insight or genuine concern about his condition. It was believed that beneath the facetious exterior he was ambitious and felt frustrated over his place in life. He made some progress in insight and improved gradually with hospitalization, but it seemed certain that much more time would need to be spent with him to effect permanent change.

P. Hypo. M:52:S:37 +4 13'2478–69 8:2:23

This patient's disorders were manifold: generalized weakness and pain in the shoulder, irritability, suicidal thoughts, and inability to work. Roughly two years before admission the patient had been struck by the branch of a tree and developed weakness and dizziness, for which he was awarded a sum in compensation. He returned briefly to an easy type of work but being still weak was awarded another sum. Twice later he reopened the case but was refused further aid both times. He became despondent and threatened suicide, claiming he was being mistreated and discriminated against even though repeated physical study revealed no persisting results from the accident.

Never an adequate person, this man held only unskilled jobs and he constantly applied for relief even though he had no family to support. In his community he was considered undependable and eccentric.

On the ward the patient repeatedly stated he would go back to work if he could "just get rid of his neck pain" and if the county would let him decide what specific care and treatment he should receive. He was convinced his symptoms were all on an organic basis and saw no inconsistencies in his attitude. The patient was of about average intelligence. He appeared irritable and rigid, disliked the hospital, and feared he might be sent to a state institution. In the last days of hospitalization he was talkative and more pleasant, but he always spent most of his time alone and the only real change reflected in his attitude toward his illness was that it was "possibly on a hereditary basis." There was no doubt that the symptomatic pattern was influenced by his hope that he might reopen the compensation appeal, and at discharge it was felt that as long as that possibility remained the patient would be unlikely to improve.

B. Psth., Path. Emot. M:52:S:119 +3 132'478–9 8:4:27
Drug Add.

The patient was admitted voluntarily to be helped with drug addiction. He promised to conform strictly to hospital routine and to other restrictions. The main pattern of the illness had appeared approximately twelve years before admission and the drug addiction was traced to physical complaints of abdominal pain. This pain had been very severe and covered various parts of the abdomen. In addition the patient had sustained minor injuries in three different automobile accidents.

Beginning as a minor sales clerk, he gradually advanced himself in a large business organization and became a successful salesman at a high salary level. He had always been an energetic, sensitive individual. He demanded that people be "honest and frank" with him and if he suspected they were otherwise he immediately cut off social relationships. He resented strongly any question of his integrity even by implication. The main driving force in his life was to accumulate money, although he spent generously for his family. He showed marked body interest and passion for fitness, and owned many lotions and types of exercisers. He used a special apparatus for enemas, the tip of which was "just the right size." These characteristics, always present, had become far more marked during the development of his illness. The drugs were at first a relatively minor part of his problem but they increased to major importance as he gradually became habituated.

In the hospital he exhibited concern over his physical condition and presented elaborately detailed accounts of the pain, employing anatomical terms. "My pain starts at the twelfth dorsal vertebra and radiates to the transverse colon and then moves over to the umbilicus." His intelligence was superior. Emotionally irritable, he was upset when his demands were not carried out. He had numerous psychotherapeutic interviews, and although it was possible to clear up his drug addiction, no real progress could be made with his basic problem. Rigid and unswerving in his certainty that there was something wrong with him physically, he rejected the idea of "nervousness." He was free of addiction when discharged but it was felt certain that he would not change his life pattern.

P. Hypo. F:27:S:50 +2 132'4786–9 8:2:24
Ps. Sz., Simple

This young woman's chief presenting complaints centered around pain in the leg, insomnia, and headache. These had begun about seven years before, according to the patient, but were not severe enough to interfere with her work and activities until a year before admission. The pain consisted of an uneasy feeling "like something moving" in the legs. Often she went to bed at two or three in the morning, unable to sleep for hours. She had anxiety dreams and was bothered by loud noises, storms, arguments, and exciting movies. Irritability developed, so that her family found the situation intolerable.

The patient did not graduate from the eighth grade because, she said, "I scalded my legs or something." Her intelligence was average. She worked in a hotel and was a barmaid for several years. An active person, she had a pleasant disposition unless crossed and then her reaction was to become self-pitying and to withdraw. At such times she cried bitterly. She had many friends and one steady boy friend.

On the ward the young woman was cooperative and apparently normal. Answering questions readily and adequately, she seemed not greatly concerned with her illness. She was dogmatic and never modified her ideas in discussion. Her own explanation for her difficulty was that it came from "nerves"—"from standing on my legs too long while working." The pain in her legs persisted but in time she reluctantly admitted that the headaches had ceased. She was treated with sedative drugs, packs, and occupational therapy. Gradually she was permitted walks, and a program was followed of rewarding her for more acceptable behavior. These efforts did not prove wholly effective, and although she was much improved at discharge, it was felt she was likely to change little.

P. Anxiety State M:31:M:22 +13 '13248–9 (37) 8:2:24
P. Hypo.

Most of the patient's complaints dated back to the previous year when he had a sore throat, accompanied by mild fever and a number of indefinite pains. The symptoms gradually disappeared, but he felt so on edge all the time that he saw numerous physicians. After two of them had told him he had a serious heart condition, he developed heart consciousness and felt his pulse every few minutes. He had a tense feeling in his throat, and at night he felt as though his heart were coming up through his chest. Nocturnal attacks of breathlessness forced him to sit up on the bed, gasping for breath. In one hospital he was given a tentative diagnosis of rheumatic fever. In the present hospitalization he was first admitted to the general medicine service, where extensive studies so reassured him his heart was normal that all his symptoms referable to a somatic condition disappeared, but he remained anxious and complained of insomnia.

The past history was not especially contributory except that he had read medical books and had imagined he had every disease he read about. When he was 23 he had had a severe itch over his entire body. An eighth-grade graduate, he had done average schoolwork and had since made a fairly comfortable living as a farmer. Even-tempered and cheerful, he was apparently normal in social behavior.

The physical studies were essentially negative. Since he had been told he had no heart disease, he accepted himself as normal. He believed his nervous condition would soon clear up, but he showed some anxiety over the fact that his gums bled readily, and he became tense and irritated when he could not answer questions put to him in the psychological examination. His insight was very superficial. Although he was friendly and cheerful, he remained anxious and tense during his stay in the hospital. Against staff advice he left the hospital suddenly before the study of him was completed, and it was felt that he would probably develop further complaints which might require study.

P. Hypo. M:31:S:20 +5 13′248–9 3:0:20

The presenting complaints for this man included paresthesias and muscular twitching in all four extremities. This had been continuous for ten years. He was partially incapacitated by the muscular twitching and complained of weakness and many other somatic ills, which he wished to have checked.

Much of the patient's life had been spent in illness. Minor physical problems with him frequently continued to a severe degree. Although he was retarded in school because of irregular attendance, he finally completed high school. For a considerable time he did not work because of tuberculosis. Owing to ill health he never did anything steadily. In other ways he was relatively well adjusted, at least until he finished high school. He never had a steady girl friend and blamed poor health for this also.

Concerned about his complaints, the patient talked endlessly of these if permitted. He displayed indifference to the fact that he led the life of an invalid, and he was unable to evaluate his symptoms objectively. Complete physical study, with strong reassurance that no organic disorder was found, seemed to help him a great deal, although he still readily developed new complaints. In the course of hospitalization and the program of reassurance he became markedly better and felt he was ready to go home and make a better life. The staff members thought it was unlikely that he would change greatly, although they agreed he might become self-supporting.

P. Hys. F:32:M:14 +2 13′24867–(41) 7:2:20

This patient came in voluntarily because of convulsive seizures which had begun a year before. The first of these followed the news that her father was being taken to a hospital for the insane. She shook and trembled, screamed and cried. Other attacks followed, with increasing frequency and usually accompanied by vertical diplopia and weakness. She experienced an aura before the attacks and at times bit her tongue. The attacks were subsiding when her husband was classified for immediate induction by the draft board and at once they again became more numerous.

Always sickly, the patient gave a medical history that included many disorders which sounded psychosomatic in nature. She had been treated at various times for asthma, cardiac insufficiency, and goiter. Below average in intelligence, she had found schoolwork difficult. She had married fourteen years before admission and had two children. Friends described her as friendly and kind. She always felt self-conscious when she went to see a physician. Once in a physician's waiting room she "saw two insane" persons. This bothered her so that she "couldn't sleep for three nights."

Fearful that someone might suspect her problem was "just in her head," the patient was upset at being in a neuropsychiatric ward although she cooperated well. With the exception of the first day or two in the hospital she had no seizures while there. The relief was effected both by drugs and by suggestion. She was immature and childish in her thinking, docile, and easily persuaded. Her moods were somewhat unpredictable. She yielded fairly well to re-educative therapy. It was impossible to get her completely remade into a mature person, but at discharge it appeared probable that she would be much better for a considerable time.

Drug Add. F:39:M:12 +2 13′249–7(49) 5:5:17

The patient was a registered nurse who had been working eighteen hours a day as the supervisor of a small hospital in her home town. She had begun to take codeine and then demerol and finally morphine. She said she had tried to hold down the amount of drugs but had had to increase the dosage when she developed pain in her ankles from being on her feet so much. She had decided to stop taking the drug four days before admission but by the morning of admission the withdrawal symptoms were so bad that she was forced to call a physician, to whom she confessed her addiction. He sent her to the psychopathic unit.

Her past history was not particularly helpful. She was in the eighth grade when her education was interrupted by her mother's nervous breakdown. After taking care of her mother for two years, she entered school again and finally received her R.N. Following her marriage she worked intermittently in order to support her husband. At the age of ten she had become very obese and she remained that way. This made her so self-conscious that her social life was affected. Her husband had recently begun to drink heavily and at the time of the patient's admission to the psychopathic unit he was in a state hospital for chronic alcoholism and drug addiction.

Upon hospitalization the patient was concerned with the withdrawal symptoms and kept asking for a "shot of morphine," although she condemned herself for beginning to use drugs because as a nurse she should have known better. It was learned that she had also furnished her husband with drugs. Her sensorium was clear. She was nervous and apparently anxious. After three days of treatment she was much improved. At first she did not get along well with other patients, but after a few days her behavior was normal. She was considered to have a good prognosis for staying away from drugs if situational pressures did not become too great.

B. Psth., Mixed F:34:M:53 +14 1326′78–X 10:3:15
Suicidal +116 3721864′–9 8:6:20

The patient was admitted to the hospital after the police had found her lying unconscious in an alley. Physical studies gave no clue to the cause of her unconsciousness. Her husband said that she had been employed as a housekeeper and that until she became pregnant about three years before admission, she had been cheerful and had done satisfactory work. After the birth of her baby she had undergone a personality change. She had become irritable; she had lost interest in her personal appearance, in her two children, and in outside activities; and she had made several rather spectacular but unsuccessful attempts at suicide. She completely rejected her husband.

The patient was a ninth-grade graduate with an average school record. After leaving school she had worked as a domestic. Her first husband—abusive, alcoholic, and unsatisfactory as a provider—had been committed for a time to a state hospital, and during this period the patient had supported their two children. After divorcing her husband the patient had continued to work as a housekeeper, finally taking a job with the man who eventually became her common-law husband. She had always been a rather unstable person who overreacted to minor occurrences. Her first attempt at suicide was made because she felt her sister rejected her for immoral conduct. The available details about her early personality were very inadequate.

In the hospital the patient complained bitterly that her second husband had mistreated her, and she went into great detail about it. She described her miserable life with her first husband and said that never in her life had she been treated with kindness and affection. She described a three-week period of amnesia preceding her present admission. No explanation of the spell of unconsciousness was elicited. She was apathetic and frequently wept, but in general she was intact in sensorium and intellect. She was cooperative, but she always insisted that her troubles were entirely due to factors outside herself. Except for frequently disturbing the ward at night by crying and complaining, she was a good patient. After extensive social service investigation of the family situation, the patient was discharged to follow a new plan for supporting her children. She intended to separate from her husband. The staff was dissatisfied with the resolution of the case, since the patient's reticence and her husband's inability to answer questions rationally prevented them from getting any real knowledge of the patient's background.

P. Hys.	F:34:S:41	+1	132'6784–9 (49)	9:4:17
P. Hypo.		+18	132'7864–X (53)	12:4:26
Ps. Sz., Simple		+19	312'7846–X (47)	10:3:24

The chief complaints of this patient on hospital admission were nervousness, aches and pains over her entire body, dizziness, blurring of vision, and weakness. Since the age of 19, following an appendectomy, this patient apparently had been in poor psychological condition. The operation had led to no somatic complications but afterward she had become tired, had lost weight, and had felt weak. From that time on she received medical treatment for countless ailments, including "leakage of the heart," back pains, urinary frequency, a goiter, and symptoms of ulcer. During the last ten years, she had also had a nervous breakdown yearly.

Each breakdown was characterized by numbness, trembling, nervousness, and stiffness, and she went to bed for most of several months.

There was much more of the same sort of material in her history. In addition to the delusions about her physical condition she had peculiar fears and thought she saw faces and heard voices. She was described as having been an adequate and fun-loving child and adolescent before age 19. Her father and mother were indulgent and it appeared possible that they had encouraged her development into a semi-invalid. Her intelligence was in the low normal range.

The patient was suspicious and evasive toward the interviewer and it was difficult to get information directly from her. Her uppermost thoughts revolved around what could be done for her aches and pains. She was clearly oriented and not obviously disturbed in intellect. Except for stretches of suspicious silence, she assumed an amused and somewhat cynical attitude. She was usually disheveled and her face was marked with pustules and scabs, of which she was sharply conscious. She quickly adjusted to the routine of the hospital and was given sedatives and occupational therapeutic treatments. However, such therapy, as might be expected, was relatively unsuccessful because of the difficulty in establishing any real relationship with her. At discharge she was little improved.

P. Mixed	F:55:M:7	+1	1326′789–4X	11:4:14
Paranoid		–68	312′9786–4X	10:5:11

Three months before the present admission this patient had spent three days in a hospital because of pain in her leg, insomnia, and paresthetic sensations in her hand. She had lain awake nights scratching her shoulders and legs until sores developed. Because of the pain in her leg she had had great difficulty walking and even turning over in bed. Aspirin had given no relief. When no serious organic disorders could be discovered she finally entered the psychiatric hospital.

Always in poor health, the patient had once spent a year in a sanitarium for tuberculosis. Her medical history included abscesses, fractures, infections, a thyroidectomy, an appendectomy, an operation for tubal pregnancy, and many other medical procedures. She claimed that she had been mistreated in one rest home.

A high school graduate, she had placed second from the top in her class. "Because of poor health," she said, she had gone no further in school but had started to work. Married at age 20, she had become a meticulous housekeeper and had enjoyed entertaining, but she had experienced periods of severe depression and had worried over trivialities. She had always been suspicious of people. She apparently had mild ideas of reference.

The neurological and other physical examination procedures indicated mild disorders, but nothing to account for the admission complaints. In the hospital the patient was disturbed over the "shame" of being in a mental hospital where everything was locked up. She fussed about her roommate, suspected the doctors of "playing tricks" on her, and, in general, was not a cooperative patient. There were no gross disturbances of intellect or sensorium. Although she was depressed and cried easily, for the most part her mood was appropriate. She, of course, was convinced that her illness had entirely organic bases. She improved markedly after the first two or three days but refused to stay long enough for any real evaluation of her case. She left the hospital to resume her regular duties.

P. Anxiety State	M:25:M		132694'78–(51)	3:7:?

This pilot, a twice-married second lieutenant, was referred to the psychiatrist by the flight surgeon. Progressive nervousness and increasingly severe pains in the back of his neck were the complaints. These were said to have appeared after a diving accident, but a physical examination and X-ray studies showed no significant pathology.

An only child, the patient appeared to have received more than his share of anxious attention from a neurotic mother. During his early life, he had been subject to nightmares and episodes of somnambulism. His school record showed no irregularities and he had finished four years of high school. Tests showed that the young man's intelligence fell in the high average to superior range. His occupational history was as regular as his school record, and he was considered a steady and diligent employee in civilian life. His first marriage had failed, he said, because his wife was always ailing physically and finally "began to drink and run around." His present marriage was said to be happy.

As the tension of precombat training increased, the pilot had developed generalized G.I. complaints ranging from abdominal pains and vomiting to explosive evacuation of his bowels. His appetite had remained good and he had lost no weight. A well-developed man although a little paunchy, he had a definite facial tic. He clearly lacked the physical and emotional stamina requisite for combat experience and disposition was made by reclassification and discharge. A. T. K.

P. Hys.	F:60:M:25	0	'1327–89 (55)	6:1:13
		+20	'31–6742 (51)	5:1:15

About six months before hospital admission the patient's voice had, in two days' time, gradually decreased to a whisper. Since she had lost her voice in association with tonsillitis on numerous occasions in the past ten years little significance was attached to the episode until it was observed that while a sore throat had accompanied the previous experiences, there was no pain with this attack. In addition, the previous attacks had lasted only four to five days, but this time the aphonia continued, with the exception of one brief incident, up to the time of admission. On the tenth day she had seen a local doctor, and besides the aphonia she had also complained of a lump in her throat, vague pains, headaches, pressure sensations when she worked hard or lay on her right side, a feeling that the right eye was smaller than the left, and a sensation of "looking through wax paper." Reassurance did not help her although she went to several different clinics. The only precipitating factor elicited was that she had been elected a delegate to a religious conference about the time of the onset of the difficulty. Frequent crying spells were the only personality change.

She had some time before undergone a hysterectomy, with unilateral ovariectomy, and, when she was much younger, a tonsillectomy in an unsuccessful effort to cure her frequent aphonias. An eighth-grade graduate at age 15, she had wanted to become a nurse but because of family responsibilities she had worked as a "hired girl" until her marriage at 18. Since then she had lived on a farm and had fulfilled her responsibilities to her home with neurotic perfectionism. A friendly, kind, and thoughtful person, she was also fairly frank, self-reliant, and truthful. Sensitive to the opinions of others, she said she had always tried to please everyone. She had wanted to have more children, but sterilization had prevented that. She was a devout churchgoer with an apparently high moral standard. Although she admitted to no sexual deviations, her husband thought she had had sexual intercourse with her brother before her marriage.

The physical and neurological examinations were normal except for the aphonia, and there were no abnormal trends in sensation. Her sensorium and intellect were intact. Her uppermost thoughts concerned the welfare of her children and financial security for her old age. She was markedly indifferent to the severity of the symptoms. She said blandly, "The doctor says its nerves. I don't know, but if it is I want to get over it." Although her manner was somewhat apathetic, she was neat in appearance, was cooperative, and made a good adjustment to hospital routine. In the second week when suggestive therapy was used her voice returned, and mild abnormalities in respiratory rhythm seemed to represent a residual of the hysterical pattern. Since she never gained any convincing insight into her problem, she was discharged as free from the present disturbing pattern with recurrence obviously likely.

P. Mixed	F:41:M:42	+3	13′2748–6 (43)	6:2:20
		+37	′231–98 46 (45)	4:3:14

The patient was admitted to the hospital because of marked vasomotor disturbances that included sweating of the palms, heart palpitation, insomnia, and anorexia. Since the first such episode at age 23 the woman had experienced four or five major attacks, and for the past four years she had felt persistent agitation and anxiety. She had been hard to live with, had spent much of her time in bed, and had been unduly harsh with her only child. She had also been unable to go in crowds because of a fear of impending doom or "of something terrible about to happen." She complained of a "tight band pressing on the back of my head."

1327′498–

She felt that her neighbors and the rest of the town gossiped too much, with a good deal of their gossip directed toward her, and some of this was probably true since she felt that no one in town was her social equal. A psychiatrist whose help she had sought had persuaded her to come to the hospital.

Before the onset of the present pattern she had been in good health, but she had always had a nervous temperament. Her interests were almost solely limited to worrying about herself. Her smile was strained, and although she said she would like to find out what was wrong with her, she was defensive about it. Her claim to have always been well adjusted sexually was not substantiated by her husband, who said she was an inadequate sexual partner, although he was more upset about her bad temper and their poor social relationship than about the sexual maladjustment.

The patient was upset about the locked doors in the hospital and felt that she had been tricked into coming to the hospital. Intact in sensorium and intellect, she was logical and to the point in discourse, but she had absolutely no insight. In spite of a verbalized desire for help the only conversation she would entertain was of a trivial and inconsequential nature. When personal subjects were brought up, she withdrew and became dreamy. No frank delusions were elicited. She was unchanged after shock therapy, and no other method of approach was successful.

P. Hys. M:25:S:112 —15 1327′498–(46) 3:6:14
P. Anxiety State +150 9′48–(53) 3:5:22

This patient came to the hospital with the chief complaint of being unable to relax. He dated this from an infantry combat experience when a shell exploded just on the other side of a wall from him, killing several members of his outfit. Following this he noticed that he was deaf in one ear, but despite the injury he was returned to combat where he remained for ten months. After his discharge he found himself unable to maintain any sustained concentration; he also began to lose weight and had some periods of insomnia. He attempted to resolve part of the tension by drinking but was afraid that he would form the habit and quit. Then he went to college where his progress was unsatisfactory, although at times he managed to do fairly well.

His earlier life had not been satisfactory since he had lived in a home atmosphere of continual parental domination. For example, when he first returned home from service his parents expected him to be home by eleven at night, even though he was 21 years old at the time. His father had continually discouraged him as a child by implying that the patient didn't have the ability to do most of the normal feats of childhood. His mother was overprotective, which also had the effect of discouraging him from developing any self-esteem. The results of this parental management showed themselves particularly during his high school years, which he recalled as being most lonely and most unhappy.

During the therapy the patient was almost childish in his emotional development. He was highly suggestible and placed a faith in the therapist that was extreme to a pathetic degree. The therapy consisted essentially of a ventilation of the guilt feeling he felt toward his parents and the army, which had been in effect a parent-surrogate. His schoolwork improved, and a month following the end of therapy he came in to show his grades, which had increased from a C— to a B— average. When last seen he had changed his major to social work and was making very satisfactory progress. A. S.

Ps. M-D., Depr.	M:41:M:53	+13	132'76984–	7:5:9
Ps. M-D., Depr.	M:42:M:18	+1	1327'869–	5:2:14
		+33 mos.	21376'84–9	5:9:14

The patient was admitted to the hospital with complaints of weakness, emotional tension, mild depression, and bizarre symptoms. This was his second admission; the detailed summary of his first hospitalization (the first MMPI above) was lost, but in general a similar pattern had prevailed. In the interim he had not been well enough to do a full day's work. From time to time he had felt pain which he described as being "in the neck with radiation in the ear." Steadily becoming worse, he had lost weight, new ills had appeared, and he had become almost completely incapacitated by the pain. "Oh, it's a terrible pain in my neck and down my side. It seems like I can't stand it any longer. I don't think I'll last much longer. Sometimes I think it's due to too much acid in the blood."

Even before the appearance of the symptomatic pattern present in both hospitalizations, this man had not been particularly strong. Of low average intelligence, he had a brief and poor school record, and he had never held a good job. Married and the father of three children, he had never adequately supported his family for longer than a few months; usually they were on relief. He insisted he didn't feel blue; it was only the pain that got him down. He appeared apprehensive and agitated.

In the hospital the patient was interested only in discussing his somatic complaints. Blaming his economic difficulties on his pains, he felt that he had never really been strong enough to work normally. Except for the delusional conviction of "something wrong with my body," he had no gross defects in mental content. One moment he cried, the next he appeared happy and sociable. Recognizing that the complaints were intensified by his own emotional instability, he nevertheless was convinced that they were based on an organic defect. When discussing any subject except his pain, he was often irrelevant and vague. His facial expression was that of an anxious, forlorn individual. On one occasion he said, "What's the use? It would probably be better if I would end it all." In the course of his stay at the hospital he gradually became somewhat better and when discharged was back approximately at his level of the four or five years before hospitalization. No basic change had been effected.

P. Mixed F:52:W:10 +5 132'78–(63) 5:3:14
−119 132'768–(63) 8:5:10

The patient arrived with a medley of complaints: nervousness, headaches, weak spells, and periods of depression and irritability. The headaches, present for many years and severer during the menstrual period, were brought on by eye-strain or excitement and could be relieved by aspirin. At times she said it seemed "as if there was constricting bands about my head." Since the death of her husband ten years before, periods of depression had occurred, with sporadic weeping and constant musing on memories of bygone days. She dreamed that her husband was alive and accompanied her to parties. During these depressions she was extremely irritable. At one time she had had a series of "fainting spells" at work. She feared she had cancer and could not be cured.

The patient's early life had been unhappy. An aunt, with whom she lived after the death of her mother, was domineering and cruel and refused to allow her to associate with other children. Her aunt also frequently whipped and kicked her, rousing in the patient deep hatred. She met her future husband at age 15 but marriage was delayed for nine years by the aunt's disapproval. After their marriage the couple lived for a while with the husband's father but here again they met unhappiness, and it was not until they moved to a farm of their own that they achieved any degree of freedom and happiness. This continued for thirteen years, until the death of the husband. The patient was a good housewife and mother and was described as having been friendly, self-reliant, and truthful, although always sensitive and at times irritable.

Although nervous and apprehensive, this patient was relatively approachable and responded well to psychotherapeutic treatments. She gained a good measure of insight into the manner in which she was affecting her health and happiness by deliberately dwelling on her husband's death. With this insight she rapidly improved and became considerably more comfortable. At discharge it appeared likely she would make a better and continuing adjustment.

P. Mixed M:36:M:60 −6 132'8–4 3:6:10

The presenting complaints of this patient were pressure inside of his head, palpitation of his heart, inability to stand heat, fear of crowds, and the like. The onset was uncertain but was vaguely placed by the patient at about two years before hospital admission. The patient at that time did not feel well. As the hot weather came on he suffered a "heat stroke," in which he felt dizzy and had peculiar feelings in his head and palpitation. Since that time he had been susceptible to heat, and whenever in the sun or in a bright light or in any muggy place he felt faint. Fear of crowds was somehow associated with these other symptoms. He also had peculiar numb feelings in his face. He recognized that he was irritable, but he came to the hospital chiefly because the relief agencies wanted to know why such an able-bodied, healthy-appearing man was unable to work.

His history before the onset of the present complaints indicated what was noted as a "strikingly uneventful" life. He had done farming, plumbing, and other kinds of work, and although a steady worker, he had stayed only a short time at each job. He had always wanted to be a farmer. He had made a relatively satisfactory marriage and had four children. Economically the family had been sound until his present disability set in. He was considered fairly stable and had shown intelligence and good common sense. A friendly man, he was well liked and reasonably self-confident.

In the hospital it was at once noted that he seemed rather unconcerned about his ailments. He did not show any special preoccupation with them except that he would detail his symptoms if encouraged at all. Emotionally at ease, he expressed anxiety to get back to work, but this did not seem very convincing to others. His tested I.Q. was 133. His behavior was conventional; he showed no spontaneity, never asked to go out or to receive any other special privileges. It was observed that he would sit in a hot stuffy room where other people were uncomfortable, but would not complain. He readily accepted a psychogenic basis for his difficulties in response to reassurance on his physical condition, and he expressed complete willingness to cooperate with any psychotherapeutic effort. However, when some genuine action was expected of him, he was not, as a rule, helpful. The case seemed unusual, with the patient inaccessible in spite of high intelligence and apparent cooperation. Discharge was made with the recommendation that he try working again, and he was given repeated reassurance about his physical condition. It was felt that recovery was uncertain.

P. Hypo. M:35:M:26 +1 132'847–9 4:3:24

This patient's long list of somatic complaints related chiefly to the skeletal and muscular systems. The difficulty had appeared seven years before when he began to pause frequently in his work to complain of his "troubles." Blaming dampness in the plant where he worked, he consulted many physicians. He told everyone he had to "drive" himself to work and he sought relief money. Then he turned his scolding to the relief board, claiming their help was insufficient for his family's needs. He was rude to relief board members and others who suggested that "it is all in my mind."

Although somewhat self-centered, this man had always been rather friendly. Throughout most of his life he had had hypochondriacal complaints. He was active in religious fields. He was readily irritable and pessimistic about his future. In handling money he was competent. In so far as he had outside interests, they included hunting, fishing, and the repairing of musical instruments, particularly violins. He had been married at 23 and had six children. His wife also showed numerous neurotic traits.

The patient's mental content centered almost wholly on his somatic complaints, and he included almost every organic system. Repeatedly he stated that the county owed him more help. In intelligence he was below average. Resistant to the idea that a psychiatric hospital or psychiatric treatment might help him, he declared his difficulty was "really overwork and from the dampness." He insisted that he was, of course, going to leave his case "entirely up to the doctor," and he did cooperate well in examinations. However, it was apparent that this role was a superficial one and that actually he was being critical at all times. Treatment was thwarted by this attitude and only indirect approaches and attempts at reassurance about his physical ills were possible. He was made more comfortable but was discharged with little real improvement.

P. Hypo.   M:37:M:14   +6   132'8749-6   7:0:23

This patient was admitted with precordial pain and low backache, the latter an almost lifelong complaint. For the previous three months, he had had gastrointestinal difficulty simultaneously with the onset of the precordial pain, which was sharp and stabbing in character. Bloating and constipation were a part of the picture also, as well as severe headaches.

At 14 the patient had completed only the fourth grade and was able to write little besides his name. His intelligence was dull normal. Before this illness he had got along fairly well in his community, and he was relatively happily married. Although his earnings were meager he was able to support his wife, his child, and himself until the onset of his illness when they were forced to accept agency aid.

In the hospital the patient dropped most of his somatic complaints and was at all times cooperative. When discharged he felt well and was eager to return to work. Apparently reassurance about his physical condition was an important factor in his recovery. It was felt that he would probably do fairly well unless new pressures in the environment began to push him beyond his abilities for adaptation, in which case he might again develop somatic complaints.

P. Mixed Paranoid   M:35:M:36   —29   132'87649-(45)   4:5:14

This patient entered the hospital with numerous somatic complaints, the principle of which were pain in his back and weakness in his right leg. Two years before he had slipped on the ice and had injured his back. Afterward he had suffered from extreme weakness and atrophy of the right leg. He had received various treatments but did not feel that he had improved; the pain had continued and he was forced to quit work and devote himself to the treatments. He had periods of apparent unconsciousness preceded by extreme nervousness and tachycardia. He also had numerous bizarre ideas.

Of low intelligence, the patient had repeated several grades in school but finally finished the eighth grade before leaving. He had held many minor jobs but usually had quit or had been fired following difficulty of some sort. He claimed that his father had spread false stories about him in the community and that this prevented him from obtaining credit. From his early years he had had paranoid ideas superimposed upon a rather pleasant disposition. He was known as a sensitive, introverted person, apparently anxious to make a good impression on people. Overreactive to disappointment, he continually sought sympathy by telling his troubles to anyone who would listen. He and his wife and seven children were on relief a good part of the time.

The patient's ideas centered around his somatic complaints and in talking about them he was voluble and rambling. A clean and neat person, he adjusted to ward life fairly well, but he was unpredictable and always craved the center of attention. He showed no marked improvement in his basic behavior pattern. Various psychotherapeutic approaches were tried and although enough improvement occurred to permit him to function at a minimal level, there was little prospect that his future behavior would differ much from that with which he had begun hospitalization.

B. Psth., Path. Emot. M:36:S:25 +3 1'3<u>29</u>78– 4:3:14
Drug Add.
Suicidal

This patient was admitted to the hospital because of suspected drug addiction and attempted suicide by taking "opium pills." A year before admission he had been run over by a switch engine and both legs had been traumatically amputated at the thigh. In the succeeding treatment he was given numerous morphine injections to relieve pain. It was thought probable that the accident had occurred when he was intoxicated. A long history of physical complaints, for which he was given various drugs, followed. At a rest home, just before the present admission, he got drunk and took four green capsules (not otherwise identified) which made him euphoric and incoherent. After gastric lavage he was admitted to the hospital in a stuporous condition.

Since the age of 12 the patient had had a hearing defect. An irresponsible person always and a heavy drinker from his late teens, he had at no time held a steady job and was an itinerant worker. Occasionally he returned home to live with his parents. He made friends easily and was usually jolly; he enjoyed hunting, fishing, and drawing. He had never been legally married, although once for six months he had a common-law wife.

After recovering from the suicide attempt the patient returned to relatively normal activity. He was cheerful, alert, and talkative. His intelligence was average. He had no recognition that drug-taking had become a habit, and his continual complaint was that he felt a sharp pain and wanted something for it. His attitude toward the hospital was reflected in his concern that he would have to "live down" the fact that he had "been in a mental ward." Superficially he cooperated well, and when there was nothing to be gained by complaint he did not mention his pain. Therapy was not importantly productive and he was discharged with little expectation that his future behavior would differ materially from that in the past.

P. Hys. F:17:S:13 +8 134′287–9 6:2:27

This girl, since the age of 3, had suffered recurrent attacks of right flank pain with associated urinary symptoms, including urgency and frequency. There had been steady weight loss and fatigue, and on the day preceding admission to the hospital she had had two fainting spells.

Following a bout of nausea, vomiting, and fever, an operation had been performed some time before and the gall bladder was found to be pathological. Recovery from the surgery was slow, and it was noted at the time that the objective symptoms relating to the somatic system were not closely tied to the psychological symptoms. The home doctor noted, for example, that when pus, blood, and other evidences of organic involvement were found in the urine, the actual pain was much less severe. Conversely, when urinalysis was negative, the pain was worse.

The patient had always been ambitious and had had high goals. In school she earned A's and B's, but only because of rigid application to her studies. She was somewhat above average in intelligence but her teachers felt that her achievement was more the result of hard work than of high ability. Athletic activities did not interest her but she enjoyed dancing and parties. Music or stenography was her vocational aim.

In the hospital the girl had a number of complaints associated chiefly with the right flank. These included numbness in the right arm and right leg, swelling of the ankle, edema of the eyelids, and pain in the abdomen. She also believed that her skin color was changing. She associated her occasional depressions with the backaches but felt she could overcome these in the future. Although convinced that her problems were related to an organic disease, she perceived that "some emotional thing" made her worse. A pleasing person to talk with, she made a good appearance. Hospitalization promptly relieved her of the majority of the symptoms, and an attempt was made to give her understanding that would help prevent future difficulty. Since it was felt that high ideals for achievement were not to her advantage, she was encouraged to make specific plans for achievement within her true capacity.

P. Mixed M:34:M:18 +1 13′428 76–9 (55) 9:3:25
Schizoid
Paranoid

This man complained of hyperirritability and feelings which can be labeled ideas of reference. A year before his admission the patient's wife had spent some days in a hospital for the birth of her seventh child. Her absence from home irritated the patient extremely. While visiting her he had outbursts of temper and weeping. At the same time he quarreled with his mother-in-law, who was angry with him because of her daughter's frequent pregnancies. He became abusive and frightened the woman, who called for help. He said, "They thought I was crazy." The family physician advised a trip and the patient and his wife visited in another state for a while. He improved considerably during this trip, but on his return he entered the hospital.

For as long as he could remember the patient had harbored feelings of inferiority and personal inadequacy. One of his statements was, "I've never had a fight in my life." In crowds he often became nervous, trembled, and perspired profusely. If anyone even spoke sharply to him his reaction was to feel "like running away." He fancied everyone was looking at him. He was emotionally labile, easily angered, always "immature."

In the hospital the patient was emotionally unstable and his immaturity was marked. He talked freely about his illness, about his feelings of inferiority, and particularly and at length about his pains and other symptoms. Gradually he gained confidence, became more relaxed, and left the hospital considerably improved. The discharge note indicated, however, that the staff felt he was somewhat paranoid and that if his future environmental situation offered many stresses he would almost certainly experience difficulties again.

Ps. Paranoid M:43:M:116 +2 '13469–(71) 3:0:18

The patient's obvious illness had its onset about three years before hospital admission when he began to suspect that people on the staff of the college where he was a history instructor were plotting against him. He thought they had planted a dictaphone in his house and were throwing bacteria-laden dust in his hair. He suspected that his maid was an enemy agent and was spreading dust around his bed to contaminate him. Before going to bed, he felt he had to sweep around the bed and put a towel over his head. He had periods of frenzy in which he would take off his clothes and shake them vigorously.

This general pattern of behavior continued until the time of admission, and there were many similar details. He was working for an advanced degree and while working on his thesis kept it locked and in a trunk in the attic. It was considered an outstanding work by the examining committee. In his oral examination the board felt that his answers were rambling and evasive but he was granted the degree. A distant cousin died and depressed by this he wrote a note to his wife, saying, "This is the end. The people at the college have done this to get rid of me." He believed that there was a black truck parked in front of his house directing X-rays into the house to harm him. To get away from these he slept on the floor. He was finally admitted to the hospital on the petition of his wife after he attempted to obtain a gun permit. Throughout the systematic development of this whole pattern very few persons realized that there was anything abnormal about him at all. Only his wife and one or two others were aware of the symptoms.

He had always developed "symptoms" whenever he had been up against something he did not want to do. For a while he was thought to have a cardiac condition and after that he would readily develop palpitation and chest pain. As indicated, he was a brilliant person; he was a perfectionist; and he was very ambitious. He was good at making friends and had many of them, although his wife said that he was inconsiderate of them.

In the hospital he appeared extremely docile and pleasant. Circumstantiality and volubility were present; obviously these were methods of evasiveness. He talked about some of his paranoid ideas but on the whole was guarded and refused to say much. The general psychometric personality picture was normal. There were few signs in the Rorschach or other tests indicating his problem. He was somewhat sophisticated in personality test methodology. At least on the surface, he was quite willing to accept therapy and underwent 53 insulin shock treatments. Active on the ward, he was usually a leader of the groups. At the time of discharge he really had changed very little in personality but had covered up what few symptoms he had shown earlier. After leaving the hospital he went on a long trip. Subsequently he was discovered disguised in another state and was brought back home where he underwent a lobotomy. After the operation he had the same ideas that he had had previously but was not insistent about them and did not act in bizarre ways. On the other hand he was definitely childish and was no longer able to occupy his former intellectual position.

P. Hypo. F:43:S:40 +28 13'49287– 7:2:24

This patient was admitted with multiple somatic complaints, many of which had been present for at least twenty years. She had prominent pains in her eyes, chest, and abdomen. Her legs ached and she was troubled by numbness and tingling in hands and feet.

Never robust, as a child she had not been strong enough to play and consequently had always been protected and pampered. Except for one year following high school graduation she had held no jobs but had led the life of an invalid. Her one job had been as a secretary, but she had found this work too tiring. Always gracious and kind, she was sympathetic and interested in the problems of others. The patient said, "I am always grateful for what is done for me," but actually, it was reported, nothing ever really satisfied her. She had many friends, kept up a voluminous correspondence, and enjoyed meeting new people.

In the hospital the patient's entire mental life seemed to be centered around her numerous complaints. She expressed a desire to live an active life but insisted that she was too weak to do the things she wished to do. She expressed thanks for everything that was done for her but resented any suggestion that her complaints might represent self-indulgence. Extremely sensitive on this point, she misinterpreted several remarks of other patients. She took no part in ward activities and showed little improvement during the days she was hospitalized. She was quite resistive to attempts at psychotherapy, making the response, "I wasn't born yesterday," to anything told her. It was observed that her mother was overly solicitous and that the patient's complaints increased sharply following each visit of her mother. She was discharged unimproved and there was little expectation that she would be different in the future.

P. Hypo. F:44:M:12 +4 1′37$\underline{246}$– 7:3:18

This patient was admitted to the hospital at the insistence of her husband. The complaints were irritability, emotional instability, generalized weakness, and "suspiciousness." According to her husband the patient over the past two or three years had shown such increased sensitiveness and irritability that she would cry about even trivial arguments between them. Her weakness became so marked that she found it difficult to do housework. She became extremely jealous of her husband. She was also suspicious of strangers, fearing they might harm her.

Her husband reported that she had always been somewhat jealous and suspicious and that her feelings were easily hurt. She had many friends, however, entertained frequently, and was active in church societies, parent-teacher associations, and other similar community activities.

When the patient was asked why she was in the hospital she replied, "My friends say I look too healthy." She considered her husband's description of her irritability and suspiciousness to be a distortion of the truth and insisted that his excessive drinking was responsible for all their difficulties. She cried easily without knowing exactly why. Depression seemed otherwise not severe, although she was discouraged about her bodily discomforts, the abdominal pain and fatigue. She was unable to relate these complaints to psychological stresses except in a superficial way. The subjective complaints subsided rapidly with hospitalization and the paranoid trend was at least no longer obvious. It was difficult to evaluate the case because of the marked disagreement between the husband's description of the problem and the patient's. There was no doubt that the patient's complaints were characteristic of hypochondriasis and out of accord with her physical condition. On the other hand the pressure at home due to her husband's behavior was assuredly also a factor in the whole pattern. While she improved some in the hospital and was discharged as much better, the marital situation could not be approached and there seemed to be no possibility of making solid plans for the future. She was repeatedly in and out of hospitals afterward.

Alcoholism F:43:M:34 +3 13′$\underline{72}$48$\underline{69}$–(59) 5:3:11

The patient was admitted to the hospital in an inebriated state with tremor of the hands, nervousness, nausea, and vomiting, the culmination of a four-day drinking spree. She had spent most of the period in bars without returning home, but she was conscious and coherent. The episode was similar to others she had had about once a month during the preceding two and a half years. She attributed the sprees to a need for escape from inner anxieties derived from marital discord. Until a few years before, she had been working and relatively independent of her husband, but after she had quit work and had become dependent her anxiety had become pronounced. She also was fighting for the control of her 14-year-old son.

Her general health had been good and she had had no psychotic upsets, although in recent years she had been in police court a number of times for drunkenness. A tenth-grade graduate, she had had no difficulty in school. She had done clerical work and apparently had been a very satisfactory employee. Her energy had always been directed more toward her work than toward her home, and she had envied men and felt inferior as a woman. Her husband was irresponsible, a heavy drinker and said to be a "big baby." The patient had given up her job when her husband got a good position and could support her and the boy. Her family had become disgusted and would have little to do with her.

The physical examination showed only minor evidences of neuritis. There were no gross disturbances or aberrations of mental content or mood. Her sensorium and intellect were intact. She was normal in stream of thought. In interviews she was inclined to be caustic and defensive, with no insight into her problem. Her nausea, vomiting, and tremor rapidly subsided, but she developed some evidences of anxiety. Pleasant and cooperative, she was mildly asocial throughout her stay in the hospital, and she was unimpressed by any need for psychotherapy. Under sodium amytal she expressed feelings of inferiority and hostility toward men. She was permitted to leave the hospital for a few hours to settle some business matters, and she failed to return.

P. Anxiety State F:31:M:27 +5 1'378– 7:1:19

This patient's chief complaints were headaches, depression, crying spells, and loss of weight and appetite. She dated these problems from a year before admission when she had fallen down the cellar steps. No clear injury resulted nor was she unconscious, but the next day she felt nervous, exhausted, and irritable, and had crying spells. At this time there were family financial troubles and also difficulties over the presence in the home of the patient's father. From the beginning of the illness the patient had received considerable medical attention.

After the patient concluded her schooling at the eighth-grade level, she held no job outside her home and she expressed no ambitions. Married at 20, she had three children. The family group appeared to be relatively stable. There was no evidence of previous personality difficulties; she mixed well and made friends readily. She was fond of her home and family life although she was not a good housekeeper.

In the hospital the patient complained of "pressure on top of the head, burning in my stomach, loose bowels, and I have been losing weight." She talked extensively of sleeping difficulties, palpitations of the heart, and many other problems. She asked repeatedly if the fall could have caused her "nervousness" or if the thyroid gland could be the trouble, and she seemed disappointed when reassured that she was in good physical condition. She said, "No one was ever as well as I and no one has ever had such a breakdown. There must be something wrong." Gradually she became better in the hospital and many of the symptoms disappeared. Headaches, however, did persist. She gained some insight into the nature of her problems, and at discharge it was felt that she had a fair chance of continuing to improve.

P. Hypo. F:43:S:40 +14 13'<u>792</u>68– 6:8:16

The presenting complaints centered around severe headaches, but there were numerous other somatic ills including sore eyes, cold feet, tender skin, and bronchitis. These appeared irregularly with no particular cause. Always in poor physical condition, she had been much indulged by her parents, and her history was a long sequence of treatments, medical and chiropractic. Almost no area of the patient's body had been free of associated complaints.

Of average intelligence, the patient was a pleasant, open person, but always immature in meeting problems. Hre social life was limited, she was not aggressive, and most decisions were made by her parents. She was sensitive and open to suggestion. She was devoted to her parents and to her siblings, who treated her as a favorite child.

In the hospital the patient's uppermost thoughts were of her numerous somatic complaints. In other ways she was well oriented and apparently not unduly depressed over her condition. She had almost no insight into the nervous background for her ills. Although a plain woman, she dressed neatly and made a good over-all appearance in the hospital. When admitted she was completely invalided, but during the course of her stay she gradually left the bed more and more, and there was some decrease in the insistence with which she advanced her symptoms. She remained immature and naive, and the overprotection she received from family members made work with her difficult. Reassurance regarding her physical problems was, of course, offered, but she got little help from this. She made no independent plans for her future and when pressed to do so she immediately resorted to talking of her ill health. Although she improved physically, the prognosis, based on the lifetime of taking refuge in somatic complaints plus the inability to gain insight, was poor.

B. Pri., Child. F:12:S:34 +3 '<u>138</u>2–9X(66) 11:5:18

The girl was admitted by order of the juvenile court because of recurrent truancy. This problem had begun when the patient first entered school. In the first grade she was referred to a child guidance clinic because of vomiting and crying spells in the classroom. The mother was judged to be feeble-minded, the father a chronic alcoholic. The succeeding years brought rejections by school authorities and numerous other difficulties. Neighbors complained that the patient and other girls were meeting boys in a neighborhood shed and performing sex acts. The patient had violent temper displays, with stiffening of the body, shouting, crying, swearing, and running through the house. These temper tantrums usually appeared when plans had been made for her to attend school or to conform in some way.

Despite a history of truancy she had advanced to the sixth grade. With her parents and five brothers and sisters she lived in a run-down two-story frame building in a poor district of the city. Much of the space in the building was rented to roomers. There was little heat. The six children were beaten frequently by both parents, especially by the father when he was intoxicated. The patient's closest friend was a 15-year-old girl who was also delinquent. Although the patient had always been insolent and subject to violent temper displays, she was well liked by boys and girls in her neighborhood. She seemed to form attachments with older girls, and she was greatly influenced by them. The mother was cheerful and friendly and her attitude was good, but, as indicated, she was of low intelligence and was unable to carry out consistent plans. If she could have provided for herself she would have divorced her husband. The girl was attached to her father though she disliked his drinking. The mother had no influence over her.

In the hospital the girl's thoughts centered wholly on leaving and returning home, even though she adjusted well to the ward. At times she was insolent and noisy but usually she expressed little emotion. When told that she could not return to her home after she was discharged, she was disturbed and cried profusely. Throughout her stay she changed little. Her contacts with adult patients were slight but she attached herself to another delinquent girl two years her senior. The etiological factors in the case were felt to be very largely environmental. The patient was thought to be at least average in intelligence although tests indicated a dull normal level. The discrepancy was probably caused by poor cooperation during the testing. The court was advised to prescribe placement in a school away from home. It was recommended also that she be given a chance to attach herself to someone who would stimulate her to attend school and form good habits. Improvement, it was felt, depended largely on these conditions.

P. Hypo. F:41:M:5 +4 1'382-96 4:2:23

The complaints of this patient were chronic fatigue, tingling sensations in her hands, feet, and scalp, and burning sensations on her scalp. The patient dated this illness from twelve years before when she had had difficulty with a pregnancy. Her husband, however, thought it had begun five years before admission when she developed a low back pain and ringing and throbbing in her ears. For these symptoms she had consulted a physician and for a while was treated for hyperthyroidism. She then had "a nervous breakdown" and suffered from cramps in her right arm. Her main reason for entering the hospital was that the fatigue had become progressively more severe.

Before the onset of these symptoms the patient had had good health. She got along well with her husband and with other people and had enjoyed social contacts until the fatigue prevented further social life. She had two children. She reported that her married life was happy and she thought a great deal of her husband; she enjoyed housework and was proud of her home.

On the ward the patient was preoccupied with her numerous complaints but did not call herself depressed, nor was she known to be suicidal. The staff, however, did not unqualifiedly accept her denial of depression; in fact, they felt that she showed a good deal of it. Her intelligence was average. During hospitalization she appeared tense and expectant. Her insight was good; she believed that her sickness was "nervous" in origin and she wished to be treated. On the other hand she disliked the hospital thoroughly and did not get along well with the personnel. This hindered the work with her and so, although she got considerably better in the five days of hospitalization, it was felt that little real help had been possible.

P. React. Depr.	F:39:M:35	+18	138 24 79′-	4:9:12
		+23	28173496′-	1:10:12

Throughout twenty years of married life this patient had continually visited physicians for treatment of numerous physical complaints. Usually no physical basis could be found. This behavior had been associated with a feeling of inadequacy. As marital difficulties became more intense the patient had crying spells with increasing frequency. In the last year she had been afraid to go into a crowd "because I might draw attention to myself by bursting into tears." In addition she was fearful that she "would go insane," and the depression became more and more marked.

The past history added little to this admission picture. She had married immediately after graduating from high school at the age of 19. A capable, cheerful individual, she entered actively into social affairs and met strangers easily. She had formed perhaps more than the usual number of warm social contacts, was a good manager, and handled money capably. In general she took her obligations seriously and was a fairly adequate person. The marital situation seemed to be an important factor in the present illness. Her husband was a spree drinker. He objected whenever the patient spent money for herself or the children, and this led to a great deal of family argument. After these disputes he was wont to vent his feelings by depriving the children of certain liberties. Resentful because his wife would not take part in his drinking parties, he accused her of depriving him of companionship. Six years before admission the patient had had an affair with another man. Harboring severe guilt about this she had sought comfort in church activities and had also tried to make up for it to her husband (even though at no time was he aware of the affair) by accompanying him to saloons. This put her in a dilemma since, if she went to saloons, she lost caste with her religious friends.

An attractive young woman, the patient appeared in good physical health. However, she complained of many somatic symptoms. She was depressed and cried easily. Her conduct on the ward was good, except that she continually found excuses to remain in bed. While in the hospital she came to realize that much of her physical difficulty was probably related to her home problems. As social service plans were directed toward providing a better environment to which she might return, the symptoms largely disappeared. She was not, however, freed of them. Discharged to live with an aunt for a while before returning home, she left the hospital apparently almost completely well.

P. Hypo. F:16:S:85 +31 13'82 4967– 7:5:21

Five months before admission this patient began to have attacks of localized abdominal pain with nausea and vomiting. The pattern recurred with increasing frequency. A detailed physical investigation indicated some physical pathology, but not enough to account for all the complaints. In spite of this, a laparotomy was performed and her gall bladder removed. This brought relief for about a month and then the symptoms recurred in almost their original form, with the new addition of "fainting spells."

Her previous health had been fairly good and there was no history of a nervous condition. She was described as placid, agreeable, good-natured, open, and friendly, and of average intelligence. She had not appeared to overreact in any fashion to difficulties, and she was apparently a normal girl in spite of a difficult home life.

In describing the course of her illness she revealed little unusual concern or preoccupation. There was no evidence of content disorder and tests indicated an I.Q. of 92. On the surface she was phlegmatic, but it was felt that she had intense deeper feelings. She craved affection and attention, and apparently her symptoms were a method of obtaining them. At admission she was depressed and cried but became happy and cheerful shortly afterward. She was languid and often did not want to get out of bed. Her personality was friendly and engaging and she was in most ways an acceptable patient. An attempt was made through psychological and social service cooperation to help her find better methods of adjustment. The family with whom she lived was instructed to divert her interests rather than make a fuss over her or pay undue attention to her physical symptoms. She continued with outpatient therapy, and it was felt that she had in time a good chance of making an adequate recovery.

B. Psth., Mixed F:37:M:32 +32 13824'976–(55) 6:11:17
Deteriorated
Epilepsy

The patient was admitted to the medical service about two weeks before psychiatric admission because of perineal itching, uncontrolled diabetes, nausea, and vomiting; she was transferred to the psychiatric unit because of inappropriateness of mood, headaches, nausea, and vomiting. The pruritus vulvae had been noticed for about six months before admission. About a year and a half before admission a similar condition had led to hospitalization for about four weeks without improvement. After this hospitalization her diabetes was recognized for the first time when she experienced a diabetic coma. Until six weeks before the present hospitalization she had cooperated well in insulin dosage and diet, but then she became irregular, and over a two-week period before medical admission she had been nauseated and there had been marked vomiting and diarrhea.

Since childhood she had had "nervous spells" which had consisted mainly of crying without apparent cause. When she was 19 y[illegible] old a convulsion had accompanied one of these "spells," and since that time the attacks had always included seizures which the patient considered to be epileptic in nature. Since there was no seizure while she was in the hospital this diagnosis could not be confirmed. She said there had been two periods when she had had "nervous breakdowns," which she attributed to too many operations (special minor surgical treatments).

In general she was a friendly person who got along well with others. Fairly intelligent, she had almost completed her second year in high school when she became pregnant out of wedlock. From the age of 12 she had a history of considerable promiscuity, and apparently her marriage at 18 to the man by whom she had become pregnant was not satisfactory. Since a hysterectomy seven years before admission the patient had detested sexual intercourse, but she had attempted to conceal the extent of her dislike from her husband. Because he had become more and more demanding, her reaction to intercourse was a source of increasing conflict.

In the hospital, regardless of what subject was introduced, her conversation always led to statements about the difficulties that arose from her intense hatred of her mother and her detestation of sexual intercourse. Although she described what appeared to be visual hallucinations, she was well oriented, and her initially inappropriate mood quickly disappeared. She usually looked worried and depressed but she kept herself neat. A final diagnosis on epilepsy could not be made. Although her diabetic condition was better controlled at the time of discharge, the general problem was not really approached, and it seemed likely there would be further deterioration and subsequent hospitalization.

P. Hypo. F:44:S:26 +1 13'8274–(63) 9:7:21

Following an infection and moderately acute lymphangitis, about a year before admission, the patient noticed increased weakness and nervousness. Something seemed to press against her skin all over, especially about her head. This aching sensation later settled in her teeth and a dentist advised removing them. This was finally completed, but still the complaint did not change. During the past year the patient had slept poorly and had lost considerable weight. Other complaints included dizziness, difficulty with vision, palpitation, buzzing in her ears, and similar sensations.

The patient had never been strong physically and her history indicated that she was prone to develop generalized complaints after attacks of influenza or other illnesses. During one period of hospitalization she was diagnosed as neurasthenic. After graduating from the eighth grade at age 15, she worked on her father's farm, where she did more of the heavy work than was common for farm women. No one ever heard the patient express ambition to live a different life, and she disclaimed any interest in men or a desire to have a home of her own. A regular churchgoer, she was in general considered emotionally stable and not irritable.

13'829–

In the hospital she appeared as a poorly nourished and poorly developed woman. She had pigmented moles and was not attractive in appearance. She was mildly depressed and the affect was flat and seemingly inadequate. Not only did she exhibit little desire to cooperate but she showed little interest in getting well. Although not evasive, her answers were vague and inadequate. She was well oriented, normal in appearance and action, and she was vaguely aware that she suffered from what she called a "nervous condition." In the hospital she preferred to lie in bed rather than to move about, and she changed little. There was an almost complete lack of motivating energy and nothing seemed to stimulate her. When she returned to her home the prognosis was judged to be poor.

P. Hypo. F:19:S:36 +10 13'829– 4:4:16
P. Hys.

For several years the patient had complained of headaches, dizziness, and blackness before her eyes; she had had frequent periods of depression and crying; and she had been regurgitating small amounts of food immediately after eating, which gave her a feeling of discomfort although the food came up without effort. More recently she had had peculiar "spells," initiated by an apparent faint, which were exacerbations of these same symptoms. Recovery from these dramatic attacks was always rapid, but afterward there was disorientation—she would be silly, talk senselessly, and repeat phrases, and relatives had to stay with her to keep her from pulling out her hair. After the first attack she had been a semi-invalid for two months; a second one had also left her weak.

She had finished the eighth grade at age 12, having done unusually well in her studies. Her I.Q. was in the average range. She had worked as a domestic but had always found it difficult to work where there was much supervision. The patient needed to excel in everything she did, and she was meticulous about her clothes and work. She mixed well and made friends easily, but there was always a barrier that prevented real intimacy. She felt considerable responsibility toward her family. She was prudish about anything sexual. As a child she had had temper tantrums when her wants were not satisfied, and more recently she had become sulky. No particular events seemed to have preceded the present illness.

In the hospital she was listless and unconcerned, answering questions incompletely with an airy indifference. She denied having any concern about her problems, although she said she was sorry to have caused her family so much trouble. On neutral subjects she was social and cooperative, but she was evasive on anything of a personal nature. She disclaimed having any improper or troublesome thoughts on any subject. Throughout her hospitalization she complained of constipation, and she felt that when her bowels failed to move they became so full that she could not take more food until she had vomited. Neither the patient nor her mother was able to accept any but an organic explanation for the illness. Discussion centered around the possibility that she might be trained as a beauty operator, which was what she wanted to do, but she felt it was her duty to remain at home. At the time she was ready for discharge she said, "I can keep swallowing and make food stay down. I'm better since I rested." Although this appeared at first to be an easy problem with which to work, the final results were unsatisfactory to the staff from the standpoint of preventing future attacks, since it was felt that the underlying cause or causes of the illness had not been exposed.

B. Psth., Path. Emot. M:40:D:12 +4 13'829– 3:3:13
P. Hypo.
Alcoholism

This patient was first seen in the general medicine service because of a complex of backache, abdominal pain with radiations to the thorax, right leg, and foot, nausea, vomiting, diarrhea, and constipation. All these symptoms were precipitated by work. Although not a specific complaint, severe alcoholism was also present.

This man had never been an adequate person. A heavy drinker, at one time he had been in a state hospital for inebriates. He had made considerable trouble for the county welfare board and had been abusive and cruel to his aged parents, who gave him all the assistance they could. He had married but had abandoned his wife. He combined an interest in sports with betting and other activities connected with horse races.

In the hospital he was demanding, irritable, unreliable, and untruthful, and he showed few evidences of a positive ability to improve. The hospital personnel were hindered in forming personal relationships with him because of his general attitude. He was a troublemaker among the other patients. Although his complaints were somewhat improved by physical treatment, profound body concern continued, far out of proportion to any physical basis. It was felt that he had a poor prognosis, and at discharge it was believed that his behavior in the future would differ little from that in the past.

P. Hypo. F:20:S:20 +6 13'847– 1:1:18
B. Psth., Mixed

This young woman was admitted to the psychiatric service from neurosurgery, where she had been hospitalized in preparation for sympathectomies to treat Reynaud's disease. The patient's particular symptom in addition to Reynaud's disease was constant sinusitis.

In ill health all her life, the patient had at one time spent a year in a hospital because of malnutrition. At age 13 she was treated for gonorrhea in a clinic. The family was exceedingly irregular. The mother was a drunkard and sexually careless. The father had disappeared. The patient was a ward of a reform school where she had been sent because of drinking and sexual promiscuity beginning at 13. The patient had never steadily followed any one line of endeavor. At the time of admission she was interested in studying medicine or in training to become a practical nurse, in spite of the fact that she had not completed high school. Emotionally she was unstable, crying without cause and sometimes elated without apparent reason.

In the hospital the patient was anxious to have the surgery and "get it over with." She described how her hands became white and then red and blue, followed by itching and tingling. She had other somatic complaints also. Actually the vasomotor disturbance had been minimal in recent weeks. Treated for the sinusitis she became a little better. On the ward she was somewhat of a problem. Not only did she talk about her troubles but she included many sexual details. Indiscretely gregarious, she was at times irritable, boisterous, and a disturbance. In some ways, however, she was likable, and she made a number of friends among the nursing staff. It was noted that she seemed much younger than her age. After the present study she was discharged back to neurosurgery with the recommendation that no surgical intervention be undertaken for a considerable time. It was also recommended that thought be given to her disposition upon discharge from the reform school, in order that the environmental circumstances might be improved.

Ps. Psth. M:40:S:49 +5 1'39428– 6:1:21
Paranoid

Seven years before hospital admission a falling tree struck the patient, knocking him down, and he dislocated a finger and received knee scratches. He went immediately to a "transient camp" expecting medical care, but did not receive it, he said, because "the manager was a good friend of my boss." Sent to another transient camp, he was finally hospitalized. After six months of idleness he attempted to work at a different job but developed a pain in his chest and soon quit. Later he felt pain in his knee. When this became worse he applied for admission to a marine hospital, was told that the knee was "bad," and advised to return home. At the outpatient department of his home town hospital, exploration of the knee was advised, but he did not come for a final examination, because "I didn't want any dumb doctor experimenting on me." The knee became swollen and sore, however, and he went to a sanitarium. There he got into difficulty and threatened to sue the hospital. Finally his right leg was amputated above the knee. Ten days later, he claimed, he had injured the stump and had had pain thereafter.

A physician said of the patient, when he was 13 years old, that he was "morose and abused his brothers and sisters." At the same time the physician noted, in writing, that the patient had a very poor home and was complaining of pain in the left side. After graduating from the eighth grade the patient became an itinerant worker. He always expected a great deal of his friends, and most of the time he felt that he had been wronged by society in one or another way. Very sensitive, he took offense readily, became angry, and was quick to say exactly how he felt. He frequently threatened to sue.

In the hospital the physical examination did show some tubercular lesions in the lung and there was evidence indicating pleuritis. The patient was, however, argumentative, demanding, hypochondriacal, and mildly paranoid. He insisted that he had been mistreated by a number of physicians and claimed that some of them were working together against him. Well oriented as to time and place, he was mentally intact except for hypochondriacal and paranoid ideas. One of his stories was that at another hospital he had "not been treated as a human being," and the nurses had refused to cover him in the morning when they entered his room. A letter from that hospital contained the information that the patient had exposed himself deliberately and had used obscene language. He advised other patients not to follow the rules of the hospital and belittled everyone who attempted to give him medical help. He was so agitated and disturbing that he had to be placed in the disturbed ward. He went on a hunger strike there for a short time and used obscene and vulgar language. Eventually he was transferred to a state hospital.

B. Psth., Asocial M:27:S:31 +1 14'38 267-(67) 9:5:23
Mental Deficiency
Alcoholism

The patient was admitted to the hospital under court order after being sentenced to jail for assaulting his sister. He had always been a quick-tempered, sensitive individual but during the past few years his temper outbreaks had been less restrained and more violent. Usually they were directed toward his sister. On one occasion he allegedly chased her with a butcher knife but was subdued by others. Apparently his attitude toward her was caused by her alleged attempts to gain control of the household and expel him and his brother from the house where she and her husband lived. His sister had also refused to care for their sick mother, who had died about two years before the admission. The patient was a heavy drinker and was irregular in his job, in his sleeping, eating, and general behavior. He complained of chronic constipation, headaches, and epistaxis.

He had been ill much of his life. In infancy he had a speech impediment that did not disappear until adolescence. He suffered a severe burn at age 3 and at age 10 was injured by an ax. At 15 he had tuberculosis which disappeared with institutionalization. He was hit on the head by a pole at the age of 20, and following that the epistaxis and headaches appeared.

He had completed the fourth grade in school at 13 or 14, having had considerable difficulty and having always felt inferior. He had been arrested for truancy and delinquency at different times and had used considerable alcohol. He had few friends and little interest in sports or hobbies. It appeared that he had been sexually promiscuous. His I.Q. was in the dull normal range.

In the hospital the neurological and physical examinations were essentially negative, no evidence of organic brain deterioration being discovered. Psychological testing, however, indicated the possibility of organic brain damage. He seemed quiet and cheerful but obviously lacked confidence in himself. He was cooperative in surface ways but clearly did not tell accurately what had happened to him in the past. On one occasion he said his trouble was due to "too much whiskey and women." The diagnostic problem was unclear in view of the indeterminate extent and effect of the brain injury. Since behavior disturbances had been noticed from childhood, however, it was felt that the chief pattern was probably independent of the brain injury.

B. Psth., Path. Sexuality M:38:D:10 +1 14 382'67–9 (59) 2:5:21

This man was referred by court order for observation to determine whether he should be classified as a sexual psychopath under the state law. His activities included writing and giving an obscene poem to a 15-year-old girl. Since the age of 21 the patient had been troubled by periods of nervousness and depression. He attempted to alleviate them by drinking but this caused irritability and assaultiveness. During one such episode he attempted to shoot a policeman. Married at 24, one year later he was divorced. Frequently lonely and depressed, he moved from job to job. He spent a few months in a state hospital from which he ran away. At that time his condition was diagnosed as schizophrenia, paranoid type. He began to exhibit peculiar behavior toward women, such as writing a letter to the wife of an acquaintance, beseeching her to intercede for him with her sister and complaining of loneliness.

As a child he had been nervous and sickly, difficult to handle. His history included frequent episodes of anorexia and vomiting, and a long list of minor physical ills. Always exceedingly dependent on his home, he had delayed starting school because of his attachment to his mother. In school he did well and finished the second year of high school before he quit to go to work. He shifted from job to job and his work record was poor. During the three months preceding the present hospitalization he used part of his spare time to write lyrics for songs, and he sent many to publishing houses but without success. Always shy and afraid to ask a woman for a date, he felt secure only with older women. The short-lived marriage was to a girl who had worked for his parents.

In the hospital the patient called his main trouble "nervousness" and admitted that the present condition was little different than at any other time in his life. He blamed his agitation on the fact that he was not married and had always been "shy with women." In regard to the obscene poems, he said that his intent was entirely different from the interpretation placed upon his writing by the court. The true meaning was really harmless, he contended, and "there are always two ways to take everything." Well oriented, he showed no other obvious defects of intellect or sensorium. During interviews he was fairly accessible and cooperative but evasive and suspicious when the discussion became personal. A sodium amytal interview revealed considerable distortion of the sexual sphere, indicating a desire to have sexual relations with young girls and feelings that certain nurses in the hospital were sexually interested in him and were making advances. It was recommended to the court that he be committed as a sexual psychopath.

B. Psth., Mixed M:16:S:19 +6 '1482–(35) 8:13:17

This boy had been stealing from his neighbors for several years, usually articles of no value to him. For most of this he could assign no reason. Usually he broke into homes alone but occasionally friends went along.

Not a good student, he had been a frequent truant, and in the eighth grade he had been expelled from school. The principal had decided that the lad was not profiting from schooling. He did not seek employment and spent all his time alone at home. Recently the neighbors had complained that he was shooting a gun near his home, and they feared an accident. The boy claimed he shot at crows and was careful not to shoot toward any building. A year before admission he had been in a motorcycle accident and had been unconscious for four hours. Otherwise, the past history revealed no evidence of physical disturbances.

Of dull normal intelligence, the youth's difficulties in school were not based wholly on lack of intellect. He had never been dependable and he was irregular in any work. A great deal of his time he spent fishing. His parents were separated and the boy lived with his father. His mother was a sexually promiscuous person. His father apparently wanted to bring up his children properly, and the patient's brother was well behaved. The father had paid for all that he could identify as having been stolen by his son.

In the hospital the neurological and physical examinations were negative. The boy wanted to "get back home and fish." His concentration was so poor that he appeared much more dull mentally than tests showed him to be. Although willing to conform he never showed any evidence of initiative and responded only in simple ways. There was no evidence of really bizarre mentation or behavior. At the time of discharge it was recommended that he be placed in a strict boarding home for long-time supervision.

P. Mixed M:33:M:22 –51 1482'36–9 4:5:15

P. Hys. M:37:M:15 +14 '321–97(53) 2:3:12

About three years before this patient came to the hospital, he, his wife, and his three children had moved into the home of his wife's parents, along with his wife's sister and her husband. There was considerable friction between the various family groups, and after the menage split up the patient accused his wife of going out with other men when she went to visit her parents. Occasionally he flew into rages for no particular reason, and at such times he would strike her, although he apparently always regretted his violence later. Because of his violence, his wife took their children to live with her parents. He frequently visited her, pleading with her to return home, and just before admission he became belligerent, demanding that she come home. He threatened her by saying, "If you don't, I'll get a gun and you'll be sorry," but the patient said that he had intended merely to scare his wife. A neighbor made the complaint that the patient habitually sat alone in the park, frequently nearly all night. There was gossip that he had taken a child into a woodshed and had held it there late into the night.

Discontinuing school in the seventh grade, the patient had continued to work on his father's farm for a small allowance. A socially withdrawn person, he had, however, several hobbies and had not been abnormally abstracted from his environment. He had always been somewhat concerned about his health and had maintained that he could not do heavy manual labor. His wife said their marriage had been compatible, and although she admitted he had treated her roughly, she forgave him and was anxious to re-establish their home. She believed that getting away from relatives would improve their situation.

The patient was mainly concerned about the injustice of being placed in a mental hospital, but apparently he held no grudge against anyone in particular. He readily discussed the events leading to his hospitalization, and he admitted that emotional rages had prompted his ill-advised statements. There was no evidence of breaks with reality or other severe personality distortions. Though somewhat withdrawn, he made a satisfactory ward adjustment. At no time did he show any insight into his own difficult personality. There was an abnormal passivity about his behavior. After plans for his self-support and for the general familial relationships had been made, he was discharged.

B. Psth., Asocial M:21:S:15 +1 14′82739–(57) 7:4:22

The patient was admitted to the hospital for study because of repeated appearances in court during the preceding decade. These had been the result of his antisocial behavior, particularly toward his family, and his refusal to work. He had first appeared in court, charged with stealing a bicycle, when he was 11 years of age. There was also a record of the theft of numerous minor articles. He was put on probation but two years later was again charged with grand larceny. Still later he was rejected by the army because of hypogonadism. Two years before admission he had been in district court for using a car without the owner's permission and was sentenced to prison for a year. Some time after his discharge he again appeared in court, this time accused of contributing to the delinquency of a minor, a girl age 16.

From the time he was about 12 years of age the patient had been very fat, especially about the hips and abdomen, and had weighed as much as 230 pounds. He had received thyroid treatment because of a low basal metabolic rate and had also been studied for pathology of the pituitary gland because of the hypogonadism. No pathology could be discovered. His I.Q. was average. He had had great difficulty in school but managed to get into the eighth grade before stopping for good. He was urged by his family to get a job but never did so though he boasted of numerous positions he had presumably obtained. Always quiet and reserved, on the whole he seemed to get along fairly well with people outside of his family. His mother said that she thought she had babied him but not much more than his siblings.

In the hospital the neurological and physical examinations did not reveal anything significant, with the exception of the underdevelopment of the gonads, a female distribution of pubic hair, and extensive fat about the hips. He was depressed and felt frustrated because he had not been permitted to marry the young girl mentioned above. He was retiring and did not talk much but when he did he was boastful, exaggerating his past accomplishments. He regarded himself a victim of circumstance in his experiences with the court. Cheerful and cooperative, he adapted well to routine and participated in activities. He was not particularly affected by the hospitalization and no psychotherapeutic regimen was instituted. It was felt that his escapes from punishment for many of the things he had done had been in no small part due to the efforts of his family to protect him. In view of his past history the prognosis was considered poor.

Ps. Sz., Hebe.	M:21:S:11	–9	148372'69–	6:5:19
		+11	18 7324'69–	8:13:18

When brought to the hospital by his brother because of peculiar behavior, the patient complained of odd feelings, muscular stiffness, and slight pains between his shoulder blades. His interest in his surroundings had gradually decreased to the point where he spent most of his time sitting in a chair, seldom speaking, getting up only occasionally to carry out some odd activity, such as making a sign of the cross accompanied by pantomime prayer, or going around and through the house, in the back door, and out the front. He also had attacks of crying associated with shaking and generalized muscular rigidity.

For the past ten or twelve years the patient had complained of organic symptoms for which no adequate medical basis had been found. He had stopped school in the seventh grade at age 15 because he didn't like school and had had trouble with his studies. His intelligence was dull normal. On his parents' farm he had been a hard worker, paying little attention to pleasure. He had no girl friends. He was somewhat interested in machinery and repaired the farm implements. A bashful, quiet, introverted man with a likable personality, he was unusually tractable and followed the suggestions of his parents and older brother without question.

In the hospital he expressed poorly systematized delusions with a marked grandiose trend, mostly religious in character. "I carry three crosses, just as Jesus did. I am the Redeemer." He had aural and visual hallucinations which usually took the form of devils who were preventing him from conquering evil. "I saw two demons, one standing on one side of me and another on the other side. My muscles became stiff. I trembled, I pushed on. I suffered terrible pain. Everyone is worried about the end of the world. I know and you know, but I won't tell and you won't tell." There was marked dissociation of mental content and mood, depersonalization, and other symptoms of personality breakdown. While stating that he was the third person of the Trinity and the Redeemer he would ask humbly for a cigarette. At times he became very active, pounding on the walls, shouting and swearing about demons and God Almighty. At other times he went through extensive rituals. There was no change during hospitalization, and he was transferred to a state hospital.

P. Mixed	F:28:M:24	+3	14 9386′27–X (55)	5:17:7
B. Psth., Path. Emot.		+6	984763′21–(63)	1:15:8
Mutilative				
Twin				

After the birth of her last child about three years before hospital admission, the patient began to have attacks of epigastric pain and six months later she developed a persistent diarrhea which a physician told her was caused by "nerves." Dissatisfied with his explanation, and wanting more medical attention, she shot herself through the foot. The diarrhea later stopped, but the epigastric pains continued. About eighteen months before admission she had another attack of diarrhea at a time when she was tired, nervous, and depressed. Hospitalized for six weeks, she got better but about three months before admission she had another attack of diarrhea accompanied by flaccid paralysis of the right arm and a bilateral convergent strabismus, diplopia, and formication and numbness over her entire body. These symptoms disappeared, and a spastic paralysis of the whole body ensued. Eventually all the symptoms except the diarrhea disappeared, and she was admitted for psychiatric evaluation.

She had had six weeks of persistent vomiting at age 18, had undergone a cholecystectomy at 22, and thereafter had had a number of other medical treatments. Her ambition to become a nurse had been thwarted because she had had to drop out of the second year of high school to help her sick mother. Always "full of pep," strong, and masculine, as a child she had climbed trees, played ball, and fought with the boys. She was uneasy in the presence of girls, but she made friends easily. She had been married for eight years to a man eleven years older than she, and although there were three children, the couple were socially and sexually incompatible.

'162394–7

In the hospital the woman showed ambivalence toward her family. She was obviously jealous of her twin sister's femininity and of her happy marriage to one of the patient's former lovers, and she resented her own husband's passivity and inactivity. In appearance the patient was overactive and masculine. She was cooperative, offering to "tell all," and while in the hospital she lost her abdominal pain and other symptoms. She was also helped with her general problems, particularly with the guilt she felt over several extramarital relationships, which had occurred because she was sexually attracted to any male she happened to like. A peculiar behavior pattern she showed for several days was judged to be hysterical in nature. Hers was considered an immature, poorly integrated personality, torn with strong emotions of various kinds, whose impulsiveness got her into trouble she was unable to cope with. At the time of discharge she was much improved, and the prognosis was considered reasonably good.

Ps. Sz., Paranoid	F:30:M:33	+3	'162394–7 (66)	7:8:11
		+13	1'2–96 (68)	6:3:13

The patient was admitted to the hospital on a court order because of peculiar behavior. She had frequently had a desire to leave home and on several occasions had done so without provocation. More recently there had been paranoid ideas: she told her mother that her husband and mother-in-law were planning to send her to an asylum; that she had to be careful what she ate around the house because they were trying to poison her; that her mother-in-law was practicing black art; and that she had had strange impulses and did "things against her nature" because her husband was putting spells on her by holding his fingers in certain positions.

A nervous, uncommunicable, sensitive, jumpy, and flighty person with a tendency to distort facts, she had always been a poor mixer, had never had many friends, and had not liked social life. She was a high school graduate and had worked as a waitress for her stepfather until she was married. Following the birth of her first child she became careless in dress and in the care of her home.

In the hospital she displayed appropriate affect, considering her ideas; she cried, smiled, joked at times, and appeared relatively normal. There was no evidence of hallucinations. Her sensorium and intellect were normal. There was improvement after nine electroshock treatments, but about three weeks after admission she became confused, got the idea that she was going to die, and again began to have crying spells. She refused to eat and had difficulty in sleeping. With this sensorium defect there was a recurrence of paranoid ideas, but after five more electroshock treatments she again returned to her normal level of behavior. Although she was anxious to be discharged the prognosis was guarded. In view of an unfavorable home situation it was felt that in the future the patient would again become psychotic.

Ps. Sz., Simple	M:18:S:21	+1	'163–97 (47)	5:2:20

At the age of 3 or 4 years the patient had shown withdrawal tendencies and had begun to stammer. He had never got along with other children, being frequently beaten up by his playmates. His school attendance was interrupted because of ill health and he had to be tutored a good part of the time. He was taken to a number of child psychiatrists beginning at age 4. His mother did not cooperate well with their recommendations. The patient had been enuretic and even at 13 he had sometimes come home from school with his trousers soaked with urine. When he was about 14 this condition was controlled. About four years before admission he began to tease his parents persistently by kicking, hair pulling, and other petty tricks. The father would beat the child and the child would then beat the mother. This continued until in the past few months the boy had been talking to himself and about two months before admission had begun pulling down all the window shades as though to hide. In the next month he had refused to take his meals with his parents. When he was first brought to the hospital, he jumped out a window and ran away.

As indicated, he had been exceedingly irregular in his school attendance though he was a junior in high school at the time of admission; he had never, however, made good grades. His I.Q. was about 118. He was timid and shy and avoided other children, he never had a date, and he spent most of his time reading magazines and staying around home. His father was a schoolteacher, a timid person, well liked but exceedingly violent in temper. His mother was aggressive, talkative, set in her ways. There was constant friction in the home.

In the hospital the patient was quiet and it was difficult to get information from him. He appeared apathetic, nervous, and antagonistic. He felt that he didn't belong in the hospital; he rarely spoke to others and often mumbled to himself. At times he would refuse to cooperate and was sullen when urged to do so. He frequently annoyed the nurses by remaining for long periods in the bathroom or by eating very slowly. He changed very little and was finally transferred to a private psychiatric hospital for further care.

P. React. Depr.	F:33:M:34	+4	163'2894–(55)	2:7:8
Ps. M-D., Depr.		+20	136'82497–(53)	6:8:13

The patient was admitted to the hospital because of depression and neurotic tendencies that had had an insidious development over a period of at least thirteen years. She had been forced into a marriage in spite of strong family objections because of premarital pregnancy. This incident, together with the fact that two of her sisters were married to two of her husband's brothers, had encouraged social misunderstanding and petty gossip. The husband and wife had had a very stormy life together. She was never satisfied with anything he did and always terminated arguments with sullenness and depression that lasted from one day to several weeks. Gradually the attacks came to be accompanied by vague abdominal and lumbar pain. Her general pattern of behavior had become progressively worse until the present admission.

There were in her past medical history numerous hospital contacts because of symptoms often apparently functional in origin. She was a sixth-grade pupil when she stopped school at age 15, after failing once and having a hard time with her studies generally. Her I.Q. was 94. She had always been backward, shy, and sensitive, but as a housewife she was able to do fairly well in caring for her seven children in spite of meager financial support from her husband. She had spent a great deal of time in recent months just sitting in her house, often crying. Her outside interests were exceedingly limited. She had always had a tendency to ideas of reference, believing that people were talking about her because of her large family and because her husband left her for short periods.

In the hospital she was neat and rather attractive. Her conversation and thoughts were centered almost entirely around her problems with her husband. She seemed to obtain great satisfaction from relating in detail minor events that substantiated her distrust of him. She had no hallucinations or delusions of a severe nature; she was well oriented and seemingly intact intellectually. She looked depressed but was pleasant and gradually began to take an interest in her surroundings and to go to the lounge with other patients. The improvement during her stay in the hospital was very slow. At first she complained of body aches and pains, and often cried herself to sleep. Attempts to give her better insight were only partially successful. She worried about her children and complained that she was tired of just sitting around and doing nothing. She was not much different from her usual personality at the time of discharge, and it was felt unlikely that she would make a better average adjustment than she had ever made.

P. Psychas. M:40:M:29 +2 1723'896–(47) 1:1:9

A fear that he would injure his youngest son brought this man to the hospital. "A voice" had told him to kill his son. The illness dated back eight months to one night at a meeting when he had felt faint and nearly collapsed. After that he had experienced vertigo, nausea, and vomiting. Later he had worried about the danger of poliomyelitis. In the last three months he had had difficulty in concentrating, had been unable to sleep, and had become sexually impotent. He found himself speechless when angry. For the past twenty years the patient had been bothered by "stomach trouble." This had disappeared since the onset of the present fear.

As a child the patient had been weak and sickly. At age 15 he finished the eighth grade and thereafter worked on farms. Eventually he became an automobile salesman. A cheerful person, he was counted easy to get along with despite the fact that he was rigid and a hard worker. His wife wondered if possibly he resented the attention she paid to the children. There was nothing, however, in the past history that seemed to explain the present episode convincingly.

In the hospital a moderate nystagmus in both eyes was observed; otherwise, the physical and neurological examinations were negative. The patient was well oriented but tense. He could not understand why the "voice" should mention such an intolerable subject as killing his youngest son. Although depressed, he laughed easily and appeared well integrated. There were no obvious disturbances of sensorium or intellect. He was pleasant and well liked on the ward. After a few weeks he no longer heard the "voice" but he still had thoughts of killing someone, although no one in particular. Later he also lost these ideas. It was learned that he had a rather dependent attitude toward his parents, and it was thought that deep feelings of inadequacy were probably covered up by his pleasant surface manner. The underlying anxiety and tension had perhaps been expressed in his "stomach trouble" and then had recently shifted from that locus to the phobia. The case was atypical. He was discharged, considerably improved, for a trial at home. The prognosis was uncertain.

P. Mixed Mental Deficiency — F:46:D:23 — +1 — 17263′48–X (55) — 11:12:5

The patient complained of dizziness, noises in her ears, burning and itching eyes, and fatigability. These were only highlights of a far wider complaint pattern.

Her past medical history was rich with details of illnesses, many of which seemed likely to have been psychosomatic. She had undergone a gastric resection for "peptic-ulcer" and later a hysterectomy was performed for "endometrioma." She was an immigrant from Norway and after coming to this country had worked, except when she was ill, as a housekeeper. She married and later divorced her husband because he drank excessively and was unfaithful to her. She complained that she had never been sexually satisfied by her husband. She was described by those who knew her as rather quiet and shy, always withdrawing from any social gathering. Her I.Q. was 72.

In the hospital she was concerned with her somatic complaints. She had very poor insight and felt that her nervous condition was a result of her physical problem. She spoke easily when addressed but preferred to stay on the subject of her physical ills. She made little progress in the hospital, though she seemed to become somewhat more at ease. At the time of discharge it was recommended that she be carefully followed by the social service worker, who helped her find a place to live and to obtain employment that would partially support her.

B. Psth., Mixed — M:36:M:16 — +3 — 17829′634–X — 3:17:3

The patient was admitted to the hospital with somatic complaints that had originally appeared ten years earlier, following an accident in which the man had been thrown against a plow. After some rest he had continued to work. Although the patient had found the pain severe, the farmer for whom he worked had not thought him seriously injured, and a doctor whom the patient had consulted had found him physically fit. Since that time he had never been free of complaints and had gone to many physicians and chiropractors for treatment.

The man had gone through the tenth grade in school, stopping at age 20. His scholastic record was poor and he had failed in several grades. Until the present illness he had worked intermittently, mostly at farm work. His ambition was to be a grocery or hardware clerk, but he never applied for such a job because, he said, "They never need anyone." He felt that it was up to his wife and the township to support him and his family until he was fit to work again. He and his wife were compatible, and they had two children, but since his illness there had been considerable strife in the family because physicians had told the wife that her husband was able to work, and the idea made him violently angry.

In the hospital he complained mainly of his pains and of his chronic inability to work. He felt that the township was unfair to him and that he was entitled to complete financial aid. He was apathetic and ready at any time to complain about a new pain or ache, but always with a smile. He remained in bed all day rather than tiring himself out by getting up. He had no insight into the possible psychological factors in his illness, and when he was asked what he would think if a doctor told him that he had nothing physically wrong with him, he simply smiled and said, "He'd be a damned liar." He acted very bored when being interviewed and obviously resented being bothered. Although he was reluctant to enter into any kind of active participation, he made a passive orientation to ward life. He insisted on leaving the hospital before any real attempts at psychotherapy had been undertaken, and it was felt that little could have been done for him.

Ps. Sz., Simple Mutilative — M:21:S:11 — +9 — 18236'74– — 6:7:16

The patient, a hired man on a farm, the night before admission had gone to town, staying at a saloon until it closed. Not drunk according to his story, he had left the place feeling all right. Arriving home, he was shot, he claimed, by an unknown party, and immediately he "went nuts." He telephoned neighbors and when they arrived they found the patient behaving in such an assaultive and destructive manner that they called the sheriff and he was taken to jail. The sheriff later said there was evidence that the patient himself had fired the shotgun, which had apparently gone off close to the patient's ear resulting in only slight powder burns. A year before this peculiar series of events the patient had wounded his foot with an ax. Treatments, including surgical cleaning and skin grafts, had not been as successful as expected and it appeared possible that the dressings were interfered with by the patient.

The young man described himself as having "always been unhappy," and he blamed this on a lack of money. He had exceedingly limited interests. Although he had liked school he had left at 15. Beginning at age 16 and for a few years thereafter he had dates with girls but later disclaimed interest in them and denied that he had even had sexual experience. The one characteristic of his past activities was a lack of interests and a poverty of experience. A moderately good worker, he had never held any jobs other than itinerary farm labor.

In the hospital the patient was at first mute but gradually, in the first six hours, began to talk in a forced whisper and, somewhat later, in a normal voice. He remained, however, uncommunicative for the most part and accounted for his actions by saying, "I went nuts. I was crazy, I guess." No marked abnormalities of behavior could be observed; his orientation and general mentation seemed normal. He would, however, laugh meaninglessly at things said and there was inappropriateness of mood and content. At times he was surly and resistive. His adjustment in the hospital was poor and he was discharged back to the court with the recommendation that he be placed in another hospital for extended study.

P. Mixed	F:30:M:33	+12	'182 374–9	7:12:14
P. Mixed Mental Deficiency	F:30:M:31	+81	84'1239–(72)	9:7:22

This patient was first seen in the outpatient department, where she complained of lower abdominal pain which had begun two days before. The pain was associated with nausea and vomiting. She also said that she had recently been experiencing dizziness and occasional diplopia. She had such difficulty in walking that at times she had to be carried. Examinations failed to reveal any organic reason for the complaints, and she was admitted to the psychiatric unit for observation.

She had undergone a cholecystectomy at age 22 and afterward had apparently never returned to her usual state of health. At 26 she had had a gastroenterostomy because of ulcers. After that she had experienced chronic constipation alternating with occasional diarrhea.

She stopped school at 16 when she was in the seventh grade. After that she did housework until 19 when she married a day laborer. The marriage was apparently congenial, but the family lived at a very low economic level. The patient was considered a good housekeeper and had taken an interest in gardening and the raising of poultry. She had never had any broader interests than these, however. She was outwardly unemotional, except that she would sometimes express to her husband a fear of death and illness.

In the hospital she was mainly concerned with her bodily pain. She felt the world was "awful" and "hopeless." In appearance she was unkempt, unattractive, and inert. Her responses were slow and she showed a poor understanding of questions. Psychological studies indicated that she was a moron. She made a poor ward adjustment, spent most of her time lying in her bed, and excused herself from activity on the basis of a generalized "ache." Her condition did not change particularly and she was finally discharged to her husband. About three months later she was readmitted. Again the chief reason for admission was an acute attack of pain and the inability of the physician who examined her to discover any organic reason for the complaint. The course of this admission was similar to the first and she was again discharged without much change.

B. Simple Adult Maladj.	M:36:D:35	+1	182736′4–(73)	7:5:20
P. Mixed		−66	276′81349–(67)	3:8:5

The patient was admitted to the hospital because of chronic fatigue, weakness, backache, and headache. Although the symptoms had been present for five to ten years they had gradually increased in severity so that at the time of admission he was unable to do even menial household tasks. There was no history of an injury. The pain, located in the lumbar region, had increased in intensity and extent over a two-year period. It was not aggravated by strenuous effort unless the patient stooped over; then it made him feel that he could not straighten up. He had always felt tired and had forced himself to work. A year before admission he had gone to a medical clinic for a complete clinical checkup that had failed to reveal any significant organic problem except for a recurrence of gonorrhea, which he had originally contracted from his wife four years earlier. In spite of the reassurance this examination offered him, there was no apparent improvement. In the last two or three years he had lost twenty pounds.

He had left school in the seventh grade at age 16 to work on a farm. He had had no particular learning difficulties. He had held many jobs of a seasonal nature. Twelve years before admission he had married a girl with whom he had had intercourse for about two years, and who was two months pregnant at the time of marriage. The first five or six years of their married life were happy, although they changed residence frequently. Gradually the couple became incompatible, and the wife got involved with another man. She transmitted gonorrhea to her husband, and both were treated. When the wife asked for a divorce the patient at first refused because of religious beliefs and because of the children. When he finally consulted a lawyer about a divorce, he felt that he was tricked into signing away some of his rights, and eventually the wife got the divorce on grounds of desertion. He assumed no responsibility for his marital difficulties, saying, "She wanted intercourse every night and all night and no man could satisfy that." The patient had paid $60 a month alimony, and when he quit, the wife, who was living with a married man, threatened prosecution. The patient had begun to go out with other women but did not contemplate marriage because, "If I want a woman, I can easily pick one up, so why get married?"

No really contributory data were discovered in the physical and neurological examinations. The patient was chiefly concerned with his organic symptoms and with the divorce and its complicating factors. There was considerable sexual content in his thoughts. He appeared to hide his true feelings behind a smile. He had no real insight into his problems. He had considerable trouble adjusting to the hospital routine, and for the first few days he stayed by himself. When he was discharged, there had been no real change and it was felt there was no reason to expect him to make better than borderline adjustment.

Ps. Sz., Simple	M:18:S:55	+3	182736'4-9X(59)	3:18:9
		+44	82716'349-(49)	5:8:9

Two months before admission the youth began to complain vaguely of trouble in breathing, headaches, and ill-defined pains in his abdomen and chest. Along with these discomforts he was worried by feelings that he was about to die and that his condition was hopeless. For eight months he had not worked, and he had spent several weeks in a private hospital. When no change resulted he was referred to the psychopathic unit.

There was no previous history of difficulty physically or mentally. All his life a quiet, shy, and withdrawn person, he was thought of as "a good boy." He had little contact with girls. All the members of his family felt a great deal of hostility to the father and this was shared by the patient. The father had had a long history of recurrent depression and alcoholism and had finally committed suicide when the patient was 15. After one year of high school the boy had worked sporadically on farms.

On admission the youth had the appearance and demeanor of a deep depression. Apathetic, he lay on his bed, covered his head with a pillow, and sobbed from time to time. There was occasional agitation. His speech was retarded and sparse. When he did speak he talked only about his somatic complaints. A voice told him that he would not get well, he said. A course of insulin therapy brought improvement and he left his bed and, to a limited extent, mixed with the other patients. At the time of discharge, however, many of the symptoms were still present, although in a less severe form.

B. Psth., Path. Emot. Schizoid	M:33:S:30	+1	'183 49-6(49)	5:3:18

The patient was admitted because of "spells" characterized by anxiety feelings and numerous attendant symptoms such as shivering, palpitation, churning of the stomach, anorexia, depression, and lack of initiative. The illness dated back to an appendectomy about eighteen months before admission. Two months after the operation he claimed he was too sick to help with the farm chores. The spells, which lasted about ten minutes, gradually increased until they were occurring about twice a week, the anxiety symptoms often being precipitated by events in the national news. Sometimes vivid dreams seemed to substitute for a spell.

Between attacks he gradually felt more and more blue, neglecting his work, withdrawing from social contacts, and losing his interest in life. Although his mother protected him, it troubled him when the family began to tease him about his "nervousness." He had periods when everything seemed to stop for a moment, and he feared that he was going to die.

He had lived all his life on a farm, graduating from high school when he was 20. His I.Q. was 117. Content to remain on the farm, he had no desire to marry, had never used alcohol, had almost no close attachments, and had never actively participated in any form of social life. A dull, stolid, and unassuming person, his general manner was described as having been shy but friendly. The family history showed nothing of particular significance.

There was no clouding of sensorium or intellect. His mental content was deep within a withdrawn personality and could not be brought out by questioning. There was a superficial lethargy. He recognized that he was nervous, but he failed to accept the true state of his problem. His stream of thought was adequate, and he cooperated passively. After a little while, when he began to mix actively with other male patients, he became excessively noisy and had to be doing something all the time that would draw attention to him. Occasionally he experienced a fear of death, and a tendency to flight of ideas was observed once in a while. At times he used foul speech, displayed a rather vulgar humor, and shouted and danced by himself to gain attention. He was given vitamin therapy. Extensive studies made to verify the possibility of brain damage were negative, and the case was never really understood. He improved somewhat and was discharged to go back to his home, but the prognosis was not good in view of the long-standing pattern of borderline adjustment.

P. Anxiety State M:29:M:138 —8 187326′49–(65) 5:12:11
Ps. Sz., Simple

This man asked voluntarily for outpatient care. His complaints consisted of peculiar sensations of different kinds which had been occurring for about six months and a ringing in his ears for a year. The ringing had first occurred in a noisy metal shop where he was employed. Leaving this job, he had obtained another that involved working at top speed for long hours during rush seasons. On one very hot day he had suddenly felt weak, as if he were "dying all over." Under special pressure for several days before this, he had not eaten well and had not sweat for 4 days. Following the initial attack of weakness he had innumerable spells of dizziness, tingling, electrical sensations sweeping over his body after urination, and "still feelings" inside his body, as if all physiological processes had suddenly stopped. He quit work and made several visits to a local physician who finally referred him for psychiatric treatment.

The patient gave little history and had nothing traumatic or unusual to report of his early life. His parents had been kind and loving, according to his description, and he had no complaints about his wife or his marital adjustment.

He did admit, however, that he had never been a person who could express his feelings. His schooling extended through high school. Rejected by the draft, he believed it was because of "nervousness."

Although the patient appeared to be cooperative and earnest in the hospital, he seemed to be lacking in affect. He made no mention of his feelings about other people and the psychotherapist who saw him for weekly interviews felt that he was totally unable to express such feelings. In therapy he talked about his bodily sensations and gave full descriptions of his complaints in a way that at times suggested somatic delusions. For instance, he elaborated on a "lightness" rising up through his body, on noises from the radio "gnawing" in his head, and on "something in the center of my head going sideways." In later interviews he also spoke of fears of dying, of feelings of unreality, and of "always waiting for something." He confided that at times he could tell what people were going to say before they began to speak. During this time the patient was given numerous physical checks and studies with no positive findings. Suddenly he went back to work and was entrusted with more responsibility than previously, in preparation for a supervisory position. Since the patient's home was some distance from the hospital, when a busy work season came along he decided to stop coming. It was felt that his somatic preoccupations were a neurotic defense necessary to his precarious adjustment and should not be attacked at a time when psychiatric treatment was not available to him. Discharged as unimproved he was urged to resume visits to the medical doctor in his own home town. E. B.

P. React. Depr. F:62:W:30 +10 '193–7 7:3:12

This woman's husband had died at the county poor farm four months earlier. Since then the patient had become increasingly depressed, and she was unwilling to stay in any one place. Leaving the county home she moved about from one institution to another, becoming dissatisfied with each place in turn. She tried living with her sister but was equally discontented there. She complained that people were laughing and making fun of her, and she refused to eat, saying, "the food isn't suitable for a woman with a bad liver such as I have." On admission she refused to eat for two days and spent hours sitting or standing in the middle of her bedroom. When spoken to she responded irritably and insisted that she be given a place "where I can live by myself."

An eighth-grade graduate, she had been a poor student and had disliked school. When she was 30 years old, she spent three months in a state hospital, apparently with a depression. After that she associated with almost no one but her husband and got along poorly with other people. All her life a selfish, tactless, faultfinding person, she showed poor judgment and a tendency to shirk responsibilities. The only positive factor in her personal history was the compatibility with her husband and her consistent attentiveness to him.

The patient was thin, small, and nervous. Examination gave no evidence of a neurological disorder. No gross disturbances of mentation or sensorium could be found. The only reason for her depression, she believed, was the death of her husband; she insisted that if she were given a room where she could live by herself she would be all right. "There is nothing wrong with me," she insisted, and denied that she belonged in the hospital. Her stream of thought was adequate and she answered questions to the point. There was no flight of ideas and only a slight psychomotor retardation. Suspicious of the examiner, she was resentful of the whole hospital procedure. She refused to associate with other patients, slept little, and had a poor appetite. As time went on she cooperated a little better and became somewhat more cheerful, ate well, gained weight, and began sleeping soundly. She was discharged to return to the county home.

B. Psth., Asocial Mutilative — M:23:D — 19′34 28–7 (51) — 1:8:9

This youthful prison inmate used a dirk knife to cut his left Achilles' tendon. As a part of the routine admission to the state prison he had taken the MMPI thirty days before.

Born in Boston, the subject was the son of immigrants. Both his parents had died when he was a young child. After completing the eighth grade he had left school to go to work. Sporadically employed, he had held jobs as a hospital attendant and a truck driver. At the age of 20 he married but was soon divorced. There was one child. The criminal records for this man began when he was 17 years old. This first sentence was one to three years in a reform school for attempted burglary. While on parole fifteen months later, he was arrested for burglary and paroled to his home authorities. His present offense was burglarizing a store, at which time he broke a rear window and took rifles, cigarettes, razor blades, chewing gum, and money. The following day he stole two pairs of boots and some petty cash. Arrest came when he was caught in the act of burglarizing a service station.

The young man's rationalization for his criminal behavior was that it had been an "economic necessity." He called himself a homeless vagabond and in fact was that. His eyesight was very poor, he claimed. A speech defect, from harelip, made it difficult to understand him. When interviewed, he was cooperative although he appeared depressed. In general he showed no stability of purpose but said he hoped to make "the most of it" while in the state prison. R. C. K.

P. Hys.	F:21:S:52	+3	1938′742–X (70)	10:6:14
		+23	1389′2764– (61)	9:8:20

After an automobile accident four years before admission, in which the patient suffered a severe blow on the back of her head, her mother noticed that she became nervous, easily fatigued, and had memory difficulties. Because of these

'2–138749

symptoms as well as extreme shyness she left school in the eleventh grade. Her attempts to work were unsuccessful because, as she described them, they were all "too nerve-racking." A month later she got several glass particles in her eye, impairing her vision; she began having attacks of complete blindness that lasted about fifteen minutes and eventually occurred several times a day. She also gave a long list of somatic complaints that would "come and go."

At age 5 she had had convulsions which led to a persisting lateral strabismus. Occasionally she had had attacks of tachycardia and palpitation, but no definite nervous upsets. A cheerful, quiet, bashful child, she had not been able to take as much physical exercise as the other children her mother said. In school she had received fair marks. Immature, naive, and submissive, she had few interests and few friends. Her only association with men had been a casual friendship with a boy from whom she had not heard for some time, and she did not know the meaning of sexual relations.

In the hospital, neurological studies revealed marked lateral strabismus of the left eye and diminished vision in the right eye. It was the consultant's impression that the other complaints had a functional basis. The patient herself maintained an indifferent attitude about her condition, saying in a nonchalant manner, "I had another attack last night when everything was black. I think it lasted about fifteen minutes." She claimed she vomited blood but no one ever saw evidence of it. She was composed but defensive and fearful, especially of men. Emotionally she was inaccessible, seldom speaking spontaneously and forming no relationships with the examiners. Her intelligence was dull normal. Regressive at first, she refused to leave her bed and had nothing to do with ward activities. Although no direct psychotherapeutic interviews were effective, she gradually appeared less apathetic and more cheerful, and became more active around the ward. The possibility of organic disorders was considered, but no real evidence was elicited. On the other hand, there was positive evidence of hysterical processes. She was improved at the time of discharge, but the prognosis was not considered good.

Ps. M-D., Depr. M:61:S:20 +8 '2–138749 3:3:5
Paranoid

This man, found wading in the river, was taken to a hospital by the police. There he claimed not to know his name or to recognize his personal belongings. Since clinical and laboratory findings yielded no explanation he was transferred to the psychiatric hospital for study. By the time he was admitted he was able to give some of his past history.

The patient said that when he had reached the eighth grade he had quit school and had worked in various places, leaving jobs suddenly without giving notice to his employers. He did not do well financially. In early youth he began to use alcohol, and his drinking increased yearly. He made few friends and had little to do with women. There had apparently been no previous psychological upsets and no outstanding physical illnesses or injuries. The patient's sister later provided the staff with further information, but she knew few personal details because he had always wandered about and kept little contact with the family.

The neurological and physical examinations at admission were all negative. The patient appeared comfortable and had no somatic complaints. He had been looking for work, he said, when "two men picked me up and started to drive me out to the country." From that time he recalled nothing until he was on the way to the hospital. He suggested that he might have been doped while drinking beer, but he did not believe he had been intoxicated. He was well oriented and normal in action. His story was consistent, and while it lacked many details which he refused to fill in or perhaps did not know, the essential pattern was constant. Making little attempt to explain the strange episode, he stated, with definiteness, that he thought it of little consequence. Although he reacted well on the ward and in general was cooperative, he always had an attitude of suspiciousness and he was reticent and evasive with the staff. He was formally polite. Much of his time he devoted to reading. The staff was unable to establish a reasonable hypothesis for the true background of the patient's admission story. He did not appear depressed; nevertheless, it was inferred that the only reason for his wading into the river was that he was considering suicide. Whether the confusion that seemed to follow (when he was picked up by the police) was true or feigned could not be determined. He did not change in the hospital but remained in appearance and behavior normal the whole time. When he left he planned to visit relatives.

P. Hys.	M:44:M:46	+16	'2–39 (53)	9:4:13

This man had "fits," in which he lost consciousness for about an hour. These were of a hysterical rather than of an epileptic nature. He also suffered from chest trouble and had not worked for a year. He entered the mental hospital as a voluntary patient.

Nothing was known about his early history.

The diagnosis was conversion hysteria in a constitutionally inferior personality, and he was treated by modified insulin therapy. He obtained lighter work at a quarry and settled down satisfactorily. M. V.

Ps. Invol. Melan.	F:49:M:37	+1	'2–47 (47)	7:3:13
Ps. M-D., Depr.		+32	'9–467 (74)	7:3:11

The patient's illness had an insidious onset about three years before admission and about a year after initial symptoms of the menopause. Her only daughter had recently graduated from high school and had begun to make plans to leave home. The patient objected to this. The family noticed that she had become indifferent to her household duties. This trend gradually increased so that she withdrew from church and community work in which she had formerly been very active. Hypochondriacal complaints began to appear and she consulted numerous medical and nonmedical sources for help. She was given a "rest treatment" in a hospital for five months. Nothing helped her. Hormone therapies were tried without benefit. The chief presenting complaints were periods of depression associated with crying, fear of suicide, fear of losing her mind, and fear of being hospitalized in a state institution. These were in addition to the somatic complaints.

At age 30 she spent nine months at a state hospital in a depression after the birth of her only child. Otherwise the past history was not particularly contributory. She had been an energetic, conscientious, industrious housewife and mother, active in community affairs, meticulous in her work, and compulsive about getting it done. She handled household finances efficiently and was considered to have good judgment, although the neighbors said that she had always worked too hard. She was overaffectionate and overprotective toward her daughter.

In the hospital she was well oriented and appeared psychologically intact. She was composed, neat in appearance, spoke quietly and adequately. Her concern was chiefly that she might lose her mind and have to go back to the state hospital. She had good insight, realized that she was ill, and was anxious to cooperate in any way that would help her. She was given seven electroshock treatments, lost some of her fears of insanity, and showed marked improvement. At the time of discharge she was anxious to return home.

Schizoid M:24:M:28 +7 '2–63 (57) 7:6:11

After his discharge from the army, this man complained of dozing off to sleep while at work. He had been masturbating excessively for the last four years, even in front of his wife after having been married only two months. He entered the hospital as a voluntary patient.

The younger of two brothers, his mother died when he was 9, and he worked as a paint-sprayer before joining the Royal Air Force (ground personnel). He was demobilized after five years. Two months before his admission to the hospital he married a divorcee seven years his senior.

No definite diagnosis was made and his illness was simply described as "schizophrenic episode, brought about by his inability to readjust himself to civilian life under somewhat difficult circumstances." M. V.

Deteriorated M:42:M:25 +16 '2–6789 (49) 5:1:16

This patient had a history of memory defect and deterioration in personality, dating back to an attack of yellow fever at the age of 39, when he was serving with the merchant navy in the Far East. He became grossly careless in his appearance and personal affairs, and inconsiderate of others. He entered the hospital as a voluntary patient.

He was the fourth of six children. His father was a master joiner. The patient joined the merchant navy at the age of 16 and worked himself up to the position of master mariner by the age of 32. He married when he was 38. Of a cheerful disposition, he was somewhat carefree, extravagant, and irresponsible, and a heavy drinker. He had no interest beyond his work and liked having a good time. He had a kind disposition and was good to his family.

He was diagnosed as having presenile dementia. M. V.

P. Psychas. F:39:M:92 +1 '2–694(76) 9:1:18
Ps. Sz., Paranoid

This patient began to complain of nervousness about four years before admission. She said that about that time her father-in-law had made improper advances to her. She gradually developed several compulsive acts; outstanding among these were washing her hands continually, cleaning the house, and keeping her clothes in order. Later she refused to eat food because she "saw dirt in it." She lost weight and was admitted to a state hospital where she was given electroshock treatments. Returning home a month later much improved, she developed the symptoms anew within a week.

She graduated from high school at age 18 and married shortly thereafter. She had never done any outside work. She was described as hard to get along with and very narrow in interests. She reacted keenly to disappointment and was a moody person. She and her husband were incompatible. The patient was described as stingy, and she continually argued with her husband about money.

In the hospital she was very nervous. She recognized her compulsive acts but could not talk freely and was quite unapproachable. She gave a story of visual and auditory hallucinations that sounded atypical, and it could not be determined whether she had had true hallucinatory experiences or not. Treated with insulin therapy, her compulsive behavior disappeared, but she was still quiet and withdrawn and felt that there was nothing wrong with her either before treatment or after it. She was discharged to go home, but in view of the brief remission she had experienced after the first shock therapy, it was not felt that she would do well.

P. React. Depr. F:37:W:11 +4 '2–861739 5:4:5

Since her husband's death six years earlier this patient had experienced periods of depression, usually of short duration. During the past two years, difficulties had piled up—chiefly financial and health problems. In her job as a waitress and cook she worked long hours for a difficult employer. As the situation became intolerable she longed to resign but hesitated because she needed the income. However, when her crying spells and self-consciousness made her conspicuous she did leave. Somatic complaints then developed in addition to feelings of depression and hopelessness. By the time she came to the hospital the patient was unable to talk without crying.

Although throughout life her health had been fairly good there were evidences of hysterical reactions. "At times it seems as if my heart would stop," she said. Headaches, pressure feelings, and dizziness had been present at various times in her life. An eighth-grade graduate, she took a job in a restaurant at 15, and after marriage continued to work. Her husband and she were compatible, and the patient had got along rather well until the husband's death by accident. At that time she had gone to bed for three months with a "nervous breakdown." That episode did not include the crying; she "just wanted to be alone and not disturbed."

In the hospital the patient showed marked improvement. The tension and weakness disappeared quickly, she gained an understanding of her problems, and she was pleasant and cooperative. She was very appreciative of all that was done for her and at the time of discharge seemed to be entirely recovered. Plans were made to help with her financial problems, and she looked forward to a new job.

P. Mixed M:45:M:49 —29 21'3–98 4:1:14

The admission complaints for this man included pain, choking sensations in his neck, tightening over his chest, and increasing intolerance to high-pitched noise. He also complained of blurred vision. This illness had begun three months earlier when the patient rose one morning feeling weak and dizzy. Certain he was going to die, he lost consciousness for five minutes, then complained of severe pain, and was admitted to a hospital where a local physician diagnosed a heart condition. Improved in the next couple of weeks, he was discharged, but had another "spell," and returned to the hospital for a week. This time more extensive studies were carried out but no organic disorders could be discovered, and it was decided that if a cardiac condition had ever existed it was no longer apparent.

Before his present difficulties, the patient had always been in fairly good health. A graduate of a business college, he at one time had been a skilled mechanic and later had made his living by teaching music. He was always exact and precise in everything he undertook, meticulous in each detail. This perfectionist attitude was characteristic of everything he did in life. When plans did not materialize in full he became upset and worried. He was described as open, friendly, kind, well mannered, and having good judgment. There were no particular contributory factors in the family marital history.

The patient was relatively intact in personality. His uppermost thoughts centered around his present illness and he was distressed and depressed. His insight appeared good. He recognized that he was sick psychologically, yet he did not feel that his pain had a functional basis and, in fact, believed that if he were treated for his somatic ills the depression would also disappear. Encouraged to mix with other patients and forget about his complaints, he gradually showed fewer signs of depression and began to make a better adjustment on the ward. Careful reassurance about his physical condition seemed to help him a great deal. At the time of discharge, he seemed to be well recovered and there appeared to be no reason for another attack if environmental pressures did not multiply.

B. Psth., Path. Sexuality M:36:M:5 +1 '21346-8(67) 3:3:15

The patient was admitted on a court order for observation because of aberrant sexual behavior and, to a lesser degree, paranoid ideas. Apparently he had begun his irregular sexual experiences at puberty; he had had sexual relations with various farm animals, and at age 15 or 16 he had acquired gonorrhea as the result of sexual relations with girl friends. After marriage, a forced one, his sex activity increased to the point where he had intercourse with his wife two or three times a day. On one occasion he allowed or forced her to have intercourse with his brother in his presence. In the last year he had suspected his wife of having an illicit affair with a neighbor, and on the basis of these suspicions, he had been unusually savage and demanding in sexual relations. On two occasions he had forced his wife into the barn, and after stripping off her clothes he had encouraged a male dog to have sexual relations with her.

He had a ninth-grade education and after leaving school he had done farm work. He had operated a small farm, which he lost because of financial reverses. As a boy he had been shy and bashful and had found it difficult to mix with and meet other people. His wife characterized him as a good husband and a fair provider, but because his moods were unpredictable and he was uncommunicative she found it difficult to understand him.

In the hospital he was considerably concerned about the future implications of his present predicament, and the possible separation from his wife disturbed him, mainly because of the sexual satisfaction she gave him. His I.Q. was 117. There was no obvious instability of emotion or aberration of thought sequence, but he did show marked abnormality in his attitudes toward his sexual life, discussing his aberrations and general sexual conduct without embarrassment, and taking pleasure in his narration to the extent that he spoke freely without questioning, even to other patients. The hospital regulations displeased him, but he mixed well with other patients, although his frankness with them made him something of a problem. In his attitude toward sex, he was not amenable to psychotherapy, and he was discharged to the custody of the court.

P. Hypo. M:20:S:74 +2 2′13468– 1:5:14

The patient had a persistent headache and was troubled by lassitude. These symptoms began about six months before admission when he had bronchitis, and they remained with him almost constantly until admission. A number of physicians were consulted about his weakness. For a brief time he was hospitalized, with the physician in charge apparently considering the possibility of a brain tumor. Worrying a great deal about his health, and largely incapacitated, he came to the outpatient clinic several times and was finally referred for study in the hospital.

There was a long history of physical disabilities, but he had had no psychotic or obvious neurotic upsets. An eighth-grade graduate, he had started high school but stopped after an altercation with the athletic coach. Thereafter he worked on his parents' farm, although farm work annoyed him. When he was 19 he inherited $3000 from a grandparent and within a year spent it all, some of it going for doctor's bills, some for a motorcycle. He was described as a sensitive person and unstable emotionally, with the sensitivity thought to be caused in part by his physical deformities, a congenitally deformed chest and thoracic spine. Stubborn and quick-tempered, he was also inclined to worry. While he was of average intelligence he lacked aggressiveness and could not compete with other boys his own age. Older people liked him. He went out with girls, claimed to have had heterosexual relations, and was particularly attracted to one girl with whom he was closely associated.

On admission to the hospital his thoughts centered chiefly about his somatic complaints, headaches, dizzy spells, palpitations, and the like, which he believed were manifestations of a serious organic disorder which would ultimately interfere with his activities. There was no difficulty in orientation or regular mentation. His measured intelligence was somewhat above average. He talked despairingly, mentioned suicide, was insecure, lacked self-confidence, and was reluctant to enter into routine activities. Although he was no problem in management, he was querulous, indecisive, and preoccupied with his symptoms, stressing that life held little for him unless he could regain physical vigor. In attempting to help him the difficulties were chiefly that he had so few assets with which to work, since it was impossible to arrange a noncompetitive world for him, and that his deep-seated inadequacies prevented an improved meeting of the problems he had to face. These considerations were explained to his mother, to whom suggestions were also made for his management.

P. Hypo. F:32:M:3 +1 213′479–(51) 6:3:6

The patient was admitted to the hospital with severe palpitations of the heart, numbness of the hands and face, and vague complaints relating to the stomach and pelvic regions. Attacks of this type had appeared about a year before admission and included also visual reduction and rigidity of the hands and knees. She often awoke and felt certain that death had come. The attacks were reduced in frequency by reassurance from her home physician, but finally she had the severe attack with which she was admitted.

At 11 years of age she had had a "nervous breakdown." This consisted of seeing ghosts on walls at night, frequent uncontrolled crying spells, and nervousness that prevented her from attending school. She rested during the spring and summer and apparently made a complete recovery. Her health since then had been good until the recent attacks.

Except for the one year she made good progress through school to completion of a two-year commercial high school course. She then held a job as secretary until she was married at age 18. Her first husband was an obscene person who abused her sexually and at times beat her. A son of that marriage became a behavior problem. After her divorce, she spent two years at home, then remarried in order to avoid living with her mother. Her second husband was described as a domineering, tyrannical individual who regarded her present illness with contempt. There were three children by this marriage. Described as having a pleasant disposition and better than average intelligence, she had always been dominated by someone and seemed unable to cope with serious problems. She was a sincere Roman Catholic until her second marriage brought excommunication. To this she was unable to adjust and it had brought grief and hurt.

The patient on admission to the hospital appeared forcibly composed, although she cried occasionally. Worried about somatic complaints, she nevertheless partially realized that her combined marital, religious, and family psychological problems could account for her illness. She was alert and eager to solve her difficulties. Her stay in the hospital was very brief but she seemed happy and rested well. It was felt that if her present situation continued, improvement or adjustment was not possible and she was discharged only because of her husband's insistence.

Ps. Sz., Simple Paranoid M:47:M:42 +22 **21'348–9 6:2:24**

Inability to work and concern about sexual matters were the chief admission complaints of the patient. Also, the county welfare board desired information about whether this man's mental disorder was contributing to his inability to work. On being told that he was no longer to receive aid from the board since he was able to earn money for himself, he had developed mild delusions of persecution. He blamed his troubles partly on his wife's use of a contraceptive diaphragm.

The patient had been admitted to the hospital five times before because of psychotic episodes similar to the present one. The diagnosis had been schizophrenia. Never a steady worker, his highest level job had been that of operator of a small town poolroom. He was considered sociable and mainly interested in money-making ventures in politics. A World War I veteran, he had begun to drink heavily in Europe and had continued for a long period.

21'3 487–6

He seemed relatively undisturbed by the hospital admission but said that he would like to get out and be strong enough to run a farm. His inability to work he attributed to the fact that when engaged in physical activities he became restless and extremely fatigued, and had marked difficulty in sleeping. He admitted that recently he had been grouchy and worried and at times had lost his temper with his wife. Acknowledging no depression, he seemed hopeful about the future. This was probably a pose. He was vague and noncommittal in his statements, but without gross irrelevancy. He was cooperative and his stay on the ward caused no difficulties. Assigning his problems to causes outside himself, he said, "In one or two years, if we continue to receive relief, we will get enough stock, and the children will be big enough to make things go." He seemed to believe that his wife had made little effort to be compatible, and that her lack of cooperation had contributed to his condition. He was convinced also that her use of contraceptives was in the main responsible for his fatigue and irritability. Apparently he was willing to stay indefinitely in the hospital. Very little progress was made in overcoming the presenting symptoms, and he was finally discharged in the expectation that he might be able to remain outside at a borderline level of adjustment.

P. Mixed	M:55:M:42	+2	21'3 487–6 (63)	1:8:11
		+26	2'134– (67)	2:6:10

For a year the patient had experienced constant intractable pain in the right side of his face with accompanying irritability. The pain, which had first occurred three years before, when he was out walking, was at first a dull ache confined to the right side. As it became more frequent and distressing, he was unable to carry out normal activities. He received a number of treatments, none of which gave relief for any length of time. He showed annoyance beyond reason over trivial things and his wife complained that it was almost impossible to live with him.

A little above average in intelligence, the patient completed high school, after failing several subjects; he attended one college for two years and was expelled for disorderly conduct, but later graduated from a large university. He worked as a reporter and advertising man but never held a job long. Regarding himself an authority on political science, he was preparing to write a book on the subject. Friendly always and at ease with others, he was described also as stubborn, egotistical, irritable, and high-strung. Subject to sudden temper outbursts, he dissipated much energy in impractical schemes. His enthusiasms were unpredictable and often went beyond good taste.

The patient was concerned about the facial pain, describing it in infinite detail and variation. His desire for an audience was keen. He was emotionally labile, showing gaiety followed promptly by depression. On the ward, his general attitude was characterized by anxiety and nervousness associated with a desire to create a favorable impression. There seemed to be no organic reason for the pain. At first reluctant to stay in the ward, he threatened to break windows if not "let out of the nut house." In a short time his attitude changed and he praised the hospital extravagantly. He began to improve markedly and not only associated with other patients but entertained them by writing skits and poetry, playing the piano, and singing. Toward the end of his stay, however, this mood passed and he complained about restrictions. On weekends when he was allowed to go home, he worked feverishly in his house. The whole pattern presented a rather unusual mixture of anxiety, hypochondriasis, hysterical symptoms, and a possible tic douloureux. It was felt that the prognosis was fairly good. He planned, at discharge, to "keep busy in the future and not sit around and brood." However, the basic pattern was probably not appreciably changed.

Ps. Paranoid F:43:M:42 +3 21'368–94 5:5:9
P. Mixed

The symptoms that brought this patient to the hospital had been precipitated by the death of her only daughter nine years before. The outstanding complaints of fatigue, spells of depression, loss of interest, and numerous pains had gradually increased in intensity. Various medications had not changed the pattern. During the last few years she had developed ideas of reference, believing that the townspeople and her family were talking about her, and she had withdrawn from social gatherings because of the assumed whisperings and gossip. She had frequent outbursts of temper in which she screamed, swore, and was destructive. More recently her negativism and misinterpretations had made it impossible for her family to keep her.

She had always been an outgoing, affable individual, capable, well liked, interested in others and in outdoor activities. She had been sexually rather frigid and had had a number of quarrels about it with her husband.

In the hospital she was mainly concerned with her widespread body complaints. Although she was reticent and vague about the ideas of reference, they were definitely present. For example, in referring to her minister she said, "He spoke of slapping people on the back, meaning that I have spoken of slapping someone's face. He said that the disciples were too tired, and that was a direct slam to hurt my feelings, because I'm always tired." The extent of her insight was that she did admit, "I know I'm too sensitive, but if I weren't so sick I wouldn't lose my temper." In the course of the hospitalization her symptoms decreased, she began to take some interest in ward activities, and she said that she had to forget a lot of her "peculiar" ideas. The social service department contacted the minister and other persons in her environment, attempting to give her every opportunity to make an adequate adjustment, but in spite of her improvement in the hospital the prognosis remained poor.

P. Hypo. F:27:S:58 +8 213'$\underline{76}$8– 7:3:5

This patient was admitted because of unhappiness, loss of interest, weakness, and multiple somatic complaints. She said that these symptoms dated back at least eight years. In addition she was stubborn and disagreeable with her family and friends; she felt that people lacked sympathy toward and understanding of her. Several physicians had diagnosed and treated her, but without success.

Never had the patient enjoyed good health. As a child she had frequently been constipated and had had headaches; with the onset of menstruation she had been troubled by dysmenorrhea. One year she missed so many days of school because of headaches that she was not promoted. At 15 she left school to do housework during the periods when her health permitted. About ten years before admission a love affair was interrupted by her parents. Her reaction to this was thought to be morbid. Next she had a liaison with a much older neighbor, a farmer. With him she had regular but unsatisfactory sexual relations, resulting in at least one pregnancy with abortion. She had been known as a sensitive, introspective individual who lacked vitality and general vigor. Her interests were narrow, and she was quiet, secretive, and rather gloomy.

The dominating trend on hospital admission was hypochondriacal. She repeatedly referred to one or another of her somatic complaints and insisted there must be something organically wrong. Her complaints always increased when she tried to participate in hospital activities. Dull normal in intelligence, in manner she was stubborn and somewhat hostile. She felt abused when any inquiry was made into her personal affairs and was so defensive that any evaluation of her, psychotherapeutically, was hampered. Never sociable with other patients, she appeared at ease with her relatives. Since she resisted the attempt to increase her food intake, her body remained dangerously underweight. She was finally discharged with little improvement. Her home physician was asked to follow her progress, but this offered little hope because of the lack of cooperation from her relatives.

P. Hypo. M:34:M:23 +1 21$\underline{37}$'68–9 4:2:16
+19 '31–94(43) 1:0:21
–155 172836'49– 3:5:14

The patient's illness had begun seven years before when he was working in a meat-packing plant. He experienced headaches and weakness, which continued without relief. He was told that he had hypertension and then later that he had active tuberculosis. A sanitarium bed was not available and he stayed at home in bed for eight months. At the end of that time X-rays indicated that the lesions were healed but his headaches and weakness continued. He finally went to another physician who told him he had heart trouble, and he took "heart medicine" for three months. This type of thing continued throughout the whole seven years, one illness after another being defined and treated. During the recent months he had become more irritable and had had spells of "blues." He lost his interest in "dressing up and going out." These factors made him come to the psychiatric unit.

He was an eighth-grade graduate and apparently did fairly well in school. After that he worked at various jobs He was described as a pleasant, easygoing fellow, of average intelligence, who was shy with strangers. He had few ambitions and was entirely regular in habits and general behavior. His wife and he were well matched, and he was more interested in his home and activities in it than in any outside activity.

In the hospital he was alert, healthy, and normal in general appearance and attitude. There was no evidence of any special thoughts or worries. He was very anxious to talk about his complaints. He believed his trouble was wholly due to organic causes and even when discussing his problems he did not appear anxious. He was given reassurance and attempts were made to help him get some insight. None of this was effective. While he was in the hospital his symptoms were partly relieved but his weakness persisted. A superficially normal attitude and manner prevented any real contact being made with him and at the time of final discharge the staff did not feel that he had basically changed at all.

P. Hypo. M:33:M:23 +7 21376′8–9 6:3:10
Ps. M-D., Mixed

This patient's own explanation at admission was, "I'm too sick to work." Soon after his marriage fourteen years before, he had begun to have "peculiar spells." The pattern was tightness, pain and roaring in his head with a dizzy sensation, choked feelings in his throat, palpitation, and a belief he was about to die. The intervals between spells decreased until the attacks were occurring a dozen or more times a week. He constantly took sedatives and demanded medicine for each new complaint. Afraid to go to work, he thought people noticed his peculiar actions. Irritability appeared, and he would at times smash furniture. He was sent to the hospital by his county welfare board.

Before his marriage the patient had been a wanderer, changing jobs frequently. At home for a few weeks, he became interested in his widowed sister-in-law. He stated with pride that when she became pregnant he "married her out of gentlemanliness." Much insecurity and sickness followed. They had four children. The patient was described as a nonaggressive person, seclusive and timid, always a weakling. Selfish and irritable, he indulged in self-pity and often said he had "never had a square deal." As a child he had preferred imaginary companions to real children and was known in the family to demand much sympathy.

He had marked bodily concern and was resentful because the doctors "can't find nothing the matter with me." "All they want is my money. They slap me on the back and say there's nothing the matter with me. Either it's my stomach that affects my nerves so that my head aches, or my headaches prevent my stomach's digestion. It's got so I don't even worry. I feel like I'm in a trance." He felt abused because his relatives thought he was crazy, and his morale was poor. As a child, he remembered feeling always "on the outside looking in." He boasted "I've only heard three talking pictures, been to two funerals in the last ten years." There were evidences of both manic and depressive spells and at times these appeared to overlap. During hospitalization a few of his somatic complaints disappeared but others appeared. His fear persisted that if he worked while having the pressure feeling he might drop dead. At discharge it was recommended that he return immediately to part-time work and then attempt to add hours until eventually he would be working full time. No certain prognosis, of course, could be given.

P. Hys. F:25:S:9 +2 213'78– 6:4:9

The patient was incompletely studied, but on admission she had pain in the lower right quadrant of the abdomen and coarse tremor in her hands, arms, and head. From the age of 15 she had always had pain with her menstrual period but about a year before admission the pain had begun to be more severe and had lasted longer. At the time of admission it was almost constant, but since numerous examinations failed to establish a cause it was felt that the pain might be hysterical in nature. A coarse tremor in her hands and in her head, which she had had for several months, was aggravated by excitement. She complained of headaches and nausea; also she had had difficulty in walking and at times refused to eat. Before the onset of the tremor the patient had become resentful over the fact that her family did not appear to appreciate the nature of her pain. She objected to medical attention and made some feeble gestures toward suicide.

Never strong, she had had two nervous breakdowns previously. During the course of the first one, which occurred when she was 16 years old, she had been in bed for months, her body rigid, her hands clenched, and unable to walk. At the age of 19 she had had a similar attack as a sequel to an abscessed tooth. A high school graduate, she had wanted to be a nurse but after one month of nurses' training had given it up because her "back gave out." She was not quick at learning and she had little energy. A shy, aloof, sensitive, and easily hurt person, she was selfish and had always had hypochondriacal tendencies. Although she had a cheerful disposition, she was a daydreamer and subject to temper outbursts. She had one boy friend to whom she wrote occasionally. There were no marked family difficulties.

On admission there were no contributory physical disorders. During the nine days she was in the hospital she stressed the fact that she had been ill since early childhood, and although she talked a great deal about her illness, little else could be obtained from her. She had no manifest distortions of mental content, and she took offense at the idea that people thought she might be crazy. She was finally removed by her family against advice. It was felt that while the patient might well recover from this attack other attacks in keeping with her personality background could be expected.

P. Hypo. M:46:M:49 +25 213'784– 9:1:14

The county welfare office asked for admission of this man in order that the eligibility of his family for relief aid might be studied and assessed. The patient's complaints centered around abdominal pain of thirty years' duration, which incapacitated him for work. During all these years he had felt "crampy pain in all parts of my body after eating." He was also constipated and used cathartics regularly. Whenever he did heavy work or stooped, the pain was particularly distressing and as a consequence during the past few years he had worked very little. Except for evidences of damage from the cathartics—a small ulcer in the anal region—medical studies showed nothing significant.

Never strong, the patient had always had somatic complaints, although there was no history of a physical illness. He grew up in a comfortable farm home, finishing the fifth grade at the age of 15. Married at 30, he ran a small farm for a while but gave that up because of ill health. From that time until hospitalization he worked at odd jobs. His wife and he managed their money economically and were proud of this. Nevertheless they went on partial relief for a number of years. Well mannered and pleasant, the patient was easily discouraged, his feelings were readily hurt. He was subject to depression and cried easily. He more than once declared his pride was wounded for having to accept charity. For this he avoided the townspeople. During his illness he became annoyed and irritated by his children. His I.Q. was measured at 91.

The patient hoped that hospitalization would help free him of discomfort and distention. "I've done all that I can do. I can't force myself any more. Hard work makes my trouble worse and I just can't do it." He recognized that he had been depressed and irritable but attributed this to his physical ills. He talked readily, cooperated, at least on the surface, and pretended to comprehend more than he really did. His vocabularly was limited. When regular attempts to reassure and help him failed, faradic stimulation was tried. This was used with an elaborate suggestive background but without result. His own summary was: "The treatments won't help me because that's for mental trouble, and I'm not mental. The nerves in my stomach just don't work right." Because he was complacent about his physical illness, and because it absolved him from all responsibilities, there seemed no clear way to help him out of his situation, and the discharge was made with a poor prognosis.

P. Hys. F:29:M:49 –1 2137'86– 3:6:10
P. Hypo. +39 2713'896–(41) 5:4:16
P. React. Depr.

The patient was admitted with complaints of severe headaches, palpitations, feelings of skipped heartbeats, and other more vague thoracic symptoms. She also had fainting spells. These various symptoms had begun six months before admission, although the first fainting spell occurred eleven months before that when the patient was told her blood could not be used in a transfusion for her sick baby. The reason given was that her hemoglobin was too low. Following this she had more fainting spells and spent some time in bed. She continued to be very nervous and irritable. Fainting spells seemed to come without particular provocation. "My blood would seem to suddenly turn cold." She would then hurry to lie down, but sometimes lost consciousness before she reached the couch. She would remain unconscious for about two hours.

Her health had always been good and there was no evidence of previous nervousness except for what sounded like hysterical attacks. She stopped high school in the third year without apparent reason, and she married at age 17. She and her husband worked hard and managed fairly well. They apparently lived a normal social life, with visiting friends and seeing shows their chief recreations. The patient had always been sociable, friendly, and active. She was somewhat sensitive. As a child she had been petted and catered to by four older brothers. Although she had had to work hard since marriage her husband was devoted and solicitous. She liked sympathy and still enjoyed being babied.

Her uppermost thoughts concerned her somatic complaints, although she also worried about her 17-month-old son. She was nervous and irritable and felt very sorry for herself. Her replies were adequate and to the point and there was no psychomotor retardation. She was rather petulant and anxious for sympathy and appeared accustomed to great dependence on others. There was rapid improvement for about three weeks during which the fainting spells and headaches decreased in frequency and intensity. However, the patient became more upset and nervous the fourth week, following a weekend of visiting, and the symptoms returned. From this setback she quickly recovered. There was a possibility but no certainty of some organic background for the problems. She was discharged feeling much better and it was expected she would recover symptomatically.

P. Mixed M:43:S:18 +1 21378′6–9 (51) 9:5:8
Mental Deficiency

The complaints of this patient were loss of pep and feeling "all shot." This last was characterized by weakness, nervousness, and countless aches and pains. A year before admission the patient had suffered a heat stroke while working in the barn of his farm; since that time he had not regained his vigor and had become increasingly depressed. He was preoccupied with his health and felt he wasn't strong enough to do heavy work. A partial list of his more specific complaints included dizziness, cold in the extremities, nausea, vague pains in his chest, and sexual impotence; at times his leg "gave out." He also complained of crying spells which came on without apparent reason.

In general his past history was free of matters of psychological import. Records showed the general medicine service had referred him to the psychiatric service ten years earlier about an "appendicitis." The opinion at that time was that his ills were chiefly "functional." He finished the eighth grade at 16, went to work for his parents, and continued as their employee from that time on. At one time he asked a local schoolteacher to marry him but was turned down. This depressed him and two weeks later the first attack of abdominal pain occurred. For a year he drank excessively but quit because "something went haywire" in his stomach. Always shy and ill at ease among people, he was oversensitive and took disappointments hard. He had no outside interests except hunting and trapping and preferred to be alone. He was of borderline intelligence.

Principally concerned about bodily aches and pains, the patient complained that he couldn't do farm work because he was "too weak." He was dull, sad, hopeless, anxious, fearful, and depressed. In the hospital a careful physical study was made and he was given reassurance which helped him slightly. Also, the routine and diversion of the ward took effect, his crying spells stopped, and he began to show more interest in things about him. He was discharged greatly improved but it was recognized that hospitalization was the chief operating factor, and it seemed unlikely that his home adjustment would be much different from what it had been before hospitalization.

P. Mixed	F:26:M:9	+1	2138′467–(43)	9:4:15
		−8	78263′14–(63)	4:6:9

The patient was admitted to the hospital with difficulty in breathing, tightness and stiffness in her arms, leucorrhea, pain and pressure on the top of her head, pain in her chest, stiffness in her neck, dryness and itching of her skin, and numerous other complaints. She had first noticed some of the symptoms after the birth of her third child about a year before admission. Thyroid medication by her local physician was stopped after a few weeks' trial because of palpitations and loss of hair from her scalp. Until she came down with influenza a few months later she managed fairly well. Since that time she had complained of various bizarre symptoms, and at the time of hospitalization she was quite certain that she was organically ill, possibly from cancer.

With the exception of a childhood kidney infection she had had fairly good previous health. Because she did not like school, and because it was hard for her, she quit when she had finished half of the sophomore grade in high school. Without definite ambitions, she had done housework until her marriage. Shy, insecure, and sensitive, she had always had difficulty making friends. Of subnormal intelligence, she had shown poor judgment and lacked the ability to handle money well. She had a poor family background punctuated with quarreling and drunkenness, and the patient had left home at 16 because she could not get along with her parents.

Primarily concerned with her illness and her numerous, often bizarre, complaints, she felt that she had malignant lesions from one or two organic diseases, the nature of which people kept from her. She showed considerable anxiety, with agitation and a tendency to misinterpret and misidentify. Her orientation and memory were intact, and there appeared to be no basic personality disturbance. At times defiant, argumentative, and negativistic, she objected to psychiatric treatment. She was always disheveled in appearance. Her adjustment to the hospital routine was slow, and she did not take much part in ward activities. Even after numerous attempts at reassurance and psychological treatment she frequently felt that she was going to die and demanded to see her husband. She was discharged at her insistence against advice, and it was felt that a change from the neurosis into an acute psychotic disorder was not at all unlikely.

Ps. Sz., Hebe. M:19:S:59 +2 213'86–9 4:2:3

The admission complaints were characterized by the patient's statement, "I'm so weak I'm all paralyzed. My food isn't doing me any good and my heart is going to pieces." About a year before admission the patient had failed a geometry course; he excused himself by saying that he was handicapped on account of his eyes. That summer he felt his body needed a change and he took a job at a summer resort. There he was considered seclusive. He spent much time in bed and complained of constant fatigue. When he returned to school in the fall he showed so little interest that he was taken to a physician, to whom he said, "School is taking something away from me." He slept poorly, talked constantly of trouble with his stomach, and made peculiar demands concerning his diet. His worries included fears that masturbation had weakened his heart and mind. During the entire period of the illness he seemed to enjoy verbally punishing his mother with the story of his troubles, not stopping until she was in tears.

Except for repeating the first grade because of a language difficulty (the family came from Sweden), he had been a good student until the onset of the present illness. His intelligence was somewhat above average. He had always accepted responsibility and had exercised good judgment about money. His only ambition had been to go into business with his father. Outdoor sports interested him and in these he was very active. He had shown keen interest in physical culture and had been overfastidious about his person. He was unpopular with other boys because he always attempted to dominate them. Stubbornness and selfishness were his two outstanding traits. He had developed no heterosexual interests but said that he had masturbated from age 15. He and his mother had been close, and she was his confidante. A nervous and irritable woman, his mother still felt keenly the fact that she was pregnant when she was married, and she wondered if her son's illness was a punishment for her. She was on the verge of tears constantly during the interviews. In general, however, it appeared that she had been an excellent housekeeper and a devoted wife and mother. She made a pleasing appearance and the three other children in the family did not complain of any particular disorders.

The patient was a neat, well-mannered boy of excellent appearance. His manner was cooperative, and he answered questions about himself eagerly. He had a distinct tendency to make much of his somatic complaints. "It seems that everything I eat just stops in my stomach and doesn't digest properly. . . . I'm always constipated because my insides are paralyzed. I know that my other organs, especially my sex organs and my heart, are practically exhausted because I'm not getting the nourishment I need." Associated with these feelings were depression and inanition. He had some insight. "Of course, naturally, my mind would be weakened if I'm not physically strong. It's a little harder for me to think than it used to be." He tended to lie in bed to avoid "tearing his body to pieces." Such statements were usually made without evidences of anxiety. He improved very slightly and was finally discharged to his mother for a try at home before state hospitalization.

P. Hypo. M:60:S:10 —3 213'867-(59) 2:6:7
P. Hys. —34 mos. 1328'7496- 2:9:9

Pain in the amputation stump of the patient's right thigh was the chief admitting symptom. There was positive evidence of tabes dorsalis, although the blood serology was negative. Medication and the usual treatments for the pain, which had been continuous for the 25 years since amputation, were ineffectual. Repeated lumbar sympathetic blocks had given considerable motor and sensory loss, but the pain had persisted. In addition there were numerous complaints such as restlessness, nervousness, poor vision, paresthesias, headaches, and poor bladder control.

A fifth-grade graduate, the man had worked irregularly until he lost his leg as the result of a fracture. About the same time, he contracted lues; after that he was never again able to work steadily and most of the time he lived on a county farm. A previous general hospital admission (earlier MMPI) had led to a diagnosis of tabes.

Very restless in the hospital, he complained constantly of pain and other somatic symptoms, insisting on frequent medical attention, although he would occasionally forget his troubles and enter into hospital activities. Plecebo tablets gave him fair relief. An intermixture of organic disease and psychological disorder was clearly apparent. The social service worker made an attempt to improve the environmental conditions which would affect the patient after he left the hospital, but in spite of these efforts it did not seem likely that anything more than relatively manageable invalidism would be achieved.

P. Hypo. F:24:M:50 +11 213'867-9X 12:6:16
Schizoid
Paranoid

Five years before admission, following the delivery of her second child, the patient had "had a nervous breakdown," the symptoms being instability, irritability, and intolerance to noise of any type. For the next eleven months she experienced tension and "hysterics" apparently characterized by episodes of rage and overactivity lasting only a few minutes. There was a gradual development of a number of physical complaints, including "rheumatism" and "swelling of the hands" which partially incapacitated her. In the present illness the patient complained of abdominal pains, weakness, extreme nervousness, and seclusiveness.

The patient had a long history of medical treatment, both physical and, in at least one case, psychological, with a state hospital diagnosis of "psychoneurosis without psychosis." She was an eighth-grade graduate who had married at age 17. She and her husband had moved to a farm and had attempted to buy it, but even though they were industrious they had not been able to keep up the payments. They finally lost the farm and became sharecroppers. Before the onset of the present illness the patient had been a friendly, agreeable person with excellent judgment, and she had had many friends. Although before her hospitalization the hypochondriacal tendencies had not been evident to the persons who described her, "nervous" traits were mentioned. For example, at one time she so feared having people see her that she hid in the attic when anyone came to the house. Earlier both she and her husband had been in the state hospital at the same time. The husband had had her committed, and her husband's brother had introduced proceedings for the commitment of her husband.

In the hospital the patient expressed numerous somatic delusions. "I have a nervous heart. My organs fall backwards. Music irritates my nerves." She also had ideas of reference. She believed that her neighbors talked about her, that they were prejudiced against her because of her religion, that they referred to her as insane, and that they warned people not to enter her home. Frequently she appeared preoccupied. She had no insight into her illness, but she talked relevantly and coherently. She was very untidy in personal appearance, did not participate well in ward activities, and spent as much time as possible in bed. Her husband finally took her out of the hospital against the advice of the staff.

P. Hypo. F:43:M:22 +1 21'387-9 (72) 6:4:21

Four months before admission the patient suffered a fall which resulted in a miscarriage. After a week in the hospital she returned home, but found she was too weak and tired to do her work, and spent considerable time in bed. When left alone one night she developed an exacerbation of these symptoms, with the addition of palpitation, headache, dizziness, and numerous other complaints. These were accompanied by a fear of death. This attack was followed by similar spells two or three times a week until the present admission. She had been in three different hospitals before the present one and had remained approximately the same throughout those admissions.

In the patient's history there was another "nervous breakdown" similar to the present one. This had occurred thirteen years earlier and had also followed a miscarriage. The breakdown lasted a year. After completing the seventh grade at age 15 she left school and worked at different jobs in rapid succession. She gave birth to an illegitimate son but apparently was not upset by that. Four years later she married and then lived on a farm until the present illness. Described as having always been emotionally unstable with a tendency toward depression, at the least mention of trouble she would begin to cry. Her intelligence was low average. Able to mix with other people and to get along with them well, she was nevertheless sensitive to what others said of her and was easily hurt. She always seemed to need a great deal of sympathy. She and her husband were sexually compatible and there appeared to have been no difficulty over the illegitimate son, who had been adopted by the husband as his own.

In the hospital the patient was chiefly concerned about her illness. She cried and showed a great deal of anxiety. Without insight into her mental condition, she sincerely believed that all her troubles were due to organic disorders. Although she was friendly and cooperative, she was difficult to work with because of her great sensitivity when personal matters were discussed. She spent most of her time in bed and complained bitterly when she was required to get up. After some faradic shock therapy, which seemed to help, she left her bed and began to take part in activities around the hospital. At discharge she was considerably improved. However, it was felt that the present episode might continue with varying severity for a considerable time.

Ps. Sz., Paranoid M:32:S:20 +2 213'87–94 7:8:16

This man was admitted to the hospital with nervousness which was expressed in tremor, diaphoresis, and feelings of general tension and apprehension. The acute symptoms dated back nine years when the patient was working his way through college. He also had ideas of reference and miscellaneous pains, and he believed he had "goiter trouble." A physician had told him that he had thyrotoxicosis. A few years later he had a thyroidectomy but the symptoms did not change; next he tried a new environment, also without good result. More and more he avoided people and showed peculiar and agitated behavior. When an uncle told him that he was "mentally ill," he voluntarily presented himself at the hospital.

The patient had a B.A. degree and until the onset of the present illness, had been a steady worker. Four years before admission he was forced to drop the level of his occupation to irregular farm work on his uncle's place. He was described as having always been shy, secretive, retiring, effeminate, and "badly spoiled." In school he had worked hard and had financed himself for the most part. Although ambitious and eager to acquire financial security, he had not selected college courses particularly adapted to this goal. He had an occasional girl friend but had never formed any close relationships.

The patient, although mainly concerned with his present illness, expressed his problem poorly. When direct questions about the nature of his difficulties were put to him he repeatedly said, "I don't know. If I could just get a job in which I could be of some use . . ." Over and over he said he wanted help and talked of vague bodily complaints and persecutory delusions. His intelligence, when measured, turned out to be surprisingly low for a college graduate. His I.Q. on the Weschler-Bellevue test was 90. He walked with peculiar short steps and a rigid body, and leafed through magazines for hours at a time. Psychologically he seemed effeminate. In spite of reassurance and other efforts to help him there was little change and he was finally transferred to a state hospital.

Ps. Sz., Cat. F:39:M:10 +2 21387′4–9 6:8:13
P. Psychas.
Suicidal

The admission symptoms of this patient were nervousness, obsessions, and suicidal tendencies. Her illness dated from three months before when she had become progressively more nervous and upset and had obsessions of doing harm. These involved, in particular, killing her children, her husband, and herself. She had hallucinations with a paranoid trend; among them was the unusual one that cattle were looking down the chimney at her and driving her to suicide. On one occasion she actually had tried to hang herself.

After one year of high school and a couple of years at a teachers' college, the patient had taught school for five years before marriage. While living with her husband and three children on a farm, she had had two previous psychotic upsets. During the first of these she was diagnosed as post-encephalitic, and in the second episode she was called schizophrenic. The patient's married life had been stormy. Abused by her first husband, she divorced him and kept one of their three children. This daughter was in a reform school at the time of the patient's admission. She later married again and had three more children. This family appeared to be getting along fairly well, in spite of poor financial circumstances.

In the hospital the patient's compulsions included breaking the windows of her room. One of her occasional hallucinations was that the devil was telling her what to do. She appeared to be mildly depressed and took poor care of herself. She had some tendency to posturize, she occasionally showed flexibilitas cerea, and she swallowed bobby pins in an attempt to commit suicide. She was finally transferred to a state hospital.

Ps. Sz., Paranoid F:26:S:21 +9 213876′4–9(57) 7:8:15

The patient said that for as long as she could remember she had had periods of depression when she had wanted to be alone and had been unable to think or accomplish anything, and as a result she had had a very irregular vocational life. Because she had always been able to lift herself out of a depression by leaving her job and going into something else, she had not previously needed hospitalization. At one time she had been very religious and had been able to quote at length from the Bible. Later she had engaged in some promiscuous romantic episodes in which she had "picked up" strange men whom she had allowed to embrace her, although she denied that she had had any sexual experiences with them. She had gradually developed delusions of reference and thought that people on streetcars and other strangers knew about her misconduct and stared at her. Sometimes a voice that seemed to be the devil's talked to her and called her names. At certain of her jobs she had delivered long dissertations on religious subjects and seemingly had been unable to stop talking even when she realized that her listeners were unappreciative. Two months before admission to the hospital she had enrolled in a night school at a Bible institute but had left when she had a depressive spell. Since that time she had stayed at home and was so depressed that she would not see anyone.

Among the evidences for psychosomatic disturbances in her past history were some brief periods of "unconsciousness." There were also complaints of headaches and a scoliosis for which she had received chiropractic treatment. She was an adopted child and had always had difficulty making friends. School had been hard for her but she had completed high school. Although she had enrolled at a business college, she had given it up because of her feelings of inadequacy. She had always had a tendency to be seclusive and to immerse herself in a religious life.

In the hospital she was well oriented and adequate in answering questions, but before each answer there was always a lengthy pause while she stared off into space. Frequently she laughed inappropriately, and she backed up her answers with biblical quotations. She said that she had been "off" for many years. In describing the past events over which she felt guilt she said that "everyone knew about it." She apparently had experienced frequent auditory hallucinations. The patient did not enter into group activities and stayed in her room as much as possible. She wanted laxatives constantly and sometimes wanted to give herself enemas. She was finally transferred to a state hospital.

Ps. M-D., Depr. F:39:M:35 +9 2′1437– 6:2:15
Suicidal

The uncommon complaints of excessive lacrimation were among the admission symptoms of this patient. In addition she had been depressed, had attempted suicide, and had complained of other somatic ills. For five years she had withdrawn more and more from social activities and had lost interest in her home. She grew thin and could not sleep. Following a tooth extraction seven months before admission her symptoms intensified. She became hypercritical, demanded attention, and developed epiphora of the right eye for which she consulted an oculist. The suicide attempt was a halfhearted one in which she was prevented from taking gas by the intervention of her husband. Frequently she refused to leave her bed. At times she imagined people were looking at her eye. One day she became agitated and cried, "I'm going crazy and I'm going to die," and requested that the minister be called. Later, however, she complained that her nephew told the neighbors she was crazy. The day before admission she again attempted to end her life and was once again rescued.

She reported that she had always been stubborn and domineering. She enjoyed playing cards and visiting neighbors, but she and her husband had few common interests and there was little affection between them. With people she was friendly but not confiding. Periodically during her life she had been restless and subject to crying spells.

Examination revealed an obstruction of the right lacrimal duct and poor tone in the musculature. Worry and discouragement over her eye, the patient believed, was responsible for her attempted suicides and despondency. She gave up card parties and other social functions, she said, to reduce eyestrain. She criticized her husband severely for his lack of interest in her activities; she was obviously depressed and discouraged, cried readily, and worried about the future and about her eye. During hospitalization she slowly gained a measure of insight. Inclined to be suspicious, she was reluctant to discuss her troubles. She avoided the other patients and was inactive. She rebelled at ward restrictions on her freedom, thought she should be permitted to come and go at will. She insisted upon eye examinations and could not be reassured. The last few days of her stay she became sociable, fairly optimistic, and more cooperative. At no time, however, did she gain real understanding of her illness, and she remained unshaken in her conviction that her eye would eventually be lost.

P. Hys. F:38:M:9 +5 '2146– 3:1:13

For the past thirteen years the patient had suffered from yearly attacks of syncope, and for the past three months she had experienced convulsive seizures that appeared to be more hysterical than epileptic. The attacks were completely relieved when she stayed in bed. About fourteen days before admission the patient had developed a transitory aphasia.

Except for the fainting spells, the past medical and psychological history was noncontributory. After going to a vocational high school for two years, she had worked as a domestic until her marriage at age 20. Always a somewhat withdrawn person, she had spent a great deal of time reading romantic fiction. When crossed, she had temper outbursts of brief duration. Since she had never discussed her troubles with her husband he had no insight of what her problems might be, but apparently the couple had got along fairly well. A serious accident six years after their marriage had partially disabled the husband. There were four children. The home situation appeared to be no more stressful than average.

The neurological and physical examinations were essentially negative. She was very resentful at the suggestion that her difficulty might be a reaction to her psychological problems, and she insisted that she was perfectly satisfied with her life situation. Aside from an immature type of emotional instability, her behavior was completely normal. A key to some of her problems came from her home physician to whom she had confided that she had been unfaithful to her husband. The date when this affair began coincided approximately with the onset of the present illness, but the patient would not discuss or bring up this matter in the hospital. The home physician after consultation felt that he could probably handle the matter when the patient was discharged.

P. Hypo. F:37:M:23 0 21637'98-(39) 5:6:6
Paranoid

This patient was admitted with weakness, speech difficulties, nervousness, and "blind spells." She had had these symptoms for approximately 25 years. For 10 years she had had increasingly severe periods of depression. The symptoms reportedly first appeared when the patient fell, injured the back of her head, and lay unconscious for a long time. No physician was seen at that time. Headaches followed this injury and nausea was present. A speech difficulty appeared, more severe during times of strain. Low back pain was described as "achey and persistent."

At 18 years of age she had suffered epileptiform attacks during which she was unconscious and injured herself. These attacks ceased after a few years. She had undergone several major operations. Her schooling went only as far as the seventh grade, and she had not desired to continue. She was a sensitive and self-conscious person. Always "nervous," crowds and excitement upset her. She envied the "prosperity" of her brother and sister-in-law. Her outlook on life was pessimistic. She had contemplated suicide but had never actually made an attempt. Temper outbursts were brought on by noises or other minor disturbances. During these outbursts she occasionally attempted to harm her husband and threw things. Her sexual life appeared to have been normal. Her youngest child was a congenital hemiparetic and this was a source of worry and nervousness to the patient. At the birth of this child the patient lost interest in her home and activities even more than before.

On admission the neurological and physical examinations were negative. Her sensorium and intellect were apparently intact. She showed very great concern about her headaches, her lack of appetite, and the pain in her back. She showed no bizarre behavior, was cooperative and open in interviews. She resisted the idea that there might be something wrong with her mind. Nevertheless she steadily improved and recognized that it helped her to talk over her problems. The staff thought the prognosis was good if home worries could be lessened. It was of course possible that the old head injury was a factor in the illness but no specific evidence of it could be found.

P. Hypo. F:28:M:12 +1 2'17346–9(51) 2:3:16

Nervousness, fatigue, constipation, and insomnia were the main admission complaints of this patient. The onset apparently dated back about three years when the patient had borne her third child. At that time she noted fatigue and irritability toward her family. These symptoms increased and two years later, when the patient "overworked herself" helping her family move to a new farm, and also had her father-in-law move in, her symptoms became still worse. She entered a hospital where for a month she was given sedatives and a concentrated diet. She left the hospital free of symptoms but within five days they returned. Later she entered a rest home but returned to her own home four days later more nervous than she had been before. She became progressively worse until the present admission.

The patient graduated from high school at age 16. Having begun to play the piano at about 30 months, she reportedly was an excellent pianist. Her intelligence was above average and she was very devout. Described as indecisive and a poor planner, she was also shy and tended to stay away from crowds. She thought people were talking about her, although she knew they were not. She worried about trifles and was very sensitive.

When the patient was admitted to the hospital she was depressed but answered questions logically and adequately. She was composed and there were few signs of nervousness, although she admitted to being very tense. She attributed some of her tenseness to her new surroundings. She believed that her symptoms were due to nervousness, but she believed also that they could be cured by symptomatic treatment such as the use of sedatives and enemas. At first she stayed in bed and exhibited all her presenting complaints; then she finally took the initiative and admitted to sexual and religious conflict. She had been practicing coitus interruptus and felt great guilt. There was also conflict about bringing up the children in her religious faith against the wishes of her husband. Reassured on some of these points, she was greatly relieved, took an active role in group activities, and became friendly with other patients. She made rapid improvement and was discharged symptom-free. Arrangements were made for her to continue in the outpatient department.

B. Psth., Path. Emot. F:35:M:26 +1 217'348–6(43) 3:6:15
Alcoholism

The patient was admitted with a pattern of heavy drinking, nervousness, seclusiveness, and weight loss, the onset of which had been insidious following an ectopic pregnancy nine years before admission. She had been under the care of numerous physicians and several psychiatrists in the last five years and had been treated in rest homes, summer camps, and private hospitals. Her main persistent symptoms were nervousness, trembling, irritability, and alcoholism, and when she went on prolonged drinking bouts, she became extremely abusive toward her mother and friends.

Small, weak, and nervous all her life, she had suffered from jaundice, shingles, a ruptured appendix, and other difficulties preceding the ectopic pregnancy. A college graduate, she had been educated in private schools where she had done average work. Although she had shown talent as an author and as a dress designer she had never developed these skills, and she had never held a job. Shy and introverted, she tended to avoid people, and her family thought she was stubborn, selfish, and intolerant of any inconvenience. Until the difficulty of getting servants forced her to cook, she had never done any of her own housework, and she complained bitterly of being "cook and bottle washer." She was seldom cheerful and obviously felt inferior toward others about her, particularly toward her sisters who could have children while she could not.

In appearance she was an unattractive, nervous woman with marked tremor in her hands. The few neurological findings certainly did not explain her psychological pattern. Complaining, cranky, and irritable most of the time, she was bossy and abusive toward the nurses and clerks. She had no real insight. Her sensorium and intellect were clear. She spent most of her time reading, and she mixed with other patients very little. Various types of therapy were tried, including modified insulin and direct psychotherapy, but although she gained some weight she changed very little in any other way. Since the present illness was merely an exacerbation of a long-standing, general pattern of behavior, it seemed unlikely that any approach would help her and she was discharged in the hope that she would be able to continue at a marginal adjustment level.

Ps. M-D., Depr.	M:47:M:52	+1	2173′6489–(47)	2:4:8
P. Psychas.		+20	172834′69–(47)	2:5:16
		+52	′17–98436(39)	2:1:12

The admission complaints for this man centered around insomnia, extreme nervousness, and fear that he might lose his mind and harm his wife and family. These symptoms had appeared three weeks before. A year earlier the patient had felt a "heart condition" marked by pain in his chest, weakness, and dyspnea associated with exertion. He also had shooting pains in his arms and gastric distress. He had received medical care during the year but without relief. Careful physical exploration revealed no positive organic disorder and he remained about the same until the present symptoms began. Fifteen years earlier he had experienced a similar illness from which he recovered (without treatment) after a few months. Aside from this earlier depression the medical history was negative.

The youngest of six children, the patient had been favored by his parents. Toward the end of the eighth grade he left school; he did odd jobs for a while and then worked as a mechanic. When he married his father gave him a farm. Never successful at farm work, he had a difficult time providing for his family. He was extremely fond and proud of his wife and children, and said he was happiest when playing with his children or when hunting and trapping. Described as even-tempered, kind, and patient, he was sentimental, friendly, and likable. His intelligence was in the high average range.

In the hospital the patient was well oriented from the beginning and showed concern about his health. That he might harm his family and also that he might lose his mind were among his most acute fears. Eagerly he described his problems and symptoms, but he had little hope that he could be helped. Whenever a reference was made to his family he cried and expressed feelings of extreme unworthiness. Considerable improvement followed a course of nine electroshock treatments. He became anxious for a discharge and looked forward to returning to his family and work. Although he appeared completely recovered from this attack, it was felt likely in view of the history of a previous attack that there might be more in the future.

P. Hypo.	M:34:S:15	+3	217′38–9 (49)	4:3:19
		−17	2′71638–9	3:6:12

The patient complained of weakness and a run-down condition which he said had been present for twelve years. He felt he had been nervous all his life. His special complaints of a weak back and backache were of more recent origin. Most of the complaints were ill defined and nonlocalized. He blamed his inability to get and hold steady jobs on his feelings of inferiority and his poor health.

His past medical history was very much like the complaints in the present admission, and there was a long list of physical conditions which he described as having been present at one time or another, but he had never had a serious illness, operation, or injury. Although he had been somewhat retarded in school because of a speech defect, he had finished high school at the age of 21. His I.Q. was in the average range. He had lived at home, had never held a steady job, had no particular hobbies, was dependent upon his family for decisions and guidance, had never gone out with girls, and had had no sexual intercourse. When nervous and excited he had experienced spontaneous orgasms. He felt he had always been backward around people, and when he tried to talk, his tongue seemed to freeze, but in spite of what appeared to be almost a speech disorder, he felt that he was well liked by people.

The patient was greatly concerned about his aches and pains and was worried about the possible effects of masturbation. He thought he was losing excessive amounts of sperm in his urine. He showed considerable insight into his condition and felt that most of his troubles were of nervous or mental origin. His speech was low, fast, and jerky, and in addition to his speech difficulty, he spoke with a slight accent and at times he had trouble finding the word he wanted to use. It was difficult to maintain his attention during an interview, and he was fidgety and nervous. The results of tests for organic brain deterioration and for aphasia appeared to be at least in the borderline range indicating a possibility of brain defect. He got along fairly well in the hospital and expressed the thought that his previous concern over masturbation and sperm loss was "foolishness." He was convinced that his was largely a personality problem, and he decided to get a steady job when he was discharged from the hospital. Although he was much improved, the basic inferiorities were unchanged, and it was felt that at best his would be a borderline adjustment.

P. Hypo. F:28:M:33 +3 21'7384–9 6:6:14

For the past year the patient had had a general feeling of fatigue, along with such other symptoms as depression, nervousness, headaches, nausea, dizziness, and burning sensations in the eyes. The patient also felt that her neighbors were criticizing her and her parents, a feeling that had some foundation in fact since her father had recently been incarcerated for illicit sexual relations with three of his daughters. Nine years before admission the patient had been admitted to the dermatology service for a chronic cervicitis with purulent discharge. Vaginal cultures were negative. She had complained of itching and crawling sensations over her entire body; and there was a mention of chronic urticaria and syphilophobia at that time.

When the patient was in the first year of high school at age 16, she quit because she thought she wasn't getting much out of it. In the private home where she had been working for room and board she had been required to get up very early in the morning, and as a result she often fell asleep in school. Although she got along well with the teachers, she exhibited poor learning ability, and she was tired most of the time. At 13 she had had numerous sexual relations with a boy about her own age, and the warning from her employer, who found out about the relations, that she could never be happily married because of these experiences worried the patient considerably. Relations with the boy were terminated at her request. After leaving school she made an unsuccessful attempt to do correspondence work for further high school credit. She described herself as a bashful child who had always found it hard to make friends. In the presence of men she had felt shy. She attributed her sex drive, which she considered to be unusually strong, to heredity, "since my father is so oversexed." The patient, who had been married at age 17, had three children, all of whom had been unwanted. Her husband was thirteen years older than she and had never had a permanent job, but the couple seemed to be reasonably well adjusted to each other. Since her marriage the patient had had a constant fear of pregnancy because of an unsatisfactory financial status.

In the hospital she was principally concerned about her physical complaints. There were no gross disturbances of mentation or sensorium. Her fund of general information was poor, and a psychological examination revealed a dull mentality. Although the woman appeared mildly depressed, she was composed and even-tempered, possibly somewhat apathetic. Her physical complaints subsided in the hospital and while she still felt uncomfortable in the presence of people she became somewhat less sensitive about her family stigma. Although heredity and early environment had contributed to the patient's doubtless low threshold for nervous disorders and although other neurotic reactions were possible, it was felt that the woman would make an adequate borderline adjustment.

P. Hypo. M:51:S:65 +1 21738′4–9(49) 6:5:16

This patient was admitted with complaints of generalized aches and pains, numbness, and "nervousness," which had persisted for two years. Numerous physicians had made various diagnoses and suggested treatments, none of which had helped. At times the patient believed he had cancer, vitamin deficiency, or ulcers. Treatment for each of these was in turn successful for only a short period. For one month two physicians treated him concurrently, one for heart trouble, the other by advice to "get out and work and forget your illness."

Born in Yugoslavia, the patient came to this country at age 18. He completed the seventh grade in Yugoslavia. In America he worked as a miner, harvest hand, and lumberjack. He lived alone in a two-room apartment in a small town. Although always "nervous and shy," he had had many friends until the onset of his illness, when he dropped a number of them because of their lack of sympathy toward his problems. He liked to watch sports, play cards, and read books. He had never married and said he had "never considered it."

Concerned with his physical ills, he nevertheless recognized that he was nervous and expressed fear that he might "become insane." Quiet and retiring, he associated little with other patients. In the hospital he became depressed. Occupational therapy, he thought, was too "simple and childish." For the most part he sat alone, occasionally playing cards with another patient. Seldom engaging anyone in conversation, he spoke well when addressed. He could not sleep, he insisted, although the record indicated he actually slept well. Reassurance brought some relief to him but this was only gradual. Eventually he came to see that his worst somatic symptoms were correlated with the "nervous spells," and to recognize the organic factor as possibly minor to the "nervousness." After a slight improvement, he was discharged to return home. It seemed likely he would gradually recover at least to his former level.

P. Mixed M:39:M:14 +6 217′3846– 4:5:13

This patient was referred to the psychiatric unit by a physician in private practice because of symptoms of depression and periods of excitability with extreme restlessness. Feelings of dissatisfaction with his work and difficulty in making decisions had been present for several months. During the past year he had had much illness, including a perirectal abscess that required opiates for the pain. The patient reported that following the hypodermics he would occasionally go out of his head and "they had to hold me in bed." He had fainting spells which were first associated with enemas but later came without apparent precipitating factors. These spells did not appear at all similar to epileptic attacks. Six days before admission the patient's foster son had left home after a scene in which he was reprimanded for carrying liquor. The patient was admitted as an emergency because of acute excitement following this episode. With admission, the excitement disappeared. Indignant at being brought to the hospital, he immediately signed out, only to return one month later for treatment because he continued to have fainting spells and to be distressingly depressed.

He had a chronic ulcer problem and several surgical procedures had been carried out to relieve bowel obstructions caused by adhesions. Leaving school at 16 to work as a laborer at odd jobs, at 19 he enrolled in a business college short course. For twenty years he was steadily employed as a white collar worker in the contracting business and worked up to a fairly responsible position. During the depression years, though placed under considerable stress, no particular symptoms appeared, but he seemed to have been rather immature and given to rationalizations and half truths. He always seemed to feel it necessary to maintain a front.

As mentioned, the patient's excitement disappeared on admission. His main concerns were his business and his foster son. He said he felt "calm on the outside" but "like exploding on the inside." Regarding his fainting spells he said, "I suppose they think I'm a neurotic old woman. They will have to give me a fancier diagnosis than that." While the patient was in the hospital his foster son was brought to court on a series of forgery charges. The son attempted suicide but later confessed it was a play for attention. When the boy was finally sent to a reform school, the patient felt considerable relief and became noticeably calmer. Although the staff advised him to remain hospitalized for several weeks he found reasons to leave. It was felt that he would probably make a fairly good adjustment.

P. Hypo.	M:25:M:20	+5	217386′-	2:12:12
P. React. Depr.		—27	2317′68–9(65)	4:6:14

The admission complaints centered around headaches, nervousness, and many other somatic symptoms which made it impossible for the patient to work. About two years before admission the patient had had a nervous breakdown which came on very suddenly while he was working. Weakness, a severe headache, and extreme nervousness were followed by malaise, chills, and fever which the patient diagnosed as "flu." As an aftermath of the illness the man became very depressed, wanted to commit suicide, and tried to get his wife and child to do the same. In the months after this attack he had many periods of depression with frequent crying spells and he became very sensitive to noise. From that time on he suffered from headaches, nervousness, palpitation, various chest and abdomen pains, and a painful sensation that radiated from the back of his neck to his head.

One of eight siblings, the patient was brought up by a very strict father who gave him no spending money and who refused to allow him to leave the farm for dates or other pastimes. His mother had died when he was very young, and the patient had been considerably neglected by a series of housekeepers and his father's second wife. When he was 10 years old he had had intercourse with his stepsister, and the relationship had continued three or four times a year until his marriage at the age of 23 to a girl with whom he was not in love. She was an intelligent, sensible girl and a good worker, and they had made a relatively good adjustment, but the wife became pregnant sooner than they had desired, and this, together with the increased work and responsibility, had helped precipitate the patient's nervous breakdown. Often irritated by his two children, he had never felt very attached to them. Never very ambitious or energetic, he had often daydreamed and had read books on "will power." Although he was religious and read the Bible regularly, he did not believe in churches. A serious and not very happy individual, he had always been ill at ease with people. Apparently heterosexual in his sexual practices to an adequate degree, he worried about masturbation and about what he thought were homosexual tendencies, although he did not admit to any actual homosexual experience.

On admission his thoughts were mostly of his illness, with some worries about debts. Recognizing in a general way that he was psychologically ill, he was sincere, cooperative, and appeared to want help, but he insisted that the basis for his complaints was somatic. Although he lost some of his nervousness and learned to control his headaches by relaxing his neck muscles, he left the hospital too soon to have made much therapeutic progress with his basic emotional conflicts, of which he had no clear realization. He was anxious to get out of the hospital and solve things for himself, and while it was possible that he might be able to work and to get along fairly well, a relapse was probable in view of the long-standing neurosis and insufficient therapy.

Ps. M-D., Depr. F:49:M:25 +15 217'3<u>86</u>–(53) 6:3:13

The presenting complaints for this woman were highlighted by depression, loss of memory, fatigue, and apathy. The illness had begun four years earlier with vague memory loss, headaches, constipation, and mild depression. These symptoms partly coincided with her son's induction into the army. After his departure she neglected housework and garden duties which she had always kept up well in the past, and she spent several periods of one to three months in bed. Partly recovered from this first attack she again became depressed five months before the present admission, went to bed, and completely neglected her duties. Except for one depressed period in her late twenties she had not experienced other attacks.

She was a little below average in intelligence, but a most adequate person. She was described as cheerful, energetic, kind, a good housekeeper. Her interests included fishing and other outdoor activities, sewing, chicken raising, and a flower garden. Married at 24, she had twin daughters and a son, all of whom were married. Her husband died after the onset of the present spell. One of the daughters had become pregnant out of wedlock and the patient believed that worry over this event had contributed to her depression.

When admitted, the patient showed marked psychomotor retardation. She offered no spontaneous speech and only after much questioning would she answer at all. She realized that she was not her usual self but the apathy was so deep that she volunteered nothing more. After a series of six electroshock treatments she became more active and took an interest in her surroundings. Just before discharge she became anxious to leave and to return to home duties. At discharge she appeared fairly well recovered from the present illness but it was believed likely that she would experience another attack.

Ps. M-D., Depr. M:47:M:52 +1 21738'649-(49) 7:8:13
P. Hypo.

The patient had experienced extreme anxiety for a year. This was accompanied by pain in his legs and abdomen and by headaches. The symptoms had gradually increased in severity as the patient, who was a truck driver, had increased his hours of work, taking little rest and eating meals irregularly in an attempt to distract himself. He began to drink excessively. He finally stopped work and developed still more physical complaints for which he was treated without success. Losing all interest in people and normal activities, he preferred, according to his wife, to sit home alone.

The patient attended school through the eighth grade and was reported to be quick at learning. He worked on his father's farm for a while and after his marriage farmed on his own until he failed; he then became a truck driver and up to the time of his illness did well, was steady, and had shown no aberrant behavior.

On admission his thoughts were chiefly centered around his somatic complaints. He thought perhaps these symptoms were due to syphilis which he might have contracted during his recent drunken period. He appeared apathetic and depressed and said that he had considered suicide. He had no insight into the possibility that his pain and other somatic symptoms resulted from anything but simple overwork. He was cooperative but slow. With time his depression gradually lessened and he became friendly and more cheerful. He was given reassurance about the syphilis, and his bodily pains decreased although they did not entirely disappear. Electroshock treatments were used along with the hospitalization and reassurance. Since he had two sons in the service, the end of the war brought relief. He began to look forward to working again and appeared quite well at the time of discharge. Except for the usual possibility of recurrence of these symptoms, it seemed likely that he would be able to continue satisfactorily.

P. React. Depr. F:25:M:43 +8 2'<u>174</u>- 6:2:17
Paranoid
Suicidal

The patient was admitted because of frequent crying spells, refusal to eat, and threats of suicide. The symptoms apparently began about two weeks before admission, on Christmas Eve, when she became irritable, cried easily, and refused to eat. On one occasion she lay in bed beside her two children and instructed her husband to pour kerosene all around them so that they "might end it all." At another time she told her husband she "would be better off dead." Before admission she improved to the extent that when urged she would eat. However, she continued to be depressed, cried many hours, and was unable to sleep at night. A year before admission she had had a similar attack which had lasted two weeks. There was no known precipitating factor for either of these episodes.

The patient graduated from high school at 18 and attended normal school for one year. For two years she taught in a rural school and then married and

'2176–98 43

became a housewife. Her ability seemed to be slightly above average and she was able to handle money. She liked to read and enjoyed singing in the church choir but her interests were narrow and limited. Known as a shy and sensitive person, she confided in no one and was extremely dependent upon her family. She gave up her religious activities, which had been quite extensive, after her marriage. She and her husband engaged in intercourse before their marriage, and the marriage followed a pregnancy. Pampered somewhat by her parents and siblings, she had led a happy and sheltered life as a child. Her husband proved to be a poor provider and kept changing jobs. In addition to financial problems there was sexual incompatibility. The husband accused her of frigidity and threatened frequently to "go out and find myself another woman." The patient professed she still loved him and she was obviously fond of the children and a good mother. Her family had disapproved of her marriage and was unsympathetic toward her troubles.

On admission she refused at first to talk about her present illness but after several interviews she did admit that she worried about finances and felt disappointment that her husband had not found work. Refusing to discuss the sexual incompatibility she believed she was being punished for indulging in sex before marriage. At first she showed delusions of reference and of persecution, and was suspicious of the entire staff. She believed the food was poisoned and that everyone was spying on her. She was, however, well oriented and in general her personality was intact. She harbored thoughts of guilt and suicide, showed psychomotor retardation, and dressed carelessly. Unless urged she would not eat. If left alone she would lie on her bed for hours without moving. One week after admission she exhibited a marked change of behavior. She entered the lounge voluntarily and seemed cheerful. This improvement lasted two or three days and then she again became depressed and sullen. For one month she refused to adjust to hospital life, sitting in her room day after day. During the next two weeks she gradually began to recover and became her usual self. During hospitalization she gained some insight into her problems but since nothing could be done to change her pattern effectively, it was thought probable her difficulties would be repeated.

P. React. Depr. Deteriorated | M:56:M:6 | +3 | '2176–98 43 | 5:1:12

A severe depression accompanied by irritability and marked anorexia, which seemed to be due to both an aversion to food and a vague abdominal discomfort, were the admission complaints. The attack began about a month before admission when the patient was charged with collusion and misappropriation of funds in connection with his job. However, members of his family and others had noticed over the past few years an increasing irritability, a tendency to complain about insignificant details, and an inability to receive orders gracefully or to carry on a concise conversation.

Some three or four years before admission the patient's brother had died, naming him administrator for the estate, and there had been some question about legal action in connection with misappropriation of funds at that time. Shortly afterward the patient was found in a closed garage with the car running, and he was revived with difficulty. Cerebral damage probably occurred at this time. The patient was born in Sweden and his schoolwork was somewhat irregular. He completed two or three grades in that country, and he continued up to the "fifth reader" after immigration. He worked at many different jobs, finally becoming an embalmer. The income from this was always sufficient to support his family fairly well, and he had sent one of his daughters through college and was preparing to send the other. He was described as having always been easily upset and subject to bouts of nausea and vomiting, with the tendency increasing in recent years. He had worried excessively, especially when someone in his family became ill. A hard, intensive worker, he had been a generous giver as far as his family was concerned, and he had many close friends.

On admission the patient seemed overwhelmed by his recent difficulties, and while he admitted that he had benefited from certain transactions he insisted that he had not meant to harm anyone. He attributed his trouble in connection with his work to his assistant who, he claimed, had misrepresented him. Much of his time he spent emphasizing his own abilities and degrading the capacities of others. He repeatedly attempted to show the examiner that he had never done anything contrary to orders. No disturbances of mentation were apparent, but he seemingly failed to recognize rather obvious tendencies toward irritability and to face his recent inefficiency at work. Although he admitted he was depressed, he thought that his run-down condition was probably the simple basis for his poor appetite. He denied any suicidal intents, saying, "What would my family do if I committed suicide? If worse comes to worse I can only be sent to a penitentiary." He was rather circumstantial in answering questions, insisting on giving the most minute details. Because of his fearfulness that the examiner would describe his difficulties to others, he had to be constantly reassured. A psychological examination indicated mental deterioration and this factor was probably important, but the whole reaction was atypical.

P. Hypo. M:40:M:22 +4 217′638–9 4:3:10

The admission complaints of this patient were irritability, insomnia, and numerous somatic symptoms. The illness began three years earlier when he gradually became dissatisfied with his work as a truck driver. Eventually he was unable to tolerate sustained work, was easily disturbed by noises, and developed aches, shortness of breath, and anorexia. His business slumped and he was obliged to accept day labor on W.P.A. Later he became uncommunicative and "demanded to be left alone." Episodically he felt depressed, "like blowing my brains out." He quarreled with his foreman and reported to the management that he "would not work under such conditions." From then on his family had to be supported by special relief. He came to demand more and more financial aid and in general projected his dissatisfaction upon the community's apparent indifference to his illness.

There was no history of a previous mental upset or health problems. He completed the eighth grade at the age of 14 and was said to have ranked in the upper part of his class. Out of school, he started to learn the printing trade but did not continue this training. Always ambitious, he wanted to be a self-supporting farmer, but most of the time he worked as a truck driver. He was regarded as honest but never aggressive; he had many friends. Before his marriage twenty years before admission he had been a tramp and "saw most of the country." He had five children and there appeared to be no significant marital difficulties.

This man showed considerable concern about his physical state. He listed his ills as "rheumatism, blue spells, a tooth ache, headaches, and jumpiness." He had trouble keeping his mind on one thing, he said, and often had a "million thoughts." People regarded him as lazy, he had heard it said. He seemed unhappy and was irritable and defensive about his reasons for failure. He was without spontaneity and was slow to grasp ideas. There was obvious tension. After two weeks he reported that "something was making him better." Gradually he became sociable and most of the somatic symptoms faded. Episodes of irritability still occurred and occasionally he made critical remarks. His complaints against his home and the relief board persisted. At discharge he was not markedly different but it was expected he would probably be able to continue at a borderline adjustment.

P. Mixed F:32:M:31 +21 2'17 64 938– 2:7:14
Drug Add.

The chief presenting complaint of this patient was insomnia. However, there were other underlying difficulties, among which barbiturate habituation was prominent. She had severe gastrointestinal upsets, which had suggested an ulcer or appendicitis. She also had spells of coughing. She became irritable and tearful on slight provocation. These complaints, while emphasized recently were the culmination of a long history of neurotic symptoms.

Above average in intelligence, the patient had been a medical student at one time before her marriage. She believed she was making good progress at that time and thought she would make a great success in medicine. Socially she had never been at ease and had not been popular with boys although she craved their company. She had a number of unusually strong attachments to girl friends. Her marital adjustment had been stormy. Her husband was also a graduate student, and while in many ways exceedingly brilliant, he was unreliable. The patient had been moody and singularly lacking in good judgment in social relationships. She obviously considered herself intellectually superior to most people, including her husband.

When admitted the patient was cooperative and pleasant, but tense and tearful at times. She readily agreed to attempt sleep without the use of sedatives. Her psychological trends were chiefly centered around personal affairs and the present illness. During the first weeks in the hospital she slept little but spent most of her time in bed. After that she began to sleep four to seven hours with occasional sleepless nights. At the end of a month she was doing well and was discharged as probably free from the barbiturate habituation at least. She had many deep-seated neurotic tendencies, however, and there was every reason to expect that the hospitalization had brought about no particular change in her basic problem.

P. Hypo. M:21:S:42 +1 2'<u>17</u>83–9 7:4:20

The chief complaints of this patient were weakness, difficulty in concentration, and loss of memory. These symptoms appeared gradually over a two-year period following a routine physical examination that revealed the presence of sugar and albumin in the urine. After this, he had immediately noted weakness and fatigue. These continued, and eventually he felt fully as unrested in the morning as at bedtime. Unable to do a full day's work, he also became listless, dull, and sleepy, nothing interested him, and he couldn't remember things. Fearing the possibility of diabetes, he consulted numerous physicians but was not relieved by their reassurances. The snapping of his joints caused him to think he might have tuberculosis of the joints, but though he would not accept the fact, this diagnosis was definitely ruled out. Concern about his physical condition resulted in periods of depression.

The patient's intelligence fell at the low edge of the normal range. All his life he had lived on one farm, ultimately becoming the sole support of his mother. Always a shy and introverted individual, he had never made special friends and had had no relationships with girls. Content to stay at home evenings with his mother or to go alone in his car to a movie, his range of interests was narrow, centering chiefly around farm work. He showed a mild interest in radio programs and movies. The mother was a mild diabetic and somewhat like the boy, toward whom she was oversolicitous. An older brother was insane.

Of fair general appearance, the patient was open, natural, and easily accessible in examinations. He seemed calm, happy, and composed, and showed a normal amount of activity. His answers to questions were complete, he appeared well oriented and smiled readily. He believed that all his difficulties were physical, that they could not be "in the mind," and he was concerned with the possible diseases he might have. In the hospital he changed little. His complaints of tiredness, listlessness, and nervousness continued. As a matter of fact the verbal patterns persisted without manifest symptoms. He was observed playing strenuous games for hours without obvious fatigue. At other times, however, he appeared listless and dull. Almost daily there was a periodic fluctuation in his temperature and the possibility of an organic basis for some of the complaints was not ruled out. At discharge he was only mildly interested in returning home, although he did express interest in resuming farm work. It was thought that if his environment could be altered, specifically if he were to separate from his mother, cultivate friends, and acquire hobbies or interests, a good share of his symptoms might be overcome.

P. Anxiety State F:15:S:23 +2 '217836–9 (57) 6:3:24
Schizoid

The symptoms dated back one month to an attack of "stomach flu" that was followed by stomach discomfort, sleeplessness, bad dreams, and loss of appetite. The patient talked in her sleep and would awaken to call her parents after a bad dream. During the day she was tired and listless, unable to apply herself to any task. She was lonely and restless. A physician who saw her could find no organic basis for her somatic discomfort.

The girl had completed the eighth grade in a country school and then had stayed at home with her parents and an older sister. She had been friendly, cheerful, active, interested in reading books and magazines; she had done well in her schoolwork but had no desire to continue further. She had always enjoyed going to parties but had had few opportunities, since she had lived in isolated places. She was the youngest of six children. The father was shiftless and a poor provider. The parents had not encouraged the patient to continue school or look for a job but seemed to have a protective attitude toward her.

The physical and neurological examinations were noncontributory. She was chiefly concerned with herself and her problems. She said she was a bother at home, was "just silly or something," and was receiving more attention than her illness warranted. She recognized that her personality had changed but could not account for the change. There were no obvious defects of sensorium or intellect. She appeared withdrawn and apathetic with occasional inappropriate laughter and smiling. There was very rapid improvement. After a few days she took an interest in recreational facilities and in her appearance. Her appetite was good, her sleep sound and uninterrupted. Her somatic complaints disappeared. She began to take an active interest in making constructive plans for the future. The staff felt that the problem had a very definite situational background and before she was discharged plans were made to get her away from the home environment in the expectation that she would then make an adequate adjustment.

P. Mixed M:34:S 217843'69–(53) 3:6:9
P. Psychas.

This veteran came to the hospital voluntarily because of "extreme nervousness," stomach upsets, insomnia, and anxiety.

Adopted when he was an infant, the patient knew nothing of his own parents. His adoptive parents, as far as known, provided a good home and were consistent and understanding in managing the patient when he was a child. Schooling, following completion of high school, consisted of one year at a business college. Until he was nearly 10 years of age he was bothered by enuresis. A friendly, agreeable man, he had for years been troubled with feelings of inferiority, self-consciousness, oversensitiveness, perfectionistic tendencies, anxiety, and guilt feelings about sex matters. He had been considerably preoccupied with sex and had never made an adequate heterosexual adjustment. Over the years since adolescence he had had a few homosexual experiences and had come to believe he must be a "homosexual."

The diagnosis arrived at was psychoneurosis, mixed type. During individual psychotherapy over a period of six weeks, the patient verbalized freely and appeared to gain considerable insight. He arrived at the conclusion that his homosexual inclinations were of a "substitute" nature. He was discharged upon completion of psychotherapy. A letter from the patient about six months after his discharge indicated that he was making a satisfactory adjustment. Although he was still bothered to some extent with stomach upsets and anxiety, he felt that he had better control of himself.

Ps. Senile Deteriorated M:53:M:18 —1 2'1786– 4:5:7

The patient's presenting complaints included bleeding from the bowels on exertion, increased nervousness, irritability, seclusiveness, and a lack of interest in his surroundings. Fourteen years before admission the patient had been told that the difficulty with his bowels was a rectal stricture. During the past three years he had insisted that the bleeding was so bad he was unable to work, although this did not appear to be consistent with organic findings. He showed increased irritability, and it had become so difficult for him to adjust to others that he had not only withdrawn from all social life, but he had become exceedingly provoked at his wife's social contacts. He accused her of intimacies with another man.

He appeared to be inferior intellectually, having completed only three years of schooling, and those with difficulty. After that he had maintained himself in odd jobs. In the last year he had been supported by his wife. He had never been especially ambitious, and he was unusually closely attached to his parents. The patient and his wife were compatible. They had four children. His home life had been fairly pleasant until the present illness.

A number of childish jokes which the patient made in the hospital, and over which he laughed heartily, seemed appropriately classified as witzelsucht. There was some defect of recent memory, and there was definite psychometric evidence of organic brain deterioration, but there were no gross disturbances of sensorium or intellect. Although the man was childish he was perfectly adaptable in the hospital situation. He refused encephalography and all other procedures that might have more clearly indicated whether or not an organic brain disease was present. During his stay in the hospital there was little if any change. He was discharged with a poor prognosis.

P. Mixed   M:45:M:30   +2   21786'34–(67)   3:8:14
P. Psychas.

The patient first became ill about eighteen months before admission when he suffered an acute pain after being hospitalized for an acid burn on his eye sustained while working as a machinist's helper. The panic was characterized by fear of death, agitation, profuse perspiration, headache, and numbness of the head; it subsided after a couple of hours, but thereafter he was subject to "crying jags," headaches, and fatigue. At times he could not work. For a while he was hospitalized and given electroshock treatment without benefit. He thought he was going insane and was irritable and subject to temper outbursts. He also developed minor somatic complaints such as "strained back." Lately he had experienced an obsessive urge to hurt someone.

He contracted gonorrhea at age 21 and apparently was treated adequately. He had been diagnosed as having a duodenal ulcer five years before admission, and he had taken barbiturates for sleep over a number of years. He was foreign born, coming to this country at age 11, and as a result of his language handicap he was 15 before he completed the eighth grade. His interests had never been broad and his social activities were definitely limited. A pleasant person, he was moderately shy and retiring. His wife said that he had many friends but tired of them easily and sought others. He had been an industrious worker until the present illness. He had always relied heavily on his mother for advice even in minor matters.

He appeared well composed in the hospital. His mental content centered around his presenting complaints of depression and sleeplessness. He expressed compulsive thoughts about hurting someone, but these were indefinite, as to both the method and the person. He was intact in general sensorium and intellect, coherent though somewhat circumstantial in speech. He appeared depressed but was friendly with other patients and in general cooperative though reluctant to join in group activities. He felt that what he needed was rest, not psychotherapeutic help. He gradually got a little better in the hospital and was discharged to his home with the expectation that he would in time probably recover from the present attack.

P. Mixed   F:50:M:47   +34   '2183 479–   7:3:14
Ps. Invol. Melan.   F:50:M:46   +14   123'8–94   7:3:9
Ps. Invol. Melan.   F:50:M:37   +27   21837'4–   7:8:15

The chief complaints of this patient were headaches, difficulty in swallowing, and hot flashes. The illness appeared a year earlier when the patient began to lose interest in things and was unable to perform household tasks. She lost weight and had feelings of oppression in her head, throat discomfort, and the like. There was also a degree of depression. She was irritable and asocial, became an almost total invalid, and developed an intense dislike of her only child.

There was a vague history of a similar attack four years before admission.

Otherwise, the history contributed little that seemed significant. An intelligent person, cooperative and helpful toward her neighbors, the patient had been sociable and had made many friends. She was said to be meticulous in her housework, tense, high-strung. Her chief enjoyment was in managing, and before marriage she had "run" a store.

In the hospital she showed considerable hypochondriacal concern, but there was no gross disturbance of personality. Although she appeared depressed there was no evidence of a deep melancholia. She was friendly and cooperative, engaged in the ward activities, and behaved in an apparently normal fashion. At discharge she seemed to be much improved and it was felt that she would likely continue to improve. Five months later, however, she was back in the hospital. Comfortable at home for a few days, she soon relapsed into the same behavior that she had shown before the last admission. At first placed in a rest home, she behaved in such an aggressive and overbearing manner that she was asked to move. Occasionally she experienced a brief normal period, but always she had a relapse. In the second hospitalization she admitted considerable dissatisfaction with her husband. She had married him late in life after she herself had had a successful career in business. Her husband was quiet and she could find little fault with him, but he had been "not at all exciting" and sexually not very satisfactory. Because her only sexual satisfaction came from autoerotic practices, which conflicted with her rather rigid code of behavior, she felt guilty. Again she improved enormously during the hospitalization and was discharged but was soon readmitted to go on to a state hospital.

Ps. Sz., Simple M:16:S:31 +1 218 47'369–(69) 6:10:15

The patient was admitted because of bizarre and inappropriate behavior following a referral to juvenile court by his parents on a complaint of incorrigibility. Since the age of 10 or 11 years he had exhibited a progressive loss of interest in his usual activities and had become increasingly seclusive and preoccupied. He was irritable when disturbed by anyone and would become agitated and yell and swear at his parents if they tried to arouse him. He masturbated openly, was generally neglectful of his appearance and developed a distorted interest in magic and mysticism. When his parents found they could do nothing with him they called him to the attention of the juvenile court and he was referred to a psychiatrist. While awaiting psychiatric hospitalization he had evident hallucinations.

The patient was an only child who had lived in rather crowded, shabby circumstances with his parents till the age of 6, when he went to live with his grandparents. He began school at 7, had to repeat the second grade, and continued to do poorly, finally dropping out after reaching the tenth grade. He was intellectually in the low normal range. After quitting school he worked at various jobs. Then his father arranged for him to attend a vocational school but he failed to report. His mother had him placed in a foster home where he remained for a week and then disappeared. He was found in a hotel after he had gone to a police station saying that he had no money and no place to stay. This led to his being taken to juvenile court. As a child he was described as "pouty and stubborn," he had had outbursts of temper, and before age 10 he had shown "peculiar" interests. Always characterized by resistance and rebellion, he gradually became suspicious of everyone.

On admission to the hospital he was found to be a thin and undernourished boy, withdrawn to the point of negativism, blocked in answering questions, and showing inappropriate affects. As a sample of his behavior, he disturbed other patients by lying awake at night, giggling and laughing to himself. He became involved in a scuffle with other patients because of this and had to be put into a disturbed ward. Extremely immature and poorly adjusted to every aspect of his environment, he could not be approached through psychotherapy and he was sent to a state hospital.

Alcoholism M:27:S 218′63–79 (49) 7:11:23

This young man, a college student, came in with complaints centered around a fear of contact with people and alcoholism. For only two periods since he was 6 years old had he been able to associate himself with others, and both of these were of short duration. During service in the navy two years before he had become so disturbed that he allegedly feigned mental illness and was sent to a veterans' hospital. For the past months he had been drinking continually and saw almost no one.

The eldest of five children, the patient had a rather drab, isolated childhood. His father was described as an extremely sensitive person, his mother inadequate as a housekeeper and mother. One sister had been surgically treated for diagnosed schizophrenia. The patient had not married and had never had a girl friend.

During the period of treatment he dressed in an unkempt fashion, apparently in an effort to demean himself so that no attention would be paid to him and nothing expected of him. At first he required alcohol in order to talk with the therapist, but later he was able to carry on an interview without this aid. Treatment consisted of approximately twenty individual interviews over a six-month period, participation in group therapy (ten sessions), and one sodium amytal interview. Some superficial improvement took place, but before the time for discharge he showed a relapse. Following his own suggestion he was transferred to a veterans' hospital and there, with "push" therapy, he again showed improvement. Eventually he was discharged and relapsed almost immediately. C. K. A.

Ps. M-D., Depr. F:44:M:43 +1 2′1873–9 (53) 4:6:15
P. Psychas. −9 683′127–9 (61) 5:9:10

This woman's complaints were depression, feelings of unworthiness, fear that she might kill herself or others, and also an unpleasant "pressure" on the top of her head. The onset of the symptoms was dated at three months before admission when she suddenly became depressed and feared she would hurt herself or her six-year-old son. She was unable to do her housework and was afraid her children would be taken from her because of her unworthiness. She told her husband she thought she was "going crazy," and she hid all the rope in the house to prevent herself from using it to harm herself or her children.

Since the age of 21, the patient had experienced periods of depression, lasting from three months to a year. As a child she was apparently normal and she completed the eighth grade at the age of 13. She enjoyed school but left it to help on the farm. Described as shy and slow in making friends, she had a tendency to daydream. Toward others she was kind and thoughtful. From her earliest years she took disappointments unusually hard. Her childhood was clouded by family difficulties climaxed by her father's suicide by hanging, following his attempt, in the presence of the patient, to shoot his wife. The patient and her husband appeared to be compatible and fairly well adjusted to each other.

On admission to the hospital the patient expressed utter hopelessness about herself. She showed marked psychomotor retardation but was attentive and neat. She was given nine electroshock treatments and these produced eight seizures. Although improvement was slight there was a steady gain, and the history of the past depressions indicated that she would completely recover, with time, from this attack. However, it was felt likely that she would have recurrent attacks, possibly of increasing severity.

P. React. Depr. F:41:M:15 +4 '23–6(47) 3:1:16

The chief admission complaint was insomnia. Although always a light sleeper, the patient had never experienced real insomnia until a year before admission. At that time she made a poor recovery from a hysterectomy, though from a somatic standpoint this operation apparently was satisfactory. The continuing symptoms centered chiefly around pains and insomnia. These were disappearing gradually until four months before admission when an appendectomy was performed. This operation was satisfactory surgically, but the patient's psychological state showed a definite relapse.

Her past health had been good; there were no evidences of instability. A college graduate, she had been a teacher until her marriage. Although active in social affairs she was ill at ease in a crowd and somewhat shy. She required a great deal of sympathy. With high ethical and moral standards, she was always punctilious in fulfilling responsibilities to home and society.

Primarily concerned with the insomnia, the patient felt that now she was in the hospital she would get well. Her explanation for the insomnia was that "nerves were cut during an operation." She talked freely, answered questions directly, and in general presented a good appearance. There was no evidence of gross personality disturbances. During her stay in the hospital she occasionally slept seven or eight hours but more often nearer to four. The treatments employed were hydrotherapy and reassurance. She was cheerful and responsive and continued to show gradual improvement to the time of discharge. It was felt that the prognosis was good in view of the relatively clear history.

Ps. Paranoid M:58:M:17 +4 2′31–(55) 4:5:14

Delusions and depressive moods had first appeared in this patient about four years before admission. He had also become unusually demanding sexually, and when his wife refused sexual relations with him, he beat her. Other manifestations of his illness included hunger strikes, frequent crying spells, and religious fanaticism. He became so irritable that when a speaker on the radio said something with which he did not agree, he pounded the radio and stamped on the floor. Three weeks before admission he had assaulted his wife, accusing her of flirting with other men. He also accused the tax assessors of being "out to get him."

The medical history was essentially negative, and he had had no other nervous breakdowns. Although he was of high normal intelligence, his education had been terminated at the third grade, and he had worked on a farm all his life. He had always been irritable and bad-tempered. He had also been very religious. Before the present illness he and his wife had been very attached to each other.

The pattern of delusions was persistent in the hospital, and he frequently cried while being questioned. He was intact in sensorium and intellect, and there was no good evidence for organic brain deterioration. Apparently there were no hallucinatory visions or voices. No specific therapy was undertaken, and he was discharged unchanged to be transferred to a state hospital for further treatment and study.

Ps. Invol. Melan. F:53:M:23 —28 231476′89–(66) 3:3:15
P. Mixed

This patient was admitted with depression expressed in frequent crying spells, loss of weight, and diminished interest in life. The depression, which had begun two years before, gradually incapacitated her in the home and upset family members so that hospitalization became necessary. The patient stated that she had exerted great effort to control her emotions, but the harder she tried the more upset she became. She also had many somatic complaints such as "soreness" on the top of her head. There were factors, such as the marriage of an only son, which may have contributed to the depression. However, it was noted that her crying spells were precipitated by inconsequential happenings, and, in general, her home environment was free of pressures.

This patient's history was remarkably clear from the standpoint of significant psychiatric findings. Described as cheerful and "always able to see the bright side of life," she had enjoyed outdoor sports and was interested in current affairs and in her family. She had never been known as moody. In the marital situation there was a mild degree of strain because of the considerable amounts of money the husband spent for alcohol. Their one son was apparently well adjusted and married satisfactorily. Her personality began to change with the onset of the menopause and since the appearance of the physical signs of this event her physician had been treating her with hormone injections and phenobarbital. As noted above, she also began to be irritable and anxious, and along with endocrine treatments she had been given reassurance suggestion.

In the hospital, she appeared drawn and haggard. She showed some appropriate affect but talked freely and clearly. Her sensorium and intellect were unimpaired. She was friendly and sociable. She had a marked fear of electroshock treatment but she was given five shocks which brought a considerable change in her behavior. She refused to take more. The history of good adjustment before these complaints led staff members to predict at the time of discharge that she might obtain permanent relief.

P. Psychas. M:48:M:2 +1 231'478–9 (57) 7:3:17
P. React. Depr.
Suicidal

The presenting complaint of this patient was pain in his back and in both legs. Ten years before admission, following an extramarital sexual experience, the patient noticed a sore on his genitals. This cleared up spontaneously, and he did not seek medical counsel. He grew to believe that he had contracted gonorrhea, and he felt guilt and shame. At the same time pain appeared which the patient decided must have been caused by the gonorrhea. He consulted numerous physicians and chiropractors, but without getting relief. Shortly before admission to the hospital his symptoms became so severe that he thought he was going to die. Ideas of suicide also obsessed him.

A mail clerk, this man had in general a good background. He appeared to be of average intelligence, was friendly, and got along well with people. He was interested in his job and family, especially his grandson. A man with set methods of doing things, he followed a definite pattern in daily activities. The marital situation appeared good and the family was congenial and happy.

The patient was entirely adequate psychologically. He was friendly, cooperative, interested in his surroundings and in the examination. Somewhat nervous and depressed, he replied when addressed but did not offer easy conversation. He had no insight about the delusory nature of some of his complaints. He discussed the problem of suicide and called it a definite possibility for him a few weeks before admission. Little progress was made with the primary pattern of complaints during hospitalization. Despite every assurance about his general physical condition and about the absence of gonorrhea his complaints persisted. After a few days the man was discharged at his wife's request.

Ps. M-D., Depr.	M:50:M:40	+3	2'31478–96 (61)	9:1:23
Paranoid		+27	89'764–2X (65)	2:20:8
Ps. M-D., Depr.	M:51:M:28	+1	2'3478– (53)	7:0:20

The admission of this patient with severe depression of about two months' duration was the latest of several such episodes, with seclusiveness, poor memory, inability to work, and somatic complaints the outstanding characteristics of the depression. When he was working, he misplaced tools; and he was convinced that people watching him noticed the poor quality of his work. He complained of failing memory; he slowed down physically and mentally; he suffered from insomnia; there was loss of appetite; and in general he lost contact with his surroundings. Lacking energy, he found it very difficult even to dress himself or go to meals. His speech was retarded and incoherent at times.

A year before admission there had been a similar attack from which he had recovered after six electroshock treatments. Until this first attack, his behavior had always been normal. His intelligence was average. A shy person, not socially aggressive, withdrawn, and moderately religious, he had always been kind and had never lost his temper. A premarital dependency on his mother was later transferred to his wife. His general adjustment to society was adequate although he was known as a "drifter," and at best he held only semiskilled jobs. Throughout his life there had been a history of cyclic mood swings in which he moved from periods of elation to periods of depression.

On admission he showed rather severe psychomotor retardation. He did not appear to be delusional. He had no paranoid ideas, nor was he suicidal. His sensorium and intellect were intact, and he had some insight into the depression. There was marked apathy, but he was cooperative and expressed the hope that he might be "well again." After shock therapy, which brought about rather marked change, he became more disoriented, careless, and talkative. He showed some regression, answered questions foolishly, and was occasionally euphoric, uncooperative, loud, and demanding. With the continuation of the shock treatments his behavior became more acceptable and five days after the last of the eleven treatments he was discharged with almost complete remission of his symptoms. At that time it was felt that he would probably have another depression. Twenty months later the patient returned to the hospital. Following his first discharge, he had been euphoric and unstable for about three months, then had begun to slip into another depression which persisted until the second admission. He was discharged after seven shock treatments and was to return to the outpatient clinic for supportive care. The prognosis about a further relapse was very guarded.

P. Mixed F:28:S:40 +7 231'64789– 7:4:17

Unhappiness, headaches, dizziness, and a "feeling of something moving in my forehead" were the chief problems of this patient on admission. This illness had begun about eight months before admission when the patient's brother and his wife came to live in a trailer next to the house in which she and her mother lived. Mingled with her jealousy of the couple was the feeling she had lost her mother's confidence. She began to sleep poorly, preferring to do needless household chores far into the night. "Fainting spells" appeared and occurred two or three times a week. Consulting a physician three weeks before admission, she was told that she might have a brain tumor. After this she became markedly overactive and apprehensive and felt that life was no longer worthwhile.

Since late childhood the patient had shown a multitude of neurotic tendencies. Most of these appeared to have been aggravated by the mother's attitude. Sensitive and secretive, the patient had never confided in anyone except her mother and her music teacher. Socially she was not completely inadequate. Well liked by members of a business girls' sorority to which she belonged, she was described as overly kind and thoughtful of others but lacking in common sense about financial affairs. After graduating from high school with high honors she obtained a scholarship for college work. She was ambitious to become a doctor. Unable to continue college for financial reasons, she took a job as a statistical clerk in which she made a fairly good salary. As a typical example of her childhood complaints, at age 15 she developed numbness and coldness of the right hand and arm. She had a "funny feeling" in her left eye and her "mouth was drawn over to the left." A physician told her that this was from "studying too hard."

The patient presented an abundance of mental content, composed mainly of references to her unhappy home life, dissatisfaction with her work, and inability to see any prospects for a good future. She said there was nothing left in life for her. She tended to be suspicious of men because her father and two brothers were "worthless." She stated that her only friend was her music teacher who "knows me better than anyone else." She still wanted to be a doctor and "do things for other people." She said that she was an unwanted child but that she was the only one willing to contribute to her mother's maintenance, and this was not appreciated. She strongly resisted accepting any psychological basis for her somatic complaints. She was attentive, cooperative, and friendly, but restless during the examination. Her tone of voice was affected.

She had considerable trouble in adjusting to the ward routine, and she had a brief period of depression in which she cried and objected to medication. In a week most of her headaches had subsided but she was still reluctant to go to occupational therapy and claimed she was unable to walk that far. Before discharge from the hospital she began to take a fairly sensible attitude toward her illness, becoming more cheerful and less irritable. She accepted some of the suggestions about her mode of life and her outlook toward the future brightened. Her mother was advised to persuade the brother and sister-in-law to move before the patient returned home. It was recommended that the patient change her occupation to one with more personal service in it. The prognosis was felt to be fairly good.

P. React. Depr. F:51:W:88 +3 231'674–(53) 6:0:16

P. React. Depr. F:51:W:141 +1 32178'46–9(51) 9:0:17
+60 61273'94–(34) 6:9:11

The patient was first admitted to the medical service because of "pounding" of her heart, increasing nervousness, inability to sleep, weakness, fatigue, tremor, and other symptoms, and after a three-week period she was transferred to the psychiatric unit. The illness, which began approximately three months before admission, had apparently been precipitated by the death of her aged father the previous month. She began to have difficulty in breathing while lying down, and complained of a crushing sensation in her chest. She cried easily, was depressed, and had a peculiar habit of sighing in a hopeless manner. Her health had always been poor. A frail, weak child, she had been babied by her parents because of her many sicknesses, and as an adult she had undergone a number of major surgical procedures. Two years before the present pattern appeared she had had a "nervous breakdown."

An eighth-grade graduate, she had enjoyed school and had done well, but she had stopped to do housework and was married at age 17. Her intelligence was average. She had always exercised good judgment in handling money and in planning. A friendly person, she was at ease with others and was well liked in her community, but she worried a good deal without being able to reveal the source of her worry to others. Those who knew her well described her as an extremely dependent and insecure person. She had been particularly dependent upon her parents, and to some extent on her husband, all of whom were now dead.

Physical and neurological examinations were essentially negative, though there was some evidence of an increased basal metabolic rate. Alert and well oriented, she appeared nervous and slightly anxious, and spoke longingly of going to live with her son. Any other prospects for the future were rejected. She did not feel that her physical complaints had any emotional basis. There was a labile emotional tone with an undercurrent of depression. Her attitude was one of complaining hopelessness. Gradually improving, she began to sleep better and to make more definite and realistic plans, and it was felt at discharge that if she could accept the reality of her situation and find needed protection she would make an adequate adjustment with mild ups and downs. A short time later she suffered a relapse, however, and was readmitted.

P. Hys. F:37:M:14 +1 23'17–94 6:5:9

For the last ten years the patient had complained of recurring attacks of numbness, weakness, and clumsiness. Treatment alleviated the symptoms, which were usually noticed about two hours after the patient had gone to bed and which tended to last for about an hour. Rubbing the upper extremities or immersing them in cold water gave her some relief.

Except for surgical correction of a congenital club foot thirteen years before admission the past medical history was noncontributory. An eighth-grade graduate, this energetic woman had always been a good manager and an efficient homemaker. It had been difficult for her to meet people, and she was uncomfortable in social gatherings. She was easily frightened. Married for eight years, the patient had two children although she had been sexually frigid.

In the hospital she gave a clear and consecutive account of the course of her illness, which she felt was probably due to nervousness, and although not positively worried about her condition she was anxious to have the etiology explained. The patient regretted her sexual frigidity and had no insight into its cause. It worried her that during her last pregnancy, two years before admission, she had had a momentary desire to kill her daughter. Seemingly a rather adequate person, she was entirely normal in all general behavior in the hospital and she entered well into activities. Talking about her problems with the staff was apparently somewhat beneficial, and at the time of discharge she was to some extent improved. Since hospitalization was not long enough to have permitted any very real change in her personality, it was felt that the attacks would probably recur.

Ps. M-D., Mixed F:38:D:49 +6 231746'89– 5:1:17
Suicidal

The patient was admitted complaining of shaking spells and rectal pains which radiated through her whole body. She feared she was losing her mind. The symptoms had begun a couple of months before admission with tinnitus, general fatigue, and feelings of tension. Concerned about her constipation, she resorted to much self-medication. All her activities slowed up, she lost weight, and insomnia was acute.

Well above average in intelligence, this patient graduated from high school at 16, then enrolled in a short business course. She did office work until her marriage, which lasted from age 22 to 30 and culminated in divorce. She described her husband as "a brilliant screwball," who came from an intelligent, well-educated family which was riddled with neuropathy. He incurred gambling debts and was an alcoholic. Their incompatibility centered chiefly in his irresponsibility. There was one son and since the divorce the patient and this boy had lived with her father. The patient contributed nothing to her income, depending wholly on her alimony. In the handling of her affairs, she was malcontent and ineffectual. She would get excited and "lose her head when company comes." She had a pessimistic outlook. She chose friends with questionable reputations and since the divorce had had a number of sexual alliances.

There was evidence of marked tension, and the patient was constantly in motion, shaking, picking at her fingers, tapping her feet, and the like. Her mental content was almost exclusively devoted to bodily concern. "I know I got too tired. I must have injured the nerves in my rectum. There's constant twitching and burning there which shoots up to the back of my head. Oh, I'm so sick. It's torture. I'm losing my mind." The mood was characterized by anxiety and apprehension. She would collapse on the floor and "flop" against the wall. She harbored the idea that she had done irreparable harm to herself, and no amount of reasoning or reassurance could shake this belief. On the ward one day she swallowed some scouring powder to "end this torture," reporting the event two hours later. Then she was certain she was going blind or that her arms were becoming numb from the poison. Another day she swallowed a straightened paper clip. Although she showed slight progress, she was finally discharged to a state hospital.

B. Psth., Mixed Paranoid F:18:S:21 +8 2317'486-9 7:8:17

Brought from a girl's reform school for evaluation of her heart condition, the admission complaints of this patient were a peculiar mixture of fatigue, shortness of breath, and bad behavior. First placed in a rest home, the girl was found to be an increasing problem as the heart studies proceeded. She kept late hours and got very little rest, was extremely uncooperative, and was a complainer. This pattern of behavior was the reason for referral to the psychiatric hospital.

The patient had her first contact with police just before her ninth birthday. She was counted a nuisance in the neighborhood, used obscene language, and could not get along with her stepfather. Unmanageable, she was placed in a county home school. Eventually she was put on probation but this was canceled when she was found guilty of stealing. In the reform school she was bitter, quarrelsome, impudent, domineering, untruthful, and vulgar. On the more positive side she was neat and showed some improvement in her work habits. Out on parole and while living in a foster home she stole money from the foster mother and engaged in promiscuous sexual activities. Again returned to the reform school she repeatedly stated, "No one loves me any more; it's no use trying to improve me." Her I.Q. was in the low normal range but her grade school work had always been poor. The only vocational history included a period as stenographer when she was untruthful and unreliable.

The evaluation of her heart condition did not justify the extent of her physical complaints although there was indubitable heart damage. Her story was that she had been sent to the reform school because her stepfather and she disagreed about her evening activities. More recent difficulties she attributed to a "heart attack." She said also that worry over her mother's health had contributed to her illness. She saw no reason for being detained in the psychiatric hospital and she heartily disliked most of the doctors. She had many paranoid ideas concerning the administrative staff at the reform school. She ate little, explaining there was "no use in eating."

Toward other patients she was kind and helpful although on the ward in many respects she was uncooperative. She gave the outward appearance of agreeing with statements that "put up a front." It was said of her that she was "fighting the world" and "suffering from feelings of inferiority." However, she continued to project her inadequacies onto others and stated that she would kill herself rather than return to the reform school. On discharge from the school at the age of 21 she planned to tour the country in the car which her mother had promised to buy for her, appearing not to comprehend that her mother could not possibly afford such a car or trip. Her dominating thoughts consisted of fantasy on ways of getting even with some of her acquaintances at the reformatory. No psychotherapeutic approaches were efficacious with this girl. It was recognized that the past few years had been somewhat better than the earlier ones and it was agreed that when she became a few years older she might possibly behave better.

Ps. Senile Deterioration M:75:M:41 +1 231′76–9(49) 8:3:16

The patient was admitted because of fatigue, depression, a tendency to be easily upset, anorexia, insomnia, and a general loss of interest. Two years before admission he had had a similar attack from which he had apparently recovered after hospitalization for two or three weeks, but he had experienced another about a year later from which he had not recovered as quickly, and the depression had continued up to the time of the present admission.

There were no previous nervous upsets in the past history. He had stopped school when he was young to go to work, and subsequently he had become a master mechanic with a considerable amount of responsibility. Five years before admission he had retired on a pension. He had always been active and had taken great interest in the things he did. He got along well with people, was friendly and thoughtful. Outdoor activities such as hunting and fishing were his main interests.

Although he was in good physical and neurological condition, he was retarded and obviously depressed. He worried about everything in general and about his somatic symptoms in particular. He was somewhat disoriented as to time, but was well oriented as to place and person. His intellect seemed affected; his sensorium was intact. He recognized that he was not well but did not clearly understand why. In about two weeks he was more willing to talk, and while he still had complaints, he was less retarded; at the time of discharge he had begun to enter into the life of the ward. He never initiated a conversation but he came to talk readily when a topic was suggested. The prognosis for complete recovery was considered poor, but it seemed likely that he would be able to continue fairly well at home.

P. Mixed F:36:M:10 +5 231′76498– 4:4:10

Eight years before admission this patient underwent an operation that resulted in an artificial menopause. She dated all her complaints from that event. She experienced a train of disorders, hot flashes, pounding of the heart, low backache, urinary urgency, weakness, nausea, vomiting, shaking spells, difficulty in walking (especially in crowds), and many other symptoms. The surgery had been carried out for the removal of a pelvic tumor. During convalescence the patient was informed that her husband was associating with a woman "old enough to be his mother." He remained away for days at a time, frequently returned drunk, and lost interest in home, wife, and children. She obtained a separation and was awarded a small alimony. Along with the development of the other symptoms she became depressed about the future for her and the children. To add to their income, she worked as a cook in a restaurant, but eventually the symptoms interfered with this and she lost energy for even simple household tasks. About this time she was told that her husband was making "lots of money." This news "upset" her, she said, for she felt entitled to more alimony, and this brought on an exacerbation of her symptoms.

The patient's health had never been good. As a child she had numerous illnesses, many accompanied by symptoms similar to the present set. Of average intelligence, she finished the eighth grade and took a job. Marriage, which came in her early twenties, represented the culmination of her ambitions and desires. She had always looked forward to a home and children. Before the separation from her husband she was active, friendly, and cheerful, not at all shy. She learned to spend money wisely and managed well. Friends described her as easy-going, even when her own rights were involved. She stated that she had a bad temper but seldom "let it go."

Concerned over her future financial situation, the patient worried about caring for her children with the meager income she received, and wondered whether her health would permit work. Underneath was a jealousy of her husband for having more money and of the woman who had been able to "take him away from me." She was obviously depressed but accessible to questioning and cooperative. It was not easy, however, for her to tolerate restrictions and she relied upon her own opinions rather than those of the nurses in any matter pertaining to her welfare. An attempt was made to help her by planning for the future and she gradually became much better. At discharge she was at least well enough to resume life at her old level.

P. Mixed F:37:M:54 +5 23′178– 7:6:18

For the past ten years the patient had had repeated attacks of pain for which various medical and surgical treatments had given no sustained relief. She was exceedingly irritable, especially with her husband, whose inability to provide an "adequate living" was a source of great annoyance. Her children bothered her, and she had frequent crying spells.

Finishing the eighth grade at age 13, she had then stopped school. After living with her parents for two years, she had done housework in a large city for eight years until her marriage. A hard worker, she had always had feelings of inferiority, chiefly because of her low economic status, but in general, she had been thought of as a sociable, cheerful, and self-reliant person. Because her husband was a neurotic, inadequate person, the patient had had to carry an unusual amount of heavy responsibility. There were three children in the family. The 11-year-old daughter had been a behavior problem, and a son had been very late in talking and walking.

In the hospital the patient talked extensively about her financial problems and about her responsibilities. She said she nagged her husband but could not help it, even though she realized that he was doing the best he could. She complained of sexual incompatibility, and she was worried about her children. She had a number of somatic complaints and a moderate depression, but no obvious defect in sensorium or intellect. During interviews she was voluble, attentive, and interested, but she continued to insist that her pain had an organic basis, and she did not accept reassurance. With hospitalization she gradually came to feel better, and she had a real desire to go home and again try to get along.

Schizoid   F:58:M:126   +15   ′23178–9X(59)   10:1:22

This patient grew restless and excitable at the age of 58, developing delusions of being pregnant by a dog. She had had three major operations for removal of ovarian cysts about ten years before, and she was much crippled by rheumatoid arthritis. She had become confused about persons and places. She entered the hospital on a temporary certificate.

She was one of a family of five. She was bright and reached the top form of a secondary school. She was married and had one son.

She was diagnosed as having paraphrenia and was treated by psychotherapy and sedatives. Her condition improved to some extent. She was no longer deluded and there was no evidence of psychotic thought. M. V.

P. Mixed   F:33:M:86   +2   2317846′–9(45)   2:10:14
Suicidal

The patient was admitted because of severe depression, with thoughts of suicide and the fear that she might harm her children. When the illness began about four years before admission she lost her appetite and became irritable and bored. After a month away from home she returned feeling much better and desired to have another child. After this child was born she again became depressed and experienced feelings of tightness in her throat. Two years before admission she received electroshock treatments in a rest home, but there was little improvement. In the four months preceding admission she went through a cycle in which she was hypomanic two days of the week and depressed for the rest of the week. Four days before admission her husband found her downstairs singing at the top of her voice at 2 A.M. She talked incoherently and resisted attempts to put her to bed.

An average student in college, she had left after three years to fulfill her main ambition, marriage. During college she had been very active and had taken a great interest in all forms of sports, but she had been so sensitive that people had to be careful not to hurt her by what they said. She had never worked except in her home. She had always been shy and had never liked her physical appearance. Her childhood had been erratic, and her marriage had been more for the security it represented than for the love in the partnership, although she had originally been very fond of her husband. That affection had turned to coldness and indifference because she felt he had not given her sufficient loving. She had never been adequately satisfied in intercourse. Because her husband had not wanted children, she had "tricked" him into having the first child by telling him that her doctor had told her it was a "safe period" for intercourse. When he discovered she was pregnant he was furious and wanted her to have an abortion. The husband was very meticulous, making her put out her cigarettes in a certain way, for example, and requiring people to wipe their feet elaborately before entering the house. He handled all the money because the patient had not used good judgment in buying household articles. Her husband had struck her many times in anger. Since her marriage she had had one love affair, and she had almost had intercourse with the man.

In the hospital she was chiefly concerned with her obsessive ideas about hurting her children. She was doubtful about reassurance and complained that other patients got on her nerves. Emotionally unstable, she cried very easily. She was convinced that her case was hopeless and that she would never get well. She was frequently found lying on her bed, crying because she was afraid she would wake up insane. She was shy, staying away from people as much as possible. When she was discharged somewhat improved, arrangements were made for a follow-up in the outpatient psychiatric clinic.

P. Hypo.	F:23:S:63	+9	23 1786′–9	2:9:12
P. Hys.		+42	231768′–94	9:5:12
		+64	237816′–9	8:7:10

This young woman's complaints of headache, dizziness, and weakness on the right side of her body dated from age 16, following the birth of a child out of wedlock. At that time there was a court hearing in which the patient's parents had attempted to prove that her brother was the father of the child. This had caused the girl great embarrassment. The earliest symptoms were insomnia and anorexia with gradual impairment of memory. She experienced falls and bumps followed by increases in the symptoms, and once or twice she lost consciousness temporarily.

Church activities constituted one of the patient's interests. In grade school she expressed a desire to continue her education and to become a teacher, or possibly to take a business course. She never made close friends and was uncomfortable with boys, usually preferring the company of older people. She considered herself fat and awkward. Her mother pampered her, especially after the pregnancy. The brother who was said to have assaulted the patient appeared to have been a rather inadequate person; on one occasion he attempted to shoot his mother and a brother. The patient's child, now 6 years old, was obese and was receiving endocrine treatment.

The physical findings, although inconclusive, were certainly not at all consistent with the complaints. It was possible there had been some head injury. The basal metabolic rate was normal. Chiefly concerned with her constant headaches and lack of ambition, the patient said, "I don't care what I do. It makes no difference to me." Her tendency to fall when she was emotionally disturbed troubled her also. She described feelings of loneliness and was pessimistic about the future. "Something is wrong with my nerves," she said, and emotional upsets, she felt, were responsible for some of her symptoms. She made an effort to be cooperative but her anxiety and apprehension were so great that it was difficult even to talk with her. With continued hospitalization she became somewhat better. One day when two teeth were extracted she had an obviously hysterical attack in which she complained of severe pain on the right side of her body and developed a rigidity of the right arm. Out for a walk one morning she said, "Every time I come to a bridge I feel like I want to jump over it." There was no real improvement during the hospitalization and at discharge the prognosis was felt to be poor.

Ps. M-D., Mixed F:38:M:12 +2 23178′64–9 (43) 9:4:21
Ps. Sz., Paranoid

The admission symptoms for this woman were anorexia, palpitations, weakness in her legs, and occasional crying spells. They had appeared about half a year earlier when suddenly she was faced with increased responsibility because of the birth of a fourth child followed by the loss of a trusted housekeeper. Fear arose that she might not be able to keep up with the household duties, and the symptoms appeared. There was a history of similar episodes, varying in severity and duration, usually related to stress of some kind.

Except for these episodic depressions the patient's past was clear of contributory factors. Well above average in intelligence, she graduated from high school at 15. She worked as a secretary until her marriage. There were four children and the family group seemed happy. The one element of significance was that she showed insecurity, requiring frequent reassurance of her husband's love.

In the hospital the patient was markedly depressed although well oriented; she showed no deterioration of sense organs. Believing she was a hopeless case she had little insight and did not consider her problem an illness. She did respond remarkably well to psychotherapy which consisted of routine hospitalization and reassurance. Her progress was good until a few days before discharge, when she became slightly manic and exhibited a few symptoms suggesting a schizoid type of psychosis. At this time her husband, without explanation, requested that she be discharged, and so, against advice, she was permitted to go home.

Ps. Sz., Simple	M:20:S:71	+1	2318'746–X (67)	10:3:19
		–22	83217'694–(76)	6:7:15

Hospitalized because of nervousness and withdrawal from social contacts, this young man's illness dated back two years to high school graduation. Since then he had become withdrawn, had stayed home much of the time, and had taken jobs for two or three days only. More recently there had been bizarre behavior when he had walked into the home of a young girl acquaintance late at night unannounced. His mother said that at home he did nothing but read, listen to the radio, and play the piano. At the time of admission to the hospital the youth wore a small bandage over each nipple. This he explained by saying that he felt erotism whenever his nipples were touched.

His past history was relatively free of any physical or mental illness. As a child he had been fretful and peevish, and had cried easily. In school he did well but never mixed with schoolmates or took part in extracurricular activities. It was said that his classmates had elected him to a high office of the sophomore class for a joke—he was the class "idiot." One year he failed two subjects but made them up in summer school. His intelligence was average, and he blamed his difficulty in school on "too many chores at home." The mother was very protective toward the boy.

In the hospital the neurological and physical examinations yielded nothing pertinent. He said that whenever he tried to work he felt weak and tired, his back ached, and the like. The cause of it all, he felt, was his frequent masturbation. He said that once he had distinctly heard knives sharpening in the kitchen even though he knew no one was there. He maintained a rather blank countenance, not varying his facial expression with circumstances or mental content. Withdrawn and inactive, all during the hospitalization he remained apathetic, at times almost to the point of catatonia. Forty-five insulin shock treatments brought no noticeable change. At discharge he was advised to find a job with simple duties and to attempt to find other activities and interests outside his home. The prognosis was considered poor. It was felt that he would make a borderline adjustment at best.

Ps. M-D., Manic Paranoid	M:45:M:5	+1	'234–7168 (53)	4:3:14

The patient was admitted in a state of acute excitement. For three weeks before admission he had been held in another hospital for observation as an aftermath of a scene in his church. He had delivered an angry, incoherent sermon and had been assaulted at the end of the services. At the time of admission to the hospital he was still hostile and aggressive. The illness he attributed to overwork and lack of a vacation. Also he had worried over the loss of a prominent and wealthy parishioner. There had been two previous episodes similar to the present one, and both times he took prolonged vacations and changed jobs. These measures brought about a remission of the symptoms. For six months before the present illness members of his church had noticed that he behaved like a "smart aleck," was needlessly tactless, and made remarks inappropriate for one in his position.

Little was known of the patient's earliest years but he stated that he was "wild" during his adolescence, especially after his father deserted the family. He began then to drink and "run around." His original vocational goal had been physical education, but he later shifted to the ministry. His wife reported that he became restless and dissatisfied if he remained in any one place for long. A friendly man with a great deal of drive to succeed in life, he was successful in the majority of his goals. He believed himself to be tolerant and to have a sense of humor, which he said sometimes got him into trouble with his more serious colleagues.

The patient was irritable most of the time. He tried hard to be a "good fellow," laughed excessively, and was friendly with other patients. A few paranoid ideas appeared. He felt that some of the people in his church had been against him during his psychotic attack. Fearing there might be a church trial, he desired to line up persons to testify on his behalf. He questioned if adequate precautions had been taken to protect him from other patients and he admitted the delusion that his urine was red. Basically his orientation and intellect appeared intact. He seemed to lack completely insight regarding his illness. In general his demeanor was flippant and his thoughts not of the dimensions expected of a man with his intellect and in his profession. He gradually lost some of his initial hostility but gained no insight whatsoever. He was finally discharged to his wife against the advice of the staff.

Ps. M-D., Depr. F:45:S:47 +8 '234-9 7:1:9
Paranoid

The chief admitting complaint given by this patient's brother was that she "stares into space, cries, and says she feels weak." This set of symptoms had appeared following a bout of influenza three years before admission. She became languid, picked at her food, and was unresponsive when people spoke to her. She complained of weakness, vague pains, and sensitivity to cold. She restlessly visited first one relative, then another. Unhappy, dissatisfied, tearful, she was suspicious of her family, believing they were forcing her to act against her will. Several times she said, "I guess you think I'm crazy." Misinterpreting friendly advances made by a male cousin, she became obsessed with the notion that she had acquired an "infection."

Although always considered delicate, the patient had had few obvious physical illnesses. Clearly above average in intelligence, she had finished the eighth grade but had no further ambition to do anything except stay at home. Sent to a business school, she quit in two weeks. Her sole interest was music but she took almost no training in that. She was inefficient and went from job to job, never remaining in one for more than a few months. Two sisters with whom she lived found it almost impossible to handle her. She was dependent, nonassertive, self-centered, gloomy, and dissatisfied; she was also described as prudish and old-maidish.

Youthful in appearance, the patient was shy and coy in manner. At the time of admission she was plainly tense and tremulous. She wept readily and expressed the certainty that her situation was hopeless. There was a poverty of ideas and an inability to assign a source to her anxiety. She distinctly had no peculiar notions, however. Throughout her hospitalization she was ill at ease with staff members but fairly relaxed with others. She improved but at times toward the end of her stay when she left the hospital for a day she became uneasy and showed relief at her return. At discharge she was back to her usual personality, which, however, was not an adequate one. In view of her past history, the present illness was judged to be a fairly mild exacerbation. It was suggested that if she continued to be unmanageable, commitment to the state hospital would be recommended.

Ps. Sz., Cat.	M:23:S:145	+16	23'46871–(71)	5:0:19
P. Psychas.		+119	23'487–9(65)	7:4:22

Several weeks before admission to the hospital, the patient, a college student, became interested in the Hindu religion and spent a great deal of time discussing truth and divinity with everyone he met. His friends and teachers noted that he was tense and preoccupied, talked too rapidly, and would listen to no one. The day before admission a program which the patient had been planning had to be canceled. Disappointed and upset, he ran through the streets in his pajamas that evening to the house of the president of the college to demand that his plans for the program be carried through. He was very excited, confused, and irrational.

As a child the patient had been quiet and obedient but very nervous. To all his mother's demands and directions he had been completely submissive. She was a dominating, aggressive woman who was constantly active and did not get along well with anyone. His father, a quiet, passive, unobtrusive man, had little to say in family decisions. The patient had few friends and adjusted poorly during the months he spent in the service. He was excessively concerned about germs and obsessed with the idea that he might catch a venereal disease although he had no sexual contacts. At the time of his illness he was doing well scholastically.

On his entrance to the hospital the young man was in an excited, confused state, completely irrational, extremely suspicious, and crying frequently. He gestured, grimaced, and behaved in a noisy, hyperactive way. Electroshock therapy was given and after four treatments (16th day) he was much improved. He was friendly, helpful, and extremely grateful to everyone. However, he was still confused at times and perplexed about why he was in a mental hospital. A course of insulin therapy was then decided on; further improvement accompanied this treatment. Three weeks after the insulin was given (119th day) he was seen by the staff which felt that he had probably regained his premorbid personality but might benefit by several weeks of psychotherapy before leaving the hospital. At that time he was cheerful and friendly in his manner but there were hints of paranoid trends in his thinking and he had a mild phobia toward germs.

At discharge he still had little insight into his conflicts. He was very reluctant to leave the hospital environment. In a follow-up study a year later the patient reported that he was incapacitated for intellectual work because he was obsessed by thoughts of masturbation. His social adjustment was poor and he was working at a laboring job. Since he seemed anxious for help, further psychotherapy was recommended. E. B.

Alcoholism M:50:S:14 +6 2′3471–9(57) 5:5:19

The complaints of this man, a priest, centered around alcoholism, a chronic problem for twenty years and particularly severe in the last ten years. He first began "taking a drink" at the age of 28. He had had intermittent periods of drunkenness since the age of 32. By the time of admission a periodic drunk would last from two to three weeks. The patient had been hospitalized a number of times for the problem.

Ordained at the age of 28 he had taught in a college for several years and had also worked in parishes. His father had been a heavy drinker all his life and there were three brothers also known to be heavy drinkers. The patient had a severe case of psoriasis.

There was no obvious disorder in the patient's mental state. He was withdrawn and did not talk freely. Inclined to feel a bit resentful that his friends and others had interfered to have him hospitalized, he was sure that he could handle his own problems. While he was superficially cooperative with the hospital routine he did not feel a need for help and spent much time in interviews rationalizing and justifying his position. It appeared that he had been an introverted and schizoid type of individual long before the first hospitalization, probably well back into his youth. No particular correlate of the alcoholism could be discovered, however. During the hospitalization he was kept away from alcohol. At his own insistence he was discharged but with a poor prognosis.

P. Hypo. F:32:M:23 +1 23471′68–9(49) 5:2:19
Alcoholism
Drug Add.

The patient's symptoms included pain in her chest, nervousness, and need for constant sedation. Dating her disorders from four years before when she had first had feelings of "tightness," she said these had been brought on by excitement or fatigue. At the time the pain was preceded by "throbbing" or "skipping" of her heartbeat. A local physician prescribed barbiturates, which helped at first, but the dose had to be gradually increased. About a year before admission she was advised to drink an occasional glass of beer. Adding to this, she was eventually drinking up to eighteen bottles daily. Without sedation she could neither eat nor sleep. If she tried to eat without sedation she suffered from nausea and vomiting. During the four years of the illness she lost interest in her duties and did little but lounge and read magazines such as *True Story.*

Before her illness the patient had been an excellent housekeeper, keeping her children and house neat and clean. She had been salutatorian of her high school class but to achieve this she had worked hard and studied many nights very late. Following graduation she had attended business school for a year. She had always been dependent on her mother but felt rejected by her even though the mother had been indulgent of her. She said that she had always been uneasy in crowds. Members of the family described her as irritable and demanding and reported that she withdrew from social contacts.

The patient displayed concern about her barbiturate craving and nervousness. Her dominating desire was to be cured and get back to her family. Anxious and somewhat irritable, she persistently believed her body was "really physically ill" and she reiterated her somatic complaints. In her general behavior she was neat, alert, cooperative, and accessible. She professed inability to eat. Frequently she demanded sedatives and insisted on a private room. She stayed away from other patients as much as possible. The barbiturates were gradually withdrawn and sedative tubs were used to relax her. With continued hospitalization her appetite gradually returned and she began to make friends. The entire pattern of complaints disappeared although once in a while she expressed fear that the staff was "keeping something from her" about her physical condition. Slowly she began to plan for the time when her husband would return from army service and she would rejoin her children and set up housekeeping again. Always, however, there was an undercurrent of insecurity. The chief psychotherapeutic effort, in addition to hospital treatment, was directed at making explicit plans for her life after she left the hospital. Unmodifiable factors in the home situation made it unlikely, it was felt, that stresses could be avoided to an extent that would permit complete adjustment.

Ps. M-D., Depr. F:54:M:45 +1 23'47816–9 (49) 6:1:20
P. React. Depr.

About seven months before admission the patient had suffered an emotional upset brought on by worry about the welfare of her youngest brother. He had lost his job because of excessive drinking and had come to live with the patient and her husband for about one month. After he left the patient was lonely and agitated. She did not know what to do with herself, lost interest in things, and did not even take care of her own appearance. After an unsuccessful attempt to fight this reaction, she went to a psychiatrist who recommended that she be admitted to the hospital for shock therapy.

Her past history did not contribute anything to an understanding of her present illness. There were no previous episodes of mental trouble. Above average in intelligence, she had successfully conducted her own business until two years before the present difficulty, selling out when a good opportunity appeared because it had been difficult to get supplies. Her past personality had not been deviant in any discoverable way. She had chosen not to have children, but she and her husband had a happy, congenial marital relationship.

Composed and conventional in behavior, she was much concerned about her condition and found it hard to overcome her depression, which she clearly recognized as a psychological problem. She had no obvious disturbances of mentation, and she was intact in sensorium and intellect. She immediately felt more secure after being admitted. When eight electroshock treatments produced little improvement, amytal interviews were tried, and they helped her relax. She began to sleep easier and was soon getting better. Greatly improved at the time of discharge, she was active and interested in her surroundings. The staff felt that with sufficient outside interests she would be able to carry on successfully, since the situation seemed to be largely a reactive one in which the problems of the home were not sufficiently challenging in comparison with those of her successful business career.

Ps. M-D., Depr. F:31:M:80 +1 23'47 861–9 (47) 5:2:19

Depression, insomnia, fatigue, and inability to concentrate were the important admission symptoms of this patient. These symptoms dated from two months before when, following a period of increased social activity, the patient had become progressively more nervous, irritable, and despondent, with crying spells and feelings of hopelessness. There was a period in which she showed improvement but then the symptoms returned in a more severe form and she became anorexic and developed insomnia.

Except for milder attacks similar to the present one, beginning at age 17, her past history was uneventful. These attacks usually were precipitated by situations in which she felt inferior (in spite of a brilliant mind). In school, the patient was considered one of the top students and, in addition, showed excellent social adaptability. The first attack of depression occurred while she was attending a private school. After her marriage she devoted herself solely to taking superior care of her home and later to bringing up her one child. She was described as gay, witty, attractive, and apparently personally secure. Except for the depressive periods she and her husband appeared to be congenial and well adjusted.

Although pleasant and cooperative, this patient was obviously uneasy about being in a locked unit. She was readily reassured about this but tenseness was still apparent. Superficially she did not appear depressed. She described her illness as a "manic-depressive psychoneurosis" and she was pessimistic about its future course. Occasionally she was emotionally unstable and had crying spells. In spite of her self-diagnosis she found it difficult to accept the depressions as typical of an illness and wistfully hoped to find some environmental factor that would account for them. She was at first reluctant to adjust to hospital routine and for the first several weeks did not improve. Electroshock therapy was then tried. She received five treatments, immediately began to improve, and continued to do so. Although her symptoms had completely disappeared at the time of discharge, it was felt likely that she would have more attacks in the future.

B. Simple Adult Maladj. F:35:M:19 +1 2348′671–9 4:5:15

After the death of the patient's father about a year before admission, she became nervous, irritable, and irresponsible, and began to have periods of depression in which she neglected her home and was annoyed by the presence and conversation of her husband. Her nervousness increased a few months later when her house burned down. She sought medical attention and was advised to obtain a job. She worked thereafter, never making much money. She often stayed out until the early hours of the morning, telling her husband that she had been drinking and enjoying herself. He said that she would leave housework or dinner to go for a ride on a streetcar or to go to a show. As she gradually became more irritable and irresponsible she began divorce proceedings against her husband. She said she was depressed and unhappy and at times wished she were dead.

Her past history was essentially noncontributory except for an apparently hypochondriacal or hysterical trend. She had persistently suffered from symptoms of what she called a "heart ailment and anemia." She had left school in the tenth grade to care for an invalid father. Not much was known of her personality or her early life, but it was believed that she had had an illegitimate child before her marriage. A quiet, somewhat sensitive person, she was very considerate and thoughtful of others. Before this illness she had been easygoing, permitting her husband practically to run her life, but she had got along well with everyone, had not been moody, and had been thought to have good common sense.

In the hospital she was quiet and well composed and did not show any peculiar behavior. She admitted feeling nervous and felt she needed a rest, but she thought that if she divorced her husband everything would be fine, providing the husband was not ill and the children were properly taken care of. She felt sorry for her children but appeared not actively thoughtful of them. Largely because of her peculiar failure to recognize the existence of a problem in her personality and conduct, it was impossible to help her, and at the time of discharge there was little change in her condition.

P. React. Depr. M:37:M:18 ? '2<u>34</u>9–7(49) 4:3:18

This man was brought to the hospital by his wife because of his excessive jealousy and his fears that she was unfaithful. She said that he had tended to be jealous throughout their twelve years of married life, but during the past eight months the problem had become unbearable. Every action of his wife he interpreted as an indication of infidelity; he became extremely nervous and created scenes over trivial incidents. He accused her of masturbation and bizarre forms of sexual behavior. Although he threatened to commit suicide if his wife left him, he said that he had no intention of actually doing it. Realizing that his suspicions were unfounded, he was, nevertheless, unable to forget them, and as the worrying and nervousness became more and more severe, he was no longer able to carry on his work efficiently.

The patient had graduated from high school at age 17; he had had no learning difficulties, nor did he have difficulties in getting along socially. Until the onset of the present illness he had been a tightrope walker and fire-eater with a circus. When he left the circus he worked first for a city firm, but finding urban life a strain he bought and operated a small farm. Industrious and always a steady, hard worker, he exercised good judgment and handled money wisely. Described as self-reliant and stable, he was not considered assertive or stubborn. His marriage was apparently happy in spite of his suspicions. The family was a closely knit and happy one.

The patient's stream of thought was logical and to the point and he was quiet and composed. Concerned about his illness, he seemed to have a kind of insight into his condition and a confidence that he could be cured. Not a free talker, he did, however, answer questions adequately and was friendly and cheerful. Interested in doing everything possible to get well, he improved markedly while in the hospital, lost his jealous feelings (at least he no longer spoke of them), and at the time of discharge felt that he had "the whole problem under control." No apparent etiology for the patient's feelings of jealousy could be discovered. There seemed to be no overt or hidden feelings of rejection or aggression toward his wife, nor could guilt feelings or inferiority ideas be uncovered. The most likely mechanism was assumed to be projection and the whole reaction was considered an immature reaction in an unstable and basically neurotic personality type. It was felt that the apparently fine improvement was not a deep one and, in fact, it seemed likely there would be a recurrence of the symptoms.

Ps. Invol. Melan. M:51:M:58 +14 2'37–(71) 7:2:16
Paranoid

This man had been depressed for about two years and had developed mildly paranoid ideas. He entered the mental hospital as a voluntary patient.

Little was known about his early history. His father was a doctor, and he was one of seven children. He received teacher's training at a university and married at 27.

237148'6–9

He was diagnosed as having mild involutional melancholia and was treated by electric convulsion therapy and mild narcosis. His condition improved and he was discharged to return to work. M. V.

P. React. Depr. F:47:M:50 +15 '237–9X 12:5:17

This woman was brought to the hospital by her husband because he feared she would commit suicide. The husband told a long story of the patient's "stupidity, incompetency, jealousy, and emotional instability." The reliability of this history was exceedingly doubtful. It was obvious that he no longer cared for his wife and that he was interested in another woman. They had been separated for some time, and every time the husband and wife had met in the past few years, she had shown a marked emotional reaction. Quite likely there had been at these times threats of suicide. The husband had also been a patient in the skin clinic of the hospital because of a hive-like eruption that occurred whenever he slept with his wife. Under hypnosis this eruption was observed to appear and disappear with appropriate suggestions. It was interesting that the patient complained of a similar eruption on occasions when she was emotionally disturbed.

The patient seemed of dull intellectual level and apparently had not completed the sixth grade. She worked as a scrubwoman. In personality she was described as friendly, cheerful, and easy to get along with. She had always cried easily and was easily excited and disappointed. Apparently the patient and her husband had been happy for the first fifteen years of their married life, but discord had gradually increased. They had four children.

Although obese, the patient seemed to be healthy. Depressed, she wept copiously, especially when referring to her marital difficulties. She said she had never really meant to carry out her suicidal threats. Beyond the obvious unhappiness about her marital insecurity, she was cooperative, pleasant, and entirely normal in appearance and conduct. After the first few days in the hospital she became stable emotionally and the crying stopped. She was discharged symptom-free and went to live, at least temporarily, with a son.

P. Mixed F:32:M:68 —160 237148'6–9 (39) 7:7:15
Suicidal ? 3142786'9– (43) 8:6:19

After her husband's departure for military service about a year before admission the patient had sexual relations with a married man on several occasions. She worried over the possibility of pregnancy and suffered strong feelings of guilt and anxiety. She developed severe insomnia, nausea, vomiting, and vertigo. In spite of many examinations and careful reassurance by physicians, she continued to believe she was pregnant. To hide her "bulging" abdomen she wore dresses appropriate to advanced pregnancy. Later she complained of a generalized throbbing pain. She was given barbiturates and began to take six to seven pills a day, becoming somewhat addicted. The pain gradually became more a "vibration" localized chiefly in her abdomen. She was pessimistic and unable to sleep, and in spite of her husband's return and forgiveness she attempted suicide with iodine.

Her childhood history indicated that she had always been a nervous person with many fears and anxieties. Her high school grades were not good because, she said, she had had "too much fun." She was said to be a sensitive, truthful, open, self-reliant person, though somewhat stubborn. Her marriage had apparently been reasonably happy although her relations with her husband had been strained because of his drinking and gambling.

On admission she was mainly concerned with her illness, cried much of the time, and was irritable, anxious, and pessimistic about finding relief for her trouble. She was firm in her conviction that her trouble was not "mental." There was no disturbance of sensorium or intellect and she was rational and well oriented. Psychotherapy was unsuccessful and she was given shock therapy, which seemed to lead to some improvement. During her hospitalization her husband decided to sue for divorce. She was upset by this but came to feel that it was perhaps the best thing. By the time of discharge her delusions had largely disappeared, on the surface at least, and she planned to live in a private home and to go to work. The prognosis was thought to be fair.

P. Mixed	F:27:M:174	—24	23'71486–9	3:4:13
P. Psychas.		+99	7238'491–	2:5:19
Suicidal				

This patient was voluntarily admitted with complaints of hopelessness, depression, suicide thoughts, and multiple bodily pains and aches. The illness had begun suddenly eight months earlier with severe anxiety attacks expressed in palpitations, choking sensations, and feelings of terror. The initial attack was followed by a quiescent period, but when a week or two later she experienced another attack, she and her husband became panicky. Because of the hysterical manifestations she was then given a thorough physical study but there were no significant findings. Gradually her outside interests lessened and she became more and more self-centered. Among her many fears was one that she might lose her mind and unknowingly harm someone—most horrible, hurt her husband or children. She lost eighteen pounds in weight. In these eight months she was hospitalized briefly three times following threats of suicide. During these panics her husband had become very upset.

As a child the patient had been docile, serious, and grown-up for her years. She had always had the feeling that no one was particularly interested in her. As she grew up, she emphasized cultural interests and worked hard toward self-improvement. This resulted in a strenuous life with little time for relaxation. When she became older, she rebelled against an aunt with whom she was living, and from age 15 she supported herself. In addition to working during this time she went to night school and studied typing and other stenographic subjects. She married when she was 19 and already a few weeks pregnant. After marriage the patient and her husband concentrated all their efforts upon acquiring a college education for him. They had two children. The patient seemed sincere in her frequent comments that married life had been the happiest part of her existence, and that she could not think of life without her husband.

The patient appeared as an attractive and intelligent woman who thought rapidly and could ignore nonessentials. She was vivacious and sparkling. Proud of her self-reliance, she was unconcerned with convention, disliked pretense, and was forthright in expressing her views. She expressed vague desires to do something "really worthwhile." She had no love for housework but desired to give her husband and children the best home possible. At times she had occasional mild panics with sharp concern about body sensations and fear that she might lose control of herself. At such times she wanted to commit suicide. There was no evidence of confusion or psychomotor retardation. On a few occasions she had uncontrollable crying spells associated with attacks of palpitations. She then gave the appearance of suffering. She engaged avidly in any form of occupational therapy and worked on several projects at one time. She expressed a marked drive for equality with men. Finally taken from the hospital by her husband, she was placed under the care of a private physician. During the hospitalization little basic change was effected.

Ps. Invol. Melan. F:54:M:75 +1 237'1648–(49) 4:3:10
P. React. Depr.

For three years the patient had been bothered by generalized weakness, glossitis, numbness, tingling of her hands and feet, and dizzy spells. These had begun with what she described as "weakness and general run-down condition." Considerable medical attention brought no relief from the symptomatic pattern. Among other treatments was a course of liver therapy for an assumed pernicious anemia.

Before the appearance of the present symptoms the patient's health had been good. She was considered a nervous person but a good mother and housekeeper. With narrow interests and few friends, she preferred reading, listening to the radio, and working crossword puzzles to social activities. Prone to mild hypochondriacal ideas, weakness was always one of her chief and most consistent complaints. Leaving high school at age 15, at the end of her sophomore year, she had worked at odd jobs while enrolled in a business course. Marriage interrupted the course at age 18. The patient's married life was apparently happy and the sole factor that obviously contributed to the illness was the unhappy marriage of her daughter.

In the hospital she was concerned chiefly with her somatic complaints and with the troubles of her daughter. Her sensorium and intellect were not obviously affected. She was depressed and dependent. She attributed all her troubles to "nervousness and neuritis." She was obviously anxious, although her responses were normal and adequate. With hospitalization she gained physically and took some part in ward activities, still preferring, however, to read in her room. At first she would not walk without strong persuasion but later she moved about the ward in a normal manner. She was treated for arthritis. On the whole she made a rapid recovery and returned home with plans to take a trip to visit in the home of a sister. The prognosis was fair for this acute episode but it was recognized that she would always be rather inadequate.

P. React. Depr.	F:26:S:62	+1	23716′48–9 (51)	2:3:9
B. Psth., Asocial		+49	2734′681–9 (47)	4:2:12
Suicidal				

A suicide attempt, nervousness, and depression were the determining factors in this young woman's admission to the hospital. She dated the present illness back five months, when she had become irritable and had begun to experience difficulty in doing work to the satisfaction of her employer. Working at that time as a cook and maid at a home for chronically ill persons, she had had trouble with her employer and had begun to feel "blue and sad." These feelings she attributed to the depressing environment of her job and to financial difficulties, for her income was barely sufficient to provide for herself and her children. A week before admission she swallowed twelve sleeping pills one night and was surprised that this dose was not lethal; then she drank a considerable amount of lysol but was discovered and treated.

The hospital summary said that she "had practically no early family life whatever," and data bore this out. Her father deserted his family, her mother was committed to a state institution, and the patient's childhood was spent in one boarding home after another. Five years before admission she became pregnant for the first time and again two years later. The first child was stillborn, the second was placed for a time in a foster home. She was uncooperative in prenatal care and admitted indulging in sexual delinquencies with many different men. She contracted syphilis, for which she received extensive treatment. In the course of these treatments she became pregnant a third time. Shortly before her attempted suicide, a widower who had promised to become her husband married someone else. The patient's intelligence was somewhat above average. Although she took poor care of herself, she attempted to give adequate care to her two sons and had few interests other than these children. She said she had no trust in people and was suspicious of friendships, having had some bitter experiences. She had always been shy and self-conscious, she reported.

In the hospital her talk centered mostly around her two children and her financial worries. She appeared moderately depressed and although she was cooperative and attentive, her replies to questions were retarded and often inadequate. The diagnosis of psychopathic personality was rejected in view of the probable influence of adverse environmental factors. At any rate, in situations relative to her two sons, she exercised considerable judgment and deep feelings of responsibility. Her close attachment to the older son was used in the psychotherapeutic approach. Considerable psychological and social service aid was given, particularly in vocational placement, and arrangements were made for her to live in a good home. It was felt that under careful management she might make a satisfactory adjustment.

P. Psychas.	F:25:S:25	+7	23716′84–	6:5:17

This patient complained of a chronic cough of fifteen months' duration, accompanied by marked fatigue and loss of weight. The cough had begun during a severe attack of "flu" which was followed for several weeks by periods of intense, nonproductive coughing. She lost twenty pounds and became a semi-invalid because of fatigue. She had numerous other complaints, concentrated chiefly in her chest and head. At times she was blue but made no suicide attempts.

Of dull intelligence, the patient had always been a quiet and unassuming girl, dependent on her family. She was ill at ease in social groups, had no hobbies, but liked home duties. Her mother described her as a "perfect girl."

Nothing was discovered in the physical examination to explain the somatic symptoms. When first seen she appeared listless, was uninterested in her surroundings, and responded slowly. The hacking cough persisted continuously during questioning or when attention was centered in any way upon her. After a very complete examination she was given reassurance about her physical symptoms. She immediately began to improve and progress continued throughout her stay. She adapted well to hospital routine but made friends slowly. The cough ceased in a week's time and did not recur. She was given medical aid for a dermophytosis and before discharge she was able to accept the presence of definite emotional correlates in her illness. Her family's solicitude, it was felt, was an important factor and an attempt was made to give her an understanding of this. She was so clearly improved and had gained such good insight that at discharge it was believed unlikely she would have further trouble, unless, of course, powerful stresses should develop for her.

P. Mixed	M:59:M:28	+1	2371′86–(69)	7:3:14
		+22	′<u>29</u>–3<u>16</u>(47)	3:2:8

The patient came to the hospital because of nervousness, depression, and a fear of returning to work. About two years before admission he had been seized with severe pains in his arm and had been forced to quit work for the day. Following this incident he consulted various physicians and went to several clinics, but no organic basis for the trouble was found. After a vacation he began to work again, but when he suffered a recurrence of the pain a physician advised him to take a few days off. He had not worked since that time; instead, he stayed around the house, lying on the couch most of the day. He felt depressed and developed a persistent cough which was annoying to other members of his family and which made him feel that he had some sort of pulmonary pathology.

There was no history of previous physical or mental difficulty, but he had always been concerned about his physical condition and had taken medicine to combat expected diseases. He had attended school for seven years and had become a barber. He made friends easily and was well liked in the community. He had been somewhat strict in religious matters. With the onset of the present pattern he had become irritable. He seemed to lack confidence and initiative, and his wife had had to push him to make major decisions.

The neurological and physical examinations were essentially noncontributory. When he was first admitted to the hospital, he was depressed and reticent. After six electroshock treatments he improved to a moderate degree, and at the time of discharge he was cheerful, and seemed to have recovered from some of his depression. The hospital summary indicated that the patient had suffered from a long-standing, mild hypochondriasis and psychasthenia, with a gradual development of depression due to his prolonged preoccupation with both real and imagined difficulties. The prognosis was not considered favorable for more than a borderline adjustment.

P. React. Depr. F:32:M:66 +7 2371'864-9 5:5:9
P. Psychas.

P. React. Depr. F:33:M:22 +13 237'1- 5:2:7
P. Psychas.

The presenting complaints of this patient centered around nervous tension, mild somatic symptoms, numerous fears, depression, and insomnia. A vague feeling of "nervousness," associated with insomnia and shifting somatic complaints which her local physician had attributed to the "change of life," had appeared about nine months before hospitalization. Although she took the medicine the doctor prescribed, she still had a fear of becoming insane since neighbors told her that nervous women often became insane at the onset of the menopause. Her fears were intensified when a spokesman for the religious sect with which she was directly associated told her that if she did not practice their tenets she would certainly become insane and that if she wanted them to save her she could not continue taking the medicine prescribed by her doctor. New fears appeared, each associated with a marked emotional depression. She was afraid that if she were left alone she would harm her children or herself; the fear that she was developing cancer became another source of anxiety.

Known as an intelligent, energetic individual who enjoyed social contacts, the patient was an outgoing sort of person who met strangers well. She had always been easily upset emotionally with small disappointments producing a depression far out of proportion to the provocation. With definite ambitions for a higher standard of living, she had always resented the fact that her choice of a husband had been dictated to some extent by her mother. Although the marriage was not a particularly unhappy one, her husband had maintained his family on a low socio-economic level.

On admission to the hospital the patient seemed in good general physical health. While her complaints were numerous, including odd pelvic sensations which she could not describe fully, she lost many of these symptoms in the hospital; she was, however, very much afraid that they would return with discharge. Although her answers to questions were spontaneous and coherent, there was a certain amount of retardation. Her recognition that she was suffering from some type of nervous difficulty did not seem to represent a very deep conviction. She spent the greater part of her time standing at the window in a dejected manner, staring out into space. With longer hospitalization her fears and somatic complaints disappeared, and she began to take an active, interested part in hospital life. While her symptoms had disappeared at the time of discharge, she still had some fear that there would be a recurrence of her trouble. It was decided to transfer her gradually from hospital to home, with a period of convalescence in her sister's home, and under this regime it was felt that she had a good chance to make an adequate adjustment.

Ps. M-D., Depr. F:60:M:32 0 2371'864-9 4:1:21
Paranoid

Agitation, feelings of hopelessness, delusions of persecution, and ideas of reference were the chief admission complaints of this patient, the symptoms having appeared about a year before admission. They had first accompanied worries over apparently insignificant incidents and had included feelings of unworthiness. Believing she had offended God, she felt that people recognized this; later she came to feel that her husband was untrue to her. She also had fears of cancer and attending death and mild auditory hallucinations. She paced the floor for hours at night and was extremely apprehensive.

Six years before admission the patient had had a similar attack, in which she was anxious and had felt severe fatigue. Following a tonsillectomy she had recovered. Described as having been a quiet, secretive individual with very few close friends, she was interested in church, home, and music. She was never cheerful but was usually reserved and had little to say. She was economical and showed fairly good judgment in home management.

Once admitted, the patient emphatically voiced her dislike for the hospital. Seeing no reason for hospitalization and no benefits to be derived from it, she was critical of the personnel (though no more so than of her family): "The nurses don't mind neglecting me." Apprehensive and anxious, she said, "I've always had trouble mixing in a crowd." She had little insight into how profoundly ill she was. Uninterested in any of the examinations, she questioned the value of them and never took part spontaneously. At times she was sullen and irritable. Within a month of hospitalization she showed real improvement and later was judged capable of returning to her home. It was felt that she had a good chance of continuing to gain and to show progress.

P. Mixed	M:44:D:19	–7	23741'86–9	4:5:11
P. React. Depr.		+15	24'317–(69)	3:1:14
P. Hypo.				
Ps. Sz., Mixed	M:44:D:28	+8	271348'6–9 (69)	5:7:12
P. React. Depr.				

Without apparent reason the patient had become blind in his right eye at the age of 10. When he was 15 years old a clinic advised that the eye be removed, but he and his father refused. On returning home from the clinic he had what he called a nervous breakdown, becoming depressed, nervous, and self-conscious. Although he thought of suicide he never seriously planned it. He apparently recovered and during the next 23 years showed only moderate signs of nervousness. About five years before the present admission he experienced a depression precipitated by a matrimonial venture which had occurred after a six months' courtship, most of which was conducted through the mails. His bride left him after a week, saying that she didn't like his mother's house, and that she was afraid she would have to live in it permanently since he had no plans for a home of his own. He had a second period of depression when his mother died within a week after being placed in a state hospital. Business difficulties precipitated another short period of depression. Seven years before admission the patient had begun to experience pain in the back of his right eyeball, which tended to recur and increase in intensity but which disappeared when he was diverted. His blind eye also caused him much emotional unrest and nervousness. Insomnia and frontal headaches were recurrent.

The patient, who finished high school at age 17, found schoolwork easy, and after graduation he studied automobile mechanics for two months. Although he wanted to be an electrical engineer he was financially unable to carry out his plans. After farming for a number of years with his father and brother he became a filling station operator. Strongly attached to his mother, he had lived with his parents all his life. Always shy and sensitive, he had had few love affairs before his marital venture and hadn't considered marriage because he thought he was financially insecure. At the time of admission to the hospital he was lonely and depressed about being single, but he felt that he was too old to measure up to his concept of marriage. In an attempt to find peace and security he had gone from church to church.

On admission the patient was indecisive about a suggested operation on his eye, worrying over such details as what anesthetic would be used and what the cosmetic result would be, but finally the eye was removed during the hospitalization with definite relief to the patient. While his mental processes were mildly slowed up, apparently because of the depression, his general knowledge and vocabulary were good; but when his problems were discussed with him he became more deeply depressed. Only passively interested in the examination and other procedures he was content merely to answer questions. While an MMPI given before and after the eye operation showed considerable decrease in depression, he feared that he would not be released as a result of the papers that he had signed for admission to the psychiatric ward. Finally discharged to return home, he was out about two months. During that time he was agitated, depressed, troubled by disturbing dreams, and careless in personal appearance. Readmitted, he was relatively little better after about 25 days during which he was given four shock treatments. Finally against the advice of the staff he was discharged to the care of his brother.

Ps. Paranoid	M:35:M:45	+2	2'378146–(73)	4:3:21
B. Psth., Path. Emot.		+43	'42378 16–(69)	4:6:20

Two years before hospital admission the patient, who was employed as a guard, had developed delusions about other employees, thinking that they were conspiring against him. Because of these ideas he was dismissed from his job. After four months' unemployment, he began to write numerous letters to authorities about the assumed conspiracy against him. He got another job but quit because he was afraid that counterfeit money would be passed to him. He also feared that some union was plotting against him. This general pattern of symptoms gradually increased in severity until he thought the conspiracy included everyone but his immediate family. The day before admission he was found unconscious in a bus depot and upon regaining consciousness he was amnesic for a period of two hours.

Before the present illness he had had no psychiatric upsets or particular physical illnesses. He had attended a university four or five years, but failed so many courses that he could not get a degree. He attempted to study stenotyping on two different occasions but soon gave it up each time. He had had various positions, but was never able to hold any of them for long, had never been able to support himself, and depended on his wife for support. He spent much of his time reading books on philosophy and concentrating on abstract subjects. He appeared as a very charming, friendly, and sociable individual who made friends easily. However, when one knew him better he was rigid and stubborn and inclined to be sensitive. Always very ambitious, he could never satisfy even modest ambitions because of his erratic behavior and his inability to pursue a course for any time.

In the hospital he showed frank delusions of persecution. He was mainly concerned with the tremendous conspiracy against him, which he felt was so widespread that he couldn't get a job any place. He elaborated considerably on abstract subjects such as duty, the ultimate, metaphysics, and the purpose and futility of life. He exhibited marked circumstantiality and volubility. His manner was pleasant and charming. He kept himself neat and in most ways was a very cooperative patient. His I.Q. was 134. Marked improvement followed six electroshock treatments. He came to admit that his delusions were a screen to hide him from painful reality. Along with this verbal insight there was a considerable decrease in at least the outward manifestations of his delusional content.

P. Mixed	F:24:S:81	−4	2378461′-(43)	8:15:10
		+23	8273146′9-(45)	5:11:13
		+55	3467281′9-(41)	5:6:17
		+64	83 74126′9-(41)	5:9:14
		+78	3481′6792-(45)	5:7:19
		+292	3718 246′9-(43)	5:8:16

The patient was admitted from a general hospital because of depression and numerous somatic complaints. The pattern of the illness had been present most of her life. She had had a particularly severe emotional difficulty about sixteen years before and during the last four years had been nearly incapacitated. She sought numerous physical examinations but considered that her problems were "nervous," recognizing that they came on when she was emotionally upset and depressed. She had completed training as a medical technician in spite of her problems and had then attempted to become a nun. After a month and a half in the convent she was transferred to a general hospital because of her somatic and other complaints and because she began to entertain thoughts of suicide. As medication she was given a sedative at night to sleep and benzedrine in the daytime to stay awake. She improved for a while but then regressed.

The past history contained numerous accounts of psychosomatic illnesses, among which were headaches, tachycardia, chest pain, nausea, vomiting, diarrhea, chronic fatigue, and many more. She was high in intelligence but was introverted and withdrawn, having little recreation and working very hard. She had forced herself to mix in social affairs and was very dependent upon religion. She said that she had had a happy childhood but had been more and more unhappy as she grew older, becoming a passive, dependent person who never found anybody to be dependent on. There was much conflict with her family in general and open hostility toward her father.

In the hospital she had many emotional feelings that she was obviously unable to express. She seemed to have guilt feelings and she was depressed to the point where she would cry on the slightest provocation. Her orientation, sensorium, and intellect were normal. There was no obviously bizarre behavior. Intensive psychotherapy and other procedures did not have any effect. In general her behavior changed little while she was in the hospital though she became less depressed and did not cry so much. The underlying conflicts, however, were obviously not improved.

Ps. M-D., Depr. F:48:M:63 +6 23′789461– 7:1:13
Ps. Toxic

The patient was brought to the hospital by her husband because of three months of persistent depression, persecutory delusions, and agitation, following the death of her 2-year-old child. A week before admission, fears of death were added, she made attempts to leave home, and she became self-condemnatory. She was heavily sedated by her physician and took additional drugs. Her general health before the present illness had been relatively good, although she had had occasional symptoms that were possibly hysterical in nature, including attacks of tachycardia.

Her intelligence was average. She married at age 21, after teaching for a couple of years. Always interested in church work, she had enjoyed being with people and was alert and active. However, her feelings were easily hurt and she often preferred solitude. She was said to be subject to mood swings. During the last five years she had become gloomy and had expressed feelings of impending calamity.

Depressed over the death of her child, the patient felt responsible, although the facts did not warrant this. She believed she was being punished for her part in the death, and she was afraid to leave home. Her orientation and sensorium generally were clear. There was a moderate degree of psychomotor retardation. She admitted no suicidal intentions and recognized that she was depressed, but she was unable to evaluate her condition more completely. Frequently she cried during examinations and at times exhibited suspiciousness. She occasionally became agitated and would leave her bed and pace around. Within a few days she made a considerable recovery. Her insight was poor and she insisted that she was well enough to go home even though the improvement was not nearly enough for that. She still occasionally misinterpreted statements made by the staff. In time she gradually became more interested in hospital activities and there was additional improvement in the general symptom picture. Her defensiveness remained, however, and she found it difficult to discuss her personal situation. She was discharged as markedly improved but it did not seem safe to predict that she would have no more trouble.

P. Hys. F:20:S:53 +9 ′2379–4 8:4:11

This young woman's presenting complaints were weakness in her left arm, depression, fatigue, and withdrawal. For several months she had shown considerable depression, had lost interest in schoolwork, and had become unusually fatigued. She had had bouts of headache and epistaxis. After failing a history examination she became even more discouraged. One day she complained of weakness, walked to her room, and for ten minutes was not responsive. This attack apparently left no residual symptoms. Several days later, while performing a light household task she suddenly complained of pain in her left shoulder and weakness of her arm. Five years before, the patient had been studied and a diagnosis of hysteria had been made. Apparently at that time she had been irritable and withdrawn for approximately four weeks, with attacks of unresponsiveness then also.

At the time of the earlier hospitalization, the patient missed two and a half years of school. In the last year of high school at the time of admission the patient found learning difficult, and she received poor grades. She held a part-time job and in addition was a great help to her parents on their farm. Somewhat shy, she seldom went out and disliked crowds. She had a boy friend with whom she corresponded. High school teachers noted that she was easily offended and that she seemed to seek their companionship rather than that of the other students. Her tested I.Q. was 80.

In the hospital the patient was bothered because she could not be at home helping her parents. She expressed concern about the health of her father and about one of her brothers. There was anxiety, also, over her inability to learn quickly and to do well in school. She was not greatly concerned about the weakness in her arm. The neurological examination showed no objective symptoms. She appeared to make a great effort to be pleasant and cooperative, and frequently ended her sentences with, "Yes, Doctor." She made little effort to associate with others in the hospital and appeared most comfortable with older women. After a rapid recovery of strength in her arm the other symptoms disappeared. So well did she adapt to the hospital that there was obviously no eagerness to be discharged. It was felt that an important part of the problem lay in the discrepancy between her measured intelligence and her level of aspiration. With this hypothesis in mind attempts were made to help her readjust. She appeared to make considerable progress in understanding the difficulty and in replanning her life.

P. React. Depr. M:32:S:7 +5 2'38-1 (74) 4:2:13

This man complained of tiredness, loss of energy, a sense of frustration, and heaviness of his eyelids. There was a facial "tic," and his eyelids drooped. He was resentful of his position as a quarryman, did not get on with his fellow workers because of their "low mentality," and claimed that he was "psychologically unsuited for quarry work." He entered the hospital for observation as a voluntary patient.

He was the older of two boys. After his father died his mother remarried, and he was not happy at home. He left secondary school and entered a quarry at the age of 15. He later studied at a university for two years, being supported by his brother, but he was "ill" when the time came to take his examination. At the start of World War II he was a conscientious objector, but he joined the Royal Air Force because of "the incompetence of the higher-ups." He later asked for his release to go back to essential work at the quarry, not realizing that he would have to stay on, owing to the Essential Works Order. He returned to the quarry at the end of the war. He had always been very ambitious and had engaged in many public activities.

He left the hospital at his own request one week after admission on the grounds that he had "self-analyzed himself as suffering from neurosis." Shortly after leaving the hospital he obtained an administrative post of some responsibility. M. V.

P. Hypo. F:47:M:30 +2 2384176'9–(45) 5:7:20

Insomnia, weakness, fatigue, loss of interest, tenseness, headaches, and body aches and pains, were the admission complaints of this patient. She had been nervous and had suffered from these and other vague complaints for 25 years; she had been treated repeatedly in hospitals and by private physicians.

Of average intelligence, she had always held jobs at the level of domestic work. When young she had been active in sports but chronic fatigue and lack of drive had thwarted her interests in this field. She was easygoing and shy, and she could not stand criticism. For years she had feared things that she couldn't describe and in general had felt the need of sympathy. Her husband complained that three years after their marriage the patient had brought an 18-year-old girl in to sleep with her. This went on for two years and eight years later a similar episode occurred with a 16-year-old girl.

Markedly preoccupied with the nature of her illness, its duration, and its effect on her, the patient believed that because nothing seemed to give relief, her complaints must be due to imagination. Extremely sensitive, it was difficult for her to discuss personal matters. When not directly under observation she was sociable toward other patients. The insomnia lessened, and she gained weight in the hospital. Although she was discharged somewhat improved to the care of her husband, there was little expectation that any important degree of recovery had occurred. It seemed, in view of the long history of complaints, that the patient would probably continue about as she had been before hospitalization.

P. Hys. F:31:S:381 +18 238'7146–(70) 8:10:11

This woman had had laryngitis every spring for some years. She was still not able to speak above a whisper six months after her last attack. The surgeon reported that there was nothing organically wrong and referred her to the psychiatric clinic. After a few interviews in the outpatient department, she was admitted to the hospital.

She was the second of seven children. The first child had died at the age of 4, so she was virtually the oldest. Her father was said to be delicate, and strange in manner and appearance. Her mother had a marked goiter and was unreasonable, generally unstable, and violent at times. All the family were said to be "pasty" and unhealthy. She had been a delicate child, had had infantile paralysis at an early age, and had not attended school until she was 8. She was timid and high-strung, not able to hold her own with others, and terrified of doctors and hospital nurses. She was antagonistic to her mother, whose domineering ways she resented. Menstruation began at the age of 16 and was always painful, with excessive loss. She was trained as a confectioner and was very good at her trade, working for the same firm for several years. She became close friends with the forewoman at her place of work, an older woman who had rigid religious views. The patient left home and went to live with her, remaining even after the older woman's marriage.

She was diagnosed as having hysterical aphonia and underwent a course of electric convulsion therapy. She regained her voice for varying lengths of time after psychotherapy given under sodium amytal and hypnosis. She left the hospital and returned to live with her friend in an atmosphere amounting to religious mania. She resumed work and remained perfectly well, according to information given by another friend. However, both women showed great hostility to the psychiatrist and the social worker. M. V.

P. React. Depr. Paranoid	F:30:M:18	+2	'238749–6 (55)	3:2:14
P. React. Depr.	F:31:M:29	+1	23'7416– (53)	5:1:16
Ps. Sz., Simple		—4	'23679– (49)	5:3:14

This woman was admitted because of a postpartum depression with claustrophobia and severe headaches. Two previous attacks of depression had followed childbirth. The first, which occurred three months after the birth of her first child (now 28 months old), had been abrupt in onset with a similar pattern of complaints. The second attack had occurred five days after the birth of her second son and had been similar to the first although milder in character. The patient attributed the second to the premature birth of her second child.

Five years earlier she had undergone the removal of an ovarian tumor and incidental appendectomy, and at the time of the second delivery a "growth" in the cervical canal was removed and she was sterilized. This last point she denied although it was in the medical record. A graduate nurse, she had been popular in school and after marriage. She liked dancing, drank moderately, and spent a great deal of time outdoors. She was a meticulous housekeeper and derived much satisfaction from doing things to please her husband.

The neurological and physical examinations on admission were negative. She was well oriented as to time, place, and person; and her sensorium and intellect were unimpaired. Although well composed she was depressed and cried easily. Her stream of thought showed no particular disorder except for the multiple somatic complaints. She was willing to cooperate. The complaints subsided quickly after admission and she was discharged entirely well as far as could be determined. The prognosis was considered good and she planned to go home and resume her regular activities. Fourteen months later she was readmitted with a similar pattern. During the interim she had been able to do her work satisfactorily, but one month before the second admission, depression and weeping became severe. Admittance was at her own request for electroshock therapy. It was apparent there was an underlying hostility toward her husband which she actively suppressed. It now was discovered that she had failed to pass the examination for registered nurses and had shown personality disorganization since that time. Paranoid trends were obvious. There was again rapid improvement and she was discharged to the care of her husband.

P. React. Depr.	F:38:S:45	+11	2416'3789–(45)	2:4:19
		+21	4'68379–(39)	4:2:25

This woman's chief presenting complaint, inability to sleep, had appeared two months earlier. The preceding six months had been filled with indecision about accepting a position with the armed forces in an oriental country. The patient and her mother argued, often bitterly, and finally the patient seemed to accede to her mother's wish that she remain at home. However, she began to lie awake nights and used sedatives that proved more and more ineffectual. She continued to work during the day but expressed feelings of hopelessness and of being "all washed out."

After high school graduation the patient attended the state university and earned a library science degree. She held jobs in several different libraries. An idealistic person, she stated that "high standards of conduct" had kept her from close relationships with men. During college years she showed independence and drive, but after her father's death, when she returned to live at home, she became deeply dependent upon her mother. Always reticent, she had desired and looked forward to marriage but she seemed to be inhibited in, or incapable of, forming new emotional ties. She had bitter quarrels with her mother, but that emotional tie seemed inexplicably strong.

In the hospital the patient expressed extreme feelings of unworthiness. She appeared depressed and reserved. There were no gross disturbances of sensorium or intellect. Although cooperative and helpful about the ward, she held herself aloof from the other patients. After three weeks in the hospital, during which she improved little, she was given electroshock treatments which brought about a marked change. By the time of discharge she seemed almost entirely her usual self. The problem about breaking ties with her mother was never resolved, since she decided to remain with her mother and make the best of things.

Ps. Paranoid	M:51:M:7	+4	'243–9	5:2:21

Five years before admission the patient had come to the outpatient department complaining of a persistent sore throat and weakness, and at that time he had been found to have a positive serological reaction indicating syphilis. In spite of continuous intensive therapy his Wassermann test had remained positive. About a month before admission he began to complain of restlessness and inability to sleep. The slightest noises disturbed him, he became irritable and impatient, and he spent his time sitting by himself worrying over the fact, as he finally confessed to his wife, that his partner at work was trying to have him discharged. He thought that the partner suspected he had syphilis, and that the partner either was trying to poison him or was attempting to have him dismissed by making him perform tests that would show he had syphilis.

Twenty years before admission the man had had an attack of nervousness, during which he had been admitted to a state hospital as a voluntary patient with paranoid tendencies of suspiciousness and mild delusions. After a three-month hospitalization, he had been discharged with a diagnosis of dementia praecox.

An immigrant who came to the United States at age 21, the patient had gone through the eighth grade before immigration and had done some informal reading and study after coming to this country. He was known as an emotionally stable, frank, and friendly person. He had always been considered very adequate; he had taken an interest in his work and in his home and for seventeen years had been employed on the same job as a truck driver. He had been married for eleven years and had one son. He did not admit any exposure to syphilis.

In this hospitalization both the neurological examination and the Wassermann test were negative. The only gross disturbance of mentation or sensorium was in the expression of paranoid attitudes toward his partner at work. Calm and composed, he showed no abnormal mood changes. Although he had fairly good insight into his condition, he felt, somewhat irrationally, that he had a good foundation for his delusions. At times he expressed his fear of syphilis. For the most part his stream of thought was logical and sequential, and he was alert, natural, and cooperative. He remained relatively unchanged in the hospital, and it was only in the one sphere that his illness could be recognized. It was felt that the disorder probably arose from worry about his luetic condition, and that he might have another attack.

Ps. Postpartum	F:27:M:46	+6	'243 71986–X (57)	15:1:20
Ps. Paranoid		+38	'9–21 43768 (57)	5:2:11
Ps. Sz., Paranoid Suicidal				
Ps. Paranoid	F:27:M:33			
Ps. Paranoid Suicidal	F:27:M:6	+1	'439–(49)	7:2:23

Shortly after her marriage four years before admission the patient began to complain of general aches that had no particular locus. At about the same time she and her husband experienced a number of difficulties including a major operation on the husband for ulcerative colitis. Shortly after this the patient claimed she also had ulcers, and she saw various physicians who attempted to reassure her. A month later she again needed medical reassurance because she was convinced she had piles. Later she became obsessed with the idea that she had a kidney disease. A few days after her first child was born, she became so worried about the baby's weight that it was necessary to call a physician. While still in the hospital she developed the idea that she had cancer of the rectum, and when she noticed a white spot on the roof of the baby's mouth she thought it had cancer of the mouth. No amount of reassurance helped her, and after writing a farewell letter to her husband she took an overdose of sleeping capsules. She was found unconscious and was taken to a general hospital where she stayed for three days before being admitted to the psychiatric unit.

There was no history of past psychotic episodes. A high school graduate, the patient had attended a business college for a while and after that had worked in a business office until her marriage. A very shallow person, easily influenced and uncertain in her opinions, she was headstrong and often unmindful of the consequences of her acts. She had never handled finances well. Very friendly, she felt ill at ease when alone. Ethically she had a very strict code.

In the hospital she was clear in sensorium and intellect and was well oriented and cooperative, but she answered questions in a glib, naive manner with considerable circumstantiality. Her stream of thought seemed normal with the exception of her delusional system, in which she felt that both she and the baby would shortly die from cancer. She was restless and constantly asked to go home, saying repeatedly that since she was "beyond medical treatment" it was cruel and useless to keep her in the hospital. After electroshock treatment she gradually became more cheerful and said she wanted to go home to take care of the baby. Shortly after her return to the hospital following a trial at home for an afternoon, she expressed the belief that her entire family had cancer. Another course of shock therapy was completed in the sixteenth week of hospitalization, and at that time all evidence of delusional content had vanished. Her memory was impaired, but otherwise she appeared to be herself. She was discharged with an uncertain prognosis to return to her home.

After a month or two the symptoms returned, and four months later she was readmitted on a voluntary basis for further treatment. She now had the feeling that certain sexual experiences had been the source of her trouble. She improved slightly and was again discharged to go home for another trial, but two months later she was once more readmitted after a suicidal attempt and assaultive behavior. She was then committed to a state hospital.

Ps. Invol. Melan.	F:57:W:48	+1	2438′1679–(53)	2:11:13
Paranoid		+46	9′8–231(49)	2:4:8

The patient's illness began about a month before admission to the hospital when she became depressed over problems arising, in part, from her inadequately controlled diabetic condition. She had had to be absent from work frequently and her boss had been angry with her because of her absence. She tried to continue working but developed paranoid ideas that people were talking about her, accusing her of doing something wrong—stealing petty cash, for example. She felt that she was being watched. The weekend before admission she went to her daughter's and said that the police were after her.

She had first been diagnosed as a diabetic ten years before admission. Otherwise, her general health had always been good. There were, however, a number of episodes in her history that indicated an hysterical make-up. These were characterized by attacks of dyspnea, palpitation, occasional insomnia, atypical sinusitis, and the like. She had had seven insulin shock reactions during one period of uncontrolled diabetes.

The patient had taken a nine-month business college course and had married a wealthy man who lost his money not long after she married him. The patient then had had to go to work in order to help support the family. Her husband died a few years later. She had always been dependent on her older sister and had gone to live with this sister during all periods of stress. In general the patient was an outgoing person who enjoyed social affairs and social activities. On the other hand her daughter described her as immature and said that she wouldn't talk to a person who had angered her and that she was in many ways rigid and meticulous. The patient's older sister was devoutly religious and seemed to dominate her.

The patient expressed definite paranoid ideas in the hospital. She was depressed, nervous, and evasive on most direct questions. She had no hallucinations. She was well oriented and a good part of the time appeared friendly and normal. She frequently sought sympathy. She had very poor insight, at least in the early days of hospitalization. Her intelligence was average. She was given twelve electroshock treatments, and the diabetes was carefully controlled. Under this regimen her paranoid ideas disappeared and she came to have better insight into her general condition. She was discharged to live for a while with her daughter and son-in-law.

Ps. M-D., Depr. F:50:M:64 +17 243817′69– 8:12:16
Suicidal

During the past three years the patient had shown increased irritability and dislike for her housework, had become easily upset, and had struck her husband on the slightest provocation. She complained of her inability to work, and she was sullen and depressed. There were also a number of physical complaints. In the last year the patient had spent a great deal of time in bed because of "polyarticular rheumatism" and had lost thirty pounds. Noises irritated her, and she said it was "not so much the noise as the spirit behind it." After she was seen in the outpatient psychiatric service her husband was told that he should have her admitted to the hospital, but he did not at first consider the problem serious enough for that. Then three days before admission she had a quarrel with her husband in which she struck him; she left home after this episode to live with her foster sister, whom she also attacked, saying, "I feel ugly." Later on the day of this attack the sister returned home to find the patient extremely lethargic and mumbling, "Goodby, be good to the kids." The sister found that the patient had taken an overdose of phenobarbital.

The patient had been adopted from an orphanage at age 2. She had gone through the seventh grade in school, stopping because of illness in her foster family. A generous, stubborn, considerate, overly conscientious person, she had always been timid in the presence of strangers, but she had been a good speaker and was well liked, active, and energetic in her community.

In the hospital there was little to support the possible diagnosis of rheumatic encephalitis. The patient was convinced that she could never be happy as long as she had to live with her husband, whom she accused of deliberately doing things to annoy and irritate her. When asked about actual incidents she said, "It isn't so much what he did, but the way he did it." She was well oriented, intact in sensorium and intellect, but she appeared generally depressed. As she became more alert, she expressed pleasure at being hospitalized, and part of the time she was fairly well behaved, but there were several episodes when she became demanding and irritable and had to be moved to a disturbed ward. On several occasions she struck nurses impulsively, but afterward she apologized. She continued to have alternating periods of regression and improvement until her final discharge, at which time she was a little better. She was discharged with the recommendation that she should have further hospitalization if she did not adjust well. It seemed unlikely that any real benefit had been obtained from the psychotherapeutic efforts.

B. Psth., Asocial M:40:M:21 +1 2467'3819–(57) 7:11:14
Alcoholism

Fourteen years earlier a box of dynamite had exploded while the patient was handling it; he had lost his right arm and a finger from his left hand and had sustained numerous other injuries. Following this experience, he said, he had experienced periods of overactivity when he could not sit still but was compelled to go out and walk in order to relieve the "tension" he felt. These periods continued, and eventually he resorted to alcohol to relieve his tension. He drank a great deal and became increasingly irritable, depressed, and abusive toward his wife. She claimed that one night three weeks before admission he beat her and threatened to kill her. She left him, taking their three children, and started divorce proceedings. One week later his tremor and general nervous anxiety became so pronounced that he stopped working and made arrangements to enter the hospital voluntarily for study.

The past history had little to contribute except for the incidents following the dynamite explosion. The patient had attended school through the sixth grade; he said he had "not been too bright" but had "gotten along." He had then worked as a filling station attendant, as a mechanic, and at other jobs, making a fair living. He enjoyed "being out with the boys" and drinking with them. Twice he had been arrested for illegal transportation of liquor. Before the dynamite explosion he had been well adjusted, he claimed. He said that he frequently relived the accident in his dreams and was afraid of explosives. According to his wife, he was sensitive and was "bothered by people," but he denied this.

In the hospital the patient was restless and agitated but coherent and cooperative. He was clear in sensorium and intellect; he seemed to be dull normal in intelligence. Greatly concerned about his nervousness, he expressed a strong desire for help. On the other hand he would not accept suggestions that did not appeal to him and he always reserved the right to judge procedures according to his own standards. He did cooperate in the hospital routine but it was obviously difficult for him to do so. He had only a superficial insight into his problem and accepted no personal responsibility for the divorce or for any of the other things that were happening. When he was discharged to return home the prognosis was considered poor.

P. React. Depr. F:41:M:14 +3 '24 6783–(55) 2:3:13
Suicidal

This patient dated her present depressed feelings and suicidal ideas from three months before, when the already tenuous relations with her husband were further strained by a series of incidents. First, she was diagnosed as having a venereal disease (a diagnosis later judged to be mistaken), and she attributed this to her husband's infidelity. At the same time, the patient suspected that attentions paid by the husband to a favorite cousin visiting with the family were amorous. Depressed and restless, she cried uncontrollably, with slight provocation. Family quarrels led to discussions of a divorce. Just at this period the patient's bedridden mother became even more ill and, therefore, more burdensome. The patient's feelings about this were mixed since she believed that in some respects it would be better if her mother died. Finally she attempted suicide by swallowing sleeping pills.

Born and raised in a small town, the patient did reasonably well in school, and following graduation she worked in a law office until her marriage. She and her husband, a farmer, worked hard to keep up financially, and they had enjoyed only a few years of security. As a child the patient had been shy and sensitive, easily hurt, and quick to resent slights. These traits she retained into adulthood. She was hard working, neat, and clean. Although she was never at ease sexually, there was no severe conflict over sexual matters. She had, however, other difficulties with her husband, centering around his dependence on his mother and religious differences. In addition the patient felt that the children preferred their father to her.

In the hospital the patient was composed, although she cried readily during interviews. She was preoccupied with the imminent breakdown of her family life.

'246879–

Her stream of thought was normal and her sensorium and intellect were undisturbed. Prone to dwell on her husband's shortcomings, she was especially bitter about never having experienced sexual satisfaction, and also about her husband's presumed attentions to other women. She fitted smoothly into the ward routine and mingled easily with the other women patients, although she had difficulty in all heterosexual social contacts. All in all she appeared almost entirely a normal person. Little definite progress was made in therapeutic sessions, but the depression and anxiety gradually decreased as the patient crystallized plans for her life after discharge from the hospital. The outlook for the future was thought to be fair.

Ps. Paranoid F:36:S:19 +11 '246879–(45) 8:4:24

The patient came to the hospital to prove her sanity. Her illness had begun about six years before. After a friend, a doctor, left for the army, the patient found "secret" messages in his letters which she believed were for the postmaster of her town. She interpreted a series of incidents to indicate a "dope ring" of national magnitude, and she thought this ring included city officials and her friends. For a year and a half before admission she felt that the ring was trying to intimidate her because of the evidence she had against them. The intimidation consisted of continuous following and observation, suggestions that "I leave town and other things." She said she had no evidence since she "foolishly threw away the doctor's letters." She was, however, certain that she could identify the people who pursued her and she thought that the ring was powerful enough to have the F.B.I. accuse her of being insane. She came to the hospital at the suggestion of a brother-in-law who was a physician.

She described herself as having always been shy socially, especially toward men. However, she got along well with people and had been socially accepted. Rather large for her age, she had been a leader among neighborhood children. She felt that she had had a better upbringing and social position than many others and that her job was below her educational and social standing. She had obtained a degree in business from a university. She had had a number of love affairs and proposals of marriage during her college years but she had hesitated so long that each boy had married someone else. She blamed herself for the way things had turned out but felt that she might not have been happy anyway.

In the hospital the patient remained by herself most of the time, preferring to read rather than to take any part in the ward activities. She believed that she was not as emotionally disturbed as the rest of the patients were. She was very embarrassed about her problem and refused to discuss it any more than was absolutely necessary. She was given insulin treatment but this disturbed her and she demanded that she be allowed to leave the hospital. She was thereupon discharged for further study and treatment at another psychiatric hospital. She had changed little during her stay.

P. React. Depr. F:35:M:14 +4 '247–(68) 5:1:9

This woman became depressed and anxious following an attack of influenza at the age of 35. She was irritable with her child, but not with her husband. She entered the mental hospital as a voluntary patient.

She was the second of four children. She reached the fourth form in a secondary school and then worked in a laundry, attaining an executive position, until she married at the age of 24. She had one child. There was a long history of nervousness (overanxiety, a feeling of being hurried, some obsessional traits, and the like).

She was diagnosed as having a hysterical depressive reaction, and her condition improved after two electric shocks. M. V.

P. Anxiety State M:25:M 2471'9638–(65) 3:2:?

This youthful air corps pilot was removed from flying status because of incapacitating nausea and vomiting associated with flying training missions preparatory to overseas duty. The only other specific complaints were a moderate, diffuse tension and anxiety.

A small, dark man, with a prominent habit of putting his thumb into his mouth, the patient was the second of three children born to Italian emigrant parents. His father made a secure living as a carpenter, but the home was dominated by his uncontrollable temper outbursts against both his wife and his children. As a child the patient had had severe feelings of inferiority and had always been conscious of being a "dago." He consorted with Negroes and first-generation Americans almost exclusively. Also pre-eminent in his history were a fear of the dark, nightmares, sleepwalking, and fainting spells. He had admitted none of these symptoms at the time of his air corps enlistment. On the other hand he had made a good academic and athletic adjustment at high school and in two years at college, and he had had an average work record in a war plant for a year before his enlistment. There was a poor emotional adjustment between the pilot and his wife, who was one year his senior. Their sexual relations were marred by the patient's premature ejaculation.

Detailed psychiatric interviews revealed the presence of motion sickness (in swings, boats, and the like) since childhood. Because he had withheld this information at the time of enlistment, the pilot was deprived of his commission and contact with him was lost. A. T. K.

B. Psth., Mixed M:31:M:19 +2 '248367–9(65) 1:3:20
Drug Add.

The particular reasons for the court order that led to the present admission of this patient were excessive use of benzedrine, personality changes, inability to study or to get a job, and threatened suicide. There was no evidence that the patient had ever in his life been well adjusted. During the past ten years he had consulted a number of psychiatrists for "inability to concentrate, mental block, and inability to get along with my wife." The present pattern began to show itself more clearly about five years before admission but was especially apparent after a hit and run driving accident a year before admission. After his arraignment on that charge he became more irritable, occasionally broke windows and doors during temper tantrums, was careless with money, and apparently was afraid to face situations and people. Unable to hold a job, he became obsessed with the desire to obtain a Ph.D. in his special field of study. To increase his efficiency he took increasingly large doses of benzedrine and caffeine. There was extreme marital discord in which the wife appeared as much at fault as the patient. The patient was also known to have engaged in various sexual perversions, some of which were homosexual.

He had always felt inadequate and when in high school had attempted to compensate by joining what he referred to as "crackpot literary groups" and the like. His mother had been overprotective toward him and he had always been given anything he wanted. He was egotistic and assumed an intellectuality that he could not back up with consistent study and learning. He was aloof, sensitive, emotionally unstable, and irritable.

In the hospital he was verbose and seemingly delighted with the opportunity to express himself. His manner, although cooperative during interviews, was pedantic and aloof. In answering a question he tended to ramble to distantly related topics and to answer only after a long dissertation. He showed mild paranoid trends, fearing that letters he wrote or information he gave might be used against him for his commitment. He was well oriented and seemed objective in a verbal way about his illness. He had an affected cheerfulness and he was overly confident that he could solve his own problems. This factor made it difficult to help him in any way. Because of the long-standing psychopathy and the relative unmodifiability of his case, it was recommended that he be sent to a state hospital for a period of prolonged care. His mother characteristically refused to cooperate in this and he was discharged to her custody.

Ps. M-D., Mixed	F:25:M:109			
Ps. M-D., Mixed	F:26:M:127	+32	2483'7-	2:12:14
		+105	2'3487-9	4:6:15
Ps. M-D., Mixed	F:27:M:131	?	'4386-1	4:8:18
Suicidal		+8 yrs.	'4386-(45)	2:6:21

The present admission (third set of admission data) was the third hospitalization for this young woman. This period showed a marked similarity to previous episodes, with ideas of suicide and threats to do away with her family as well as herself consistently present. She expressed extreme feelings of self-depreciation, saying over and over, "I shouldn't be here; my family and I are a burden to society. You're wasting your time and money." Not only had she contemplated various means of suicide, but she had twice, for several days, refused food for herself and her two children. During part of the time between depressive episodes the patient experienced mild manic states.

Attractive and intelligent as a child, the patient had made an excellent school record and she had expected to attend college. However, in spite of her own keen desire and interest in college work, and her mother's pride in the girl's academic abilities, the family was financially unable to send her to college. After several unsuccessful efforts to earn her way through college the patient accepted a marriage proposal as an escape from her mother, a shrewish, domineering woman. The man she married was a graduate student, and while the two had expected to continue together in the university, a pregnancy forced them to alter this plan. Again the patient's ambitions were frustrated. Living in impoverished circumstances in order to provide for her husband's schooling, the patient had her first depression and was hospitalized for three months. Well for a few months, she again became pregnant, and the cycle was repeated. During her "well" periods the patient, a most attractive and socially acceptable young woman, lived actively and ambitiously, showing many traits similar to those of her mother. She had a persistent desire to mold her husband into a suave and polished gentleman.

When admitted to the ward the young woman was sullen, withdrawn, and tense. Sitting quietly, staring into a corner hour after hour, she answered in monosyllables only. She felt that she was obnoxious to others because of body odor (a delusion) and because "I am so horrid." The future looked hopeless to her. "They [the husband and children] can never amount to anything because I have ruined their lives. They aren't well trained, they haven't been fed right, and I don't know what to do. My husband can never amount to anything." This attitude continued for several months, with improvement very gradual. At a later date she said, "I find myself taking an interest in things in spite of myself." Shortly before her discharge the patient went out for little trips unaccompanied, and she had changed to the extent that she was hypomanic. Subsequent to this hospitalization there was another depression period in which she turned on the gas in an attempt to kill herself and her children. The attempt failed because of a gas explosion. Following this episode there was another "normal" period. A number of situational factors were eased and altered, and considerable effort and time was devoted to psychotherapy, but because of the regular recurrence of the depressive episodes and the severity of these periods, little optimism was felt for this patient's future.

B. Pri., Child. M:14:S:19 +1 248371′6–(51) 7:10:17
Ps. Sz., Simple

The patient had been a behavior problem since his birth. Even in infancy he had been slow in development, had tended to "live within himself," and had been apathetic. During his early childhood there had been two episodes of convulsions following his recovery from whooping cough. In school he was unable to make friends and felt inferior to other boys. Completely lacking a sense of responsibility, he seemed to have no remorse about his behavior. On one occasion he ran away and attempted to rob a filling station. Finally, as a last resort, he was referred to the psychopathic unit for study and recommendations.

His intelligence was in the dull normal range. He had had great difficulty in school and had repeated the fifth grade. He had constantly had to compete with his older brother and his younger sister, who were both normal, well adjusted, and intelligent. Compared with other children, he was quiet, slow moving, depressed, and apathetic. Because of a low basal metabolic rate he had been given thyroid medication; he had discontinued this three months before his present admission.

In the hospital there were physical evidences of moderate hypothyroidism. Psychologically he showed no spontaneous conversation and answered questions slowly with the fewest words possible. He was expressionless and remained immobile in his chair, showing no curiosity or interest in anything about him. He had spells in which he would stay in his room, lying down and staring into space. The withdrawal symptoms became more and more marked; he avoided other boys in the ward and refused food. When reprimanded for childish behavior he remained silent or just smiled. He did verbalize some anxiety and insecurity by saying that he did not eat because he could not compete with the other boys in the ward and "couldn't stand to be teased." He said he was afraid to "lick" the other boys because it "would be held against me," and asked to be put into a disturbed ward to "get away from those other boys." When the nurses did not give him the sleeping pills he demanded, he threatened them. Toward the end of his stay in the hospital he became a little more cooperative and began to associate with the older men at least. He was discharged with the general recommendation that an uncomplicated environment be arranged for him. This probably indicated institutionalization.

Ps. Sz., Paranoid M:30:S:280 +10 24'87–9 (59) 5:8:9

This man was invalided out of the Royal Marines on account of "psychoneurosis," and the medical report described him as "Retiring, seclusive, untrainable and living in a world of his own. Thinks contemplatively of suicide, and rumination of schizophrenic nature was evident." He frightened his family by strange and aggressive behavior to the extent of threatening their personal safety. He was admitted to the hospital as a voluntary patient.

He was the youngest of four children. His family was of a good social and intellectual standard. His father had committed suicide after some years of periodic melancholia. The patient had been a bright child, but shy and solitary. He went to a public school [corresponding to an American private school] but was expelled after a knife attack on another boy. After this he engaged in freelance journalism, without success. He became a farm student shortly before the war, then served with the Royal Marines until his discharge.

He was diagnosed as having schizophrenia, and he underwent a course of modified insulin therapy and electric convulsion therapy. His condition improved and he left the hospital to take up farm work. M. V.

B. Psth., Mixed F:33:S:35 +2 24′876193– 4:10:8
Schizoid —4 yrs. ′469 728–1 1:4:7

The present admission of this patient was the fourth for the same difficulty; the last admission had been eight months before. After discharge at that time the patient had gone to work in another city as a nursemaid, but she had lost the job because she was unable to control the child, and in what she said was a suicidal gesture she had taken ten sedative tablets. Since the last admission she had had sexual intercourse a number of times. The original symptomatic picture was not clear. Usually the patient was brought to the hospital by her aged father, a minister, whose complaints were that the patient was intractable, had engaged in stealing, and was going about with undesirable companions. It was known that she was untruthful, drank to excess, and engaged in a rather promiscuous sexual life, but her parents, who had had difficulty with her from her late teens, knew very few details about the patient's behavior. She was so unreliable and secretive about her activities that there was no way of knowing exactly what she had done, but her difficulties had not brought her to the attention of law enforcement authorities or other public agencies. She had had a number of affairs with older married men, all of whom were very inadequate persons.

Her school record was irregular, and she had been expelled from college after a brief attendance, mainly for failure to go to class and for breaking dormitory rules. She had started a nursing course at another university but had been dropped after two months. The same pattern was repeated at still another university. She had never been able to hold any job for more than a short period. Early in childhood she had begun to show unstable traits, with frequent temper tantrums, and she had always insisted on having her own way. She was exceedingly selfish and appeared to be more amoral and asocial than antisocial. In an attempt to control the girl, the parents had showered kindness on her.

In the hospital she appeared as a somewhat obese, moderately attractive person. During previous hospitalizations she had never shown distinct psychotic signs, but in the present period she experienced clear-cut delusions of persecution and possible visual hallucinations. She did not usually appear unduly depressed or upset, and she always seemed normal in behavior except for the complete unreliability of her conversation. It was impossible to tell when she spoke the truth and when she was lying, and it was better to assume that she was telling a falsehood. In some desperation the staff recommended her transfer to a state hospital.

B. Psth., Asocial M:21:S 24'8<u>763</u>-(51) 4:7:10
Mutilative
Mental Deficiency

This youthful prisoner performed self-mutilation as the result of a compact with three other prison inmates. He had used a dirk knife to sever the left Achilles' tendon. The prisoner was among those who, at an earlier date, had been given the MMPI as a part of an experimental program for the classification department of the state prison.

The young man is at present serving a life sentence for murder. His first sentence at the state penitentiary was for burglary. Granted a conditional pardon, he was later returned as a violator. During the same year he escaped from a prison farm but was soon apprehended. One year later he was discharged after other unsuccessful attempts to escape. Throughout his present term, he has also made a series of escape attempts, all unsuccessful. On one occasion, he participated in a mutiny, resulting in loss of good time and privileges; two weeks later he received 142 hours of solitary confinement for possession of a dirk knife; five months later he received 120 hours of solitary confinement for refusing to work; one month later he participated in another mutiny and subsequently mutilated himself by cutting his Achilles' tendon.

The youth had been brought up, with one sister, by both parents. He apparently had been residentially stable. His education went as far as the fifth grade and his grade placement on a standardized test showed a grade of 4.1. His I.Q. was 75. Employed as a common laborer, chiefly as a lumber checker, before his imprisonment, he had been rated as occupationally stable. A veteran, he had been honorably discharged from the navy. He was classified as a maximum security risk, "probably dangerous and vicious." The man's own version of his present offense was that it started when he was drinking beer with a friend who carried a revolver. He borrowed the revolver and hired a taxicab, ordering the driver to take him to a deserted spot. There he told the driver to stop, "get out of the car and start walking." He then fired three shots into the driver's body. Unable to explain why he had killed this man, he swore that he had not known him previously and had no reason for disliking him. He deserted the taxi one mile from the scene of the crime. When he was arrested four days later while at work, he promptly admitted his guilt.

Since his return to the state prison, the prisoner has been sullen, depressed, and uncooperative. After the mutilation act, he was placed in an isolation cell. The circumstances surrounding the mutilation compact are being investigated.

R. C. K.

B. Psth., Asocial M:18:S:13 +1 24'8<u>79</u>-(57) 3:8:11

The patient was admitted on a court order. The admitting problem was an intensification of personality trends that had resulted in a series of burglaries by this young man. Above normal in intelligence and with other assets, the patient had no guilt feelings about his crimes, saying that he had committed them only "for the heck of it"; he was not concerned about going to prison; and he was completely indifferent about his future. With the exception of this indifference no gross personality defects were noted. He had burglarized a manufacturing company, had broken into a hotel room, and had committed other similar offenses for which he had been sent to a reform school about sixteen months before admission. In eight months he had been paroled, and it was while on parole that he had committed the series of offenses leading to the hospital observation.

There was a long history of enuresis and encopresis. He had had childhood temper tantrums with foaming at the mouth. Truancy and occasional alcoholism were also a part of the pattern. He had been rejected from the army because of poor vision. He had a bad family background and had never been happy.

Overtly pleasant and cooperative during the hospital admission, the patient answered questions with seeming frankness and was not at all reticent about his deeds. He seldom talked for long without mentioning his crimes, often in a boisterous manner, and he was self-confident to the point of egotism, saying, "It would be a snap to get out of here." His I.Q. was 120, but his school history was bad because of truancy and other misbehavior. He seemed almost too alert. With the exception of the lack of concern about his general situation, which seemed to be more bravado than anything else, there was no obvious defect of personality. He always seemed to enjoy himself immensely and resisted any implication to the contrary. During his time in the hospital, he changed very little, and he seemed to be unconcerned when the sheriff came to take him back to court.

Alcoholism M:42:M:30 +7 249'7836–X (55) 1:16:4

This patient had suffered from daily narcolepsy attacks, lasting from a few minutes to half an hour, since the age of 21. He had also taken alcohol excessively for the last two years and was admitted to the hospital in an alcoholic confusional state.

The unwanted child of an overstrict father and an ineffectual mother, his family life had been unhappy. He received a public school education [corresponding to an American private school education] until the age of 16, but he left school without passing his examinations. He joined the Royal Air Force and was hospitalized in Trans-Jordan three years later, following an earthquake, in what apparently was an acute anxiety state. He then worked his way up to become manager of a department store, a position he left owing to differences with his employers. He later became a licensee of a public house and was successful. He had married at the age of 26.

The diagnosis was acute alcoholic state and his condition improved after psychotherapy. M. V.

Ps. M-D., Depr. M:69:M:104 +1 '26-483 (59) 3:4:8
Paranoid

Ten days before admission to the hospital the patient had experienced a sudden onset of tenseness, nervousness, insomnia, hyperirritability, and depressive anxiety. He said that he had "just gone to pieces." He had a sense of impending disaster and his head felt light. There was no precipitating event that he could identify.

The present attack was similar to two previous ones ten and five years before. During those attacks he had been hospitalized and did not know how long they had lasted, but he said, "it took a long time to get over it." His wife said that there had also been a period of manic behavior about nineteen years before admission. Except for these spells the past history was not contributory. He had had few interests outside of those connected with his work. He was a college graduate and had taught science at a university until ten years before admission when he was discharged "because of his political views." He had always worked hard and had provided well for his family. Friendly and at ease when well, he was suspicious of others, irritable, and nervous during his spells.

In the hospital he was belligerent, anxious, and suspicious, and he did not cooperate well. He said, "I don't want to talk to anyone. Go away and leave me alone." He would sit and pick his head and say "I don't know. I don't know," to anything that was asked. He seemed to know that something was wrong with him but he could not tell what it was. His sensorium was clear but there was evidence of an intellectual defect, chiefly in recent memory. He was given electroshock treatment and after a few shocks he became affable and cooperative and began to take part in group activities. He improved until his discharge. It was felt that his recovery from the present attack was certain but it was also likely that he would have recurrent trouble.

Ps. Invol. Melan. F:54:M:56 +1 26'13748-9 (41) 3:4:13
Paranoid

The patient had been perfectly well until four years before admission when she began to hear "rocking" noises and to feel rocking sensations in her body. At first she paid little attention to these queer ideas, but gradually she began to blame upstairs tenants who she felt were intentionally tormenting her by making the noises with a mechanical rocker. When these tenants moved, the sensations ceased, only to return when other people moved into the apartment. She said the sensations were "like vibrations running through my body, and a feeling of worms and ants crawling over me." She used various devices to get rid of the sensations, such as locking herself in the closet, doing her ironing in the woodshed, and wearing a cotton-lined aluminum pan on her head. Her invalid husband, for whom she had to care, gave her no sympathy, and when he intimated that she was insane it greatly upset her.

A high school graduate, she had been an average student and had enjoyed school. She had worked as a bookkeeper until she had quit at age 30 to be married. She had always got along well with others but was shy, somewhat sensitive, and afraid of doing or saying the wrong thing when she was in the company of others. Her interests were reading, listening to the radio, and playing cards. Until the onset of the present difficulties she had been active in social affairs. She said that she was short-tempered and held a grudge for a long time. During the past few months she had been depressed. Her husband had a bad heart, and for three months before the onset of the illness she had had to care for him hand and foot. Although she had been a very good manager, he scolded her for trivial things.

In the hospital she was chiefly worried about the noises and vibrations, and she firmly believed her tenants to be the cause of them although the present tenant was the third since the onset of her illness. Her ideas were not well systematized. She spoke slowly, there was no flight of ideas, her sensorium was clear, and her intelligence appeared to be well above average. She had no insight, except that she believed her nerves were giving her trouble. She was alert, calm, and cooperative. Occasionally she appeared to be depressed. She was given electroshock treatment and got a little better. At discharge she still felt her delusions were real, but she could talk about them somewhat humorously. It was hoped that she would continue to improve, and arrangements were made for outpatient contacts.

P. Mixed F:19:S 2613'7489–(43) 2:6:8

This young woman came to the clinic because she felt she was "in need of outside aid in straightening emotional entanglements." She had lost weight in the previous two months, could not eat, and complained of a general lack of energy.

From her earliest years, the client, an only child, had been warned by her mother that people are not to be trusted; even after she grew up her mother continued to seize every opportunity to point out possible infidelities on the part of the girl's friends. The mother was a domineering woman who enjoyed the martyr's role; her attitude toward her husband resulted in constant tension within the home. When the girl was very young, her mother repeatedly forced her to eat excessively and then waited for her to vomit; when she did, the mother beat and scolded the child, complaining that she was just a slave whose life was nothing except cleaning up after her child and her husband. Of superior intellectual ability, the girl did well in school and was preparing in college to be a teacher. She was engaged and planned to marry when she finished school.

Good insight into her own problems was manifested by this client. She felt that much of her difficulty might have been ameliorated if she could have left home and been free of her mother's influence. In the meantime, however, she determined to do something about her situation, and in spite of her meager funds, she had arranged one visit to a psychiatrist. In view of her financial cir-

cumstances, the clinic recommended that she take advantage of the psychiatric services at the student health center, and the client left (after two interviews) planning to do so. She did not return for further counseling. M. V. B.

B. Simple Adult Maladj. F:31:M:22 0 264'1783–9 4:5:12
P. Hypo.
Paranoid

The illness of this patient had had no definite onset, but the events leading to her admission had begun about five years before when her husband had been sent to prison. She taunted her husband by telling him about her interest in other men and she openly carried on affairs in her home town. When her husband was paroled she refused to live with him and obtained work on a nearby farm, but she got into financial trouble and had to go back to him. There was much haranguing back and forth and it was difficult to determine which of the two was the deviant. Local welfare workers had the patient admitted to the hospital for observation considerably against her own will.

The patient's general health had been good. Two years before admission she had been told that she had gonorrhea and had been offered treatment but did not accept it. There was no definite history of a previous nervous breakdown. She had reached the eighth grade in school but had then quit and had worked at home until her marriage. Her intelligence was average but she never applied herself steadily to anything, being interested only in dancing and in movies. Always a sensitive person with inferiority feelings, she was distant and did not make friends readily. She was also described as stubborn and suspicious and having a quick temper. She had five children after her marriage at 18. Her husband had been considered a good citizen until he was found guilty of embezzlement and was sent to a prison. However, the couple had begun to have marital troubles before this event.

No signs of gonorrheal infection were found in the physical studies; the neurological and physical findings were essentially normal. She told the story of her marital and other troubles in a way that placed most of the responsibility on other persons. Clearly on the defensive, she evidenced no definite delusions of persecution or reference. She had various somatic complaints that were indefinite and general; she seemed unhappy; and at times she cried when speaking about her problems. She talked fairly readily about neutral subjects but always withdrew when more intimate problems were approached. This aloofness, which was very resistant to psychotherapeutic approach, made it difficult to work with her. Appearing reasonably content with being in the hospital, she nevertheless obviously suspected that she had been falsely brought in. She had no definite plans for the future and showed no disposition to make any while in the hospital. Her condition remained unchanged during her stay although she did finally decide to take steps toward divorcing her husband, and she planned to take her five children to live with her parents.

P. React. Depr.	F:29:M:16	+2	26'4378–(43)	4:4:9
P. Mixed	F:30:M:41	+1	24738'6–(43)	4:5:16
		+35	'43–(39)	7:2:19

Although her present illness, which consisted of feelings of total inadequacy, depression, unreality, and hostility in conjunction with jealousy and fears, had begun only six months before admission, this young woman's whole life seemed to have been leading to just such a breakdown. In the past two or three years a number of things had upset her. One Saturday night while she was attending a party a drunken driver ran into her car and damaged it. Already filled with guilt for being at a party instead of entertaining her mother-in-law (as she had done weekly since her husband left for the army), the patient regarded the accident as a punishment. Also, her husband ran over a little girl when, at the patient's insistence, he was driving his mother-in-law on an errand. After a stormy pregnancy the patient delivered a six-month stillborn child. She felt as though she was in some way responsible for this.

There was a never ending progression of minor "crises" in the patient's home life. She became unable to make decisions, and when the husband finally found a house in which they could live, she could not make up her mind; first she wanted it, and after they had signed the papers she decided it was a mistake. Never interested in housework and cooking, she now found herself totally unmotivated to do these jobs in that "horrible" house. Finally, a week before admission she broke down completely. Driving home from a baby shower, she completely forgot directions and much later when she reached home, she lay awake and cried for the rest of the night. The husband could do nothing with her and took her to her mother's home where she stayed for one week until admission. Exceedingly depressed during the week, she kissed her mother goodby several times and said she was going "to end it all." She did not actually attempt suicide, however. She did attend a dance and while others thought she enjoyed herself she said she was "only pretending."

The past history included no really severe illnesses but there were a number of episodes of a hysterical type. In one of these her appendix had been removed and several doctors had examined her for pain in the abdomen without discovering a reason for it. Menstruation had always been accompanied by great difficulty and by depression.

After two years in college the patient had been unable to continue because her eyes seemed weak and her doctor told her to quit school. Next she did secretarial work. Even after her marriage the patient liked to work and was successful. She was thoughtful, at ease, and friendly with others. In general she was a passive, dependent person who let other people solve many of her problems. Full of energy, she led an active life. Although she usually handled money well, she had recently played the stock market and had lost heavily. She felt badly about this. In general she had been marked by high drive and ambition but had had basically little resilience.

In the hospital she seemed composed and showed only moderate anxiety and mild depression. She was friendly and could apparently forget her troubles completely when engaged in some activity such as playing bridge. She was intact in sensorium and intellect. At first she was kept in the disturbed ward because of agitation and depression, but improvement came quickly and proved to be steady. She talked freely and expressed feelings of hostility and resentment toward both her husband and her mother-in-law. It appeared that many neurotic qualities had been present all her life but that she had always kept up a "surface" which had successfully hidden them. The gain in perspective was clear, and she developed a great deal of insight into the nature of her problems. The outlook at discharge was felt to be good. Four months later she was readmitted. She had been in a private hospital for a few days in the interim and had left against advice. She then got steadily worse and was readmitted with symptoms similar to those of the first admission. She again got better and was discharged to return to her home.

Ps. Paranoid F:48:S:29 +1 264781'3–(49) 3:13:11

The patient was admitted with paranoid delusions and vague generalized somatic complaints. About a month before admission she began complaining that a woman in a downstairs apartment was intentionally making noise to disturb her. She said that by overhearing a conversation between two girls who also lived downstairs she had found out about a machine by which the woman was spying on her. The patient thought that sound traveled from floor to floor in the house, and that in some way unknown to her this was encouraged by neighbors for ulterior purposes. Investigation of her occupational history revealed that the patient had quit several jobs because she believed that people in the office were reading her mind and talking about her. She entered the hospital not because of any insight into the delusional nature of her complaint but because her sister asked her to.

An eleventh-grade graduate, the patient had held various positions, mostly at the clerical level. Her social life had been mainly within her family. She had never married and denied ever having had any sexual experiences. A quiet, easygoing, capable person, she was overly suspicious and sensitive. Her complaint that she was overloaded with responsibility apparently had some foundation because she was accustomed to working twelve to fourteen hours daily, but it was not clear whether this was in part by choice or whether it was required by her employer.

Her sensorium and intellect were clear, and she was well composed, conventional in behavior, cooperative, and logical. Only with regard to the delusions was she obviously maladjusted. Average in intelligence, she was passive in bearing and manner, participated poorly in group activities, and was not able to associate comfortably with other patients. After shock therapy, the delusions persisted but were less troublesome because she at least accepted the behavior she still assumed present in people about her. However, she gained no insight into the fact that her ideas were delusional, and there was little basic change in her. When she was discharged to her family, it was with the feeling that she would continue to make a marginal adjustment only as long as she was within the family group.

Ps. Invol. Melan.　　M:60:M:8　　+2　　2'67–1(61)　　2:4:10

The illness of this patient began about three years before admission when he complained of a backache for which his physician could find no organic basis. He was a dentist and, simultaneously with the appearance of the pain in his back, he began to have arguments with his patients. He blamed their failure to appreciate his work for his depression and insomnia. Later he became disturbed about an affair that his wife had had before their marriage. His sexual desire increased markedly, and he was very uncomfortable until he finally went to a state hospital as a voluntary patient. He stayed only three weeks, complaining that it was cold and depressing there. He did receive some electroshock treatments. At the time of admission he was moderately disturbed.

There was nothing outstanding in his past medical and psychological history, although he had a few hysterical symptoms. He was reserved and had never sought friends. He had prided himself on his virtues and ideals. He was a slow but hard worker and had earned his way through dental school. He had married after graduation. He described himself as somewhat stubborn, irritable, pessimistic, nervous, and easily depressed. He had occasional periods of rage, during which he would rant and rave. He depended on his wife to bolster his self-esteem.

In the hospital he was depressed, continually making such statements as these: "People don't care about me," "People don't appreciate my work." His worries centered around his misfortune in being conscientious and hard working when people did not appreciate him. He felt that he was passing through the male climacteric and that this was the cause of his upset. His intellect, orientation, and general mentation were intact. Emotionally he was fairly stable though depressed. He spent almost his whole energy worrying about his insomnia, which appeared to the staff to be only moderate. The patient was unable to grasp the fact that the insomnia was the symptom of a broader personality disorder. His family became alarmed because he did not appear to be sleeping as well in the hospital as he did at home and in cooperation with the patient they took him from the hospital against advice.

Ps. Invol. Melan.　　F:62:W:26　　+1　　26'7 13 48–9(61)　　6:4:14
Deteriorated　　?　　271'3684–9(51)　　7:6:14

After the death of this woman's husband five months before admission, she had become depressed. As the condition grew consistently worse, she lost interest in things, neglected her housework, and was nervous, self-conscious, and afraid to make simple decisions. After study in the outpatient clinic she was admitted for more intense treatment.

Seven years earlier a period of depression had followed an accident in which she had broken her hip. Apparently at that time she had been agitated and had had paranoid ideas. She had recovered without hospitalization, and no further details were available on it. The patient's past physical health was described by her as having "always been poor." For years she had been subject to vague gastrointestinal complaints and to food idiosyncrasies.

2671'4398–

At the age of 16 she had finished the ninth grade and had begun taking care of her mother. From that time on she had worked as a housekeeper. Her social interests were limited and she made few friends. Somewhat high-strung, and with a worrisome and complaining nature, she was meticulous but efficient in the management of her household.

The physical and neurological examinations were negative. She was cooperative but showed psychomotor retardation. She was chiefly concerned with her personal problems. There were no obvious delusions or hallucinations or suicidal tendencies. She was untidy in appearance but well oriented. There was no clearly demonstrable defect of sensorium or intellect. Her only explanation of her illness was "nervousness." After electroshock treatment she became more active, entered into ward activities, and showed more interest in her personal appearance. At the time of discharge she was cheerful and looked forward to returning to her usual activities. The prognosis was thought to be good.

P. Hypo. F:40:M:19 +2 2671'4398– 7:3:10

P. Hypo. F:41:M:7 +3 2137'64– 8:4:11

At the admission of this patient there were symptoms of cholelithiasis and also headaches and diminished hearing. The patient had been told thirteen years earlier that she had syphilis and had been treated for it. Although she had been reassured that the treatment was adequate, she continued to worry. As she began to have more and more headaches, she decided these were due to the syphilis. Married seven years after the diagnosis of this disease, she had not told her husband about it, and this became a source of anxiety to her. She complained of diminished hearing which became progressively worse until she was barely able to hear a distinct voice.

The patient had attended a country school and at her mother's insistence had finished one year of high school although schoolwork had always been difficult for her. Then for a while she did housework and later became a waitress in a hotel restaurant. At 25 she was married and did not work again outside the home. Her "sick headaches" began many years before admission. Always shy, bashful, and sensitive, these characteristics decreased somewhat as she grew older. She was given to daydreaming and spent considerable time reading. She held grudges for long periods of time and had strong likes and dislikes. A self-reliant person, she had few friends. She was usually not deceitful. She exercised good judgment in money matters and described herself as "stingy." She claimed that the premarital intercourse which led to the syphilitic infection was by force. Most of her symptoms and personality changes dated from this experience. She harbored considerable guilt over not having discussed the episode with her husband. She and her husband were congenial.

The physical examination revealed a typical Argyll-Robertson pupil, bilateral partial nerve deadness, and other neurological findings consistent with a nervous system disorder. There were also signs that the cholelithiasis was a definite condition. There was no evidence of progressing nervous destruction from the syphilis. She appeared anxious and worried and found it hard to accept the findings indicating that her headaches were not due to syphilis. She was somewhat voluble and gossipy. Open and accessible on most subjects, she was, however, evasive about the background for the syphilis. She got along well with the other patients and with the personnel. With careful reassurance, she gradually came to accept the fact that syphilis need not be the "terrible disease" she had always felt it to be. She still refused, however, to tell her husband about it. There was considerable improvement, and at discharge it appeared probable that she would make a reasonable adjustment.

Ps. M-D., Depr. Suicidal	F:25:S:5	+1	2'6743-	4:4:17
Ps. M-D., Manic	F:25:S:7	+4	'4679-1	3:3:14

The illness began about a month before admission when the patient, a teacher, began to fear that she might not have done as good a job as she should have, and that her pupils might not be able to pass their examinations. This worry and depression progressed to the point where she made one definite attempt on her life (by hanging), followed by another questionable attempt at suicide. She also said once that she wanted to take her life. Within a relatively short time the depression shifted to a hyperactive elated state. When she was alone she talked to herself. She entered the hospital as a voluntary patient.

The patient was born with the congenital absence of both arms below the lower third of the upper arms and the right leg below the lower third of the thigh. She also had a withered and useless left leg. She had learned to walk with artificial limbs and had learned to write, eat, dress, and take care of most of her personal needs by using her arm stumps. Apparently she had adjusted well to her physical abnormality. She had no apparent self-consciousness about it, and it bothered her only because of the problems it presented for her future success. A university graduate with a very high standing, she had done work toward a master's degree. Socially she had been very adequate, and taking her handicap into consideration she had taken more interest in a variety of activities than one would expect. She read and wrote extensively, and until the onset of the present illness she had been a cheerful, stable person. With the exception of her physical disabilities she seemed to have been an entirely normal person.

In the hospital she was able to cover up her depression nicely, although she cried a little. Neat, conventional in behavior, clear and logical in everything she said, she had good insight into the fact that she was sick. She had some fear of failure, and a slight tendency toward self-depreciation. Her elation had apparently disappeared. As nearly as could be determined, the illness had run its course before admission. Five months later she was readmitted in the latter stages of a manic phase.

P. React. Depr.	F:61:M:46	—20	2674'8139–	2:15:6
P. React. Depr.	F:64:M:47	+1	2867'1493–(63)	8:13:10

Seventeen years before admission the patient's husband had become totally blind from glaucoma. From that time, taking care of him and meeting financial difficulties had placed a great burden on the patient and she had become increasingly worried and depressed. She had repeatedly attempted to get her husband to go to a state school for the blind, but he had refused until the admission of the patient to the hospital, when he simultaneously went to that school. The patient and her husband had both been upset and nervous, which had precipitated frequent quarrels.

About twelve years before admission the patient had developed dermatitis, which had been chronic since that time in spite of many medications. This rash was the patient's chief complaint because it led to a great deal of physical discomfort and to insomnia. She also complained of tinnitus and deafness of the left ear and said that these conditions made her more nervous. She had a number of other somatic complaints and had noted an increasing defect in recent memory. She was taking digitalis for "heart trouble" at the time of her admission. An immigrant, the patient had attended school in Bohemia as far as the third grade and had come to this country when she was in her teens. After arriving in America she had worked as a housekeeper and as a maid. Before her illness she had had many close friends and had been happy and satisfied with her life, although she had always been somewhat unstable emotionally.

In the hospital the physical and neurological examinations indicated the possibility of some senile changes. There was no specific evidence for severe organic deterioration, however. The dermatitis appeared as leathery patches at the sides of the neck, on the anterior chest, and on the arms. The patient was neat, friendly, and talkative, especially when the conversation concerned her illness and her troubles. She gave the impression of being fidgety and nervous and never stayed in one position for long. She was sad and was worried about her dermatitis and about her husband. She wept readily and appeared resigned to the fact that she might have to live with the dermatitis for the rest of her life. She felt that the rest in the hospital would do a great deal for her. In fact, she did get somewhat better, though not markedly so, and at the time of discharge she and the staff had made plans for some changes in her home situation to give her more security, and for follow-up visits to the outpatient department. Three years later she was readmitted to the hospital. Her husband had stayed in the school for the blind for only seven weeks and had then moved back with her. Under these conditions her previous symptomatology gradually reappeared. She was discharged to go to a rest home with the strong recommendation that she live apart from her husband.

Ps. M-D., Depr. F:58:M:43 +1 26794′183– 8:10:8
Paranoid

About six months before coming to the hospital the patient developed multiple joint pain, and subsequently she gradually became depressed, nervous, agitated, and irritable. At times she alleged that her neighbors and some relatives were talking about her, and that they were not treating her right. When her care became too much of a burden for her husband and her sister, she expressed suicidal ideas, and she was referred to the hospital.

Since childhood she had had annual spells of depression lasting for a few weeks, during which she became agitated, lost interest in things, had difficulty in concentrating, and showed paranoid trends, but in the last few years before admission the attacks had increased in frequency and intensity. There were no manic intervals. Only once during this series of attacks had she been hospitalized. The patient had taken some normal school training and a few summer courses at a university, and she had taught country school for about twenty years. After one unhappy love affair she had married a man who was ten years younger than she and a not very successful farmer. Their economic insecurity troubled her, and she did not find farm life satisfying. She was described as an intelligent, hard-working, sensitive, stubborn, impulsive, and unusually religious person. Never open or friendly, she tended to brood over her problems and to blame others for her difficulty.

Symptoms such as weakness and joint pains were presented in the hospital, and she also complained about her depression. There were no gross defects of sensorium or intellect, but she was convinced that her relatives had colluded against her. A cooperative person, she made a good adjustment in the hospital and was usually open and accessible for discussion of her problems, although there were times when she was unaccountably defiant and recalcitrant. Her attitude and manner made her unpopular with the other patients who found her irritating, and she accused the staff of having her "on the spot," implying vaguely that she was being held for some ulterior purpose. On one occasion she ran away from a group while they were out walking, and she was returned by the police who had found her making her way toward the home of relatives in a nearby city. Psychotherapeutic measures and reassurance aided her little if at all. Although the staff felt that she should stay in the hospital for a longer period, she had to be discharged because she was such a disturbing element. Since her husband did not want to take her to another hospital, she was sent home on trial to see if she could make an adequate adjustment.

B. Psth., Mixed F:33:S:15 +6 ′268 14 37–9X(55) 10:6:17
Ps. Sz., Simple
Paranoid

The patient had always been dependent and insecure, definitely inferior to her siblings in scholastic and social attainment. She had never gone out with a boy and had twice attempted to become a nun but was dismissed—once possibly for physical reasons and the second time apparently because of her inability to make an adequate adjustment to the order. She became seclusive and began to wear old-fashioned and odd clothing. Eight days before admission to the hospital she allegedly stole a cake from a bakery shop and was taken to jail. Three days later in the attorney's office she had what was apparently an attack of hysterical fainting.

There were no previous psychotic episodes, though there had been a period when she was thought to be a hypothyroid case. Her intelligence was average or somewhat above. She seemed to be basically unhappy and thwarted. Her social adjustment was inadequate since she was restricted to her family and her interests never led outside of her home.

In the hospital the most marked feature of the patient's illness was the frequent, inappropriate, and silly laughter which punctuated her speech. She repeatedly denied having been guilty of stealing; she was depressed over her failure to become a nun and felt that it exemplified her inadequacy. Openly hostile to an older sister, she expressed poorly defined ideas of persecution but was obviously trying to give the impression of being cheerful and normal. She felt that her problem was summed up in the fact that she had lost weight and had been very lonely since her mother's death. Her appearance was unkempt and she was slightly aggressive. She had no hallucinations or marked delusional ideas. She changed little on the ward and mixed with the other patients in a noisy and restless manner, frequently criticizing their behavior and thus becoming unpopular. A psychiatric follow-up program was organized for her, including an attempt to encourage her to make broader social contacts. She was improved at discharge but the prognosis did not appear to be good.

Ps. Paranoid F:29:W:38 +8 2683'7194– 4:5:12

This patient's personality had always been poorly organized, and there was no sharply separated episode of illness. As far back as four years before admission attempts had been made to arrange for a psychiatric investigation of her. Her behavior had been irresolute and erratic. She had unfounded objections to people and situations and showed paroxysmal rage reactions. Some of her feelings were described as "delusions of persecution" by the social service reports on her. A physician described her as an "early dementia praecox." She was a problem for the welfare workers who had to supply her with aid of various sorts. Her appreciation of this help was very limited and her cooperation poor.

She had had ill-defined physical complaints for a long time. There were, however, no previous episodes of mental upset. At one time she was given an intelligence test by a state psychologist and was found to have an I.Q. of 70. He classified her as a moron and put her on a waiting list for admission to a school for the feeble-minded. In the meantime she graduated from high school and completed a two-year normal course in a state teachers' college. She taught for two years but lost her job, apparently because of incompetence. After this she remained at home until her marriage, occasionally working at odd jobs but never doing very well. Defective in judgment, she was considered shiftless and irresponsible. She had narrow interests, was self-conscious, and made friends slowly. Her marriage had occurred when she was 23 to a man who was dull, impecunious, poorly adjusted. They had lived on a shabby farm and had received relief, but there had been no gross discord between them. There were three children. Four years after the marriage, however, the husband had committed suicide by hanging, and it was said that he was mentally unbalanced at the time. It was difficult to estimate the influence of this factor upon the patient but the faultiness of her adjustment did become more pronounced. The family was helped by the welfare board, but the patient could not adjust herself to the conditions imposed by the board.

In the hospital the patient talked at length about her problems and difficulties. She showed no well-formed delusions, but there was a definite suspiciousness. Her talk was vague and rambling. She complained of tiredness and said that if she could rest she would probably be all right. Her orientation was good and there was no marked disturbance of intellect or sensorium. Her I.Q. as determined in the hospital was 117. The contrast of this finding with the earlier one and with her life history was obviously marked but inexplicable. There was an emotional blunting, although for the most part she was pleasant and friendly and cooperated very well in ward activities. Occasionally she showed some concern about her children, but never any real anxiety. She said she eventually wanted to go to work and to try to make a better life. After arrangements were made for her to begin work and a place was found for the family to live, she was discharged.

Ps. M-D., Depr.	F:53:M:43	+25	2'687-9 (68)	5:8:8
Schizoid		+28	<u>26</u>'<u>78</u>3-9 (55)	5:8:12

The patient had been overly religious most of her life, but in the four weeks preceding hospital admission this had become extreme. She frequently recited irrelevant quotations from the Bible and preached religion to her family. She told her family and her neighbors that the people of the city had been watching her and were going to harm her. She said that workmen who had been repairing a neighbor's roof had looked into her window and bathroom. Some days later she became still more preoccupied with religion and said that she could see God and the angels. Four days before admission she became excited, paced the floor, waved her arms, and sang religious hymns in English and German. She called houseflies "bats" and was afraid of them. This acute period was followed by one in which she became depressed and denied that she had done any of the things mentioned. This melancholia increased until her admission to the hospital. Twelve years before, she had apparently gone through a similar episode of depression that had lasted about four months.

The patient's interests were limited to her home and to church affairs. She was quiet, shy, aloof, and sensitive. Her intelligence was dull normal. She was described as hot-tempered. She and her husband appeared compatible, and they had one daughter who was 17 years of age.

In the hospital the patient was depressed and reserved, looked unhappy, and answered questions very slowly if at all. She cried occasionally and covered her eyes with her hands. She was well oriented and seemed psychologically intact except for the depression. She gradually improved until the time of discharge but always preferred to stay in her room rather than to mix with other patients. The depression had obviously not left her at the time of discharge.

Ps. Psth. P. Hys.	F:27:M:33	+31	26871'34–	4:5:15
Ps. Psth. P. Hys.	F:27:M:70	+69	4836'712–	5:2:18

The patient was admitted to the hospital because of peculiar spells of marked agitation and depression and talk of suicide. The illness began when the patient realized that she was pregnant as the result of a casual sexual episode. She became despondent, centered all her attention on her predicament, lost her appetite, and was unable to sleep. She had attacks of marked restlessness when she threw herself on the floor, kicked, and screamed. Her talk during these episodes was a constant repetition of these ideas: "I want to die. I don't want to live. Why don't you kill me? I can't go home or I would kill my daughter."

The patient was of dull normal intelligence and had had considerable difficulty in school, which she left at age 15 after reaching the seventh grade. She had never been able to earn money but had assisted on her parents' farm. Interested in outdoor sports, she was reticent and bashful around people. From an early age she had been "boy crazy." She first became pregnant at age 22 as a result of promiscuous sexual relations. Marriage was forced upon her by the man in this case and by her parents, though she would have liked to marry another. She had two children by this husband, who finally left her for good. They were not divorced. After the separation the patient continued her promiscuous affairs. Her alliances with men appeared to have been on a very superficial level and her sexual behavior seemed less determined by her sexual desire than by passivity.

In the hospital she exhibited a psychomotor retardation. She tended to lie on her bed, continually poking and kneading at her abdomen. When pressed she complained of feeling "blank and empty." She said she didn't know what the hospital personnel were going to do with her and that she was sure she couldn't "recognize people." She described her spells by saying, "I'll fall on the floor and kick and scream. I feel as though I would have them as long as I live. I know what is going on but I can't stop myself." She blamed all her troubles on her pregnancy. On the day of admission she had two of her "spells," in which she threw herself from side to side screaming, "Take my baby so I can die." She was a difficult hospital patient, meeting suggestions that she take part in activities with such excuses as, "I don't know where the kitchen is, or what my duties are." The confusional state seemed to be a defensively assumed attitude rather than a real disorder.

She was sent home to her sister but was readmitted a couple of weeks later, having been unmanageable while she was out. This time she had stereotyped mannerisms, picked at her face, and disrobed. She showed negativism and had to be fed by tube. Much of the time she was almost completely inaccessible. In the course of the seventy-day second hospitalization she gradually got better. Toward the last of her stay the child was born without complication. In cooperation with the social service she made plans for placing the child in an institution. She showed no evidence of concern about this: "I know my folks can't take care of another one of my children." She insisted that she was going to be all right and the main reason was that she was "going to stay away from men from now on."

P. Mixed　　M:19:S　　26'8749–(65)　　5:6:13

This college student was referred to the clinic because he had been troubled by sleepwalking over the last five years. This had become more frequent and he had recently lacerated his hand severely during one of the episodes.

He was the only child of a family that had been broken by the suicide of his mother (in a mental hospital) when he was 7. The father appeared to have been an irresponsible, psychopathic person. The patient was brought up by a maiden aunt to whom he was tied by feelings of great indebtedness and of guilt because of his hostility and desire to be independent. He was a very intelligent boy.

During treatment it rapidly became evident that he had many compulsive defenses, and a considerable amount of masochism was evident in his sexual fantasy. He also complained of frequent mood swings in which depression was more prominent than elation. The patient was seen in 21 individual interviews and 12 group interviews over a period of about nine months. He responded well to this relatively intensive treatment and lost many of his obsessive characteristics. He became freer and more tolerant of himself and of others. The depressive spells were less frequent and he made progress in working out his relationship with his father and his aunt. The sleepwalking disappeared as a symptom.

C. K. A.

P. React. Depr.　　M:47:M:40　　+5　　2'6973–　　4:2:7
P. Psychas.　　+39　　'964–873　　6:3:7

Two months before admission the patient suddenly became depressed. He said that he did not feel well, and his reaction was to cry. He had a fear of impending insanity, and a fear that he would harm someone. He worried about financial matters and about his work. Visitors upset him. He had periods during the day when he was fairly comfortable, but he would suddenly become overwhelmed by his fears and worries. About a year before the present illness he had had a similar depression that had lasted for two weeks.

After dropping out of school in the fifth grade he was employed in sawmills and harvest fields as an itinerant worker. A rigid, poorly adjusted, sensitive, and easily offended person, he felt resentment toward his family, and he had a tendency to carry grudges against people. He worked hard, never taking time for recreation; this work drive was apparently compulsive behavior. After marrying at age 21 he had difficulty providing for his wife. They were fairly compatible, but his wife would have liked to have had more social life. There were no children.

In the hospital he worried about financial matters. He said that his wife's friends and relatives came to visit him in the hospital at all hours of the day and night and that it interfered with his work and with his sleep. The conduct of some of the young people disgusted him. He wanted to get back to his home and work. When questioned on psychiatrically significant material he became anxious and depressed, expressing ideas of hopelessness, but he was cooperative, and his stream of thought was adequate. He was intact in sensorium and intellect. He felt that his troubles were due to his difficult life. He seemed to get some benefit from the free expression of his antagonisms toward his wife and her friends, and the bland routine of the ward helped him. At the time of discharge he was relaxed, and slept well, and it appeared that he might make a very satisfactory home adjustment. The likelihood of improved behavior was greater because a number of mild physical disorders were cleared up during his stay in the psychopathic unit.

Ps. Sz., Simple	F:23:S:72	+1	'27-3 (53)	3:9:9
		+22	'9-13 (53)	2:11:11

This young woman had apparently been normal until two years before admission. At that time she had been working regularly until suddenly one day she had appeared, exhibiting peculiar behavior, at her sister's home in a distant part of the state. Placed in a mental hospital for three weeks, she was then returned to her own home. Throughout the interval before the present hospitalization there was a marked social withdrawal. For hours she would sit in a corner and stare into space. At times there was inappropriate laughter. She ventured infrequently from her home. In dress and behavior she appeared to be in early adolescence. Except for the presence of severe dysmenorrhea and gastric distress all her life the past physical history revealed little.

After high school graduation the patient had worked at five different jobs before the onset of this illness. During the first year following high school her parents insisted that she live at home. It was suspected that while living by herself just before the beginning of her illness she had done a great deal of dancing and drinking. There were also stories of a boy friend, but details were few and the sources unreliable.

In the hospital it was impossible to establish rapport with the patient. She answered all questions, after a long hesitation, with monosyllables. At times she showed evidences of hostility toward her family. There was inappropriate laughter which she explained by saying that she had "funny thoughts." Her sensorium and intellect were intact. She appeared to be no older than a 15-year-old girl. Throughout her stay she remained withdrawn and she frequently smiled to herself. Extensive insulin treatment resulted in a somewhat more normal appearance, but the difference was not great. She was discharged to return to her family. It was felt that her behavior was not severely abnormal, and that she would cause no real difficulty. Several months later her family had her committed to a state hospital.

P. Psychas.	M:50:M:92	+4	2'7–9	3:1:11
P. Psychas.	M:59:M:15	+4	732816'4–(55)	5:0:21

The patient was admitted to the hospital with a disabling fear of all germs, especially tuberculosis, which led to continual hand washing and crying spells. The trouble had begun about a year before admission when he became obsessed with the idea that his food was contaminated. Soon afterward he began bringing his barbering tools home to boil them. As the condition became worse, he was almost continually washing his hands and the compulsion to sterilize his tools prevented him from doing his barbering. In his insistence on cleanliness, he kept his wife constantly washing clothes and household furniture, so that her hands became macerated. Just before admission he began to fear that he would go insane unless he could be cured.

A barber from about age 16, the patient was known to be overly meticulous about his personal habits and belongings. Although he had always been dependent upon his family for emotional security, he was a thrifty person and had never had to worry about finances. He was accepted in his small community and had been the village treasurer for twenty years. He was considered a nervous person, and he had suffered from nervous indigestion. Of average intelligence, he was somewhat stubborn and rigid, but in spite of these characteristics he was a likable person. He was happily married, and the couple had one married daughter.

In the hospital the patient took a calm, rational attitude toward his problems; he recognized that there was no reason for his feelings about germs, saying that although he knew it was foolish for him to wash his hands incessantly, he was most uncomfortable when he did not. A great deal of time was spent in attempts to re-create earlier experiences and to obtain insight into possible guilt feelings, but such techniques as free association and hypnosis were unproductive. He was somewhat better when he left the hospital, and he and his wife spent several months in a small cottage in the woods where he cut the firewood and did other strenuous work. When he went back to barbering, he was well and for about eight years was his old self. Then the symptoms came back with an almost exact repetition of the original pattern. He went to a private psychiatric clinic where he was treated with electroshock. This did not help and he was readmitted to the psychiatric unit. The second hospitalization appeared to have no more beneficial effects than did the first. He was discharged again to try his own methods for recovery.

Ps. Invol. Melan. Paranoid F:60:M:17 +2 '27–9(47) 5:1:13

When admitted to the hospital, this patient showed erratic behavior with fright, melancholia, weakness, inability to swallow, and other somatic signs. Five months earlier she had begun to have spells of "nervousness" characterized by excessive sweating, palpitation, apprehension, indecisiveness, and emotional outbursts. She was afraid to go out, and once on a shopping trip she had to be taken home because she was suddenly seized with shaking and apprehension. For a while she felt that the food she ate was not entering her stomach. She confided to her husband that she thought she was going to die. She never made any suicidal attempts.

The patient graduated from the eighth grade at age 14; she had been a fair student. Her family and friends described her as stubborn, self-depreciating, shy in the presence of others, and easily hurt. She had been neat and clean about her person and, in general, had been thought of as "dutiful." She was a devout Christian Scientist. A fairly cheerful person, she had been a good mother and housewife, and there were no obvious factors in her background that fitted in with the recent exacerbation of symptoms.

On admission the uppermost thoughts in the patient's mind were centered around her family. She appeared to have hallucinations. Among her gross delusions were the beliefs that she was to be sent immediately to an asylum, where her head would be shaved, and that the doctors were annoying her on purpose. She appeared apathetic and depressed and made many self-pitying remarks. Her insight was poor, and she showed marked psychomotor retardation. She was slovenly and generally neglectful of her appearance. Day by day she became steadily more apprehensive and upset, and finally electroshock therapy was begun. After five treatments she appeared considerably improved and seemed almost normal. There was a slight regression, but at discharge she was in good condition. However, she seemed unwilling to accept the problems of her age and the fact that her family was growing up and leaving home. It was felt that she had only a moderate chance of making an adjustment without further attacks, and in fact she was soon readmitted with another acute spell. She received shock therapy and again improved markedly. Admitted a third time only twenty days later, she was finally sent to a state hospital.

Ps. M-D., Depr. M:52:M:54 +27 27'1–4 3:4:5
Suicidal

The patient's admission symptoms were excessive worry, irritability, inability to concentrate, abdominal pains, and spells of weakness during the previous twelve months. A crop failure in the summer following the first appearance of these symptoms had aggravated the condition. He had sudden outbursts of temper, crying spells, and compulsive acts which prevented him from working, and he talked of driving a car into a train since he was "no good anyway."

From the time he had left school in the sixth grade, he had worked at numerous occupations including truck driving and farming. At one time he had been diagnosed as having stomach ulcers, and although he had gone on a farm to avoid hard work, he had found farming more exhausting than the other things he had done. Very much a family man, he was devoted to his wife and children, and he had always been well liked by his neighbors and fellow workers. He had always been easily offended and had taken disappointments unusually hard.

In the hospital the patient had a marked tenseness revealed in tremor, perspiration, and occasional crying spells. His mental content was chiefly concerned with his conviction that he was an abject failure. "I'm blue and all worn out all the time. I have spells when I feel like I could fly into a thousand pieces. I can't make up my mind what to do. I let my wife boss me all the time. The easiest way would be to have a train wreck. I'm a whipped man. I've worked hard all my life, and now I haven't anything." Among his somatic complaints, a severe pain in the abdomen was the main one. Soon he began to gain weight and to take a more hopeful attitude toward life. His wife was advised to dispose of the farm, and before the patient was discharged his son-in-law had agreed to help him for a while, his wife had taken another house, and plans had been made for him to do light farming which would relieve him of much of the responsibility that had previously so depleted his morale.

P. React. Depr. M:48:M:24 +5 271348'69–(61) 1:4:13

The patient's difficulties had begun just before his dismissal from his job six months before admission, with the onset characterized by apprehension about his future. After he was laid off from his job he went for a vacation to a lake; while there he noticed "gas on his stomach." There was also a fluttering of his heart and short periods of rapid heart beat. He consulted a local physician who prescribed small amounts of whiskey. This was ineffectual and he consulted another physician who advised cathartics. Still another physician told him he was "going to die of coronary thrombosis very soon." This disturbed him so deeply that he was admitted to a veterans' psychiatric hospital, where he was placed in an oxygen tent and heavily sedated for a period of about six days. After a few days at home in bed he became so nervous and irritable that he could sleep only with sedation. The situation became unbearable for his daughter, his son-in-law, and his grandchild, who lived with him, and for his wife, and he came to the hospital in the present admission.

The patient had attended high school for two years, and while he had not actually failed he had not liked mathematics. After going to a mechanics' school for two years, he worked as a mechanic for a while and then worked at various partially skilled jobs. His interests were chiefly in passive sports such as fishing and hunting. At ease with strangers, he was known to be cheerful and stable but rather secretive. His wife and he appeared to be well matched and there were no evidences of marital difficulty.

On admission to the hospital he was very worried about dying, about his debts, and about being in a mental institution. He was well oriented and his memory was apparently intact. He was depressed and resigned to some fate about which he was not at all clear. His tested I.Q. was 111, but he had very poor insight and was slow in speech and retarded in behavior. Irritable and disliking questioning, he was disgusted with hospital routine, and no real progress could be made with psychotherapy. In an amytal interview he stated that his present illness began when on two occasions he had pain in his penis during intercourse. The most important general causes of his difficulties appeared to be the insecurity about his financial future and the problems of aging. He was somewhat better at discharge, and it seemed likely that he would probably continue to improve.

Ps. M-D., Depr. M:36:M:67 +9 2'71368–9(47) 9:3:14
Paranoid +30 '934–(35) 6:1:19

About four months before admission to the hospital the patient was involved in a peculiar incident which evidently precipitated this illness. His brother had sold some unclaimed cattle, and apparently the patient had been an innocent onlooker to the affair, which was shady in part. The sheriff had investigated, going so far as to take the patient's child out of class to question her. Immediately, the patient had begun to show changes in behavior. These included paranoid ideas that members of the community considered his brother a thief, suspiciousness of the motives of others, agitation, and depression. He became mute and spoke abruptly if at all. Placed in a rest home, he showed no improvement and was finally brought to the hospital.

The patient was of average intelligence. At the end of the seventh grade, when he was 16, he left school to go to work on his father's farm. At the time of admission he owned a large farm of his own and was well-to-do. Before the illness he had been capable in managing his own affairs and had been known as a hard and conscientious worker. A quiet man, he was sensitive to criticism but friendly. He had a high sense of responsibility toward his work and his family.

In the hospital the patient was well dressed and neat. He showed a marked psychomotor retardation and was practically mute except for occasional short-phrased, abrupt, and often incomprehensible answers. He was apparently well oriented and relatively coherent. He got along well with the other patients and seemed interested in their activities but did not join in them. Following six electroshock treatments, he began to show gradual improvement. He talked more freely and took part in the social activities of the ward. However, he still would not discuss himself or his problems. After four months of silence on these subjects, he suddenly began to talk freely and in retrospect admitted to delusions of reference, suspiciousness, and feelings of guilt and hopelessness. Improvement, however, continued to be very slow. At the time of discharge he was definitely not well, but it appeared likely that he would be able to adjust with reasonable adequacy to his home environment.

P. React. Depr. F:25:M:22 +22 2713̲6'84– 4:6:12

This young woman suffered depression associated with insomnia, loss of interest, anorexia, and dislike for her 6-month-old child. Following the delivery of this child the patient had shown a marked personality change. She lost interest in the baby, spoke of abandoning it, became depressed, and complained of loss of appetite. All her "normal feelings" seemed to have disappeared or changed.

Before the illness, the patient had been an active, energetic person, interested in social activities. There were no particular difficulties in her physical development or her history. A high school graduate, she worked as a domestic until her marriage at age 23 to a man fifteen years her senior. The marriage followed a six-year courtship, and she said she felt "it was the thing to do" after such a long period. At 16 she had had a lover whom she had never really forgotten. Emotionally dissatisfied with her marriage, she tended to dwell upon "what might have been" had she married her early suitor. The family was very poor.

In the hospital the young woman complained bitterly that she seemed "unable to enjoy anything," that her emotional responses seemed blunted. In spite of feeling tired, she slept poorly, and most of the time she felt despondent and hopeless. She looked depressed and moved about only after much urging. She gradually showed improvement and eventually took a fairly active part in ward activities. Her physical condition improved and she felt more her "normal self." The whole pattern appeared to be a type of reactive depression, and although she was considerably better at discharge, it was felt not unlikely that she might have a new attack if she later experienced stresses.

Ps. Invol. Melan. M:58:M:83 +5 2713'84–9 4:8:10

This patient was admitted to the hospital because of extreme nervousness and a mild depression of five years' duration. The nervousness had forced him to discontinue work and prevented him from holding a job. He had pulled out nearly all his hair; he stuttered; and he complained of a dull headache, indigestion, and paresthesias. The onset of these symptoms had coincided with financial difficulties and other circumstances that required major readjustments in his life. He had resigned from his position and had moved from a large home to a small cottage. This simplification of his life helped his condition for more than a year. Then he experimented in some minor business activities and after a series of failures and disappointments in these he again became nervous and began to pull out his hair. This and other symptoms increased until admission.

The patient had previously been in good health all his life; occasional headaches were almost his only physical complaint. A good student, he finished the eighth grade and would have liked to continue school but was forced to take a job for financial reasons. He developed skill in "white collar" commercial work and remained with the same firm until the onset of the present illness. Of average intelligence, he was well liked, friendly, and at ease in most situations. He belonged to several fraternal organizations and was, in general, a "perfectly normal individual." His wife and he were unusually close and engaged in many activities together.

The patient, when interviewed, recognized that his illness was caused by "some factor in the mind." He wished very much to be well again. At times he was quite depressed and was seldom hopeful, although he did not contemplate suicide. In manner he was friendly and attentive; nevertheless, one felt that he was occupied within himself, and he appeared agitated, his hands being in continual motion. Day by day he became less excited but remained depressed, reserved, and quiet. Reactions and stories of some of the other patients agitated him at first, but gradually he came to accept hospitalization. He still pulled at his hair, which, however, began to grow again. After a relatively long stay he was sent to a state hospital.

P. React. Depr. M:26:S:35 +8 27138'4–9 (73) 5:13:10

This young man became depressed and lost interest in everything after his discharge from the Royal Air Force. He felt unable to concentrate, to carry on with his work, and to attend to the daily routine of life. He dated the beginning of his symptoms from the time when he had been given increased responsibility during his service with the Royal Air Force in Rangoon. He felt at that time that he was not able to shoulder the responsibility and this depressed him to the extent that he had suicidal ideas.

He was the only child of working-class parents. Leaving school at 16, he passed a civil service examination at 17. Subsequently he left home to live in lodgings. As a child he had been lonely and resentful of his family's low social standard in speech and manners. Psychometric tests showed him to be of superior intelligence. After serving in the ranks of the Royal Air Force for four years, he had been commissioned, without asking for it himself. He did not mix with the other officers. He became engaged, broke this off twice, and finally "just let it drop." After the war he returned to the civil service.

He was diagnosed as having a depression and he was treated by psychotherapy. His condition improved and he decided to work for a science degree. He married and on a follow-up visit seemed well settled in his work. M. V.

P. Mixed F:43:M:19 +1 2'713846–(53) 4:2:15
Suicidal

Tiredness and depression were the outstanding complaints of this patient. She had functioned satisfactorily until six years before admission, when she had an experience in which she was embraced by a man other than her husband and "found it quite thrilling." She said that she had not been well since and had been afflicted with tinnitus, vertigo, paresthesias, and headaches. Her menstrual flow became excessive and a hysterectomy was performed. She entertained suicidal ideas and one night took a mild overdose of sleeping tablets. On one occasion she threatened to kill one of her sons. Her appetite increased as did her desire for erotic pleasure, although at times she became negativistic and refused food. During one of these latter periods she spent three weeks in a state hospital.

Of average intelligence, the patient finished the eighth grade and then quit school to help on her parents' farm. At 17 she married to get away from home; the marriage appeared to be fairly successful. There were six children. Although she had apparently always been somewhat unhappy she had led a fairly successful social life before her illness; she had once been president of the local P.T.A. and had always had numerous friends.

On admission the patient spoke in a whining tone and her general behavior was that of a complaining, depressed person. She was so dissatisfied with little things that she found life almost unbearable. She was rigidly meticulous. The first week she resisted any type of therapy and spent most of the time demanding special privileges or asking to leave. When she finally agreed to stay, attempts were made to discuss her problems. She came to recognize that she had severe feelings of hostility toward her husband and her family and that these might be related to unfulfilled pleasures and ambitions. With this approach the depression subsided to a great extent and she was discharged. The discharge note stated that if the patient retained her insight and the family aided her in finding some new pleasures in life her prognosis should be good.

Schizoid M:33:M 27138'46–X(59) 6:19:2
7821463'9–(63) 2:15:9

This man was a machine operator who came to the counseling center to ask advice about changing his job. He complained that it was monotonous and that he did not fit in with the other men at the plant. He had taken aptitude tests in another city several years before but had been dissatisfied with the results. He reported no difficulties at home with his wife or his children.

Vocational aptitude examinations suggested he probably would be much happier doing carpentry or cabinetmaking, or assisting an interior painter or decorator. These findings were in line with the earlier vocational recommendations, but he was so poorly adjusted emotionally that he could not make constructive use of the suggestions.

In several interviews he talked readily, expressing feelings of depression and anxiety, fear of going to the hospital for a recommended hernia operation, fear of moving his family and working somewhere else, fear of being unsuccessful on a new job. Some additional training and the hernia operation were necessary before he could work at any job which seemed more desirable to him. An actual shift to a new field was difficult to manage financially and otherwise. He decided to explore the possibilities, but asked in leaving if we could refer him to a psychiatrist. This was done and we had no further contact with him for thirteen months.

The psychiatrist reported at the end of the year that he considered the man a "schizophrenic personality" and not accessible to psychotherapy. He reported he had given him supportive treatment at three-week intervals.

The client returned to the center some time later to discuss a new job he was considering. He said he felt a little better but got discouraged sometimes. The second MMPI profile was obtained at this time. No essential change had been made in his environmental situation, except for an expansion of his hobby interests which could relate more directly to his activity interests than did his job. He remained on the same job, and for several years this man supported himself and his family, giving the outward appearance of stability, but enduring great personal anxiety and unhappiness. He returned for an occasional interview but no therapy was effective in relieving him or in improving his adjustment to any marked degree. D. F. C.

P. React. Depr. M:32:S:33 +1 27138'46-9(51) 2:7:16

For eight or nine months this man had noted a gradual onset of depression. He had difficulty in concentration and some psychomotor retardation; accompanying problems were insomnia and anorexia. In addition he had become more seclusive. Having some insight, he made a tremendous effort toward his own rehabilitation. Beginning a college course as part of this rehabilitation program, he did poor work, and as his symptoms increased in severity he was forced to withdraw. During this period he was receiving psychiatric advice. He also had a number of somatic complaints that included a hypersensitivity to odors, an awareness of heart beat, and a sense of pressure on his head.

A college graduate, the patient had completed specialized professional training. In his childhood he had been overprotected and had developed a strong attachment for his mother. There was a lifelong history of reacting to stress with neurotic symptoms. He was described as having been rigid, self-conscious, sensitive, and somewhat seclusive.

In the hospital the patient was depressed, anxious, and retarded. He had vague feelings of guilt with occasional suicidal ideas, and he was obsessed with the idea that he was suffering a psychotic attack. There were no hallucinations or marked delusions. During the first two weeks in the hospital the depression deepened, but then he began to improve and had moved well along the way to recovery at the time of discharge. It seemed certain that he would recover from this episode, although later difficulties were considered probable.

Ps. M-D., Depr. F:38:S:59 +11 271'3864–9 (53) 6:1:18
Paranoid
Suicidal

Depression and psychomotor retardation were the outstanding symptoms of this patient. Approximately a month before admission she had had an upper respiratory infection from which she had failed to make a good recovery. Fatigue, headaches, backaches, and a rapid heart beat had been her chief complaints. She consulted a physician who examined and reassured her, but soon she began to show evidences of depression. Things seemed unreal to her and she complained of thoughts of death. She had a marked fear that she might lose her mind.

While the patient had always looked upon herself as frail and easily fatigued, her previous health had been, in general, good. At one time a diagnosis of goiter was made because she suffered from a rapid pulse and exhaustion; removed from school, she recovered after resting for one month. After she graduated from high school, her mother felt that she was not strong enough to attend the university; and after a rest of approximately a year, enforced more or less by her mother, she was sent to business college. When she had completed the course, she was employed by a bank. She disliked this work. Next she attended a teachers' college but after graduation disliked teaching so much that she took employment in a bank where she worked for thirteen years and was considered a satisfactory employee. Her mother almost completely dominated her life; and while some of the patient's siblings attempted to break this attachment, they had limited success. She had few interests outside her home, and only after a great amount of pressure did she even learn to drive a car.

On admission to the hospital she was quiet and reluctant to talk about herself. Slow and indecisive in manner, she had little interest in others about her, was unable to concentrate, and complained of loss of pep and difficulty in sleeping. Hopelessness was outstanding in her mental content. Her face appeared blank and she was rarely able to smile. Occasionally she expressed feelings of guilt, saying, "I could have prevented it. I always planned to care for my mother, and now I am a burden to her when she needs me most." She gradually improved; but as she became able to talk more freely, she occasionally revealed paranoid tendencies and suspicions which were particularly directed toward her physician, who she felt was making fun of her and keeping her in the hospital to get her money. During the last three weeks of her stay, she showed definite improvement. Although she was far from well, she was so anxious to go home that her family finally agreed to a trial. This was permitted after the dangers of suicide and relapse had been thoroughly explained to them.

Ps. M-D., Depr. F:43:S:70 +8 271'4836– 7:3:13

P. Hypo. F:46:S:24 +1 267'138– 5:4:12

The patient was admitted with incapacitating multiple somatic complaints (which she attributed to medication and to her own wickedness), psychomotor retardation, and thoughts of suicide, all of which coincided fairly closely with the beginning of the menopause six months before admission. At that time she complained of tremors and jerking of her extremities, she had obsessive thoughts that she was suffering because of her past sins, and she began to feel that her food and medicine were poisoned. She would not move out of her bed, but would lie crosswise with her head hanging over the edge. She paid no attention to her appearance and said, "I want to die so I won't have to live and suffer." Relatives found it impossible to keep her at home, and she was finally taken to a private hospital from which she was transferred to the psychiatric hospital.

A chronic invalid for twenty years with many medical studies and operations, she had always been unobtrusive and dependent on others, and her poor mental health had been her excuse for not taking up nursing or running a rooming house, two things she claimed to want to do. Without strong interests or drives, she had always overreacted to small complaints and had been fearful of many things, including such a strong fear of draughts that she would stuff windows with rags and keep the doors tightly closed. She was gullible and would send money to faith healers for mail-order treatments. The longest time she had ever held a job was for six months when she earned \$3 or \$4 a week. At that time she had lived as the common-law wife of her bachelor employer, and although they were in love she had felt that she could not marry him because he also had poor health. Through misinterpretation she came to believe that she had syphilis, and in consequence she had a persistent feeling of sinfulness.

A dull, disinterested, and depressed person, she regarded her situation as so hopeless that only her religion kept her from considering suicide. Her one concern was with her bodily complaints, which she felt prevented her from leaving her bed. "I have taken poor care of myself and misused my body when I was younger. I often worked too hard and ate improper foods," she said. She worried about the salvation of her soul. Of average intelligence, she lacked practical ability. At the time of her hospital discharge there was some improvement, but when she was readmitted about three years later with a similar pattern, except for more concentration of pain in the abdominal region, she was discharged to a state hospital.

P. React. Depr. M:31:S:15 +5 271486′3– 5:2:15
P. Hypo.

Along with depression, anorexia, and insomnia, this patient had numerous somatic complaints. These symptoms for the most part dated back a year to an automobile accident in which the patient had suffered a back injury. At first he had continued to work, but as increasing pain and multiple ills developed he was forced to quit. Placed in a cast for a while, after it was removed he found that he was no better and claimed that it had been removed too soon.

Before this illness the patient had been known as a "friendly and happy" young man who liked to be with friends and to go out on dates. Born to a poor farming family, he had worked his way through high school, finishing at age

18. He had held many jobs; he had been a cement worker, a carpenter, and during the war a ship fitter. There seemed to be few or no factors in his past history that could be identified as particularly applicable.

In the hospital the patient was mainly concerned with his bodily health, his inability to work, and his rejection by the army. He fretted also because he could not accompany his brothers to Alaska. Although he appeared depressed and anxious, he was cooperative and friendly. He said he realized that most of his trouble was "in my head," and due to his worried and anxious state of mind. He readily accepted reassurance about his numerous physical complaints. After a thorough X-ray study and other checking for the sources of his pain, and after careful reassurance that his back injury would not physically incapacitate him, he showed much improvement. At the time of discharge he seemed to be back to his usual self, and there was every reason to expect a good outcome.

P. Hys. M:16:S:18 +2 '2718–94 3:2:16

When the patient was about 8 he began to have periodic vomiting spells lasting several days and accompanied occasionally by what appeared to be a stupor. Frequently he had a temperature of 103. Although he received considerable medical attention no organic basis was ever discovered for these spells. At age 14 he developed a speech disorder that showed itself as a peculiar hoarseness, at times preventing him from speaking above a whisper. This became worse after his father's death two years before admission, and he was also examined extensively for this disorder, but again no organic pathology could be discovered. The present admission was chiefly motivated by the speech difficulty since the vomiting spells had practically disappeared as the speech problem became worse.

The patient was in his second year of high school where he was making fair grades. He had never been physically well. Early in his life he had shown evidences of nervousness. He was described as a very dependent boy who needed considerable affection and who dramatized all the situations in which he moved. He was interested in collecting stamps and other outside activities. His associations were with boys of the more effeminate type. He disclaimed any actual sex experiences or interest. He had always been a reliable and well-liked boy.

In the hospital no neurological or physical findings that appeared related to the symptoms could be discovered. He spoke in a high-pitched voice which at times quavered. He discussed his personal problems and the situational factors freely. The only symptom he complained of was the dysphonia. No definite psychological conflict could be discovered in the conscious field. He was lonesome but showed no other deviation in his behavior. During his hospitalization his condition remained unchanged. He was given reassurance and encouragement, and attempts were made to discover deeper conflicts, but no one formulation could be selected definitely as the causative pattern. The patient did get somewhat better and the improvement in voice control was accompanied by some decrease in what was at most a mild anxiety over the matter.

Ps. Invol. Melan. **F:40:M:43** **+33** **27183'64–(59)** **9:7:19**
Suicidal

The patient was admitted because of a fear that she was insane and that no treatment could help her. The onset of this pattern was indefinite but was at least two years before admission. She had always been a nervous person and had worried about things of no great consequence. Recently she had had frequent crying and dizzy spells in which everything went black. At the time of admission she was disorganized and delusional. She believed she was in an airplane and wanted to jump out.

There was no record of previous nervous upsets. She had had fairly good health. She was a high school graduate and had worked until the time of her marriage. After her son was old enough she again worked to help support the family. Her one goal in life had been to save money enough to buy a home. Her husband and she were happy in their married life. She made friends easily and had frequently taken part in social activities. In general there had been no abnormalities of behavior until the insidious onset of the present difficulty. As indicated, she had always been nervous and in the last few years people about her had noticed that she was increasingly worried and concerned about things. She had worked at a job of checking cans in a production line and had felt a compulsion to recheck every can, spending long hours at this tedious job.

The patient was chiefly concerned with leaving the hospital to go to a state institution. She thought she was insane and wanted to commit suicide. She was poorly oriented as to time and place but her sensorium and intellect were clear. She said she thought everything was hopeless and she didn't care what happened to her. There was no marked retardation and she gave complete answers within her ability. She was uncooperative at first, would not do as she was told, and attacked the nurses. She had many bizarre ideas. She was started on electroshock treatment and began to improve. She experienced a brief relapse at about the time she took the MMPI but then again improved until the time of discharge. Her general reaction to therapy had been good and in view of the adequate past history the prognosis was felt to be good.

P. Mixed M:25:S:41 +7 2718364'–9 9:13:18
P. Psychas. –8 2718346'–9 9:9:17
Schizoid

The presenting complaints for this young man, nervousness, seclusiveness, and facial pain, had first been noted four years before when he was employed in a hardware store. Bothered by a severe sore throat, the patient underwent a tonsillectomy at that time, without relief, and some time later he developed nervousness, tenseness, and facial pain which could not be relieved by dental treatment. He became unable to work and withdrew from society. Upset and trembly, he could not sit still and went for five- to six-hour walks. Calling himself unworthy and a burden to his family, he often said, "It would be better if

I would just wander off and never come back." No overt suicidal behavior was noted.

Described as having always been rather retiring, he had occasionally formed close friendships but had never had many acquaintances. He was considerate of his family and frequently expressed his obligation to them. He was described as sensitive and easily hurt. He had always felt social insecurity, partially because of his rigid code of ethics and morals. He had not been accepted well by others because of this code, which had kept him from participating in childhood pranks. Of good intelligence, he made the honor roll in high school, was a conscientious student, and had contemplated admission to a theological institution. He had been steadily employed until the appearance of the present illness. There were no girls in whom he had more than a casual interest.

The patient was much concerned with his illness and showed clear hypochondriacal tendencies. He was self-depreciatory and expressed his unworthiness for the consideration shown him by members of the staff and by his family; he appeared markedly depressed and seemed to have no insight into his illness. With psychotherapy he made a little progress, chiefly in the verbal understanding of his problems, and was finally discharged. It was felt likely that if he were again admitted he would be diagnosed as having schizophrenia.

P. Mixed F:33:S:105 0 271836'4–9(45) 1:8:8
Schizoid

This woman's original complaint consisted of weakness in both legs and a feeling that they could not move. This had first been noted about ten years before when she was returning from the funeral of an aunt. At that time her legs "gave way" and she fainted. A similar experience occurred on her first day at a new job, and during the next few years these episodes gradually grew more frequent. At first she associated the weakness with her menstrual periods and thought little about it, but in the four years before her admission to the hospital she began to consult doctors. She became afraid to walk because of the weakness and she had periods of depression and crying. At times she had vague fears, when she scarcely knew what she feared. One physician gave her prostigmine and diagnosed her condition as myasthenia gravis. The drug helped, she thought, but the condition slowly became worse. After she discussed some of her fears with the doctor, he referred her for psychiatric help.

The patient's mother was Negro, her father white. She had been raised by her maternal grandmother, who was described as cruel and temperamental. As a child the patient had been shy and fearful of everything. At the age of 11 she was sent away to school. Although she had always got along well in school she had never made close friends. After junior college she held various jobs such as personal maid, typist, and, at the time of her present illness, clerk. She refused an offer of marriage because she feared she might faint while taking the vows, and she was afraid also that she might die in childbirth.

2731 48′6–

A dark-skinned young woman, the patient presented a neat appearance and was pleasant and cooperative in the interview situation. While she tended to wait passively for questioning, she answered readily and to the point. Her mood was somewhat depressed. Although she mentioned anxieties she did not appear anxious and it was difficult to evaluate the amount of insight she possessed or the amount of subjective concern that was present. She did express some fear of insanity and was embarrassed and self-conscious when speaking of her physical ailment. However, in general, she was very poised. A physical examination at the beginning of psychotherapy revealed a ptosis of the upper lid but no other evidence of myasthenia gravis.

The patient was seen for outpatient psychotherapy once a week. She pictured herself as a person who had never established close relationships. Over the last few years she had become increasingly apathetic and socially withdrawn. Gradually she made a tenuous, positive transference to the therapist (a woman), and probably on this basis made some effort to renew social contacts. However, after four months, she dropped out, explaining that she had to work overtime and could not find an hour to come in. The case was closed and she was considered unimproved. Three months later she called again requesting a renewal of interviews. When arrangements were made she did not carry through, perhaps because she was told that she would not be able to see the same therapist as before. E. B.

P. React. Depr. Twin	F:31:M:2			
Ps. M-D., Depr. P. React. Depr.	F:31:M:13	+1	2731 48′6–(47)	5:6:19
Ps. M-D., Depr.	F:32:M:45	+8	27318′64–9 (37)	2:5:12
		+28	23′17 468–(41)	4:2:15

The patient was admitted to the hospital because of insomnia and depression that had begun five weeks before, in connection with the birth of her second child. During the latter part of the pregnancy she had suffered considerable anguish because she felt unable to keep up with her household duties and could not get help. She complained of tightness in her chest, "butterflies" in her stomach, loss of appetite, and a general feeling of hopelessness. She cried often and easily over simple tasks. She was self-accusing and self-depreciatory.

With the exception of brief episodes of depression she had previously been an emotionally stable person. A trained nurse, she was above average in intelligence and had always shown good judgment. Although she had always felt inferior to others, she was usually energetic and had prided herself on her efficiency in her household tasks. She was somewhat secretive and did not confide in her husband because she felt that he had enough worries.

Her chief concern was with returning home. There was no evidence of an acute break with reality. Well oriented, she appeared composed and cheerful, and she seemed to have very good insight to her problem. She said that she felt somewhat tense, but that the tenseness was abating slightly. She was open and natural, interested in the proceedings, and very cooperative. After a brief study she was discharged and her recovery was expected, but 28 days later she was readmitted to the hospital with a similar pattern of symptoms. In the interim she had been in another hospital for a few days. Increased feelings of inferiority and self-condemnation had developed, and she was much more irritable. There was steady improvement during her 13 days in the hospital, but about seven months later she was again readmitted for a 43-day hospitalization. During the interval, she had identified herself with an identical twin sister, who had developed an almost directly comparable illness, for which she had been admitted to the hospital. Once again there was marked improvement, and the patient was discharged with a reasonably hopeful prognosis.

Ps. M-D., Depr. M:32:M:66 0 27314'86–9(55) 1:6:20
P. Psychas.

The patient was admitted with multiple complaints. He feared that he might harm his wife or children, or possibly attempt suicide; he harbored thoughts of death, had trouble sleeping, was bothered by palpitations, gastric upsets, and severe depression. The main pattern had begun about half a year before admission when the patient took a job in a noisy plant. With little to occupy his mind, his thoughts gradually turned to morbid subjects—death of himself and his family, suicidal and homicidal urges, and concern about his own bodily health. He felt tired and dizzy, developed nausea and crampy abdominal pains, and finally became deeply depressed. When compulsions to seize a sharp instrument and kill himself and his family became acute and frequent, he voluntarily came to the hospital for protection of himself and his family.

The patient's past personality can be characterized in part by an event which occurred when he was 17. At that time he read a depressing book and immediately suffered gastric and cardiac pains and had an acute fear of death. After several months this condition cleared up and he and his brother "hoboed" about the country for three months. From that time on his history was one of frequent changes of job, no high aspirations, and no great financial problems. He was mildly superstitious and by nature pessimistic. Friendly and easy with people, he was, however, oversensitive to slighting remarks. He was known as stubborn and methodical and showed minor compulsive behavior in certain daily activities. In spite of his depressive thoughts he was not subject to excessive worry and always gave the outward appearance of being entirely normal and well adjusted.

On admission to the hospital his mental content was made up chiefly of thoughts of disease, killings, and death. Other peculiar ideas were also revealed, such as the fear of leaving a building by the same door he entered and the compulsion to use the same street going to and from work. His fear of insanity and his compulsion to violent action were resisted with obvious effort. In spite of the deep depression and the obsessive thinking, his attitude and behavior seemed to be essentially normal. The first days he showed rapid progress but later slipped back into the somatic complaints and fear of impending death. He was well liked by the other patients and entered well into the ward activities. He was discharged as improved but without assurance that any genuinely deep change had occurred.

Schizoid	M:26:S:58	+8	27'31846–X (67)	10:3:16
		+243	27148'36–9 (67)	8:6:20

After this man had become violent and aggressive and had attacked people, he was admitted as a certified patient into the hospital, where he underwent a course of electric convulsion therapy and deep narcosis. Before this admission he had been a patient in another mental hospital for five months. He left the hospital and worked regularly as a tram conductor and driver for about five years. He was readmitted (present admission) as a voluntary patient six years after the first admission. He complained of depression and lack of concentration and had ideas of reference. However, on the surface, he showed no psychotic trends.

He was the oldest of three children. Nothing was known about his early history, except that he had been considered average in intelligence and had received an elementary education.

On admission he was classified as having schizophrenia, but on discharge his diagnosis was modified to depressive state. He was treated by psychotherapy on a superficial level. He left the hospital after a few days, but returned subsequently on three occasions, none of his stays exceeding 24 days. M. V.

P. Hys.	M:39:S:29	+23	2731'846–9 (55)	8:4:26

The patient had been near an exploding bomb at the age of 33, and he dated his anxiety symptoms, palpitation, overactive mind, fear of insanity, and the like, to this incident. He began to brood and to ponder on past experiences. He entered the hospital as a voluntary patient.

Nothing was known about his early history.

He was diagnosed as having anxiety hysteria and was treated by psychotherapy under sodium amytal. His condition improved considerably. M. V.

Ps. Invol. Melan. M:46:M:61 +3 2731'86–9(57) 2:1:12
+12 27318'4–9(57) 2:4:16

While at work about a year before admission to the hospital, the patient had a dizzy spell and suffered pain in the back of his neck after, he said, "something snapped in my head." Since that time the patient had not been well although he continued to work most of the time. During the latter months there had been a marked personality alteration with crying spells, dizziness, pressure sensations in his head, weakness, and feelings of "electric shock" in his stomach. When a physician assured him that there was no physical disorder, the patient changed jobs in an unsuccessful attempt to help himself by varying his work. The progression of his symptoms and a drastic weight loss took him to a psychiatrist who recommended hospitalization; and when the depression persisted, his family could no longer delay taking this step.

There was no history of previous upsets. Of average intelligence, he had demonstrated his learning ability by being able to go back to school to train himself for a new job when the war eliminated the demand for his former trade. While he had a pleasant disposition, he was known to be shy and was rather readily irritated. He did not have many friends but was fond of sympathy. A truthful person, he never hesitated to express his convictions. He had been a fairly steady drinker for ten years, but liquor suddenly became distasteful to him and he gave up the habit completely. He had married a woman considerably younger than he, and apparently they were relatively compatible. Aside from quarreling during the period when the patient was drinking, his wife had never nagged at him in spite of his shortcomings. Their five children were relatively well adjusted.

On his admission to the hospital one could easily have been misled by the patient's apparently affable manner. While on the surface he was somewhat preoccupied with his somatic complaints, his attitude was very acceptable, he was cooperative, and he immediately entered cheerfully into ward activities, which he seemed to enjoy. On closer observation it was obvious, however, that he daydreamed at any moment that he was not occupied, and at such times he appeared extremely depressed. He was unable to sleep without sedation and complained of headaches and dizzy spells. Electroshock therapy produced some improvement, but the underlying depression appeared relatively unaffected. He was discharged to return to his home where it was felt that he would probably slowly improve, making a good adjustment to society.

P. React. Depr. M:42:M:10 —1 2734'16–(65) 6:7:18

The complaints of this patient, nervousness and insomnia, appeared five or six weeks before admission and day by day increased in severity. The patient usually went to sleep immediately, but many nights he awoke three or four times and lay for hours worrying about his job. In an attempt to dispel his fears at these times he talked aloud to himself. Shortly before admission he began to complain of pain, tenderness, and tenseness in all his muscles. Although very fond of pipe smoking, he gave it up.

There was no evidence of a contributory illness or upset in his past history. An immigrant with college training in Europe, the patient took further college work after he arrived in this country, and he became a graduate engineer. Although he was successful in his work, the psychological pressure on him increased enormously during the war. He made an attempt to enlist in the army and then the navy, but his vision was inadequate. A submissive personality with a good disposition, the man had always been told by someone what to do since childhood. He usually consulted his wife before making decisions. Introverted as a child, he had had a domineering father who restricted his activities. A fearful individual, with fears of dentists and hospitals outstanding among his apprehensions, he considered himself a very sensitive person.

His inability to sleep was of great concern to the patient. In spite of a dislike for the hospital, he was quiet and at ease there even though he felt that hospitalization was a mistake. In his opinion there was nothing that seriously wrong with him. He showed little insight. An attitude of superiority was evident, and he felt he was deserving of more than he was getting. He displayed the same attitude toward his job even though he had a feeling of insecurity about it. He made such remarks as these: "A fellow shouldn't have to worry about his old age. A person can't save. If you've got a dollar you've got to keep up with the Joneses." He was given bed rest and sedation. Under this regimen he improved somewhat and became anxious to leave. At discharge he planned to make a try at returning to his job. The prognosis seemed good.

B. Psth., Path. Emot. M:31:M:56 +15 2734'816– 4:2:15
Schizoid

The admission complaints of this patient centered around excessive sexual activity, including masturbation which the patient believed had depleted his strength and injured his nervous system. The onset of these feelings had been gradual over approximately a two-year period. He complained of weakness and inability to work as hard as he previously had done. Any loud noise, such as a door being slammed, startled him unduly, and he was disturbed by a compulsion to work much faster and to accomplish more than he was physically able to do; consequently he tired himself unduly. All this was associated with a gradual falling off of interest in outside activities, particularly social affairs.

A marginal itinerant worker who had completed an eighth-grade education with great difficulty, the patient had lived in his parents' home until his marriage at age 26. Never particularly ambitious, he was apparently satisfied with living in a tar-paper shack. Until the time of his marriage he was a heavy drinker of the spree-drinking type, but after his marriage liquor became relatively unimportant to him. He complained that he had practiced masturbation from an early age and had had frequent sexual relations with Indian girls of the neighborhood. During the first year of marriage he demanded sexual relations with his wife five or six times daily. The fact that in the past year this sexual desire had greatly decreased appeared to be one of his chief sources of worry. The patient had always been a compulsive type of individual; and if he started a task, he could not rest until he had finished it as quickly as possible. When things did not go as he had planned them, he was upset. There were three children.

The patient, who was chiefly concerned with his weakness, fatigue, extreme nervousness, and feelings of tension, attributed his difficulty to excessive sexual activity, particularly masturbation. He had no insight into the possibility that he was mentally ill. His answers to questions were usually relevant and coherent although if he continued to talk, one sometimes had difficulty in following his line of thought. At all times conventional in his conduct, he adapted well to ward life. During his hospital stay he changed very little; and he was discharged against advice. It developed that he had come to the hospital more in the hope of demonstrating his family's need for relief aid than to get help for his own symptoms.

B. Psth., Path. Emot.	M:38:M:73	+6	2'73486–(74)	6:2:24
Alcoholism		+77	4782'6913–(76)	4:4:25
Ps. M-D., Manic	M:42:M:9	+1	4698'3–2(45)	2:8:16
Alcoholism				

Admitted for study because of a four- to five-month history of depression, nervousness, and feelings of inadequacy, the patient was brought to the hospital on a court order secured by Alcoholics Anonymous. Although he had engaged in drinking sprees for years, the bouts had been more frequent in the past seven years. Joining Alcoholics Anonymous, he had responded to the efforts of the organization so favorably that he had found a job and had abstained from liquor for several months before admission. Past falls from grace had been preceded by the admission pattern of symptoms.

When he was a child, his indulgent family had given him everything he desired, and he had had few family responsibilities. His mother had made excuses for the boy's errors and had fussed over him when he was sick. Finishing high school near the top of his class, he went on to college for about three years, quitting because of his father's ill health. Although he had worked at various jobs, usually as salesman, bookkeeper, or clerk, the longest time he had ever held one job was three years. In the army for several months, he was discharged because of alcoholism. While he got along with others, he was never a leader and always became uneasy if decisions were thrust upon him. He refused a promotion at one time because of this trait. He took many jobs not because of any interest in a particular line of work but because it was the line of least resistance. He had no hobbies, but he liked to write poetry. Afraid to have sex relations before marriage, he had masturbated since childhood, using a woman's shoe as a fetish. He was compatibly married to his wife who had always forgiven him for his misdeeds, and there had been no extramarital relationships. Following an alcoholic episode he had always wanted punishment from his wife. During the entire period of his marriage, his mother had lived with or near them. They had a 9-year-old son.

No unusual mental content or abnormalities of affect were apparent on admission. While he felt ashamed of the "dirty deal" he had given his wife and wanted to prove to her that he could settle down, he felt that his entire problem arose from the fact that he had been overprotected as a child. Through alcohol he had been able to continue to escape from responsibility. Depression such as he experienced at admission had always presaged a drinking bout, and he had come into the hospital in an effort to stop the sequence. He appeared cheerful and carefree, exhibiting no detectable mood swings; his insight was felt to be largely on a verbal level. Well liked by everyone, he was very cooperative and interested in other patients. His self-confidence, which apparently had increased on admission to the hospital, was a rather severe bar to any psychotherapeutic aid. He was discharged feeling very confident that he could get himself in hand and would not need help much longer; but there had been no real change in the underlying problem, and the prognosis was not good. About four years later he was readmitted with a similar set of complaints. He had been fairly well behaved until a month before the second admission. In this admission he was judged to have a manic psychosis and was sent to a state hospital.

P. Hys. Epilepsy Suicidal	M:36:M:23	+3	27′36 184–(53)	6:1:16
P. Hys. Epilepsy	M:36:M:24	+1	2′137–(43)	4:1:14

The patient was bothered by periods of shaking and nervousness, and episodic failure of memory. Personality changes had begun about five years earlier when he became moody and unhappy, "did not seem to be myself," and experienced insomnia. About that time also, one morning after leaving his home for work, he was found outside of town wandering in a corn field with a big knife and had to be overpowered. He remembered nothing and had no knowledge of how he arrived at the spot. Committed to a state psychiatric hospital, he remained there for three months and was diagnosed as manic-depressive. Released from the hospital, he tried to shoot himself with a .22 rifle and was returned to the hospital. He was released two or three months later. Still nervous and irritable, he could not be controlled by his wife, and he entered the state hospital a third time for a short stay. On the way home he drove his car into an underpass and suffered a broken jaw and ankle. When he recovered consciousness in a doctor's office, he did not know what had happened. A new development before the present admission (first MMPI) consisted of sudden attacks of shaking followed by two-hour periods of deep sleep.

Before the present series of episodes the patient was said to have been a happy person, apparently normal in almost every way. He was active socially and physically. A farmer, he had at one time moved to a small town but had returned to the farm because "he did not like town life." As clearly as could be determined, he was happily married.

There was no satisfactory evidence that the patient's spells were epileptic or in any sense organically caused. Well composed, well oriented, and very cooperative, he appeared cheerful most of the time, and his intellect was intact. He had no insight, however, and no recognition of any psychological problem. He expressed fear of returning to the state hospital. Tests showed him to be somewhat above average in intelligence. His adjustment to the hospital was good; this was reportedly true of his previous hospitalizations also. The prospect of being discharged made him very happy. The diagnostic category was unsatisfactory because, although he became symptom-free, there was little reason to believe that he would remain well. The poor prognosis was justified, and three months later he was back in the hospital with a similar pattern of symptoms. Further study did not add to the understanding of the patient. Again he made an immediate and excellent adjustment and within the hospital situation behaved in a normal fashion. After a few weeks he was permitted to return home with, of course, a very poor prognosis for a long-time or complete recovery.

B. Simple Adult Maladj.   M:43:M:3   +2   2'73648–1 (80)   2:2:12
P. React. Depr.

Until about eight months before admission to the hospital the patient had lived a relatively normal, happy life as a small town businessman. At that time he began an affair with an 18-year-old college student, a girl whom the patient considered attractive although most other people had the opposite opinion of her. It was known that she had been expelled from several colleges, that she had had other affairs, and that she indulged in homosexual activities. As a further complication, the girl's parents were good friends of the patient and his wife. The love-making apparently was of an immature high-schoolish type and took place mostly in parked cars. Because he was endangering his family life, the patient resolved to terminate the affair, but after making this decision he became extremely nervous, was unable to concentrate, and, in addition to insomnia, suffered attacks of hay fever and asthma which resisted treatment. Before he could terminate the affair, it all came to a restricted public light. He then told his wife everything, threatening suicide because he felt that his world was tumbling about him. The threat to his business of a public scandal precipitated an acute reaction in which the patient became hysterical. Taken to a local physician, he was given sedatives; and it was suggested that he be brought to the psychiatric hospital.

While the patient considered himself slow in making friends, what friends he did make he always enjoyed deeply. One meaningful adolescent friendship very nearly became homosexual in character. An immigrant who had been very successful in his own country, the patient had been forced to seek refuge because of the advent of a political system of which he disapproved. He spent some time in a concentration camp where he had been subjected to various forms of torture. In all ways he was a very intelligent and accomplished person. Known to be strong-minded, a leader rather than a follower, he was, however, always very dependent upon sympathetic advice from his wife.

Soon after admission to the hospital the patient learned that he had been forgiven by his business associates for the notoriety he had brought on them. When first seen, he was almost arrogant in manner and felt that now that everything was settled the only thing that remained for him to do was to go back and work as best he could. Further interviews made it apparent that he could not understand how he could have been so irresponsible and that he was worrying about living with himself and with other people. He was troubled about what others would think of him and whether he would ever again be able to concentrate. He had considerable insight and was exceedingly anxious for reassurance that he could overcome his impulses. In the few days that he was in the hospital his attitude changed from that of arrogance to one of complete cooperation in which he spoke freely about his problems. When his wife was brought in, the two worked both together and individually with the therapist in a sincere effort to work out a course of action; and when it seemed to be adequately planned, the patient was discharged from the hospital. It was felt that there would probably not be any further difficulty.

Ps. Invol. Melan. F:43:W:43 +1 27'36481–9 (63) 6:1:13
P. React. Depr.

The patient exhibited marked depression, irritability, insomnia, and hypochondriacal trends. About two years before it had been noted that she seemed to be preoccupied most of the time—her mind seemed to wander and often she failed to respond when addressed. A year before admission, following an attack of "flu" which lasted for two weeks, marked personality changes had occurred. She was nervous and downhearted, lost interest in her appearance and in her children, and had crying spells. Gradually these symptoms became more pronounced. She was suspicious of the activities of her children, began to open their mail, and in other ways pried secretly into their affairs.

A high school and business college graduate, the patient earned good grades and was on the honor roll throughout most of her schooling. For six years she worked in two different banks, then married and kept house for seven years until her husband was accidentally killed. She took a job with a real estate company and stayed at that until the present illness. A friendly person, she was at ease with people and was known to be conscientious and trustworthy. She had no hobbies; she was secretive, independent, and inclined to be stubborn. Her readjustment following her husband's death had been rapid. No hypochondriacal tendencies, daydreaming, or absent-mindedness had been noted before the onset of the illness. Her previous health had been good. She was known to have strict ethical and moral ideals.

In the hospital the patient worried about her health and the care of her children. Depressed about feeling incompetent and unable to concentrate or think, she wept readily. Mentally she was clear but she complained of loss of memory for recent events. She was somewhat retarded in speech but her replies were pertinent and coherent. Under general routine ward care and psychological reassurance she improved slowly, became less agitated and confused, cried less frequently, and began to take part in the activities of the ward. At discharge she was markedly improved but far from well. It was felt there might be a long period before her complete recovery.

P. Hys. F:25:M:42 +7 2'73681-(57) 6:9:5

The onset of the patient's complaint of inability to swallow was about three years before admission following the birth of her first and only child. A feeling that a lump in her throat obstructed the passage of food had originally given her difficulty with coarse food only, but the trouble had increased to the point where it was difficult for her to swallow even liquids in quantity. About a year before admission she had noticed a soft mass in her neck and when iodine therapy had not helped her, she had undergone a thyroidectomy which had exaggerated the symptoms. Recently she had become extremely irritable and she had had crying spells at least once a day.

Her previous history contributed nothing pertinent. She had always had a poor appetite. After one year in high school, she had begun at age 15 to do housework, and until her marriage at 21 she had worked in several homes. She had liked drinking and dancing before her marriage, but her social life had become extremely limited because, although her husband had also liked night life before marriage, he had become so religious that he no longer approved of such diversions. Her judgment was poor, and she had always relied upon either her husband or her mother to make her decisions. As a housewife she tended to be nervous and to worry excessively. The patient was pregnant at the time of her marriage.

In the hospital she was mainly concerned with her trouble in swallowing and other related symptoms, and there were somatic trends in all her conversation. In spite of repeated and careful reassurance she was convinced that the obstruction in her throat had an organic basis. Her sensorium and intellect were clear, and she was well oriented. She was nervous, and it was obvious that she did not reveal all the problems that were bothering her. Amytal interviews elicited nothing pertinent to the situation other than the fact that the husband was more strongly sexed than she was. While under the amytal she had no difficulty swallowing. Since no approach was discovered that removed the dysphagia for more than short intervals, a diet permitting her to live primarily on liquids was worked out.

Ps. M-D., Depr. F:20:S:35 +1 273'6849–(45) 6:4:17
Suicidal

Two years earlier a boy with whom the patient was in love had become engaged to another girl and since that time she had had recurrent periods of depression. At the time of the engagement she had felt so generally depressed and had found it so difficult to concentrate on her studies that she had spent a week at home in bed. Even after the boy's marriage he had continued to show interest in the patient, taking her to his home and seeing her on numerous occasions. The following spring she had had crying spells that lasted for three or four hours and her ability to concentrate on her studies had suffered so much that she saw her family physician who gave her sedatives and benzedrine. Several months later she had a severe depressive episode during which she saw a psychiatrist, and when marital difficulties developed between her parents, the mother's threatened suicide put the patient under even more strain. Several months before admission the patient took an overdose of sleeping pills, and just before the present admission she was inhibited in an urge to commit suicide by the fact she did not have any sleeping pills.

A graduate student at a university, the patient had strong interests in music and literature. A friendly, cheerful, and capable person, she had shown nothing particularly deviant in her personality before the present pattern.

On admission to the hospital she was labile emotionally, and during the initial interviews she frequently broke down and cried. Her sensorium and intellect were intact. Her thought was logical. She tended to control the interviews, revealing only what she wanted to tell, and obviously many facts were omitted. Her response was superficial, and she concealed her true feelings. After a series of electroshock treatments her improvement was so accelerated that at the time of discharge, when she planned to continue graduate work, she was in an optimum state of mind. Contacts with outpatient psychiatry were to be continued. It was felt that she was likely to have more attacks in the future.

Ps. Toxic F:42:M:51 +19 27381'4–(47) 3:10:10
Alcoholism
Drug Add.

On admission to the hospital the patient was in semicomatose confusion. She had been using alcohol excessively for some time and in increasing amounts. A week before admission she entered a general hospital with signs of early delirium tremens and she received extensive bromide treatment.

Until the last three years the patient's health had been good; then she began to consult numerous physicians, seeking relief from nervousness and anxiety. She was a graduate nurse with specialization in anesthesiology. As a child she had been somewhat shy and aloof and less a member of neighborhood groups than the other children in her family were. As she grew up, she was narcissistic and timid in interpersonal relationships. Her parents were indulgent and her childhood had apparently been a happy one. She married an engineer whose jobs required them to move often. There were two children who, the patient felt, occupied too important a part in the family. During the first years of their marriage the patient got along fairly well with her husband but gradually more and more conflicts arose, many over the patient's unsatisfactory management of finances.

Within a day or two after admission a fairly clear Korsakoff's syndrome developed. With proper medical treatment these symptoms gradually disappeared. As she recovered from the effect of the alcoholism, the person emerging was narcissistic and self-centered, unable to form much of a personal relationship. These factors militated against an active therapeutic approach, and the patient herself did not feel the need for one. She was accordingly discharged with marked improvement of the presenting complaints but without any particular change in the underlying emotional problems.

P. React. Depr.	M:33:M:73	+5	2738<u>1</u>'46–	4:6:10
		+29	217<u>38</u>'96–	3:6:11

The patient was admitted to the hospital with complaints of headache, backache, and depression. A particular intensification of the illness followed a series of misfortunes beginning approximately a year before admission with the death of the patient's only son. Next, in the process of changing jobs, he had an illness which left him without either his old job or a new one. Working briefly at a job considerably beneath his abilities, he then shifted to specialized training with a company. During the preliminary stages of this he had symptoms of feeling cold and nauseated. Reporting to the office for instruction, he "didn't know what they were talking about, although I could hear voices." Since these occurrences his depression had become gradually more marked.

His physical complaints dated back as far as ten years before admission. The patient was a congenital syphilitic who was treated with apparent success when he was 8 years old. His home broken by divorce, the patient had lived with his mother, an unstable woman. They changed residence frequently and in general his boyhood had not been happy. At 15 he left school in order to support himself and his mother. He was married at age 22. During the first two years of his married life he was happy, but later financial problems arose to mar this. He was always somewhat shy and retiring but engaged in normal activities and sports and was genuinely interested in games.

At the time of admission to the hospital this man was very depressed. His mental content was chiefly centered around his financial problems and his difficulties in solving them. He said he felt "as if I am cornered." He was tense and nervous. His general insight was good, and he was alert and cooperative. During his stay in the hospital he had a number of minor surgical operations, such as the removal of epidermal cysts from behind his ear. He took these procedures well and made continual progress during his hospital stay. At the time of discharge he appeared completely recovered. An attempt was made to help him meet his problems and it seemed likely that he would make a good social recovery after discharge.

P. Mixed M:38:M:35 +1 27′38146–(49) 4:1:17

The patient's condition at admission was characterized by a 25-pound weight loss over a period of two years, chronic insomnia, and many somatic complaints referring chiefly to the intestinal system. The illness dated back several years to a gradual onset of multiple somatic difficulties. A barber, he had gradually lost business when many young men left his community to enter the army. He developed the habit of leaving his shop to go next door and drink coffee—eventually as much as 25 cups a day—when he should have been waiting for customers in his barber shop. At home he presented more and more nervous complaints.

The patient had been brought up by foster parents and relatives. He had had operations for gall bladder, appendix, and hemorrhoids. He had completed two years of high school and had left at the age of 16 to work at odd jobs. Later he took an apprenticeship and learned the trade of a barber. In school he had been a good student and was described as an "ambitious boy." He married a schoolteacher, with whom he was apparently fairly well adjusted. There were three children.

On admission to the hospital he appeared to have a clear intellect and sensorium. He had a superficial insight into his problems. He showed a moderate amount of retardation, appearing depressed and anxious. He had frequent episodes when he stayed in bed, cried, and discussed at length his somatic complaints. Given superficial reassurance and phychotherapy, he gradually improved to a considerable extent. It was felt that he had always been introverted and had never made a really good adjustment to life. At discharge, arrangements were made for him to continue visiting the outpatient clinic.

P. Mixed M:23:S:100 +7 273′8146–9(69) 5:6:12
Schizoid

This young patient was seen by a neurologist because of occasional jerking movements of his head, arms, and legs. No organic basis for them was found and he was then referred for psychiatric help. His complaints at the time he was first seen by a psychiatrist were these: he felt he looked peculiar and comical to other people; people laughed at him; his home life had been very disturbing to him for several years; and he had lost confidence in himself and needed vocational help.

From an Irish Catholic family, the youth had been reared for the first ten years of his life by an indulgent maternal grandmother whom he preferred to his own parents. He could remember little of his early childhood and reported only that nothing unusual had happened to him and that he had "got along average." He described his father as a dominant, successful man who drank too much and caused his mother to have nervous spells which upset the whole family. At the time the patient came in for treatment he was living with his parents and spending his time lying around the house. He had never been a person who planned for the future, and after graduating from high school he had drifted from one job to another without ever holding one for any length of time. He explained, "I'm the kind of guy who keeps his mouth shut and then I pull out cause I can't take it."

The patient was a tall, unattractive young man, with large protruding ears, actually somewhat comical in appearance. He had a dull, stupid manner which caused his therapist to suspect borderline intelligence. However, when an intelligence test was administered, it indicated high average ability. He came in for eleven psychotherapeutic interviews, presenting each time the same dull manner, and needing frequent prompting to give information. He resisted the suggestion that his head-jerking had an emotional basis and in general seemed to lack insightful concern about himself. He did show physical manifestations of anxiety.

The therapist felt that he was never able to establish a working relationship. When the patient did speak spontaneously, it was to tell about his parents' quarrels, which he believed were the primary, if not the sole, cause of his own unhappy state. Expecting direct advice about his parents, he was disgruntled when this was not forthcoming and he began shopping around for other doctors. It was suggested that he was not really interested in continuing therapy and he readily agreed. Although he was considered unimproved at the time of discharge, a short time later he was reported to be feeling more encouraged and to have obtained a job. E. B.

Ps. M-D., Depr. F:34:M:42 +10 27381′64– 8:3:17
P. Psychas.
Suicidal

The admission complaints of this patient were emotional depression associated with inability to make decisions, fear of insanity, and apprehension that she might harm her infant. Apparently well until a year before, she had suddenly become obsessed with the fear that she might do injury to her 3-month-old child. This obsession was associated with feelings of depression that gradually increased and became so marked that the patient, feeling hopeless, made an attempt at suicide with sleeping pills. Interest in her work, in her personal appearance, and in her general activities lagged. Attempting to find emotional quietude, she tried living with her relatives, but this failed. For one week her husband stayed home from work and devoted his time to her. During this week she was much better, but afterward she went to bed and became a helpless invalid.

The patient, it was said by friends and family members, had always been a "big baby." Although she had graduated from high school, she had never been economically independent—she was supported by her parents until their deaths and then until her marriage by a sister. The sister said that the family had not only always pampered the patient and supplied all her desires, but had expected nothing of her. She had had many minor illnesses and made much of each. Her affairs had never been handled in a mature way. Her husband was seven years her senior, and it was she who had insisted on the marriage. Her husband worked sporadically and the family existed at a low socio-economic level. There was one child. Unknown to her husband, the patient had become involved with another man, and this had continued for the last several years.

The patient often spoke of herself in the third person, saying, "This is not the real Doty. The real Doty loves her husband and baby." So depressed and withdrawn was she that the nurses had difficulty inducing her to eat or to remain active. She was retarded and at the same time seemed to be in a mild panic. She picked out her hair, rubbed areas of skin from her ears, and swallowed a number of pins and other small metal objects that had to be surgically removed. Throughout her hospital stay, she continued to be depressed, anxious, and retarded, and she showed depersonalization. She once attempted suicide by strangulation. No real contact could be made with her and finally she was discharged to a state hospital.

Ps. Invol. Melan. F:43:W:52 +7 2738'1694– 6:8:16
P. React. Depr.
P. Psychas.

Six months before admission the patient's daughter was married and left home, leaving the patient with elderly parents. At this time the patient began to notice insomnia and she frequently woke up so frightened that she would spend the remainder of the night in her mother's room. Often she wept on her mother's shoulder and poured out whatever happened to be "preying on my mind." She had persistent "bothersome thoughts," such as "bad ideas" when passing men on the street, or "swearing thoughts" just before receiving communion, which made her feel unworthy of the sacrament. She began to call her daughter to come home for frequent short visits. She described a pressure "working all through my head."

Although physically healthy, the patient had always been nervous. At 21 she had had a "nervous breakdown." She quit school before the eighth grade because, she said, "The work was hard for me." Her husband had died eight or nine years before admission, leaving her with five children, and after that she lived on a widow's pension. She had never held a job, her entire life having been spent on a farm. Although she had few outside interests she was friendly and thoughtful toward others, and in general got along well. Religion played an important part in her life. She was usually cheerful and calm, but at times she tended to brood about her sorrows and disappointments. She was always a "mama's baby." Her married life had been harmonious except for some difficulty with her husband's family. This had worried her a great deal before and since the husband's death.

On admission to the hospital the patient complained almost constantly about being "lonesome and nervous" and feared it would lead to insanity. She fretted about her body, asking for examinations and medicines. She was obsessed with "bad swearing thoughts," which she thought might "influence other people." She was well oriented, and she appeared otherwise mentally intact. Her thinking capacity and general knowledge were poor. She whined about her troubles and paid little attention to logic. She considered loneliness not to be a factor in her sickness and had no true insight. She got somewhat better and admitted that her "nerves" were steadier, but the head sensations and the fear of insanity were still present. Finally discharged to return to her former environment, it was not felt that the prognosis was favorable.

P. Psychas.	F:43:M:29	+1	273'8614–(51)	4:6:14
		+3	2<u>37</u>'18–<u>49</u> (45)	7:2:12
		+441	<u>872</u>361'4–(51)	7:14:12

The patient was troubled by depression, insomnia, and ideas that she might harm her young daughter. She said that she had been feeling well until about seven months before admission when during one evening as she was entertaining a group of friends she suddenly felt severe pressure in her head, accompanied by nervousness, apprehension, and depression. It was difficult for her to remain with her guests for the rest of the evening and for three weeks she continued to be upset, nervous, and depressed, she had difficulty sleeping, and she took barbiturates. She could not comprehend the reason for this attack. Her physician offered reassurance which helped her temporarily, then the depression returned. Life wasn't worth living, she felt, and the world was a dismal place—it was best for her to die. Although she made no actual plans, she thought of taking her own life. She could offer no reason or explanation for these feelings. Later she feared that she would harm her children, and she was afraid to be left alone with them. She entered the hospital in a highly agitated state, bewildered and worried as to why she should have such thoughts.

A rather sickly person all her life, the patient was diagnosed as having a goiter at age 8. At 18 she underwent a subtotal thyroidectomy. A number of operations followed. She described herself as a "nervous person, high-strung." For the greater proportion of her life, she had suffered from indigestion, weakness, and periodic "migraine headaches."

She was satisfied to leave school after the eighth grade. Her intelligence appeared to be average. Liked by everyone, she was well thought of in the community. She went with her prospective husband for nine years before marriage. Sexual intercourse was never a source of enjoyment to her. She realized that this was somewhat unusual but insisted that she loved her husband just the same. A daughter had been sick at regular intervals and seemed to be following the patient's pattern.

Uppermost in the patient's mind were concern and perplexity about her ideas, and over and over she said, "I always loved my daughter so and took such good care of her during her illnesses. How can I think such bad thoughts about her now?" She was cooperative and her attitude and manner were satisfactory. The fear of hurting the daughter remained throughout most of her hospital stay. Ten electroshock treatments gave her some relaxation, and she became a little more cheerful. Not only was she reassured that many women have ambivalent feelings toward their children, but she was given some help in improving her marital relationships. Much better at discharge, she was to continue in the outpatient department.

Ps. M-D., Depr.	M:44:M:54	+1	274′136–9 (57)	4:3:11
P. Psychas.				
B. Psth., Mixed				

For the previous eleven years this man had had periods of excessive worry and depression. The present illness began two weeks after he was sentenced to prison for grand larceny. He developed a defensive type of psychosis, lapsed into a dreamlike state, "suffered from horrible unnatural feelings," and was horrified at the prospect of waking up in the morning. His own face in the mirror frightened him, he said, and the prison guards became for him "terrifying indescribable objects." After a year in prison his psychosis and loss of weight resulted in his transference to a hospital for the criminally insane, where he remained for another year. He gained his weight back, was returned to the prison, and was then given parole. For a time he worked with a section crew on a railroad and was fairly well adjusted, but increased family expenses, feelings of insecurity, and fears again took hold. He lost his job but obtained another which was the best he had ever held; it was terminated one day when his employers learned of his prison record. The succeeding history was a cycle of obtaining jobs, losing them, and developing depressions.

The patient had completed the seventh grade; he apparently was able to learn but had trouble with teachers because of mischievousness. He quit school when his parents were divorced, and he was left to shift for himself. He became a swindler, at times a bootlegger. He married at 24 against his parents' wishes, set up a small restaurant of his own on borrowed money, but soon failed. The prison sentence came as a result of a robbery, in which, according to his own story, he had been used as a "fall guy." At that period he was drinking heavily and, while he had no psychotic upsets, was certainly an inadequate person. Known to be friendly and confident, he was at ease with people and liked to be the life of the party. He showed poor judgment in handling money and often bought expensive things merely because of what they cost rather than because they were attractive or useful to him. He appeared to be compatible with his wife and they had six children.

On admission to the hospital the patient was neat in appearance but had an anxious and troubled look. Much of the time he paced the floor and was possessed by oppressive thoughts and fears. His past record of drinking, gambling, thievery, prison, and improvidency served as a constant source of shame and anguish to him. He was clear mentally and showed what was termed a "smiling depression." If drawn into a conversation he talked and gave adequate answers; in every way he appeared alert and not deeply depressed. However, his behavior and his mental content when it could be obtained were adequate evidence of the depths of the true depression. If encouraged he talked at length, dwelling always upon his fears. A number of methods were used to attempt to free him, including narcosis therapy and electrical stimulation. The effects of these approaches were transitory, if any effect occurred at all. Finally regular electroshock therapy was begun and there was steady improvement. After five shock treatments, it was felt that although he was not completely well he was ready to leave the hospital. In view of the long-standing illness and the incompleteness of recovery, prognosis was guarded. It was hoped he might make a fair social adjustment.

P. React. Depr. M:39:M:31 0 27'43–(55) 6:2:18

This man's life was marked by numerous episodes of depression, usually transient, moderately severe, and responding readily to changes in the environment. His present symptoms were depression, with feelings of insecurity and inadequacy, and insomnia. Severe for two weeks, the feelings actually dated from a period of difficulties in the patient's family some time before. While one of his two sisters was being treated by a psychiatrist for convulsions following childbirth, the other committed suicide. At the same time the patient felt that his wife's community activities were robbing him of companionship. Dissatisfaction with his work and the home situation mounted, and finally he sought psychiatric help.

As indicated, the patient had always shown a tendency to develop symptoms from time to time, and apparently he gradually became dissatisfied with any given mode of life. At the age of 5, following a three-month attack of paralysis, he had had to learn to walk a second time, but he completely recovered. The patient had broad interests and good intelligence; he was a university graduate. He was discharged after only a few months in the army, probably because of psychoneurosis or a psychotic episode. For ten years he had been employed steadily in legal work. His own statement was that, between periods of depression, he was never free from feelings of inadequacy. Disappointment with his lot in life was voiced in such comments as this: "My background and experience would entitle me to greater achievements."

In the hospital the patient showed concern about his depression but continually minimized the importance of the attacks. Recognizing that these occurred in response to stressful situations, he nevertheless seemed to be more ashamed of "weakness" than motivated to recognize the recurrent depressions as a problem that he should attempt to solve. He was somewhat nervous and ambivalent in his desire for psychiatric help. In general, however, his behavior appeared quite normal. After electroshock therapy he seemed somewhat better. Nevertheless, he still rigidly maintained the old pattern of "doing the right thing," in an immature fashion, and wanting to overcome his problem "right away," without effort and without recognition of the need for prolonged effort. Although at discharge there was obvious improvement the outlook was considered doubtful.

Ps. M-D., Depr. M:53:M:25 +3 27431'86-9(61) 4:2:19
P. Psychas.

The principal symptoms of the patient were depression and insomnia, which had had a sudden onset about three months before admission when his son developed an epileptiform seizure. At that time the local physician so impressed the patient with the seriousness of his son's condition that the patient became depressed, could not sleep at night, was unable to work, and could not stop worrying. A similar period of depression following some financial reverses eighteen years before the present admission had lasted about six months, disappearing gradually without medical care. While there were no other psychotic episodes, the patient said he had always been "nervous and high-strung."

Although he had liked school, the prevailing custom in his community was to "get on the farm and work," and after finishing the eighth grade, he had left school to work on his father's farm. A respected man in his community, he had served in several public offices and had done well financially. Known as a perfectionist who did over anything that did not meet his high standards, he was very quick to criticize and to condemn anyone who did not meet similarly high standards or who failed to measure up to his strict ethical code. In spite of this, he thought that he was able to get along with people very well. His management of the farm and his good judgment in planning were evident, and he was progressive in his work, adding modern conveniences as they became available. The patient had a strong desire to have his son work on the farm, and for that reason the son's illness and his desire to go to college were matters of great concern to the man. In addition, the farmer was troubled by the fact that his son was what he called a "high liver" who did not subscribe to the patient's rigid code of duty. The man had very strong feelings about his son, and apparently it was difficult for him to accept the fact that he was unable to impose his will on the boy.

Although on admission to the hospital the patient freely admitted that he felt depressed, he was well composed and acted normally. He was above average in intelligence; his general knowledge was about what would be expected from his limited formal education. He was cooperative and appeared willing to try to understand his problems. He was given seven electroshock treatments and showed some improvement, but he remained depressed. Against the advice of the staff, he decided to leave the hospital because he felt that he was needed on the farm during harvest time. While the possibility of further episodes was present, it seemed probable at the time of discharge that he would gradually recover as he had from his first attack.

Ps. M-D., Depr. M:50:M:2 +1 27436′18–9 (53) 5:5:19

The complaints of this patient on admission were depression, seclusiveness, and loss of interest in his family, his business, and his friends. A fairly successful businessman, the patient had begun to change in personality, without particular inciting factors, about ten months before admission. He had felt that he was going through a change of life and this had depressed him even though he was reassured about this. The early part of his illness was marked by periods of crying, though this symptom later improved somewhat. He had a number of somatic complaints also. In general, he had recovered to some extent before the present admission but had come to the hospital for electroshock therapy which he hoped would speed his recovery.

He had had a previous attack of depression when he lost heavily in the stock market in 1929. His intelligence was good. His interests had been limited chiefly to his family, his business, and his intimate friends. He had always been high-strung and impatient when resisted. He had been sexually well adjusted and maritally compatible except that in the past year his wife had been away because of illness and his depressed mood had emphasized a decline in his sexual drive.

In the hospital he was obviously tense and somewhat anxious, but he was clear in sensorium and intellect, answered questions intelligently, and was concerned about his desire to get well quickly. The hospitalization did not work as he had hoped. He actually began to get somewhat worse. He had expected that he could conduct his business by telephone while in the hospital, and when this could not be done, he became irritable and immediately requested discharge. He left with the intent to get shock therapy at a place where he could have his own way.

B. Simple Adult Maladj. M:39:M:10 +5 27436'189– 2:3:12
P. React. Depr.
P. Psychas.

This man, a pastor, came to the hospital seeking help for marital incompatibility, depression, restlessness, and general feelings of inferiority. Since adolescence he had had personality problems, marked by short periods of hyperactivity and overwork, followed by longer periods of irritability, depression, and compulsive behavior. The patient and his wife had separated eight years before admission after he had begun to project his own inadequacies upon her. He still brooded over having lost the love of his children and his wife, and he harbored thoughts they had turned against him. Recently he had considered suicide, and during a visit with his family he became markedly depressed and had temper outbursts in which he paced the floor, mumbled to himself, talked loudly, and accused his wife of being the perpetrator of all his difficulties. Three days before admission he had received a letter from his wife in which she suggested that he see a psychiatrist.

Always, as indicated, the patient had been subject to mood swings. At one time he spent four days in a state hospital for depression but at discharge was considered "not sick enough to be in a mental institution." Throughout his life the periods of depression had prevented him in various ways from progressing normally. For example, several times he was compelled to withdraw from school. Finally, after many starts and stops, he did complete his course in a small college, prepared for the ministry, and for the next few years preached in small rural communities. One of his "lifelong" difficulties, he said, was in thinking or concentrating, particularly when under pressure. He felt that his friendships were superficial, and that he "was never treated like a human being." Particular and neat in dress, and overly conscientious in all his actions, he was angered by any disturbance of his normal routine. He had few interests outside of his work and family. He believed himself to be strong in sexual drive. At one time he had masturbated frequently, but he felt masturbation was "neither a vice nor evil."

Once settled in the ward, the patient immediately expressed his wish for diagnosis and for counsel about his home situation. His wife was totally unsympathetic with his problems, and he had never been able to confide in her, he said. He was self-derogatory, and although sure that his wife was responsible for some of the difficulties he recognized that he had personality problems. Of these he spoke openly and seemed almost to appreciate the situations which aggravated his symptoms. He frequently praised the ward routine. Although he appeared to derive considerable relief from long interviews, he made little progress in psychotherapy because of an underlying rigidity covered over with elaborate acceptance of everything. At the time of discharge he still said that "people in this town wouldn't stand for me if they knew how things were." The patient's course in the hospital seemed encouraging and there were indications that some of his conflicts might be resolved after the hospitalization. He was appreciably recovered from the depression and irritability, but there was no assurance that he would remain so. At discharge he planned to take a vacation before he returned to his congregation.

Ps. M-D., Depr.	M:48:M:48	+1	274'3819-(41)	8:6:15

The present illness of this patient had begun after a gastric resection three years previously. Ten days after the surgery he had had an acute three-week episode of confusion and disorientation. Because of complications from the wound, he was incapacitated for four months, and a few days after finally returning to work he developed further complications including a draining sinus that persisted almost to the time of admission. He also had a chronic tired feeling and never felt well. He changed to an easier job, became careless of his appearance, lost interest in his former hobbies and activities, and described himself as just "too tired to do anything." He came to the hospital at his employer's suggestion.

He had had a chronic pain in the pit of his stomach since he was 16 years old, but in other respects his health had apparently been good. At least there were no obvious psychotic or neurotic upsets. He had had a cholecystectomy 25 years before admission and an operation for adhesions about 15 years before. It appeared possible that hysterical factors had contributed to these. He was an eighth-grade graduate and had had to repeat three grades; he quit school when a good job was offered to him. Always withdrawn, he preferred going off by himself for recreation. He had never been particularly cheerful and tended to worry. Dissatisfied with his social and economic status, he said he wished he had finished school so that he could get a better job and more adequately support his family, but he had apparently quit one job to take another at a lower salary so that he would not have to get up early. His intelligence was low normal.

In the hospital he was extremely depressed and retarded, giving answers slowly and reluctantly and rarely speaking spontaneously. His facial expression was dull, anxious, unsmiling, and he did not seem interested in anything around him. Although he was well oriented, there appeared to be some inexplicable impairment of intellect, chiefly in recent memory. His chief concern was to get out of the hospital as soon as possible. Twelve electroshock treatments brought some improvement. He finally persuaded his wife to take him out of the hospital against the advice of the staff. There were indications of an organic component to the illness but nothing that would fit this hypothesis could be demonstrated objectively. The prognosis was poor.

P. React. Depr.	F:32:M:81	+4	$\underline{27}$'4$\underline{38}$ $\underline{19}$-6	5:3:17
		+36	'247-8	4:5:14

P. React. Depr.	F:32:M:72	+21	7'23148-69	3:4:12
P. Psychas.		-35	'24-698	3:1:15
		-50	'74238-69	3:2:15

Ps. M-D., Depr.	F:35:M:61	+3	728$\underline{41}$3'$\underline{69}$-	4:11:15
P. Psychas.				

The patient was first admitted to the hospital with complaints of depression, anxiety, general dissatisfaction with life, and mild hypochondriasis. Fairly well until about seven years before admission, she had then begun to note increased nervous tension and a tendency to worry excessively about small matters. This had coincided with the end of a second pregnancy. The birth of the child brought relief but as time went on she was bothered by somatic pain. Reassurance by a physician helped temporarily, but one night eight months before admission she experienced a real panic reaction. She suddenly awoke, trembling and crying, feared she was "losing her mind," and believed everyone had forsaken her. Similar attacks occurred two or three times weekly; she wept a great deal and worried lest she harm her husband or her children. Following advice to take a complete rest helped somewhat, and by the time she was admitted to the hospital she was markedly improved.

An outgoing person, interested in social activities, she had at the same time always been cyclothymic, having "blue spells" in which she wept copiously. She was known to be sentimental. Because of her dislike for school she stopped at the end of the eighth grade, worked a couple of years in a factory, and then began a business course which she did not finish. Until her marriage she held a clerical job. She was apparently fairly compatible with her husband, although she felt that her sexual desires were greater than his and she craved more attention and affection than he provided.

On admission the patient reported that she had been "feeling much better" but still felt depressed and that the night panics were still present. She expressed dissatisfaction with her husband. In addition she was disturbed about religion, since she now had doubts about her faith. She appeared depressed but showed no obvious psychopathology in mental content or sensorium. On the ward she adapted well and was cooperative. During her hospital stay the night panics disappeared and she became relatively cheerful and happy. At discharge the prognosis appeared good. However, she was comfortable for only a few days and quickly developed depression and anxiety again. Within a month she was readmitted to the hospital. Again she was given considerable attention and psychotherapy, was a good patient, and appeared to make splendid progress. After the second discharge she seemed well for one year, then the symptoms reappeared, and gradually she slipped back into the old pattern. This was extenuated by a new pregnancy. After delivery the symptoms continued and she was readmitted to the hospital, this time for two months. She was now more worried, fearing that she would eventually become permanently insane. Again she improved and was, as before, a "good patient." Two shock treatments seemed to help, but at this third discharge she appeared not as obviously well as she had at the previous discharges.

B. Psth., Path. Emot. M:29:D 2746′1983–(69) 3:4:?

This man, a first lieutenant, had been in the army fifty months at the time of his referral. Demotion procedures had been instituted against him for drinking and for general irresponsibility. Stripped of his commission, he had been returned to civilian status.

The patient was a small, dark-haired person. He appeared in a soiled uniform and unshaven in spite of the late afternoon hour of the psychiatric interview. Ingratiating and unctuous, he was insincere in his attitude. The family history was pathological in that his father was a chronic alcoholic whom his mother divorced. She supported the children and was described as overly indulgent. The childhood history gave many evidences of early neurosis including bed-wetting, sleepwalking, and recurrent bad dreams. These had been specifically denied at the time of commissioning. The psychosexual history was characterized by inadequate adjustment. His promiscuity dated from the age of 16 and repeated marital infidelities resulted in two attacks of gonorrhea. In contrast, his school and occupational attainments had been good. His schooling, which continued to the end of two college years, showed no irregularities and his work record was equally steady.

The officer's performance in the air corps was adequate until immediate precombat training was reached. He then developed severe anxiety which could only be allayed by drinking. He was hospitalized three times for "nervousness" (tenseness, anorexia, insomnia) in the few months preceding his separation from the service. No follow-up material was available. A. T. K.

Ps. Invol. Melan.	F:51:S:33	+1	27'463891–(53)	3:1:13
Paranoid		+25	'6–39184(59)	3:5:9
Ps. Invol. Melan.	F:51:S:25	+3	2734'681–9(45)	4:10:10

Anxiety, depression, agitation, and excessive worry brought this patient to the hospital. These symptoms, all severe for the past six months, were more or less correlated with difficulties at her place of employment. Advised by her employer to "take a vacation," she did and returned feeling much better but was then told that the vacation was actually a discharge. Abruptly the symptoms returned and became progressively worse. She felt incapable of finding a new position and worried constantly about financial matters. Three weeks before admission she fell down a flight of stairs, and, while no injury could be discovered, she continued to have pain. Her mother became so concerned that the patient's brother was called in, talked to her briefly, and then left to consult the family doctor. She followed her brother all the way to his home, believing he planned to kill himself in order to avoid the responsibility of caring for their mother, since she herself was ill and could no longer do it. The brother quieted her and brought her to the hospital the following day.

Although she had always been friendly, the patient had never been an outgoing person. She had inferiority feelings regarding her abilities and social standing. She had a few close friends but never many. A strict Roman Catholic, she attended church regularly. Of superior intelligence, she had graduated from a business college and then had worked for several different firms, changing from one job to another in the hope of advancing her status. The job she finally lost was one that she had held for many years.

On admission to the hospital the patient was agitated and depressed but well oriented. She was fear-ridden about her financial problems and the impossibility, as she saw it, of obtaining another job. Although somewhat evasive she really seemed to want help. She recognized that she was ill. She did not readily accept the hospital routine and avoided other patients. There was a paranoid aspect to her thinking. She was frightened by sedative packs but accepted the electroshock therapy well and improved rapidly under it. There seemed to be a slight euphoria at the time of discharge. Seven months later she was readmitted with similar symptoms. After leaving the hospital she had taken a new job, had settled down, and had appeared to be happy. But soon symptoms appeared in much the same fashion as before. In the hospital this time she was more uncooperative and suspicious than formerly, in fact, markedly so. Again, with electroshock therapy, she improved gradually. At the end of three weeks she was discharged with the recommendation that she continue in the outpatient department. The prognosis was guarded.

P. Psychas. M:19:S:62 +7 274'86–(73) 4:8:13
Ps. Sz., Cat.

This boy was referred by his parents who felt there was a possibility of a relapse into the catatonic condition which had previously caused him to be confined in the state mental hospital for a year. He had been out of the hospital for a year at the time of the initial interview. His parents felt there was a recurrence of the hostility picture which had preceded the original breakdown. Actually little, if any, hostility showed itself in the interviews. In fact, the client stated in the first interview that he didn't believe there was a possibility of a relapse. The picture he presented was one of severe feelings of inferiority: he doubted that he would be able to finish high school; he felt himself incapable of making an application for a job; and although he could manage himself well in a social situation, he felt that his social contacts were always on a superficial level. He regretted the passing of his childhood and approached the growing-up process with a great deal of apprehension. He worried about the age of his parents, feeling that they would leave him alone to face the world.

The developmental picture was one of close home ties; there had been few children with whom he could play. Following the death of his mother, and the remarriage of his father, he had begun to feel isolated even from his home. For a while he identified himself with two siblings, but they finally moved away. He never felt any resentment toward his stepmother, but he did not feel free to turn to her with many of his childhood problems. In high school the results of this pattern of isolated living began to take effect. He had always been a meticulous boy, and when he could not keep up with some of his studies it bothered him. His tension mounted and eventually he found himself moving in a vicious circle: he needed scholastic success to give him a feeling of self-confidence, the need was so great that it caused anxiety, the anxiety decreased his efficiency, and so on. The problem resulted in a "nervous breakdown" toward the end of his junior year. He was hospitalized, with the diagnosis of catatonic schizophrenia, and at that time he was given a series of electroshocks. The family was unable to meet the expense of a private hospital, and he was transferred to the state hospital. This hospital continued the convulsive treatments for a short time; afterward their care of the patient was essentially custodial. After a year's stay he returned home and went to a vocational school, which he graduated from one year later, shortly after the beginning of the present therapy. At the time of his release from the state hospital it had been felt that the prognosis was poor.

The boy responded well in the therapeutic situation, quickly establishing insights, although his over-all demeanor was naive. He faced the problem of growing up with some reluctance, but he eventually came to accept this as one of the "breaks" of life. Because of his charming manner, his sincerity, and his willingness, he was a delightful person to counsel. At the end of the counseling he still remained somewhat naive in his interests and attitudes. He discontinued the therapy spontaneously, feeling that he was now making a satisfactory life adjustment. Shortly after, he obtained a clerical position. He later registered at the university, although when therapy first began he had rejected the idea of further education, believing that he lacked sufficient intelligence and maturity to do college work. A. S.

P. React. Depr. F:26:M:20 +21 27486'31– 7:9:14
P. Hypo.

Until the delivery of her last pregnancy four months before admission, the patient had felt well; but following the delivery she began to complain of fatigue, restlessness, headaches, backaches, and insomnia. Becoming depressed and finding it difficult to do her work, she gradually became more and more irritable, with the symptoms being especially severe whenever she was reprimanded.

There had been no previous medical or psychiatric disturbances. She did not start school until she was 9 years of age, and she was dull normal in intelligence, a slow learner. After finishing the seventh grade at age 16, she did housework for neighbors. Her chief hobby was sewing. In the presence of strangers she was ill at ease but not outstandingly so. Her husband was a farm laborer of limited intellectual ability, and the two had been married for five years. There were two children.

On admission to the hospital the patient felt that many of her difficulties were in large part due to the unsympathetic attitude of her husband's employer. Much concerned with her insomnia, irritability, and weakness, she appeared moderately depressed and cried during the course of the examination. She was shy and ill at ease on the ward. While the nature of her complaints indicated that she had some insight into the fact that she was mentally ill, she never elaborated to any degree in telling about her troubles, and she felt that the symptoms were due to her enlarged but medically benign goiter. There was some psychomotor retardation. At the time of discharge she was much improved, and in the hope that some of the strain would be relieved, particular efforts were made to improve the home and social situation generally.

Ps. Toxic	M:24:S:22	+1	274981 36′–X (59)	1:17:8
Alcoholism		+15	94′187 26–(59)	0:13:11

This young man had learned to drink during high school but at that time it was not a problem for him. Later, while he was in the merchant marine his engineer's license was suspended for being drunk on duty and allowing a cargo to be spoiled. When he returned home from the service he was restless and nervous. Just before coming home he had considered taking his life but could not go through with it, he said. During the summer before admission to the hospital he was drunk most of the time. His average was two "fifths" a day. Noisy, surly, and abusive toward his parents, he pushed his mother around but did not strike her. His father, who was 79 and feeble, he did strike. Apparently, he was in a toxic delirium and he suffered from delusions about having three guns in his suitcase. It was finally necessary to have him taken to a jail and from there he was sent to the hospital.

A graduate of high school at age 17, he had had no learning difficulties. Tests indicated his I.Q. to be 128. He had been an eagle scout. Except for the scouting activities, however, he had few friends and no other interests. As a child, he had been quiet and well behaved, always somewhat withdrawn, and he had never had a girl friend. His mother could not recall that he had ever taken a girl out. She described him as kind, gentle, and generous. Apparently, however, he had felt dissatisfied with life and depressed enough to wonder if life was worth living. His mother was a rigid, domineering, matriarchal person, oversolicitous and possessive toward her son. She was devout and extremely intolerant of drinking and smoking.

In the hospital the young man showed evidence of an alcoholic neuritis. By the time of admission he was oriented and was beginning to recover. Cooperative and attentive, he showed a willingness to answer questions but never talked freely about himself. He admitted that his drinking was a problem for him, and he realized that he had never been able to curb it. However, he was obviously not interested in obtaining help for the problem. With the other patients he was aloof. This withdrawal prevented any approach for psychotherapy, and his attitude was that he could handle the problem himself in his own way. At the time of discharge he was physically recovered.

Schizoid M:46:S:64 +61 '276–9(69) 2:2:11

This man had become depressed at the age of 30 when he was a theological student. He developed strong feelings of guilt and unworthiness for his calling. He made several attempts at suicide and had at the same time a constant fear of immediate death. He had persecutory ideas. He was at that time a patient in the hospital for five months; he came in again for six weeks ten years later. In the present admission he came as a voluntary patient.

No information about his early history was available, apart from the fact that he seemed overprotected and excessively attached to his mother. He had become a nonconformist minister but still considered himself unworthy.

He was diagnosed as having depression in a schizoid personality. He was treated in his third admission by a course of electric convulsion and modified insulin therapies. He improved, though he still lacked insight. According to the psychiatric social worker's report after his discharge, he preached occasionally but had no regular work. He seemed very anxious to obtain some clerical work instead of continuing in the ministry. His appearance was upkempt, and he gave the impression of being lonely and unhappy. M. V.

Ps. M-D., Depr. F:37:S:41 +15 276'138–9 7:3:11
Suicidal +40 27'63148–9 7:3:12

The patient's complaints centered around nervousness, lack of interest, depression, and withdrawal from activities, but the onset of the illness was difficult to define since she had always been moody and depressed. About four years before hospital admission she had met a rather nervous young man, and during the time she associated with him she was less nervous and took a more lively interest in life than she had at any previous time. After the date of their wedding was set, the man was unable to go through with the marriage because of his nervous condition, and although the ceremony was postponed indefinitely, the patient apparently took this in a rather matter-of-fact way. About three weeks before the patient's admission her fiancé either committed suicide or accidentally shot himself, and the incident precipitated a marked depression characterized by weeping, insomnia, and loss of appetite.

Never a robust individual, the patient described many illnesses and symptoms which went back into her earliest memory. An eighth-grade graduate with an average scholastic record, the woman had been a telephone operator in a small town near the family farm until she had been placed in a hospital for tuberculosis. Upon recovery she worked as a maid in a private hospital, but she was discharged from this position, in part because of her general weakness and depression. She was described as having always been a shy individual who took little part in family activities. On encountering minor difficulties she had always withdrawn into herself, never discussing her problems with anyone.

At the time of her admission she stated frequently that she had nothing to live for. Although she attributed her depression to her "great sorrow," it was felt that her depression dated from before her meeting with the young man.

Questions were answered relevantly and to the point, but she never spoke spontaneously, her speech was slow, and she spent her time by herself weeping. During the time in the hospital she improved only to a slight extent. At the time of discharge she was still very depressed, and because she had become more active she was considered a great suicidal risk. She was discharged for a trial at home with the possibility of further institutionalization suggested to her relatives.

P. React. Depr. M:41:M:10 +1 27'63489–1 (59) 3:6:6

The patient was admitted to the hospital because of periods of nervousness and feelings of inadequacy over eleven years. The first episode had lasted about a month. One of the two other episodes of similar character had occurred eight years before admission, and the other three years before hospitalization. The episodes began with feelings of inadequacy and increasing irritability toward his wife and children and depression, weeping, and suicidal threats followed. By getting away from his work and his usual surroundings for a few weeks he had recovered from the first two attacks, but after his last attack there had been only partial recovery, and the present admission represented an exacerbation of a pattern that had been present in part for three years.

A college graduate, he had done very well in business and had lived at a high social level in his small town. Easily influenced by others, especially by his mother and by his brothers and sisters, he was a sensitive person who always tried to please everyone, and who customarily felt inferior to many people. There was no open conflict in his marriage, which was on the whole fairly satisfactory, but he was having difficulty in his business because his mother and his siblings were attempting to control him in opposition to his wife who also wished to dominate him.

In the hospital he was well oriented, was intact in sensorium and intellect, and had good insight into his problems. He appeared to be an ultraconscientious person who had good contact with reality and high integrity. Simple psychotherapeutic interviews and the opportunity to work out his problems away from his family were very reassuring to him. His improvement was rapid, and at the time of discharge the prognosis appeared to be very good.

P. Anxiety State M:40:M:46 +19 2'7683–9X (65) 10:2:19
Ps. M-D., Depr.
Schizoid

The patient exhibited increasing signs of anxiety, lack of confidence, and inability to concentrate, with insomnia and irritability, while serving with the

Royal Air Force in India. He had had a stable record previously and his symptoms were regarded as due to "conscientious obsession in a highly intelligent personality." He recovered and carried on with his duties. Later he again became depressed and agitated, could not concentrate, and harbored suicidal ideas. He heard his own thoughts spoken and had a tendency to shout out. He was admitted to the hospital as a voluntary patient.

He was one of nine children. He joined the Fleet Air Arm at the age of 17, changing to the Royal Air Force during the war, in which he served as an instructor in navigation. He married at the age of 26.

He was diagnosed as being manic-depressive (depression in a schizoid personality) and was treated by modified insulin therapy and electric convulsion therapy.

M. V.

P. Psychas.	F:28:M:8	+1	278134'69–(53)	5:8:12
		−19	278134'6–X(63)	2:16:11
		−46	2781463'9–(53)	0:11:13
		+68	278'13496–(59)	2:8:7

About a year before admission to the hospital and at a time when the family was staying with her husband's parents because of the housing shortage, this young mother of two children developed an acute fear of poliomyelitis, which placed her under considerable strain. After this abated she began to fear sharp knives. When she read a book about diseases, she felt that she had each one she read about; and she had attacks in which she suddenly became faint and perspired profusely. Someone told her that in order to solve her problems she would have to retrace her childhood, and in attempting to do this she concentrated on herself to the exclusion of everything else. As a result of reading about fear and its consequences she developed a fear of dying. Two short hospitalization periods did not give her much help.

There were no previous psychotic upsets and nothing in the past history contributed clearly to the present picture. Average in intelligence, she had completed the tenth grade. Nervous and dependent with severe feelings of inadequacy, she had difficulty in school apparently because she was unable to assert herself, showed no ability to plan, and lacked special interests. Her school attendance had been irregular because the family had moved frequently, and afterward she had held several jobs as clerk and typist from which she had been discharged for unknown reasons. Since early childhood she had taken an excessive interest in her own bodily functions, as did her mother and an aunt who had lived with them. The patient had been married about six years before admission, and she and her husband were relatively compatible.

Pleasant and cooperative, the patient smiled frequently, despite a marked feeling of depression and a conviction that everything was hopeless. While she recognized that she had an emotional problem, she also felt that something must be organically wrong with her. Although there was no apparent disturbance in her thoughts or orientation, she was troubled by such marked fears as that death was impending or that her heart would stop beating. Her condition changed very little with hospitalization, and she made no attempt to mix with other patients. The possibility of using active psychotherapy was complicated by the fact that she continually wavered between staying in the hospital and going home where she claimed to feel better. She was finally discharged, against the better judgment of the staff, and it was thought to be highly doubtful that she would be able to solve her basic problems while she remained in her home environment.

Ps. M-D., Depr.   M:34:M:38   +5   2781′364–9   7:7:10

The patient had been constantly "doctoring for his nerves" over a two-year period, and at the time of admission his depression had been increasing in intensity for the last few weeks. His symptoms included many hypochondriacal components, but extensive medical examinations and prescriptions had helped him very little. Until the onset of the present illness he was said to have been in relatively good health, and there was no evidence of any previous psychotic disorders.

The patient had emigrated from Sweden at the age of 16, where he had finished the eighth grade. He had gone to night school in this country and had eventually become a skilled workman. A steady worker who had made a fair living for his family, he had always been sociable and "full of pep and fun." Although he expressed dislike for his work, he did not appear to suffer particularly from it, and he had no other specific ambition. He and his wife seemed to be well adjusted, and he was fond of his children. No precipitating factor was discovered to explain his illness.

On admission his main concern was with his physical condition: "I can't work. I can't concentrate. I have a pain on the top of my head. I am in utter despair. What is the cause of all this?" There was a definite loss of interest, his speech was slow and lacking in spontaneity, and there was psychomotor retardation, but no feelings of guilt or ideas of reference could be elicited. His eyes frequently filled with tears, and he sat slumped in his chair without change of his facial expression. Gradually he began to take part in the hospital activities, and he developed a liking for a young boy, also a patient, with whom he seemed to enjoy playing games. He took an active interest in occupational therapy, and by the time he was discharged he had a real desire to go back to work. It was recommended that he engage in some outdoor activity before actually taking up his occupation again. While the long duration of his illness seemed to be against a permanent adjustment, considerable optimism was, nevertheless, felt about his future.

Ps. M-D., Depr.	F:31:S:78	+7	278'14396–(49)	4:11:8
Ps. Sz., Simple		+55	287139'46–(45)	2:10:8
Ps. Sz., Simple Ps. M-D., Depr.	F:32:S:44	+5	7824136'9–X(49)	10:18:19
P. Hypo. P. React. Depr.	F:32:S:65	+2	9172 48'36–(55)	1:6:9

The patient entered the hospital with an acute depression. For two weeks also she had been unable to concentrate. She had been in more or less chronic ill health and had experienced bilateral femoral venous occlusions about a year before admission. At the time of hospitalization she was unable to walk more than a block or two before severe pains appeared in both legs. She felt that "life was not worthwhile" unless her physical condition could be improved. All her leisure time she spent at home in bed crying and complaining of severe headaches.

About two or three years before admission the patient had had dyspnea and palpitation, and a diagnosis of mitral stenosis with regurgitation and fibrillation was made. In addition to the femoral occlusions she had suffered from mastoiditis and ultimately a left lumbar sympathectomy was performed. She had had numerous other surgical operations during the ten years before admission. Throughout this entire complicated medical history it was recognized that she was a neurotic person, but no one was ever certain to what extent this contributed to the problem. The patient had been a skilled worker; but since she changed jobs and lines of work frequently, she never progressed far along any particular line. Of average intelligence, she had managed, before this illness, to be fairly independent. She had few close friends. For recreation she bowled and swam. She never showed any interest in men and associated almost entirely with girls.

At the time of admission there were physical scars of her numerous operations and some physiological effects of the removal of the lumbar sympathetics. The findings were all medical, however; no neurological signs of anything contributing to the present illness could be noted. Very uncooperative, she cried continuously and complained of headaches. She refused to talk with people and would simply say "leave me alone." After some time she was a little more cooperative but remained deeply depressed and relatively uncommunicative. She became slightly better and was finally discharged to the care of her sister. About three months later she was readmitted for 44 days with the same pattern. Varied diagnoses were considered but since nothing could be done with her she was committed to a state hospital where she improved. Discharged from the state hospital, she was again admitted with the same pattern at a later date.

P. Psychas. P. React. Depr. Suicidal	M:34:M:79	+2	27'831–9(59)	3:4:10

P. Psychas.	M:35:M:75	+7	287'<u>36</u>1–(71)	1:8:9
Schizoid		–15	2783'169–(78)	2:7:10
		+74	2'673–94(61)	2:2:7
P. Psychas.	M:35:M:11	+2	278'<u>36</u>41–9(78)	2:4:11

Impulsiveness, depression, and low back pain were the admission problems of this patient. He believed that a fall six months earlier, which had resulted in an injury, was responsible for the depression in that it had created nervous tension and mental anxiety. Foremost among his worries was his impulse to do bodily harm to himself, to his family, and to others; and while he realized that these impulses were dangerous and unnatural he had an intense fear that he might not be able to control them. He lost interest in his work and in people and became more and more emotionally unstable. He grew careless in his dress and felt that his absent-mindedness had progressively increased. Because he thought he might hurt them, he was afraid to play with his children. The history showed at least three periods in which he had had similar troubles, always connected with a wrenching of his back, the first happening when the patient was 17 years old. The pain in his back, dull and aching in nature, was localized in the lower lumbar region. Reassurance, at first somewhat helpful, finally lost its efficacy. In his opinion the pain was "too real to be due to my imagination."

Above average in intelligence, he had skipped from the seventh grade to high school and had later enrolled at a university with the intention of becoming a dentist. Forced to discontinue this course because of financial difficulty, he had been employed since then by large concerns. The fact that he always did more on the job than was expected of him made him angry at himself. He had been a stubborn, likable, sensitive child, and had always read a great deal. A marked characteristic of his entire life was conscientiousness and perfectionism in his work. Known as self-reliant, fair, sensitive, and self-confident, he had never been very religious, and until the present illness, he had always been emotionally stable. Happily married, he had three children.

Well aware that he was mentally disturbed, the patient was eager for help, and spoke readily about his condition, with his thoughts mostly centered around his almost irresistible impulses. Although his stay in the hospital was an up and down affair, he was alert, thoughtful, and conscientious, giving the impression that he wanted to be completely accurate and honest. While at times he felt "better than I have in the past six months," for the most part he was depressed. Four electroshock treatments seemed to help the depression somewhat. Psychotherapy, directed at bringing out some of his latent hostilities and at giving him better insight into his perfectionist tendencies, was somewhat productive. During the last two weeks in the hospital he became optimistic, planning actively for a normal future, and at the time of discharge it seemed likely that he would make an adequate adjustment. Approximately two years later he was readmitted. In the interim he had alternated between periods of relative comfort and periods of severe depression. Once more he was discharged with some improvement, but three months later he was again admitted with the usual history of ups and downs during that interval. Shock therapy failed to bring improvement, and it was felt that he was a good subject for a frontal lobotomy. With this operation in mind, he was finally discharged for voluntary admission to a state hospital.

Ps. M-D., Depr.	F:41:S:42	+1	278316'4–(34)	7:9:13
Suicidal		+39	'712389–(30)	4:2:17

Four years before admission to the hospital the patient had noticed that she was inefficient and unable to concentrate on her teaching duties, and she thought she was going insane. A few weeks before, her aunt had died and she had stayed with her uncle against her own wishes. Following an attempt at suicide with sleeping pills, she was hospitalized and after electroshock treatment, she improved. About two years later when her mother had a stroke, the patient felt that her own suicide attempt had been a precipitating factor, and late that year it was necessary to give her shock treatment for an illness that lasted two months, during which she again attempted suicide with sleeping pills. When she was discharged she again began to teach, but she had a roommate who was not compatible. As she continued teaching she gradually lost interest in outside activities, felt tired all the time, and found it was necessary to drive herself to her duties. Shortly before admission to the hospital with the present illness she had received four more electroshock treatments.

The past history was noncontributory. In high school she had failed in several subjects because of a lack of interest, but she had graduated from college, and since getting her degree she had taught school although she had not liked the job. Twice engaged, she had broken the second engagement because she insisted on delaying marriage until she had paid off her father's debts. She had also assumed responsibility for her mother's support. She had become increasingly rigid and had driven herself to live up to religious and ethical standards of a high level.

The patient was depressed and preoccupied with thoughts of her failure to marry, her mother's and aunt's illnesses, and other happenings from which she derived considerable guilt. She was resentful about not having married. She realized that she was sick and needed help, but she had little insight beyond that. Her sensorium and intellect were normal. There was little spontaneity and she was not especially accessible. For the first four weeks she showed little interest in other people or in her surroundings, and she was resentful because she had been brought to the hospital. Improvement was rapid after electroshock treatment. She was literally bubbling with excitement at the prospect of being discharged, and it was apparent that she was recovered from the present attack although, obviously, future ones were likely.

P. Mixed	F:26:M:46	—20	278'3194–(41)	4:9:9
Suicidal		—53	18327'6–(45)	2:10:7
		+42	28713'946–X (49)	3:15:5

P. Mixed Schizoid Suicidal	F:26:M:20	+3	82769413'–X (51)	0:21:5

The patient entered the hospital because of severe depression and many somatic complaints. She had just taken an overdose of sleeping tablets. The illness had been progressive for the past five years and had been severe for about six months. In a sanitarium for six weeks, she thought she was getting well and returned to her husband but gradually she became worse again and began coming to the psychiatric outpatient department. Childlike and immature, she had made the present suicidal attempt because a cat she had been very fond of had died. At the time of admission she was still in a semicomatose state as a result of the overdose of sleeping pills.

Four years before the present illness she had sought admission to a general hospital for treatment of "swollen joints and eyelids." She was not admitted but was found in the street soon afterward apparently in a coma. The husband said that they had made a diagnosis of rheumatic fever and that this was the real beginning of the whole series of difficulties. It was never determined whether she had been hysterical at that time or whether some more obviously organic illness had caused the difficulty, but it was most likely hysteria. Later she had a premature baby delivered by caesarian section and with another pregnancy underwent a therapeutic abortion and was artificially sterilized. Her intelligence level was in the average range. She had always been easily upset emotionally, moody, and unstable.

An orphan at the age of 2, she had led a very irregular life from that time on. When 15 she was employed by an elderly woman who committed suicide after many threats while the patient took a one-day vacation. The patient had an illegitimate child at age 21 and married at age 22 but to another man than the father. The marriage was not a compatible one and she claimed to have been unable to care for her child because of her ill health although it was adopted by the couple after their marriage. With reference to the therapeutic abortion she had undergone, she said at the time of admission that she felt like a "murderer."

In the hospital she was high-strung and unstable, as evidenced by her distractibility and frequent tears. Her sensorium and intellect were normal and her stream of thought was rational. She could apparently not approach her own problem; whenever the subject was brought up or any personal reference was made she would become exceedingly hesitant and answer in monosyllables. There were periods when she was uncooperative, refused food, threw medication on the floor, and the like. At first there were some schizoid signs with posturing but these disappeared very quickly. She was discharged to be followed in the outpatient department.

Two months later she was readmitted as an inpatient because of her continued symptoms. She had obviously taken a sedative or had been drinking when admitted the second time since she was staggering and her conversation was irrelevant and facetious. During the interview she constantly toyed with a small pocket knife and suddenly she attempted to slash her wrists. When the knife was taken away from her she slumped to the floor and began to act in a hysterical manner. She spoke vaguely of taking pills and later apparently became comatose. She was not disoriented but as she recovered from the sedative she spoke of eyes peering at her through the ventilator and was greatly disturbed if anyone touched her. She was finally transferred from the psychiatric unit to a state hospital.

B. Psth., Mixed F:22:S:67 +2 278'3416–9 6:5:14
+50 mos. 278643'–9 5:7:16

The patient entered the hospital as a voluntary patient because, she said, "I've been depressed all my life and lately I've felt I wanted to die." There had been no definite onset of the symptoms, the present problem being merely an exaggeration of previous personality defects and feelings of inadequacy created by unfulfilled ambitions. The immediate problem centered around her inability to concentrate on her schoolwork and to comprehend simple statements. She was also annoyed with the idea that she was inferior mentally.

With the possible exception of a period of convulsions when she was 21 months old, her past medical history indicated nothing of importance. Her I.Q. of about 92 was in marked contrast to her ambitions. Although she had graduated from grade school on the honor roll, upon entering high school she had immediately found that she learned slowly and she had felt this inadequacy so keenly that she had discontinued school at the end of her freshman year. Four years later her ambition to be more than a housemaid—she wanted to be a beauty parlor operator—had taken her back to school, but she had found the sophomore and junior years extremely difficult. In her junior year she had been made class president but, she said, "It wasn't because they wanted me, but because I was the oldest one in the class." At the beginning of her senior year she had been unusually depressed, and it was during this time that she had come to the hospital.

The patient had always been extremely neat and clean, and she was described as having always been seclusive, sensitive, overly modest, prudish, and given to daydreaming. While the girl had always been personable, with many friends, she was bashful with strangers and found it difficult to confide in others. From interviews with the patient's mother it became obvious that the woman had entirely rejected her daughter, and although the mother refused to accept the idea that the girl would be better off in an environment other than her home, it was obvious that she was relieved to have her daughter hospitalized. Especially in her early teens the patient had demonstrated considerable religious fervor, and even as a child when she had been naughty she had worried about going to hell. In recent years she had considered going into a convent, and religious matters had been of great concern to her. While at one time she thought that "God is capable of knowing innermost thoughts," she said, "it doesn't bother me as much as it used to." She was very shy in the presence of men and denied any desire to be married.

Her mental state was of great concern to her, and she feared that the depression had finally affected her brain so that she was going insane. In her discouragement she had considered taking lysol but her fear of a life hereafter had been a determent when her moods of depression led her to consider suicide. The idea that she was mentally lower than average was an obsession with her. Cooperative and pleasant in attitude and manner, she gratefully accepted the interest of others. During hospitalization she was passively willing to stay almost any amount of time in the ward. In examination she was guarded about her fundamental problems and showed a great inflexibility about readjusting her concept of herself in relation to her ability. She was discharged to return to high school on a restricted schedule in the hope that she would be able to graduate. With the proper emancipation and encouragement, it was felt that the patient might be able to make a fairly good adjustment in spite of the poor organization of her personality, and the marked immaturity, insecurity, and unhappiness dating back to her childhood.

Ps. M-D., Depr.	F:57:W:64	+26	2783'416–9	4:6:15
		+30	'2437–9	4:0:11

This patient was committed by the court because of symptoms chiefly characterized by agitation, anxiety, feelings of depression, and invalidism. The pattern had begun two years earlier when she showed excessive worry over inconsequential matters and complained of headaches, loss of appetite, eye strain, and abdominal discomfort. She spent an increasing amount of time in bed, was anxious and depressed, and felt that the future was hopeless. Motor signs of restlessness consisted of purposeless movements, picking of fingers, slapping of thighs, and the like. Similar periods had occurred from the time of her husband's death six years before admission. The attacks always began in the spring and usually lasted from "two to six months." Others had been less severe than the present one. Most of the attacks terminated suddenly, and for the previous ones she had not been hospitalized.

The patient's education had been terminated in the sixth grade at age 14. Her first marriage ended after one year with the death of her husband. Left with a baby son, she was forced to alter her scale of living radically. A second marriage was also interrupted by the death of the husband, and she and her son then went to live with her parents in a single room over a tavern. Her income was restricted to a mother's pension and a small amount of insurance. A well-liked, friendly person, she enjoyed social gatherings and took pride in presenting a good appearance. She tended to be selfish and impractical in money matters, was always dependent on others, and never really accepted the responsibilities of motherhood. She was a devout Catholic.

On the ward the patient appeared depressed and agitated. She constantly moved her hands and feet, rubbed her elbows, tapped her feet, and picked at her nails. Over and over she said, "I'm sorry I ever came. I can't stand the noise." She was concerned with the details of her illness and her recent inability to gain weight satisfactorily. She showed marked restriction of interests and preoccupation with her own affairs. After a few days she began to improve and adjusted well to the hospital routine. Gradually she took more interest in her surroundings and became more normal in her activity and mental content. At the time of discharge she was nearly recovered and it seemed likely that she would recover from the present episode. It was felt, however, that future episodes might occur.

P. React. Depr.	F:25:M:100	+1	27834′61–9 (45)	3:8:18
P. Psychas.		+72	2′673–9 (34)	6:3:14
Suicidal		+107	′276438–9 (49)	3:10:18

This young woman was referred by her husband after she attempted to commit suicide. Following the birth of a baby she had taken forty tablets (twenty grains) of phenobarbital. The suicide attempt was made deliberately; in fact, she had failed once before and wished to "make sure" this second time. During the initial contact with the therapist she expressed no confusion, depression, or anxiety, but she did present the picture of a rigid personality, was meticulous in speech, dress, and thought. She talked fairly calmly of her attempt at suicide and there was a general flattening of the affect.

The woman's early childhood had been marked by unhappiness and privation. She described her mother as self-centered and garrulous. The father played little, if any, part in her life. He was kindly and intelligent, and the patient identified herself more with him than with the mother. When she was 15 she married one of her high school classmates, and both finished school the following year. Her husband proved to resemble her father in kindliness and intelligence, and, also much like the father, he was endowed with little economic drive. Thus, the client had felt that she was under financial pressure, and she had worked until the coming of their baby (in the ninth year of marriage). Although she did not consider herself to be a good housewife, she managed to keep the home always immaculate.

During treatment the client continually tried to place the burden of the responsibility for help in the hands of the therapist. After two weeks her husband became apprehensive about the possibility of a third suicide attempt and arranged for her to be placed in the state hospital. There for a period of six weeks she received nine electroshock treatments. Shortly after she left the hospital she resumed therapy and showed continued improvement. During this time she took a job and invited her mother into the household to take care of the baby. Although she had previously rejected the baby, now she began to form a slight emotional attachment to him. When the husband was seen a few weeks after the termination of therapy he reported continued improvement. His wife was happier, he said, she was finding it easier to make friends, she was accepting the baby more and more, and there was a marked improvement of adjustment in the sexual area. However, she did have an occasional period of despondency stemming from her chagrin at having been in a mental institution. A. S.

Ps. Sz., Paranoid Suicidal	M:40:M:32	+1	27836941′–(55)	5:11:10
Ps. Paranoid	M:41:M:84	+30	23178′4–9 (57)	7:7:10
		−91	278631′49–X (65)	5:19:14

This man had formerly been hospitalized elsewhere after a suicidal attempt. In the present admission he showed anxiety about his thoughts and complained of palpitation and "burning of the heart and left arm." The illness had been insidious in onset. Gradually he had begun to worry more and more, particularly about world events. Two years before admission he had become markedly depressed following the suicidal death of a sister. Later, after the death of a friend, he complained of excessive tiredness, brooded a great deal, and talked little. As the symptoms progressed, he lost interest in his home and his activities and developed insomnia. In the ten days preceding admission, he heard the sound of airplanes and automobiles constantly and believed they were purposely annoying him. When he was well rested, these hallucinations did not occur. He also saw "the Holy Ghost" one night.

Although the patient had complained of palpitations for many years, no organic heart disorder was discovered. There was no evidence of previous psychotic episodes. A printer by trade, he had been a good worker. In personality he was described as shy and sensitive but friendly, kind, thoughtful, and truthful. He was said to have always reacted excessively to disappointments. He also was pessimistic and required sympathy. In general, however, he had fulfilled his responsibilities to his home and to society. His father had been sent to a state hospital and one of his sisters had, as noted, committed suicide. His marital life had been relatively satisfactory.

On admission to the hospital the patient's concerns were with his family's welfare and with his own condition. He had prominent religious trends. He was only partly oriented, his memory and retention were defective, and he appeared perplexed, anxious, and somewhat elated. In the hospital he improved a great deal and made a good adjustment. He showed interest in ward activities and made friends with other patients. He became able to discuss the stresses which he felt had precipitated the need for hospitalization, and he came to feel that he could handle the problems that faced him. He was given four electroshock treatments during this period. At discharge it was agreed that he had made significant progress in handling his situation. He remained at home and active for about seven months and then suddenly developed a similar pattern of symptoms and was readmitted for treatment. The pattern of improvement was repeated during this second hospitalization.

P. React. Depr. M:35:M:20 —60 278′436–(65) 3:2:12
P. Psychas. +150 –741 (63) 3:2:12

This man came to the clinic with the pretext of vocational advisement, but he quickly brought up the fact that he was going through a period of considerable anxiety concerning his chosen profession, his marriage, his social relationships, and his self-confidence. He felt that he was not in a satisfactory profession and because of his age it was imperative that if he was going to change, he should change immediately. It was found later that his wife also had a serious emotional problem. Their two problems were of such vastly different natures that there was constant conflict. Rather curiously the sexual adjustment between them was excellent, probably the result of their having previously sought professional advice in this area.

The history of this patient contained almost every adverse element that could be conjectured for the son of a very idealistic small town minister. As a child he could not fight because one was expected to "turn the other cheek." As an adolescent he felt himself an outcast. There was an almost continual conflict between sex and religion. Fortunately, in high school he found himself adept at sports and he further capitalized on this at college. In college, however, his dissatisfaction with his inner self could not be completely overcome. He was undecided about where to turn professionally, and his decision was finally determined by the intense attachment he felt for one of his professors, who played, to a certain degree, the role of a father-surrogate. There was some sexual activity during college, but always attended with great guilt. He married somewhat hastily, chiefly under the impetus of a guilt feeling. He interpreted being married as a handicap because he no longer would have the freedom to direct his own mode of life. He did continue working toward the doctorate, which he obtained about five years after his marriage. He then served in the navy, enjoying it very much. Following his discharge the unhappy family situation came to a crisis, and it was during this time that he got some psychiatric assistance for his sexual problem. This improved the marital relations but there was still friction from the clash of the two maladjusted personalities.

This patient came to the clinic only after spending approximately six months "sizing up" the counselor, but when he actually came for consultation he worked into his problem almost immediately. The unusual thing about this case was the extensive way in which he would trace down every emotion. He was not content to permit himself a single emotional statement unless he carefully traced it to its roots. Because of this the counseling was a long and tedious process involving biweekly contacts over a period of approximately eight months. He was always prompt, always courteous, and he pushed himself terrifically to make sure that none of the implications of his problem eluded him. Counseling was terminated by mutual consent, although it was felt that there was still much ground to be covered. He continued to progress uneventfully following the cessation of counseling but returned regularly every three months for a checkup. Approximately four months after the termination of counseling, both he and his wife went to a marital counselor. This vastly improved the family relationships, although the friction was never completely eliminated. In all probability the continuing friction in the family was due in a large part to the emotional maladjustment of the wife who was never able to admit that even a part of the problem was hers. A. S.

Ps. M-D., Depr. F:26:S:149 +6 278′436–9(55) 8:12:16
Suicidal

At the age of 23 this patient had been admitted to the hospital, as a certified patient, with acute mania, following treatment for a goiter in a general hospital. She was extremely violent and noisy; she refused food; and her habits were faulty. She improved and left the hospital after five months. She re-entered in the present admission as a voluntary patient after an attempt at suicide by cutting her throat.

She was an illegitimate child; her mother later married and the patient had a younger sister. She received an elementary education and passed a scholarship examination to a secondary school; she did not, however, continue her schooling. She worked as a domestic servant, changing her place of employment fairly frequently.

She was diagnosed as having a manic-depressive psychosis, and her condition improved considerably after she received a course of modified insulin therapy.

M. V.

P. React. Depr.	F:19:S:33	+3	278′46–(41)	6:7:16
Schizoid		−31	2478′63–(34)	6:10:13

Upon returning home from college four months before admission, the patient had found it difficult to carry out her routine duties. She was nervous, insecure, and seclusive toward her friends. She had long crying spells, and she became bitter and resentful toward her parents. She attempted to return to college but was so upset that she had to stop immediately, and she requested admission to the psychiatric service.

Her past health had been exceptionally good and she had made a fairly satisfactory personal adjustment until the present episode. She maintained a high scholastic average and was serious and conscientious in her schoolwork. She had always enjoyed reading. She had been a little uncomfortable in crowds but this had not been outstanding. Her mother had been in a state hospital since the patient was 3 years old. Her present stepmother was a fairly adequate person but the patient had always feared that she herself would have a mental illness like her mother's.

In the hospital the patient was composed and conventional in behavior though at times she appeared depressed and sobbed uncontrollably. She was unable to explain what it was that started her on these sobbing spells. She was clear in sensorium and intellect and there was no evidence of hallucinations or delusions. She recognized that she had personal problems but she tried to minimize these and to convince herself that she was ready to go back to school. She mixed very well with other patients and in the course of her stay in the hospital gradually seemed to be freer from depression. It was difficult to evaluate the case. Some schizoid trends were felt to be present although the depressive factor was predominant. She was definitely improved at the time of discharge, and she went back to her home after arrangements had been made to continue the psychotherapeutic interviews. She planned to remain at home for a time before attempting to return to college.

Schizoid M:53:M:48 +19 27861'3–9X(41) 10:10:11

This patient had been gassed in World War I; he had been depressed for some time after that, and he thought he had never been the same since. Complaining particularly of an inability to concentrate and insomnia, he again became very depressed at the age of 53 and entered the hospital as a voluntary patient.

He was the fourth of five children; his father was said to have been very strict. He had an elementary education and had started working in a quarry at the age of 12, remaining there for forty years. There is no information about any abnormal trends in his childhood. He married at the age of 27 and had two children.

He was diagnosed as having a depressive reaction with schizoid features. His condition improved after he received one electroshock. M. V.

Ps. Sz., Simple M:19:S:183 +7 2786'134–9(71) 8:10:11
P. Psychas.

This youthful patient's chief complaints were insomnia, confusion, feelings of unreality, and phobias of "going into nothingness," of being unable to sleep, of dying, and of being unable to defecate. For years earlier he had felt "nervous," and at the age of 15 he had sought psychiatric help and had tried a short period of hospitalization without benefit. The present symptoms had begun about two years before he applied for help at this hospital.

A shy child always, the patient left school after the eighth grade because of his nervousness. He had no friends and spent most of his time at home except for occasional gardening jobs which he and his younger brother took to support themselves and their mother. The mother was described as "kind and understanding but nervous." The father, who had died recently, was a braggart, and when drunk and in a bad temper he beat his wife and sons. The patient felt he had contributed to his father's death by his own illness and by "acting up."

The youth impressed the therapist, who saw him weekly for interviews on an outpatient basis, as being an extremely passive, dependent individual. Treatment was largely supportive and consisted of continual reassurance about his many fears. He slowly began to talk more freely about himself and told of lifelong insecurities and current arguments with his mother. After transfer to a new therapist, made necessary after fourteen interviews by a change of personnel, the patient claimed that he felt worse than when he started and that he was on the verge of a breakdown. He reported many severe compulsions, such as having to reread whole pages of a book for fear he had missed one word, and having to check an entire tree for fear of missing one piece of fruit. It was felt that little or no progress had been made. The patient seemed to be actively enforcing his dependency by insisting on his illness and by inviting sympathy. Since maintenance therapy was of doubtful value he was discharged as unimproved, and he and his family were advised to seek state hospital care if he could not adjust at home. It was hoped that he might continue to work at simple jobs and get along, but the prognosis was considered guarded. E. B.

Ps. M-D., Depr. M:56:M:161 +25 2786′314–9 8:7:15

This man was admitted to the hospital with severe anxiety and feelings of guilt. The signs of his tension, which had been increasing for a year and a half, were tremor, headache, fatigue, and a thirty-pound weight loss. He also had numerous vague somatic complaints and a psychomotor retardation. A week before admission he had developed extreme restlessness associated with guilt feelings and hopelessness about the future.

A graduate of a teachers' college, the patient had always lived in a cultured and sheltered atmosphere. For fifteen years he had worked in a position well adapted to his unaggressive nature. Then, after marrying an ambitious woman who was thirteen years his junior, he shifted to another business in which his income was raised. However, they were "on the edge of having too little." A hard-working, self-effacing person, he adhered stubbornly to what he considered "proper standards," and he was exacting in details. In completing "big deals," he usually lacked audacity. He never confided his financial problems to his wife and often borrowed in order to pay for things which she probably would not have ordered had she known the true state of the family finances. He regarded himself as unsuccessful in life. He was meticulous about his person, staunch in religion, and intolerant of relaxation in himself. Toward his wife and children he was affectionate and devoted.

In the hospital the patient was quiet, but there were constant restless movements, picking at his lips and fingers, and pacing the floor. Negative toward all suggestions, he would disregard the answer and continue with his own stream of thought. He showed ridiculous delusions, and slight faults became crimes requiring a life sentence for absolution. For example, he recalled signing his wife's name to a check three or four years before and interpreted that as meriting grave punishment. His idea that the psychiatric unit was a federal board of investigation set up to try his case was based on many misinterpretations. Often he said, "There never was such a terrible case." He was never assaultive or suicidal, and his sleep was not severely disturbed. He spoke only in whispers. He was discharged to another hospital where it was expected that he would receive insulin therapy.

P. Hypo. M:28:S:39 +1 278634′9–(67) 6:4:13
P. Psychas.
P. React. Depr.

The presenting complaints of this patient were inward nervous tension, excessive worry, slowness and indecision in thinking and acting, general apathy, and depression. The symptoms dated from fourteen years before when the patient had developed an irresistible urge to masturbate. Several times his nervous tension had resulted in spells of violence during which he threw furniture and became almost maniacal. Leaving school in the tenth grade because of his illness, the patient had entered the hospital for eleven days and when he was discharged was told to get as much outdoor exercise as possible. At about age 20 he had formed an intimate relationship with a 35-year-old widow; and for five years, until she broke off relations with him, he became somewhat better. When the affair was terminated, he became progressively more nervous and indecisive; in spite of much medical advice his symptoms continued, with the addition of such somatic complaints as sick headaches, backaches, and blurring of vision. The continuance of his desire to masturbate was a constant worry to him.

The patient had been slow in school but had had no real trouble until the ninth grade. His family social level was middle class. Never a skilled worker, the man had done odd jobs but had held none of them for any length of time. His judgment was fair, and he had saved some money; but he was never energetic, had no interests, was shy, and did not enter games readily. A sensitive person, he was easily disturbed by teasing or jokes. Although he was rather selfish and self-centered, he was honest and truthful.

In the hospital the patient had an anxious facial expression and appeared nervous. Although he was interested in his own condition and in his own problem, he completely lacked confidence in himself and he was afraid that he could not do anything right, especially if someone watched him. He believed that there was something wrong with his mind, but he had no understanding of what it was. He appeared to have had auditory hallucinations on several occasions. His intelligence measured 104. There was marked retardation and difficulty in thinking. He kept himself neat. He was natural and open although his personality was inadequate and his outlook on life immature. His past love affair was constantly on his mind. Electroshock therapy brought little change although he mixed somewhat more with other patients and did some occupational therapy work. He was finally discharged slightly improved to the care of his family. The long duration of the neurosis and its early onset, combined with the fact that the patient had few assets, offered little hope for future improvement.

Ps. M-D., Depr. F:25:M:32 +6 2786'41-9 2:11:8
Ps. Postpartum
Suicidal

The patient was admitted to the hospital with depression associated with a fear of venereal infection and ideas of reference. During the last two months of her first pregnancy about a year before admission the patient became depressed and irritable, and expressed a delusion that people were talking about her and laughing at her during radio programs. At the time of delivery she refused to enter the hospital where she was employed as a stenographer, going instead to a private hospital, where she felt that the nurses neglected and ridiculed her. After leaving the hospital she refused to live with her husband, whom she accused of infidelity, and she went to live instead with her mother. Her depression continued and a few months later she attempted suicide. Shortly after that she improved considerably, recognized that many of her ideas were unreal, and went back to live with her husband. The old symptoms returned in connection with a second pregnancy, and she resigned her job, insisting that she had gonorrhea in spite of reassurance by physicians. Rejecting her husband, she felt that her mother was the only person capable of caring for her children. As the depression became more marked, hospitalization became necessary.

The patient had spent her life on an Indian reservation. After graduating from high school with a satisfactory record, both in curricular and extracurricular activities, she had studied stenographic work and had then obtained a civil service position, where she had made a satisfactory work record. Always an active and energetic person, she was considered a social leader. Although her husband, with whom she was well adjusted, wanted her to stop working, the patient objected to this loss of financial independence and to the loss of her own individuality which would naturally be associated with such a change.

In the hospital the patient expressed ideas of reference, particularly concerning radio broadcasts, and while she did not attribute this to any special group, at times she spoke vaguely of some theatrical organization. She said she believed that she had acquired gonorrhea during a premarital relationship with a man other than her husband and that because of this infection her last child was deformed. Appearing depressed and taking no active part in ward life, she preferred to sit by herself staring dejectedly into space. There was moderate psychomotor retardation; and while at times she appeared to be on the verge of tears, at other times she concealed the depression with a smiling countenance. Although her answers to questions were relevant and coherent, the patient seemed rather perplexed and often her replies were inadequate. During the hospitalization there was no change in her manner; and when she was discharged, it was with the recommendation that her husband prepare for a long hospitalization. Although the interim history is not known, the husband did apply for her readmission three years later.

Ps. Sz., Mixed M:23:S:98 +45 27'8916–(73) 1:5:8
P. Psychas.
Suicidal

Although the patient had for some time shown increasing agitation and negativism, a fall from a second-story window on the afternoon of admission had actually precipitated hospitalization. Brought to the hospital by his parents, the man himself complained only of low back pain. While in the navy he had had feelings of inadequacy and a fear of responsibility. When he began to complain of gastrointestinal symptoms, he was hospitalized and was given a medical discharge. It was said that a diagnosis of psychoneurosis had been made. When he returned home he lacked initiative, became preoccupied, and was relatively uncommunicative. Attempts to help him reorganize himself on a civilian basis were passively resisted. All he would say about himself was that he had "an ulcer," but a physician to whom he was referred failed to find supporting clinical evidence. He wanted to enter a university and scored very high in the entrance examinations, which he actually managed to take, but at registration time, he procrastinated so long that he could not begin the term. Concerned about him, his father tried without success to force the boy to enter the university.

Shortly before admission the father had asked the patient to take the family dog, the boy's pet for fourteen years, to the Society for Prevention of Cruelty to Animals to be killed. Several times the patient refused to carry out his father's wishes. When he finally acceded there was a great increase in his agitation, and the patient spent all his time by himself pacing the floor, wringing his hands, and pulling at his hair. When his father followed him in an attempt to talk to him, he would retreat from room to room. On the day of admission he "fell" from a second-story window, landing on his feet seemingly uninjured. For a few minutes he was entirely lucid, for the first time in months. He said that he had been trying to fix a loose storm window, and that in the attempt both he and the window had crashed to the ground.

The patient was described as having always been a sensitive, shy, retiring individual, who had never been able to assume responsibilities. He was passive, docile, well behaved, entirely noncompetitive and nonaggressive. Extremely conscientious, he took great pains with the things he did. Although he did superior work in school he took no part in extracurricular activities. In the navy he was successful and was several times promoted, but with each increase in rank he became more and more apprehensive about his ability to assume responsibility. This apprehension had increased until his discharge.

Agitated and resistant on admission, the patient refused to remain in the ward, saying, "I don't want psychiatric treatment. I want something done for my back." Other than this he said practically nothing. Consistently blocked or completely negative when spoken to, his affect was entirely flat and colorless. Refusing to remove his clothing when taken to his room, he paced up and down, wringing his hands, and plucking hair from his head. He was well oriented, and apparently he was not experiencing any hallucinatory visions. The only statements he made were such remarks as these: "Dad is always one or two steps ahead of me," or "If only I can get out of the mess I'm in now, I may be all right." This condition remained unchanged during the first week after admission. His resistance to the beginning of electroshock therapy was so violent that this approach was temporarily abandoned. Two narco-analytic sessions loosened him up to the point where he talked readily, but nothing very helpful was elicited. Subshock insulin was finally initiated and he received seventeen injections. After two weeks electroshock treatment was begun, alternating with the insulin. Five shock treatments brought about a marked alteration in his behavior; he became somewhat euphoric, talked readily, and took an interest in his surroundings to the point of playing ping-pong and bridge with other patients. For a week after the treatment was discontinued he was well, but he regressed almost completely. After five more electroshock treatments, he lost some of his agitation, but he did not get markedly better. He was finally discharged to a veterans' psychiatric hospital.

P. React. Depr. F:23:S:10 +9 2791'8346-(51) 4:6:8
Suicidal

The presenting complaints of this patient were withdrawal, loss of religious faith, and lack of desire to live. The onset of this pattern was gradual. The patient was a college student and had lost interest in her studies, her friends, and her social activities. Discussion in her Bible study class conflicted so with her religious concepts that she lost all faith in religion. She felt so depressed and confused that she sought help from a teacher who suggested that she find new outside interests. She tried this but it did not help. She had thoughts of suicide but she was afraid to make any attempt because she believed it was wrong. There were periods in which this depression lifted and she was overly gay, active, and sociable. Depression predominated, however.

About a year before, she had seen a physician who found that she had achlorhydria and he prescribed for it. This brought on a worry that she might have cancer, more acute since her grandmother and another relative had recently died of cancer. Other than this there was no contributory information in her past medical history. She had had a three-year nurses' training course and had worked as a nurse for a while, but she quit because she tired too easily. She then went back to school until the development of the present problem. She had always been an A student, but in recent months her schoolwork had deteriorated. She was a cheerful, friendly, easygoing, but immature person. After the onset of the present illness she became moody, unfriendly, and easily angered.

In the hospital she showed no unusual behavior; she was intact in sensorium and intellect. She maintained a pleasant smile most of the time and showed no deep emotion. Her chief concern was about the loss of her religious belief. She was sure that she had no ability and could not accomplish her goals in life. The depression noticeably lifted after the first few days in the hospital, and she entered actively into ward routine but was not particularly social, preferring to be alone. She was given ample opportunity to discuss her problems but did not elaborate on them where they touched on psychologically sore points. Apparently she had led a sheltered life because of generous and oversolicitous parents who had wanted to make life easy for her. All in all the problem seemed to be in large part a generalized immaturity. The patient was suffering from the conflict of this immaturity with the steadily more demanding society about her, in which she was being forced toward independence and self-sufficiency.

P. React. Depr. F:29:M:16 +3 '2794-1X(68) 11:2:8

Five years before admission to the hospital the patient had had a period of depression, following the birth of her first child, in which she had lost weight and had been melancholic, irritable, and tearful, but the attack had cleared up spontaneously. Several months before the present illness, while the patient was in the latter stages of pregnancy, she had again become depressed about the "weight of the baby," about financial problems, and about the promiscuity and excessive drinking of her husband, and the depression had continued until the birth of the baby. After delivery the patient was interested only in the baby and in herself. Two weeks before admission she had developed so severe a weakness and depression that a physician had been called, and her husband had been sent home on furlough. Her spirits rose until the time for his departure approached, and she became anxious about the possibility of his being sent overseas and not returning. A physician at this time recommended a rest home for her.

She had been a sick, weakly child, but she had had no definite nervous breakdowns. She had failed the eleventh grade and had then stopped school, marrying at age 18. Her only ambition had been to have a family, and the only work she had done outside her home, as a nurses' aid, had been too hard for her. She had never shown any interest in others or in community affairs, and she was thought of as a flighty, emotionally unstable person.

She was poorly developed and undernourished, with skin pigmentation. Cheerful and at ease in the hospital, she talked freely and was cooperative at all times, but at the time of admission she was very apprehensive and demanding of attention. She continually wanted to leave the hospital. She gave the appearance of great activity, asked many questions, and ran after other patients or nurses. After four electroshock treatments she quieted down to some extent, but it was apparent that her anxiety to get home and her rather generalized lack of assets made it unlikely that she would perform at anything better than a marginal level.

Ps. M-D., Depr. M:33:M:4 0 27'94 836-1 (76) 1:7:10

Chiefly as a result of frustration and disappointment, the patient had experienced over a period of about thirteen years repeated mild depressions characterized by decreased motor and mental activity, disinterest, tension, and insecurity. The present admission had apparently been precipitated by numerous difficulties relating chiefly to his feelings of inferiority in attempting to fulfill his duties with an insurance company.

A graduate of a large university, the patient had varied interests and was described as an intense, driving person, who always worked too hard and played too little. All his life he had felt inferior, insecure, and incapable of making decisions. He was prone to exaggerate his problems and to have excessive concern about small matters. Although the patient said his current problems had been present for only thirteen years, in reality they were apparently lifelong.

The patient was well oriented, cooperative, and intelligent. His main concern was in getting well and in finding out how he could achieve it. He spoke at great length about his previous conflicts, especially his feelings of insecurity. He also expressed anxiety over financial obligations. While objectively he did not appear to be depressed, he said that he felt depressed. He looked insecure and agitated. The treatment in the hospital was abruptly interrupted by the patient's desire to join his business friends in a tour. He felt that the trip and the congenial company might be good for him. He also did not want to receive electroshock therapy. For these reasons he was discharged with his condition unimproved. While it seemed that the present attack of depression might eventually improve, there was little expectation that it would not recur.

P. Mixed	F:30:M:55	+3	27'98631–(51)	5:6:8
Ps. M-D., Mixed	F:30:M:87	+20	87'261439–(59)	4:10:18
		+75	69'438271–(53)	2:15:12

Various fears and somatic complaints were the difficulties of this patient. The present episode began a month after the birth of a daughter; her husband thought the symptoms were probably related to a vaginal pack which inadvertently had not been removed during delivery. Much upset by the odor, the patient began changing clothes several times daily, refused to be close to people, and became increasingly nervous with frequent crying spells. She was beset with fears that she would harm her two children and was afraid to remain alone with them. Her other complaints were throbbing pains in her head, tingling sensations, nausea, vomiting, headaches, insomnia, diarrhea, and the like. There had been a gradual personality change toward depression, forgetfulness, and confusion.

During her first pregnancy, the patient had had toxemia and during the second, an illness similar to the present one, although less severe. After graduation from high school at the age of 17 she had worked as a telephone operator for five years before her marriage. After her marriage she had lived in a small farming town. There were no financial difficulties. She was described as a person of abundant energy, pleasant but always busy. In manner she was natural and open but hypersensitive to the opinions of others and subject to noticeable mood swings. She had a marked tendency to compulsive neurotic behavior, and she was described as a "dirt chaser."

On admission to the hospital the patient was well oriented and showed no evidences of mental confusion. She expressed feelings of utter hopelessness and depression. Mainly concerned with getting well, she felt, nevertheless, that there was a good possibility she could not be cured. At first she was relatively inaccessible and showed a tendency to circumstantiality. Her intelligence was average. During the first three weeks she showed steady improvement; but when she was about to be discharged, she developed marked feelings of guilt and said that she had attempted to murder her children and also had caused other patients to be sick. She had paranoid ideas and again showed obvious depression. All these symptoms came on suddenly. Shock therapy was not considered advisable since she was obviously suffering from an acute psychotic reaction. Recovery from the setback occurred within a few days and she was released. Two months later she was readmitted. She had done well for a month; then she wrote the F.B.I. saying that she should be in prison. She shaved off her hair in preparation for the penitentiary. She was given electroshock treatment and became hypomanic for periods. She got well enough finally to try living at home.

P. Mixed F:52:M:43 +4 2813746'9– 3:10:9

Fifteen months before admission to the hospital the patient had become greatly upset when she found evidence that her husband had had relations with another woman; since that time she had shown marked nervousness with frequent attacks of impaired consciousness, headaches, tinnitus, insomnia, anorexia, fatigue, inability to concentrate, and severe depression. Her social interests disappeared, and she was unable to perform her household tasks. Numerous physicians were unable to help her. The previous medical history revealed a rather long list of surgical operations, including a cholecystectomy and a hysterectomy. Symptoms such as "hot flashes" during the past five years had been attributed to the menopause.

She had begun working when she was 18 years old, doing practical nursing and housework, at which she was very good. Her management of her financial affairs was good. She had many friends and was easy to get along with. As hobbies she played golf and the piano. She was married for the first time when she was 18, and her first pregnancy was characterized by nausea and vomiting throughout the nine months. Of the other pregnancies with this husband, one ended in spontaneous abortion, and at least nine other abortions were induced by a physician because of the severe nausea and vomiting associated with them. Six months after she divorced that husband because of his drinking, she married a man ten years younger than she. He drank but she loved him, she said, because of his many "admirable traits." Her daughter and her first husband had both objected strenuously to her second marriage and had frequently written derogatory letters to her. Her sexual life had always been unsatisfactory, and she had rarely experienced orgasm. She and her present husband had been fairly compatible although at times he had been irritable and mean to her.

On admission she was worried about losing her mind, she wondered what made her have all her symptoms, and she was concerned about her husband's drinking and presumed infidelity. Although depressed, she was well oriented, open, and cooperative, and she appeared intact in general mental ability. The idea of suicide had occurred to her but she had made no known attempt to take her life. In her opinion menopausal changes and organic factors contributed to her illness. She expressed the belief that 50 percent of her marital discord was due to sexual incompatibility. There was rapid improvement, and as most of her symptoms subsided, she became more cheerful, looking on the future more hopefully. When she was discharged she felt she could cope satisfactorily with her problems.

Ps. M-D., Depr. F:42:M:118 +3 281736'4–(61) 9:6:15
+51 281763'4–X 10:7:17

The present episode began a year before admission when the patient experienced extreme pain in her head and spine and had numerous other complaints of pain and paresthesia. Approximately every two weeks spells of dyspnea, tachycardia, palpitation, and inability to walk or talk occurred. At such times she felt that her heart was "no longer beating," her body "no longer alive." She stayed in bed much of the time and slept only with medication. She claimed she could not see things clearly and said "it is as though I am looking through a thin curtain."

Since her marriage 25 years earlier the patient had had numerous somatic complaints, for which she had consulted many physicians. Previous periods of acute depression (three in all) had each lasted from six to seven months. Each attack had been related to a pregnancy. The present illness had begun with a hysterectomy; for a short time after the operation she was "mentally better," then the symptoms reappeared. An eighth-grade graduate (at age 16) the patient had worked for a while as a maid in a hospital, had quit because she "couldn't stand the sights." After marriage she was a housewife, apparently adequate in that role. Hypochondriacal traits were, however, always present, and her reactions to disappointments were usually greater than normal. She was described as emotionally unstable. Her own opinion was that she had been a failure as a wife because of her increasing frigidity during the past eighteen years. With each new pregnancy she had worried about supporting another child.

In the hospital the patient showed numerous somatic delusions and complaints. She felt "slowed" up intellectually, appeared to be severely depressed, and apparently had lost interest in her surroundings and personal appearance. Gradual improvement took place, and after she had spent several months in the hospital, she was given several electroshock treatments which seemed to hasten recovery. At the time of discharge she was comparatively well, and it appeared that this particular attack was over.

Ps. Invol. Melan.   F:52:M:34   +35   28316′74–(63)   5:5:10

The symptoms had begun about two months before admission after the patient had undergone a pelvic repair in another hospital. There was restlessness, disinterest in her work and home, easy fatigue, depression, nervousness, and the feeling that no help could be given to her and that she ought to be in a state hospital for the insane. She was given twelve electroshock treatments, with some improvement in all the symptoms. However, they recurred shortly thereafter. Another series of shock treatments was given with only slight improvement; eventually she relapsed and was admitted to this hospital.

Twenty-six years before admission, the patient had had a "nervous breakdown." Apparently she had recovered after a few weeks. She was described as a "high-strung" and nervous individual who worried about trivial matters. As a child she had cried for everything she had wanted, and she had always been dependent on people. She was a devout church member and had been active in church affairs before the present illness. She had gone to high school for two years but had then stopped because her mother was sickly. She married in the next few years. She and her husband had six children and were always on the borderline of financial trouble. The patient carried a great deal of the responsibility of the family's farm.

On admission to the hospital the question uppermost in the patient's mind was how she was going to get well. She felt that she would never be completely cured of her symptoms. This feeling made her anxious and concerned. She was in other ways oriented and cooperative. Her thinking seemed to ramble at times but always centered around her own condition. She was given ten electroshock treatments with moderate improvement. But when she knew she was to be discharged she again regressed. She gave the impression of being addicted to hospitalization. She was finally discharged to the care of her husband, and the recommendation was made that she be taken to a state hospital if she could not remain at home.

Ps. Sz., Paranoid F:26:M:46 +8 2831'76– 2:4:6

A year and a half before admission, coincident with the birth of a second child, this young woman had become tense and depressed. She doubted that she loved the child and feared she might harm it. Over a six-month period the symptoms gradually disappeared so that she was fairly comfortable and appeared recovered. However, six months later, having missed two menstrual periods, she began to fear another pregnancy and the tenseness, nervousness, and emotional depression returned. One of her numerous convictions, without a factual basis, was that her husband had remarried and planned to take the children to live with their new mother. People were talking about her, she claimed, and at times she said that radio programs pertained directly to her. If she heard a train whistle she said that she would soon "turn into a train," and when she saw men working with cement she feared she would "turn into cement."

Her history included no other attacks of this character. An eighth-grade graduate, she had worked as a domestic until her marriage at age 19. After that she worked as a restaurant employee. Active and energetic, she enjoyed social activities; she was somewhat stubborn and apt to indulge in mild emotional outbursts when thwarted. These were more frequent after her marriage, and they usually occurred when she desired amusement or diversion which the husband felt they could ill afford. For the most part the patient and her husband (who was thirteen years older than she) were compatible. She apparently enjoyed homemaking but was resentful over pregnancies.

The physical examination in the hospital revealed the possibility of cerebral atrophy but a definite diagnosis could not be made. The patient expressed ideas of reference and delusions, but it required considerable persuasion to induce her to describe them. She was apathetic and did not cooperate well, preferring to sit alone. Her facial expression was apathetic. The psychological examination did not yield evidence of deterioration but did show her to be dull normal in intelligence. In time, she became somewhat better and was finally discharged to the care of her husband.

Ps. M-D., Manic Schizoid   M:31:M:71   +21   '28349–(65)   2:7:20

Six days before admission to the hospital the patient became talkative and overly enthusiastic. His wife noticed also that he would become extremely interested and absorbed in an idea, would read all the books he could find on the subject as well as talk about that subject constantly. This latter tendency had been increasing even before the present acute episode. The subjects in which he would become completely engrossed varied from time to time and were always of a generally scientific nature. Four days before admission he became acutely excited, and he displayed great physical hyperactivity, flight of ideas, and the like.

His past health had been good. He had had one previous attack similar to the present one which had occurred nine years before admission and had required six months of hospitalization. The patient was a student in law at the time of his present illness and had been doing well. His past personality presented, in general, a milder picture of his present illness. He had always been competitive and an extrovert, "the life of the party." He had been married a year and the marriage was a happy one.

In the hospital he needed heavy sedation for the first two days and was then given four electroshock treatments. His excitement diminished rapidly; his mental and physical activity slowed down by the eighth day in the hospital. He was quiet and seemingly ready for discharge. He gradually became excited again and developed a flight of ideas. He then began to show a more schizophrenic type of illness with catatonic posturizing and schizoid ideas alternating with hypomania. He was again given electroshock treatments and became apparently normal. He was discharged to go to his home after it seemed certain that he would recover from the present attack. It seemed likely, however, that he would have more attacks in the future.

Schizoid   F:20:S:192   +62   2'83674–(74)   5:3:16

This girl became depressed at the age of 20, with much crying and insomnia. Her menstrual periods stopped. She was withdrawn and retarded, but she had a voracious appetite all the time. She spent two short periods, not exceeding a fortnight, as a voluntary patient in a mental hospital. She entered this hospital as a certified patient after becoming violent and grossly careless of her appearance and daily routine.

Little was known about her early history. She was the seventh of eight children. A bright child, but with a solitary disposition, she received an elementary education and became a children's nurse on leaving school. She had left her last position shortly before the present admission.

She was diagnosed as having schizophrenia and underwent a course of electric convulsion therapy and modified insulin therapy. Her condition improved.

M. V.

Ps. Paranoid F:46:S:28 +3 28 371'46–9(59) 4:6:16
Ps. Sz., Paranoid

The patient's admission complaints were depression, weakness, loss of appetite, insomnia, auditory hallucinations, and inability to concentrate. The onset of these symptoms was insidious. A year before, the patient had received numerous telephone calls actually meant for another person with the same name. These calls disturbed her greatly although she could give no reason for being so bothered. Simultaneously she became tired and "run-down"; she consulted a physician who advised a vacation. At this time also she quit her job because of the antagonism of other employees toward her, an attitude she could not explain. For a while she visited friends but noted that "people said insulting things" about her. The exact words she did not remember, but she was sure they were "antagonistic." Much of the time she was tired, and she was frequently uncomfortable because she felt that she was the center of attention and "being watched." She became afraid to go out of the house; and, as time went on, she began to hear people talking when she was alone. This happened usually at night and "the people" were neighbors or friends. She believed that she could communicate with her friends by mental means. More and more frequently she suffered attacks of palpitation, muscle twitching, and salivation initiated by slight noises such as the refrigerator starting.

The patient's past health had been fairly good. She finished the eighth grade at 13, worked as a housemaid, then attended business college for six months. For a time she did office work; then she held a job as switchboard operator and other similar jobs until the present illness. She had several hobbies, mainly sports. Although she was considered shy and sensitive, she enjoyed people.

On admission to the hospital the patient was concerned and depressed about her illness. The delusions and auditory hallucinations were evident. Recognizing herself as abnormal, she nevertheless was sure that the hallucinations represented realities. On the ward she was neat, alert, and cooperative but appeared anxious and apprehensive. There was no gross defect of mentality and she was well oriented. She was given sedative tubs and electroshock treatments. The hallucinations and delusions of mental communication disappeared soon after the beginning of the shock treatments. However, she still did not believe that the delusions and hallucinations were entirely "mental," and she said it was difficult to believe that some of them did not happen, "they are so real." At discharge she appeared happy and friendly and readily discussed her past illness. The condition was diagnosed as a typical paranoid state, which would usually have a good prognosis. However, in view of the patient's lack of insight it was considered unsafe to predict that in the future there would be no recurrence.

P. Hypo. F:27:M:33 +18 283716'4–9 4:3:16
P. Hys.

This young woman was admitted for "hysterical spells," nervousness, epigastric distress, headaches, paresthesias, weakness, depression, and fear of losing her

283716'4–9

mind. The illness apparently began five years before admission with what was called a hysterical spell, in which she cried, complained of discomfort, and appeared to faint momentarily. This was followed by weakness. Similar spells occurred intermittently during the following year with the physical symptoms increasing in severity. She then developed paresthesias, and it was noticed that when she was thwarted the symptoms tended to be worse. Gradually the somatic complaints were present almost constantly, and she became weak, restless, and irritable. Greatly concerned about her condition, she used numerous patent medicines and consulted one physician after another. She feared insanity and at times felt deeply depressed.

The patient had finished the eighth grade; she had been a fair student but had stopped school to work at home until her marriage. She had few interests outside her home and never traveled beyond the state border. A quiet, reserved, introspective, colorless person, she was somewhat immature and inadequate, fearful, shy, easily offended, and not gregarious. In her home, she did her work satisfactorily and was relatively happy. Her judgment was poor; she allowed herself to be dominated by people about her; and she retained a childlike attachment to her mother. She did not adapt well to marriage, for example, and refused to go on a honeymoon trip. Later she began to think that her husband's relatives did not care for her, became suspicious of her husband (possibly with some justification), and preferred her mother's counsel. Her religion did not permit the use of contraceptives and she was somewhat troubled by a fear of pregnancy. There were three children. The family's poor economic situation did not appear to be an important concern to her.

On admission, the physical examinations revealed little except that she was rather anorexic; she was described as a "droopy, dreary, asthenic woman of a hundred and two pounds." She said that her illness appeared when she developed strong feelings against and dissatisfaction with someone or something. At first some of her difficulty was tied in with religion. During the second period of the illness problems were more centered around her husband, and the final stages involved her parents and her husband. She could not account for the antagonistic feelings she had at these times and was anxious for an explanation. Her attention was strongly centered on her symptoms and, also, on the details of her sex life. Religious prejudices and personal wishes were in sharp conflict and she was unable to resolve this antagonism to her satisfaction. Restless and depressed, she lacked energy and vitality, had a hopeless outlook, and feared insanity.

In the hospital she took little part in activities unless strongly urged and paid little attention to her appearance. At times she cried. She introduced the subject of sex in conversation with examiners at every opportunity. Her dreams frequently were of sex. She often discussed her dread of becoming pregnant again as soon as she returned home and her distaste for sexual relations, as well as her jealousy. There was little improvement, and she remained more or less miserable, although she ate and slept well, and her physical health was obviously better. She was finally discharged to her husband, and although it was felt that she might become somewhat less miserable there was little expectation of ultimately good adjustment.

P. Anxiety State F:20:S:42 +1 28′$\underline{37}$64–9 (51) 3:6:15
+50 ′$\underline{783}$– (55) 5:2:16

This girl's complaints centered around her inability to explain an anxiety attack which she had experienced following a motion picture. After the movie she had returned to the college dormitory. She became mute and remained in this condition for approximately four hours, crying much of the time. Following this she experienced depression, which she related to her inability to make an adequate vocational choice. Although she attempted to forget the anxiety attack, it "kept coming back," and she worried that her friends might think she had a "nervous breakdown." Until this time, she believed, she had been making a satisfactory adjustment, both socially and emotionally.

The client was an only child of fairly well-to-do parents. There were no obvious causative factors in her background except that for one period of several months when she was 6 she had lived in a neighborhood in which there were no other children and she had been left to amuse herself. Her scholastic progress was uneventful. Sheltered by her parents from most of life's hardships, she had never faced any disturbing situations. Until the time of the attack her life might be best described as humdrum.

In the therapy interview this girl took no initiative, nor was she capable of sustaining a conversation longer than three sentences. As a result, therapy was directive and resulted in a series of questions and answers. Despite this treatment, she enjoyed the therapy sessions and refused to terminate them early. When the school year ended and the contacts had to be discontinued she was disappointed. The emotional upheaval apparently resulted from her feelings of inability to meet a real life situation which was forced on her by graduation. She compromised by taking graduate work, for she felt this would give her time to prepare more completely to face a reality for which her uneventful childhood had given her no training. A month following the conclusion of the therapy she wrote: "Things are quite changed since I last saw you. I have been dating regularly. Lately my moods of depression have been closer together but of brief duration." A. S.

P. Mixed F:32:S:19 +7 $\underline{284}$37$\underline{16}$′–9 6:10:13
Mental Deficiency

This woman's symptoms were weakness, multiple somatic ills, and occasional acute attacks of a hysterical nature. The onset of the symptomatic picture was not clearly defined. Apparently the patient had never been entirely free from the symptoms, at least according to family members and friends. The patient herself was a poor witness, since she appeared to be of low mental ability, but she dated the difficulties back ten years to a sexual experience when she had been infected with a venereal disease. Although she had been treated adequately, she felt she had never completely recovered. She had had no serious illnesses or major operations.

Although school was difficult for her, she finished the eighth grade at age 16.

She attributed her slowness in school to physical illness. For a while she worked as a domestic but could not hold jobs long and became a relief case. She always tended to feel that people mistreated her, that she was overworked and underpaid, and that the welfare board was inconsiderate of her. The welfare people reported that if plans were made for her she interpreted them as an attempt to swindle her. This suspiciousness made it difficult for the worker. When pressed the patient always sought refuge in physical illness. The entire family appeared to be backward, although their farm was fairly well managed.

Although obese, the patient was in good physical condition, and repeated tests and examinations were all negative. There was no evidence of the supposed venereal infection. Nevertheless, the patient complained bitterly of physical discomfort and insisted that she was too weak to work because of the venereal disease. She admitted having sexual relations with a number of men but claimed that all of these were forced and that she had been promised marriage in each case. Bitter over these disappointments, she accepted no responsibility for her present condition. The patient lived with her family and was on poor terms with them. Her I.Q. was about 75. She was careless in physical appearance and insisted that she was too weak to take an active part in ward activities. No essential change occurred in the hospital, and she was discharged scarcely improved. It seemed that the hospital could offer little to this patient, and that social service before admission had been as adequate as possible, although with negligible results. It was suggested that she be placed outside the home, and she was discharged to the care of the welfare worker.

B. Psth., Asocial M:50:M:30 +1 2846731'9–(59) 3:15:13
Alcoholism +18 4321'786–(43) 2:5:18

Seven years before admission to the hospital the patient and his wife had begun having difficulties. The patient became egotistical and drank excessively. He was mean and temperamental when he came home intoxicated. His use of alcohol increased. He became irresponsible about his debts and was regarded by the community as a nuisance. He himself noticed that he had become more "nervous" in the past seven years and said it was a reaction to his wife's irritability and her attitude of independence and unwillingness to forgive. In connection with the surgical repair of a hernia, he was seen in the psychiatric service and admission to the psychiatric unit was advised.

He had apparently been in good health in spite of his symptoms. Finishing the eighth grade at age 14 he worked for a few years on farms; then he became a salesman but was discharged from the company because he owed them money. He was able to get other good jobs later but tended to lose them in this way before he had held them for very long. In the last year he had served two terms in the workhouse for beating his wife. He always appeared easygoing and weak to a casual observer, although he was really very much the opposite. It was strongly suspected that he had numerous extramarital relationships. His wife claimed that the marriage had been relatively successful until the last eight years. She blamed the change on his egotism over a temporary business success. She was considered to be his superior by people who knew the couple.

The physical examination was essentially negative. The majority of the patient's statements in the hospital were directed at the examiner in such a way as to put the patient in the best possible light and to throw blame on others. He had average intelligence and showed no evidence of organic brain deterioration. He was cooperative, cheerful, apparently humble, and anxious to make a good impression. There was definite evidence of his laziness, but he showed no resentment when this was pointed out to him. He was apparently immature emotionally and had little insight into his responsibilities to his family or to society or even to himself. There was little change in the hospital because he offered no avenue of approach to the basic problem and appeared relatively rigid when any opening was found in his armor.

Ps. Invol. Melan. M:58:M:64 +16 2847'1639–(74) 2:7:14
Suicidal

The present illness first became apparent six months before admission when the patient was transferred from one high school in which he was a teacher to another. He had taught for 26 years in the high school he left. The change may have been related to the present illness because it was arranged by the superintendent after the patient did not cooperate well with his principal. In any case the patient was deeply distressed, had difficulty in keeping discipline in his classes, became nervous, restless, and brooding, and blamed himself for the loss of his good position. After school was out he attended summer school but showed marked irritability and nervousness. The symptoms continued and greatly troubled him at the beginning of school the next term. He slept little, smoked incessantly, and treated his wife badly. He expressed the fear that he was going insane and spoke of "ending it all" for himself and his family.

There was no past event that appeared contributory. He had been a successful teacher and had written a number of books that were used widely. As a small boy he had been shy and sensitive because of his size. He had always had feelings of inferiority and claimed that his good grades were obtained mostly by bluffing. He was very secretive with his wife and never confided in her. An egocentric individual, he frequently started new things with great enthusiasm but seldom completed them and was said to be rigid, stubborn, and talkative. There was considerable bickering between the patient and his wife at all times, but their home life was on the whole fairly satisfactory.

The patient presented a neat appearance in the hospital but was agitated and restless. He paced the floor a considerable portion of the time, was depressed, and worried about what his family and friends would think. He described himself as a "failure as a father." He talked at great length and would tell his story over and over again in great detail. He considered himself headed for a state hospital and suspected that his wife would have him committed to obtain their property. He often asserted that "three lives depend on me," and he would then proceed to elaborate on the poor financial condition of his family. He was caught several times obviously falsifying things purportedly told to him by the staff. Shock therapy was refused by the patient and his family. He did not improve and was discharged against advice to the care of his wife.

P. React. Depr. F:40:M:37 +1 286'3471-9 (55) 8:13:12
Ps. Postpartum
Suicidal

Less than a month before admission this patient had given birth to a baby girl about three weeks ahead of the expected delivery date. The baby, her sixth child, was born in the family car on the way to the hospital. The night was cold and damp, and the mother suffered considerably. After five days in the general hospital she was discharged. The following day she told her daughters that they would have to take charge of the family since she wanted to die. Her impulse was to choke the infant. Psychomotor retardation was noticeable to her family and she appeared to have guilt feelings, but her immediate improvement was so great that the family was reluctant to have her admitted to the hospital.

Possible contributory factors in the past medical history to the present symptom development were a short leg due to an early fracture and a thyroidectomy the year before admission which had not lowered her basal metabolic rate. She had finished the ninth grade, quitting because she found school hard and uninteresting, and until she married at the age of 25, she did general housework. At the time of her marriage she gave up Catholicism at her husband's insistence. Interested in other people, thoughtful, kind, and open in manner, she was active in several women's organizations and was described as a good mother and housewife. The children, especially the oldest daughter, believed that the parents were unjust, inconsiderate, and too strict in that they did not allow the children time, opportunity, or permission for recreation. The husband, who ascribed his use of alcohol to the failure of contraceptive techniques, was described as shiftless and lacking in understanding of the patient's problem.

The physical examination on admission disclosed a normal metabolic rate. The other findings were also normal. Depressed and worried, the patient was quiet and difficult to interview. She was oriented and while she complained that her memory was not as good as it had been in the past, she did not appear affected in sensorium or intellect. When she did reply to questions, her answers were direct and adequate. She realized that she was not well, but she was confident of her ultimate recovery. Except for the apprehension there were no peculiarities in her attitude or manner. Gradually she began to take part in ward activities. Cooperative and pleasant to all with whom she came in contact, she showed steady improvement, looking forward to going home and caring for her child. While she was not tested, it was felt that her mental level was probably dull normal. In addition to the low intelligence (which was felt to be an element in her problem) other background factors to be considered in the psychiatric condition were physical disability, religious conflicts, and family conflicts. The absence of previous mental difficulties, the sudden onset, and her quick recovery made for a good prognosis.

B. Psth., Asocial Mutilative	M:27:D	286417′93–(61)	4:8:6

This prisoner had mutilated himself four times in the past four years, each time by cutting the Achilles' tendon. At the request of the prison administration he was given the MMPI. Later his sentence was terminated and he was discharged.

During his childhood the subject's parents moved frequently because his father was an oil field worker and truck driver. The young man reported that he completed the sixth grade in school and then quit because he "made bad grades." On a standardized achievement test his grade placement was 4.2. He worked at odd jobs as a common laborer. He was married, but after three months he and his wife separated; there were no children. In 1940 he joined the army and went permanently AWOL eleven months later. Following his civilian conviction he received an "other than honorable" discharge.

The first official record of criminality for this young man consisted of two convictions for armed robbery by assault with firearms. For these he received seven- and five-year sentences, to run concurrently. The plea on both counts was "not guilty." Released on conditional parole, he was returned as a parole violator. He participated in a mutiny and was punished for mutilation. Later he escaped but was recaptured. Following the recapture he "jumped squad" and mutilated himself again. A year later there was another instance of self-mutilation. After still another mutilation he was punished for abusing a guard and for crushing a wash basin and commode at the prison farm. When the prisoner's sentence ended and he left, the warden remarked: "I hope he left the state; otherwise, I'm sure we'll get him back. He is permanent lock-up case, not capable of profiting from past experience. He was a constant troublemaker, agitator, and to a certain extent a leader among other inmates. He was responsible for a number of plots and schemes that created a serious problem." R. C. K.

Ps. Invol. Melan.	F:59:S:57	−14	28647319′–X(39)	7:18:9
Paranoid		+22	82476139′–(39)	4:13:14
Suicidal		+50	2837416′9–(51)	4:8:12
Ps. Invol. Melan.	F:61:S:61	+3	28471369′–(51)	3:10:17
Suicidal		+25	8214 736′9–(66)	5:10:12

The patient was admitted to the hospital because it was felt that she was possibly suicidal. She complained of feelings of uselessness, hopelessness, insomnia, and intermittent pain. The onset of these symptoms could not be identified.

They had developed very gradually, chiefly in the past year. A few days before the admission she had been very agitated and had had prominent paranoid ideas.

She had visited numerous physicians in the last eleven years and had been studied at least fifteen times in different medical clinics, but no good organic basis for her complaints had ever been discovered. In spite of her very long history of somatic complaints she had been able to work and hold a job without difficulty and was a fairly adequate person in her social contacts.

In the hospital she was depressed, complained of pain in the abdominal region, and was nervous and anxious about trivial matters. She received nine electroshock treatments and improved slightly as a result. After somewhat different living conditions had been arranged for her she was discharged, although the prognosis was considered to be very poor. Two years later she was readmitted with a similar pattern of complaints.

Ps. Invol. Melan. M:50:M:6 +2 286'731–9 (65) 5:9:15
Suicidal

The patient had last been well about a year and a half before admission. At about that time he had developed feelings of worthlessness. He thought people were acting differently toward him and this worried him. He lost interest in his farming and could not do his work. He felt he should do something but did not know what. He made several attempts to commit suicide. During this time he was a voluntary patient at three different hospitals. Each time he signed himself out against advice. After each hospitalization he was improved for a short time but always relapsed. Occasional headaches were the only obvious physical complaint. Before the present illness there were no apparently contributory events.

He was described as a rather bashful and sensitive individual. He had many friends, always got along well with everyone, and was known to be easygoing and careful about hurting other people's feelings. He had temperate habits and was average in intelligence. A good farmer, he had followed that trade after finishing the eighth grade at age 14.

In the hospital he exhibited ideas of self-depreciation and reference. He believed that people were trying to make him feel "no good." In manner he was worried and irritable. He was also aggressive, though he maintained that he was never angry. His general sensorium and intellect were intact. He had little insight since he felt that most of his difficulties were due to the attitudes and actions of others. No clear hallucinations or more obvious delusory patterns could be elicited. Again he left the hospital after only a few days.

Ps. M-D., Depr. F:38:M:42 +6 286'7341– 8:6:13

For two years the patient had complained that she never felt tired enough to sleep, and although she did sleep, she found no comfort in it. Following an illness and financial difficulties involving her family, her condition grew worse and she was admitted to a private hospital (where she stayed until she came to the psychiatric unit) with anorexia, depression, and inability to work. Treated in that hospital with typhoid vaccine, she developed distressing paresthesias throughout her whole body, which she interpreted to signify the death of her nerves.

At the age of 21 she had felt ill for a year and had been briefly hospitalized. Depression and insomnia had characterized this first illness and two others that preceded the present admission.

A high school graduate, the patient had taken a business training course and then had worked as a stenographer. She was a religious person and was thought to be uprighteous, earnest, practical, hard working, and reliable. Her judgment was good. Quiet and reserved in manner, she was said to be easily excited and tearful, but she got on well with people and had many friends. She had had no obvious hypochondriacal or inferiority feelings. She had married about twenty years before admission, and apparently she and her husband were compatible. There were three children, and before her illness she had been an adequate, devoted mother and wife.

On admission to the hospital she repeatedly alluded to the numbness and loss of feeling pervading her entire body, and to the fact that it was impossible for her to sleep because she was never tired. She felt that these symptoms indicated that something terrible had happened to her nervous system and in her opinion the only thing that was functioning properly was her mind. Although she never elaborated upon her ideas of what caused these feelings, she felt that this attack was more severe than others she had experienced, and she was so convinced that she could not get well that she expressed the desire to die. Beyond this there were no obvious disturbances in mentation or orientation. She was quiet and talked relevantly when interrogated, but she was underactive and lacking in spontaneity. For most of her stay in the hospital she remained about the same, and efforts to get her to cooperate in the ward activities were only partially successful. She steadfastly refused to accept the idea that there was anything mentally wrong with her. Although she often repeated her wish to die, her only suicidal gesture was a threat to stop eating. When tube feeding was suggested, she abandoned the idea. Psychotherapy could not be very active, but a careful routine of health-building and rest brought about physical improvement. She was discharged to her home against the advice of the staff who recommended state hospitalization.

P. Mixed F:23:S '28674–(43) 6:4:19

The client, a university student, was referred to the clinic because of her deviant responses in a routine administration of the Mooney Problem Check List. Both in response to the check list and in the preliminary interview, she expressed feelings of inferiority, fear of marriage and sexual relations, suicidal ideas, and anxiety toward new situations in general. Among other things she said, "I'm not sure that I have a right to bring children into the world when I wish I hadn't been."

The young woman was inclined to ascribe her fears of marriage to the unhappiness she had witnessed in her own family—her father was a chronic alcoholic who came home only sporadically, and eventually her mother had obtained a divorce. Furthermore, she regarded the marriages of her siblings as unsuccessful.

During the client's schooldays she had made few friends and had spent most of her time in reading. Her original ambition was to be a nurse, but she did not get along well in nurses' training. The nursing school authorities felt that she was immature and could not take criticism, and they finally expelled her for coming in late. This the client felt was unjust and was based on inaccurate reports of her activities. Following this keen disappointment, she became an attendant in a state hospital, where she remained for a year. When she found she was showing irritability toward the patients, she left the hospital to join the WAC.

At the time of her referral here, she was in the first year of a premedical course. In a scholastic aptitude examination the results were as follows: verbal, 99.6 percentile; mathematical, 13.0 percentile; social studies, 78.0 percentile. Although her grades during the year of treatment were mediocre, she remained determined to achieve her vocational goal. At the beginning of treatment she had broken her engagement to a man who was four years younger than herself, because she felt that medicine should come before marriage in her life. She harbored fantasies of eventually combining marriage with a career and pictured herself practicing only four or five hours a day. She attributed her interest in medicine to her belief that it, more than any other possible vocation, would prove an all-absorbing occupation, one in which she would be able to "forget everything else."

Throughout the course of the interviews with this girl, the contrast between her willingness to discuss even the most intimate *facts* of her life and her evasiveness concerning her *feelings* was striking. The therapeutic plan was to provide for the expression of feelings in a permissive setting and to encourage fantasy and free association so as to lead to some understanding of the repressed wishes which seemed to contribute to her difficulties. The girl became blocked whenever it was up to her to initiate discussion, and she would sit wringing her hands and crying. She was completely unable to cooperate in the Thematic Apperception Test, for example. The resistance encountered was so great that it was the therapist's impression that only through psychoanalysis could this client be reached. Although she was superficially cooperative, broke few appointments, and always came on time, there seemed to be much underlying hostility and essential unwillingness to enter into the therapeutic situation. At the end of the treatment period, the client felt herself essentially unimproved, with as strong feelings of inferiority, depression, and apathy as she had previously had. The therapist agreed.

M. V. B.

P. Mixed	M:37:M:32	+1	2871346′–(59)	4:7:13
Schizoid		+27	2781346′–9 (55)	2:7:14
		+3 yrs.	2781364′–9 (61)	5:9:9

The episode in which the patient was admitted to the hospital had begun six months earlier when he was employed on the night shift and, unable to accommodate himself to daytime sleeping, became nervous and run-down. He had numerous somatic complaints, lost weight, became forgetful, made mistakes, and believed his work was inferior to that of co-workers. He lost his former interests, such as having company, and he became indifferent toward his two children. After a while he made no effort to work, was content to remain at home, and became progressively worse until admission.

His previous health had never been good. In his early twenties he had had a nervous breakdown and, in fact, had never been completely free from nervousness. An ulcer had been diagnosed at one time. He had also had medical treatment for chronic prostatitis and an appendectomy had been performed when he was 21.

Because his father needed his help with the farm work, he left the fifth grade at the age of 12, and he lived with his parents until his marriage eight years before admission. After that he lived with his wife's parents in homes provided by the W.P.A. Once he moved from the country to the city so that he might be close to the relief office. He refused several jobs offered by the W.P.A., and social service reports indicated that he was overly willing to accept relief and was considered a loafer. He showed little energy to plan or ability to meet adversity. The marriage was apparently a good one, and he liked his home and was particularly fond of his children.

On admission the patient frankly stated that he was depressed and could not get certain thoughts out of his mind. At every opportunity he discussed his complaints at length. There were no gross delusional or other disturbances of mentation and his intelligence was tested as average. One felt that his depression, reflected in his behavior, was much more severe than the psychological signs indicated. In the hospital, he was cooperative, polite, and noncomplaining. Much of the time he spent in his room just sitting, and he seldom took part in group activities except for an occasional game of checkers. He made almost too good an adjustment to hospitalization and when it was near time for his discharge he began to worry. He said he would like to go back to work but was afraid he "couldn't stand it." Through social service he was given help in making plans for the future and every effort was made psychotherapeutically to help him gain better insight. Although little could be done there was some improvement, and it was believed he would make a somewhat better adjustment than he had before.

P. Mixed Mutilative	F:43:M:45	+1	28713′6–9 (34)	3:10:12

P. Mixed	F:43:M:70	+14	28371′469–(39)	3:9:11

P. Mixed	F:43:M:8	+79	$827'9\underline{61}3$–(55)	3:12:9
P. Mixed	F:45:M:145	0	$2783'\underline{146}$–(49)	5:11:12
P. Psychas.		+34	$82\underline{37}'\underline{16}9$–(43)	3:11:8
P. Mixed	F:45:M:5	+4	$2\underline{78}316'$–(43)	3:9:11
P. Mixed	F:45:M:26	+2	827316′94–(39)	2:10:12

The first of six admissions for this patient was caused by severe itching in the inguinal region and "nervous headaches" which had been present many years. The inguinal itching dated from the birth of a son. The patient's husband felt that the illness was due to a deep-seated resentment against his joining the armed services. Since his return from the service they had lived in a small apartment where there were many inconveniences. They were on the point of leaving this apartment for a newly built home when she developed nausea and vomiting and severe headaches. As the headaches diminished, her skin became more irritable and she scratched incessantly. She became hysterical and wanted to give her child away because she thought she was an inadequate mother. Hospitalized almost continuously for six months, she received both electroshock and insulin shock treatments. After this the attacks were mild and intermittent until the present admission. With the onset of the attacks she had difficulty focusing her eyes and became dizzy and confused. Unable to sleep, she was depressed, anxious, and tense, and there was daily nausea and vomiting.

Although she had been a "sickly and delicate" child there had been no frankly psychotic episodes. A very intelligent person, she was a university graduate and an honor student. Following her university years she worked as a practical nurse. Her outside interests were varied and normal. She was, however, sarcastic, unsympathetic, and difficult to get along with. According to her associates, she was also intolerant and overcritical. As a child she had been petted and dependent, but as she matured she learned to make decisions when necessary. Sexual intercourse was painful for her and was carried through only to please her husband.

On admission to the hospital she was found to be depressed and tense. The emotional conflicts obviously present centered around her husband's political and social beliefs, her feelings toward her son and toward her father, and her attitude toward her illness. She recognized that these conflicts were important to her illness; nevertheless, she was unable to resolve them adequately. On the one hand she believed herself to be a neurotic, on the other she could not really accept that diagnosis. When first admitted she was in agony from the constant itching and an extreme headache. She cried frequently and was unable to stop scratching until she was restrained in order to prevent further excoriation. After a few days she was removed from the restraints and was more rational and accessible. She adjusted to hospitalization with difficulty and was tense, haughty, and sarcastic. Her own view of herself as an inadequate and unsuccessful mother disturbed her enormously. After a few weeks she was free of symptoms but the basic psychology was little changed. Discharged to the care of her husband she was to be followed in the outpatient department.

One month later the patient was readmitted, having been free of the symptoms for only a week. Unable to adjust to her new home, and even to select decorations for it, she found household tasks too difficult for her to handle, and she became resentful about the monotonous daily routine. At this admission she was semilethargic, having taken 75 grains of nembutal in the preceding four days. During this hospital stay she had several severe relapses when she had to be restrained, and she was given parenteral fluids because of excessive and persistent vomiting. These exacerbations seemed to begin after permitted visits to her home—both she and her husband remarked that she must be allergic to her home and her husband. Before this discharge she was well for several weeks and remarked, "I'm beginning to know myself and live with people. I realize that all of us have got to be disciplined somewhat and finally I'm getting a certain amount of satisfaction and pleasure talking about everyday happenings and beings." The patient and her husband were interviewed together and the patient was dismissed, again to be followed in the outpatient department.

Six months later the woman was again admitted with similar complaints and also, this time, with suicidal ideas. Her condition had changed little. Now she said, "I know my troubles are functional and why they occur, yet knowledge does little to lessen their intensity." While she was in the hospital this time her husband left to go into the navy, which hurt her very much. A sodium amytal interview was undertaken, in which she reiterated some of her past history. Nothing new was brought out, except that her mother had taught her that all men were vile and interested only in their own personal pleasure. Again she improved and was discharged. Five months later she was admitted for the fourth time, in a semicomatose state from barbiturates. After two more similar hospital admissions, the patient was finally sent to a state hospital.

P. Hypo. M:40:S:6 +4 2'87139– 6:5:11

Thirteen years before admission the patient had spilled lye on his left leg and genitalia, and although this lesion had healed uneventfully and without leaving an obvious scar, since that time he had been relatively impotent because it was difficult for him to get an erection and his scrotum felt drawn up. He imagined that he had a chord running from his heart to his testicle which "wasn't working right," and that his "semen was not powerful." The condition bothered him, particularly because he had been forced to curtail greatly what had previously been frequent sexual relations with local girls and prostitutes, and he had sought considerable medical treatment. Neither medication nor manipulation by way of therapy had brought relief. There were no other medical events that appeared contributory except that about ten years before admission he had had gonorrhea, from which he had apparently recovered completely.

The patient was a high school graduate although the quality of this training was questionable since it had been completed by correspondence with a New York school. School had been hard for him and his grades had been low. People in his community considered him lazy and inefficient, although he was active in community affairs and popular. In personal contacts he was pleasant, cooperative in disposition, and mild-mannered.

There was nothing obviously abnormal in his behavior, and there were no obvious abnormalities in his mentation. The general physical examination showed no contributory abnormalities. He dwelt constantly on his worry and concern about his impotence and the strange drawing sensations that he experienced in the region of his genitalia. He had an I.Q. of about 95. His answers on tests were characterized by carelessness. He was unusually limited in general knowledge and interests. His insight into his condition was distorted by his notion of a chord running from his heart to his testes. Although he recognized that his complaints might not have wholly physical bases, he resented any implication that his problem was entirely psychological. Cooperative and friendly, he appeared anxious for help, but he was so well protected underneath that no one could approach his somatic delusion. He did not improve and was discharged to continue as an outpatient.

P. Mixed Schizoid   M:46:M:24   +1   287′1463–9 (45)   3:8:7

The illness of this patient had had a rapid onset, beginning six days before admission when he created a disturbance in church by opening and closing the windows. The next day he became ill with the "flu" and was in bed for three days. He returned to work the following day but complained that he was unable to concentrate. He came home and spent the rest of the day doing odd jobs about the house. That night he complained that his mind had become "foggy." He began having hallucinations that the room was smoky and that there were red lights flashing in front of his eyes. He trembled and shook and screamed at the top of his voice. He forced his wife to play the piano and then made her stop. He demanded a cup of coffee and then refused to drink it. He paced from one room to another continuously. He finally slept for a few hours and when he awoke he was confused. He was then admitted to the hospital.

His previous history did not appear to contribute anything, except that he had been impotent for the past ten months. As a child he had been thought somewhat sadistic. He would purposely hurt his mother's feelings and then would feel sorry. He completed high school and one year in business college. After that he worked for one company until the time of admission. He was likable and got along with others. He had always had periods of depression followed by periods of euphoria. There also were hypochondriacal trends. His sexual behavior was somewhat unusual in that he would demand sexual intercourse with his wife in strange places such as the garage or the basement. The impotence had caused him to be even more cyclothymic and irritable than he had been previously.

On admission to the hospital the patient was somewhat confused and markedly depressed. He was primarily concerned about his feelings of inferiority, his inability to advance in his work, and his impotence. The confusion did not prevent his being well oriented and was more evident in a clouding of the sensorium than in any outright disturbance of mentation or orientation. His attitude and manner were not markedly abnormal, although he was inaccessible. He was contented and cooperative. He adapted well to the ward and said that he felt better than he had for ten years. With reassurance he seemed to get a great deal better, and he became optimistic about the future.

P. Mixed M:35:M:41 +15 287164'39– 0:13:4

Three years before admission to the hospital this man had begun to have spells of nausea and vomiting; he was put on an ulcer diet and since then had lived chiefly on crackers and milk. A great deal of his distress, which included "burning sensations," seemed to be unrelated to meals; in fact, he was bothered mainly at night. During the last two years the patient had been in constant trouble in his business affairs. According to his wife he was using very poor judgment, borrowing money unnecessarily, running up bills, and the like. He acted impulsively, showing little responsibility. More recently he had done very little work and had developed a number of new somatic complaints including occipital headaches, numbness, tingling of his hands, blurring of his vision, and palpitation. His wife thought that he had amnesic episodes and said that at times he talked continually, threatened to kill himself and others, yelled, and ran until exhausted. The patient denied that he was amnesic for these periods.

The patient had never been well; he was chronically afflicted with stomach trouble and rheumatic fever and said he had been "nervous" all his life. His early home life had been psychologically unhealthy. At the age of 14 he quit school in the eighth grade and left home. He was married at 24 after a premarital relationship had resulted in pregnancy. The family lived on the same farm for nine years, doing fairly well at first, later running into debt when beset by crop reverses, fire, meningitis, and other troubles. The patient's wife had contracted poliomyelitis a year after their first child was born. Her recovery was fairly complete and the two led a reasonably good life for a few years. The patient was known as a pleasant and frank person with considerable poorly directed energy. He was dominated by his wife. Quick-tempered and uncontrolled in speech, he considered himself "the black sheep of the family" since he was always in trouble. However, other members of the patient's family appeared to provide competition for this role. His father had been permanently committed to a state institution after it was proved that he had had incestuous relationships with a daughter, and most of the brothers and sisters were either in an institution or on relief.

On admission the patient showed vague concern over his family and economic troubles. He was a believer in mental telepathy and in general was strongly interested in occult matters. On the other hand he harbored a fear of religion, saying, "I never would have anything to do with it on account of it's what made my father crazy." His multiple somatic symptoms referred to all systems and there were obvious depressive trends. There was an overproductivity in his stream of thought with much circumstantiality. He tested average in intellectual ability. Toward anyone willing to listen the patient showed an unusual frankness in discussing the intimate details of his life. He spent much time discussing the past and his troubles with his wife. Quick to accept a suggestion, he was just as ready to reverse the acceptance. His opinions vacillated from hour to hour. His outstanding characteristic seemed to be anxiety. During the weeks in the hospital he changed relatively little and was not accessible for psychotherapeutic help. No good diagnostic formulation could be made.

Ps. M-D., Mixed F:57:M:87 +21 2873'1469– 2:5:9
Suicidal

About nine years before admission this patient had experienced her first "funny spell" in which she became so depressed that she "couldn't see the bright side of anything." She felt a sense a guilt, which she could not account for, and this was very irritating to her. This episode, lasting for about six months, was followed by a remission and then a six months' relapse. Six years before admission she had been well only for three months of the year and in the past three years she had been cyclically ill every three months. The present episode, of six months' duration, was marked by a sense of guilt; she believed that she had cheated a magazine company out of some money and that the police were after her. She blamed her neighbors for flashing lights in her window and for winding up her garden hose in a "funny way." Why they did this she did not know, but she believed that the government was probably to blame. Many times she had thought of taking her life, but she had made only one halfhearted attempt. She had a fear of becoming insane. She believed that her teeth were coming through her lips and that her saliva had lumps in it. At times she refused to eat and had to be fed by tube. Between her depressive periods she showed marked overactivity. Just before the onset of the present illness, the patient had been in good health.

A tenth-grade graduate, she had learned easily in school. She had previously exercised good judgment in the handling of money. A friendly, energetic person, she liked to go to movies and to entertain friends, but with the onset of the present illness she became more introverted. The patient and her husband were maladjusted. The husband assumed the attitude of "king" in the home, and he was much more interested in sexual activities than his wife was. He had a bad temper and had knocked the patient down on numerous occasions. There were five children, and the family's financial situation had never been good.

On admission to the hospital the patient was found to be markedly adipose, especially in the lower extremities. There were scattered neurological findings that could not be summed up as contributing obviously to the problem. The psychological symptoms included a sense of guilt, delusions of persecution and other ideas of reference, and somatic delusions. She appeared calm and well satisfied, but she complained of nervousness, tenseness, and inability to sleep. She was relevant, logical, and in general made a very good appearance. At first she complained constantly, insisting that she was not being treated properly; as the complaints subsided she became generally quarrelsome, finding fault with everybody and everything. Hyperactivity and a mild euphoria developed, but these symptoms in turn subsided, and at the time of discharge she was apparently in remission.

Ps. M-D., Mixed F:37:S:75 +41 287316'49– 5:12:13

It was difficult to date the onset of symptoms for this woman since they had gradually progressed during a year. Even earlier the patient had felt that she had failed in her chosen work and had decided to change her occupation. To facilitate this she took a year of special training and began to work in a new job. It was noted that she was nervous, worked under great tension, and obviously lacked confidence in her work. Because of fatigue and tension she gave up this job and in the next week developed insomnia and numerous somatic complaints. Finally, believing that she was a hopeless failure and the cause of many of the world's problems, she became seclusive and felt unworthy of any form of attention from anyone. Before the appearance of this pattern of symptoms she had been relatively well.

After high school graduation the patient attended college and made a good though not outstanding record. Then, until her recent change of occupation, she had taught high school in various small towns. Overly conscientious and self-sacrificing toward her family, she worked steadily with no time off for vacations. After one love affair, she said she would never marry and devoted herself unselfishly to looking after her family. The latter came to depend heavily on her. She was reserved, cheerful, and a meticulously orderly person, who never made any warm personal friendships. She showed no mood swings, partly because of her inability to express inward feelings.

On admission to the hospital the patient was obviously suffering from delusions of guilt and self-depreciatory ideas. "All the buildings are cold. I am the only person who is warm. No one but myself is being fed. Food is set before the other patients but they don't eat it. I have caused all this trouble." She spoke hesitantly and in a low voice. Her answers to questions were inadequate and drawn out, so that it required considerable effort to talk to her. She did not care to eat or to take part in ward activities, and she rejected aid of any kind. Spending most of her time in her room, pacing up and down and wringing her hands, she never gave expression to any of the ideas that were disturbing her. She was discharged to go to a state hospital.

P. React. Depr.   F:28:M:13   +3   28731'694–   3:8:10

Following the death of her only daughter about nine months before admission, the patient had become depressed, taking little interest in her surroundings. A severe weakness prevented her from doing her duties as a housewife, and she was troubled by insomnia. About seven years before admission, she had had a "nervous breakdown" with a similar pattern of symptoms. Six years before admission she had had an oophorectomy and a bilateral salpingectomy.

An active, sociable individual, the patient had always been eager to have a good time and had enjoyed dancing and other night life, but she had always been somewhat hypochondriacal, showing marked reactions to slight discomforts. Impatient and headstrong, she insisted on having her own way and was unable to accept graciously any sort of compromise. She had completed the eighth grade with an average scholastic record and had worked at odd jobs until her marriage at age 15 after an unusually short courtship. The marriage was not too bad a one except that the patient was not satisfied with the family's socioeconomic level.

A rather attractive woman who was obviously on her guard against appearing ill, she said that she had come to the hospital for a rest and to overcome the grief which she felt because of the death of her only daughter. The woman was concerned with the difficulty that she was having in adopting a little girl to replace this daughter. She thought that if she could adopt a child her difficulties would completely disappear, but she treated the adoption somewhat as one might consider the purchase of a pet. The only obvious depression was exhibited when she talked about her deceased child or when the requirements for adopting a child were discussed with her. Although she worked well into the ward life, she was antagonistic toward the examiner and resisted psychotherapy. An immature person, she was obviously "running away" from problems and responsibilities that she had never learned to face, and although she was entirely normal in her ward behavior the basic pattern was not changed by hospitalization.

Ps. Sz., Simple   M:20:S:52   +10   2873614'9–(63)   7:9:15
P. React. Depr.

About nine months before admission to the hospital the patient was classified 1-A in the draft and his induction into the army appeared to be imminent. Soon after this he noted a feeling of discomfort in his chest, characterized by a "turning, circling sensation." This depressed him and he worried considerably. He was working but felt that he would be more essential on a farm. Therefore, he obtained work on a farm and was reclassified by the draft board. There was a marked improvement in his symptoms, but a month later he again became worse following a sexual experience with a married woman. He became anxious about the possibility of a pregnancy. When this no longer was likely he again became somewhat better for a time; then his employer noted that he wandered aimlessly about the farm and got little done. The patient consulted a physician who told him he had a nervous breakdown and prescribed some "pills." He stopped working and returned to his home. There he sat about the house, staring into space much of the time. Sometimes he would cry aloud and say he hoped he would get well. He often remarked to his mother, "I wish I had gone into the army with the rest of the boys. Everything would have been all right then." He avoided meeting people whenever possible. When visitors came he would hide in the basement. He explained this by maintaining that he had a choking sensation which accompanied his chest symptoms and prevented him from speaking. He was very sensitive to any inquiry about why he was not in the army.

Before the onset of the present illness he had apparently been a well-adjusted, normal adolescent. He was cheerful and friendly and mixed easily with others. He was interested in sports and went out with many different girls without having a "steady." He had had a number of sexual experiences before the one related to the present illness without undue concern over them. He was somewhat above average in intelligence.

On admission to the hospital he was markedly concerned about his inability to talk to people as he formerly had. He believed that others resented him because he was depressed. When asked why he was no longer cheerful he replied, "It's just not in me any more." He had prominent feelings of guilt about the army. He was well oriented and appeared essentially normal in sensorium and intellect, although he consumed an inordinate amount of time answering questions and showed much more than a normal perplexity. He believed he had a nervous breakdown and was well aware that his behavior had changed. He was suspicious, distant, and rather evasive. He adjusted well on the ward although he remained by himself a great deal of the time. There were definite evidences of anxiety and tension. Throughout his whole hospital stay his behavior changed very little and he showed no evidence of a desire to leave. He would avoid the staff doctors by going into his room and shutting the door as they walked through the hall. He was finally discharged to go home for a trial before possibly entering a state institution.

Ps. Sz., Cat. F:39:S:23 +1 287 3641′9–(68) 4:9:13
P. React. Depr.

The onset of the admission complaints of this patient was insidious. They included marked weakness, excessive worry, and depression. For about a year before her mother's death from diabetes the patient had administered insulin under doctor's instructions. Her apprehension about this responsibility was enhanced by her mother's expressed desire for death. Many times the mother had asked her daughter to forget to give her the insulin, and about four years before admission the patient claimed that as a result of her failure to give the shots her mother had died in a diabetic coma. This began a periodical cycle of depression and weakness with nine severe attacks before hospitalization. Although various physicians treated her, mostly for somatic complaints deriving from her physical symptoms, the pains amounted to somatic delusions. Among them were ideas that she had cancer and syphilis. While she had suicidal ideas, she had never made any attempt on her life.

Even as a child the patient had been unable to control the movements of her left eye, but aside from this weakness she had enjoyed good health up to the age of 17 when she began to suffer from recurrent weakness and fatigue. Presumably because she was helping her mother, the patient had had to repeat the eighth grade; and at the age of 16 when she completed this grade in a rural school, she discontinued her education. Apparently she had average learning ability and in general was thought to have very good judgment. Stubborn and at the same time very sensitive, she worried excessively about minor matters. Always nervous and weak when "put to a test," she tended to be secretive, never confiding in anyone. She was somewhat worried over the fact that she had masturbated from childhood. While she had never gone out with a man, a neighbor had once asked her to go out. Feeling that he had "been put up to it" by others, she refused; but she told of hallucinations and dreams concerning her marriage to this man.

Appearing tired and haggard on admission to the hospital, the patient would close her eyes whenever she was asked an emotionally charged personal question. Worrying constantly about her health, about sexual difficulties, and especially about events in the past which were expressed as strong guilt feelings, she was hopelessly depressed and often felt that life was not worth living. She tended to be seclusive, remaining by herself most of the time. Although it soon improved, her weakness on admission was so severe that she had to be supported when she walked. Once she became accustomed to the hospital routine and realized that she had no personal responsibility for her own care, there was marked improvement and she began to mix with the other patients, but her underlying feelings of inferiority and "queerness" remained unchanged. She was discharged to a state hospital.

Ps. Sz., Paranoid M:23:S:9 —36 '2874–69 (74) 2:5:16

Four years before admission when the patient was a university graduate student, he went to a psychiatrist with plans of suicide based on supposedly inadequate scholarship and poor social adjustment. It was recommended that he withdraw from school and do manual labor for a while, and there was marked improvement until he attempted to return to school. Since entering college as a freshman he had been in the habit of taking from 25 to 100 milligrams of benzedrine in tablets a day, and when legislation restricted the availability of the tablets, he said, "I was caught. And so one usually turns to the next most logical stimulant, alcohol." His involvement with a young woman graduate student, to whom he proposed marriage during one of their drinking parties, made him panicky (he had had a number of homosexual experiences), and he again canceled out of school, this time to enter a "mental rest hospital," from which he was discharged in a few months markedly improved. He entered another graduate school where he again began to use benzedrine. He was soon in another psychiatric hospital where he received 25 insulin shock treatments, with 6 subsequent electroshock treatments. After his discharge he was employed as a day laborer until his seclusiveness, his untidiness, and his usual compulsive psychotic behavior patterns again made hospitalization necessary. A diary was found in which there were many self-observations, including possibly hallucinatory and delusional experiences, all meticulously set down.

He had been a brilliant child and a mature, frank, and social adult before the onset of the trouble, but he had always been rather rigid and in need of support whenever he was under tension.

At the hospital he was depressed, tense, and restless, and he wondered about the outcome of this "disaster." He was passive and ambivalent. He thought benzedrine was the etiological factor in his illness, but he realized that "it was a little bit more involved than that." His speech was meticulous, his sentence structure was very stilted, and there was some depersonalization. He was clean and neat, and as he improved he gradually entered into ward activities, but he was still so obviously ill that he was transferred to a state hospital.

Ps. M-D., Depr. F:32:M:38 +4 287′61349– 7:12:13

The patient attributed her illness to a combination of factors. She and her husband had "never got along," partly because of his failure to provide adequately for her, and also because he was of a "lower intellectual level." The marital discord led to a clandestine affair with another man, a close friend. Before leaving for the army, this man wrote repeatedly asking her to get a divorce and marry him. The patient worried about this decision and became progressively less able to keep up her activities. She wanted to be alone, cried with little or no provocation, and was self-depreciatory and self-accusatory. Finally she was taken to a medical clinic, but no organic basis for her troubles was found and she was told to "mix with people." Her condition remained static until admission to the hospital.

The patient's past history contained many suggestions of the present problems. As a child she had preferred to be alone and had often worried excessively and unnecessarily about trivial matters. She had always kept things to herself. At one time she was told that she had a low metabolic rate and was given thyroid for several months without apparent effect. A high school graduate, she did above average work throughout school; she attended a university for a while but stopped because of an acute depression. A year later she took a business course but never used the training because of inferiority feelings which prevented her from looking for work. After her marriage she occasionally worked for brief periods. She appeared intelligent and cheerful but in the background were always the self-depreciatory and depressed feelings. These would come to the surface periodically. She had some insight into the fact that she was mentally ill, and she appeared to be intact in orientation and mentation. In appearance she was attractive. Obviously tense, at first she adapted poorly to the ward but later did well except for brief depressed periods. During these she felt that she would never get better and wished to return home. In five weeks she left the hospital against advice because her husband was to go out of town to work. At discharge she was somewhat better but still had periods of agitation.

P. Psychas.	F:30:M:51	+1	28763′149–(55)	5:13:11
P. Hys.		+33	723′18694–(53)	6:4:14
Paranoid				
Schizoid				

The present illness of this patient had begun about sixteen months before when she was living in another state with her husband. First she received news of the death of her husband's mother, to whom she was very attached. This was a severe blow, since she felt she could have prevented the death if she had been present. Two weeks later she heard of the sudden death of her brother. To this she reacted violently, running from the house, rubbing snow on her face, and doing other peculiar things. She had seizures that appeared to be convulsive in nature. She came back to her home in this state and continued to have symptoms, prominent among which were attacks of dizziness and fainting which left her weak for about fifteen minutes. These spells became more and more frequent and she began to change in her attitude toward other people—for example, becoming antagonistic toward her father whom she had formerly liked. She took so many sedatives that she was practically stuporous part of the time. She finally went to a private hospital where she was taken off sedatives but she continued to have her spells. Immediately after her discharge she began taking just as many sedatives as before and returned to the hospital for some shock treatments. These did not work and she changed to whiskey instead of sedatives until her mother made her give this up. She visited many physicians during this time. Occasionally she had delusions of persecution and reference.

Before the present illness the patient had been in apparently good health. She attended school through the tenth grade and then left because, she said, most of her friends were leaving. She had had no difficulty in school and had always got along well with her friends. Her sister described her as strong-willed and stubborn, but she was said to be charming and vivacious socially. The patient and her husband were doubtfully compatible. The patient had an undue allegiance to her mother and her husband disliked her mother intensely. The patient had also been much drawn to another man, who had married her sister. This marriage to her sister had occurred before her own marriage and it was possible that her present husband represented a "rebound."

On admission to the hospital she was restless and apprehensive. She had indescribable and overwhelming fears. She had feelings of guilt about taking the sedatives and said that she had fought her fear until she had no strength left. Her mood was labile and she was unable to be constantly attentive to any one subject. At one moment she would be hopeful, at another deeply depressed. She had very poor insight. She spent most of her time during the early part of her hospitalization pacing up and down the corridors. Gradually she responded to therapy and became somewhat better. There were enough evidences of decay and possible paranoid ideas to justify consideration of a diagnosis of paranoid schizophrenia. On the other hand there were obvious hysterical and neurotic features.

Ps. M-D., Depr. M:38:M:95 +1 2876′341–(61) 3:15:11
Suicidal

The illness had begun about six months before admission when the patient had been discharged from the navy where he had been chief of a large medical service. He associated himself with another physician and got along well for a time but then felt that he was merely an assistant and that the other physician was dissatisfied. This made him fear that he would lose his job and not be able to support his family. He lost confidence in his abilities and dreaded even minor responsibility. Obviously depressed, he talked of suicide. Treated with electroshock he returned to work and got along all right for a while but his associate canceled the contract between them. This was a severe blow and things seemed to "close in on him."

The patient had had two previous periods of depression. These had each lasted about three months. In both there had been some inciting stress in the environment. He had been a top graduate in his class and for a while associated with a man from whom he learned a specialty. He then took over a small country practice but thought it was a "dog's life" and entered the navy. He was a studious person, exacting and critical of his own work. He had many friends, however, and was easy to get along with. He considered himself somewhat introverted and always worried about financial problems. His wife and he are well matched and happy together.

On admission to the hospital the patient was mainly worried about his own lack of worth. He was self-accusatory and troubled about his family. He had good insight. He was nervous and irritable and very sarcastic. He would pace the floor. Occasionally he felt like his old self, but these periods lasted a short time only. He was considerably better at the time of discharge and arrangements were made for him to take up his medical practice gradually. The prognosis was felt to be reasonably good, at least for his complete recovery from the present attack.

Ps. M-D., Depr. F:35:S:37 +9 2876413'9– 4:10:11
Ps. Sz., Paranoid
P. Hypo.

The present illness of this patient began about two and a half years before admission and followed the breakup of a love affair and the commitment of a favorite brother to a state hospital. At first her major complaint was low back pain; this was the verbalized reason for a series of medical treatments. Other symptoms appeared, including headaches, insomnia, loss of appetite, constipation, paresthesias, pounding heart, and vaginismus. She began to make statements that she was "blue" and "depressed," and "would never be any better"; she called her case hopeless and declared that her back was permanently injured. She was resentful toward her family for having her brother committed. For short periods she was much better, but most of the time she was incapacitated. So complaining, dictatorial, and disagreeable was she that she jeopardized the marital happiness of her sister, with whom she had gone to live. Before the present illness she had been in good health. Her sister requested that she be admitted to the psychiatric unit.

Because her father wanted her to take business training, she stopped high school in the tenth grade. She went to business school, worked for several years as a stenographer, and then finished high school. Her ambition had been to enter nurses' training, and she had enrolled but had not finished because of a love affair. Next she worked for a family where she became overly attached to the child who was placed in her care. Discharged from this job, she relaxed into semi-invalidism. The love affair had been with a married man and had persisted for ten years, despite attempts by her friends to convince her of his insincerity and lack of affection. During this time she felt that she must be sophisticated to keep the man interested and she pretended to like smoking and drinking and other "smart" activities. Intelligent, she was always interested in self-improvement, enjoyed poetry, and liked to read in the field of social science. Friends described her as self-conscious, vain, haughty, and jealous of the opportunities of others. She was always stubbornly blind to whatever facts she chose to ignore. Attractive to men, she was for the most part indifferent to them.

When she was admitted to the hospital it was recorded that the patient was "tall, blond, and meticulously dressed." Her major concern was with her body, and she commented, "They said that I had an intervertebral disc and then that I had arthritis. That creeps up and gradually paralyzes a person. What about the way my heart pounds? What about the pain in my abdomen? And the terrible pressure in my head?" She also had ideas of reference: "People can see by my eyes that I'm not right. They talk about me." There was depression, hopelessness, and psychomotor retardation. The orthopedic brace she wore was removed and she gradually worked into the hospital routine. She clung to her ideas tenaciously and haggled over minor variations in the routine. She became overly attached to a few of the patients, started feuds with others. Slowly there was an amelioration of some of the symptoms, but the patient's basic rigidity made it difficult to help her. She had a horror of state hospitals and was anxious to remain in the psychopathic unit rather than risk living at home for fear that that would lead to a state hospital. She was discharged to return to the home of a sister. The prognosis for recovery from the acute phase of the depression seemed good, but it was believed that the patient's personality problems were unalterable.

Schizoid M:24:M 287'9136–(43) 7:12:8

The soldier, a radio operator–mechanic, was referred by his base surgeon and his commanding officer for not discharging his duties adequately because of spells of loss of memory and confusion. He was bothered also by severe headaches and backaches.

The only child of his mother's second marriage, he was the youngest among six half-siblings. Although his childhood was "happy," it was characterized by feelings of isolation from other children, frequent "bad dreams" of falling, severe nail-biting, and an uncontrollable habit of hair-pulling. He disliked school, kept away from his schoolmates, and entered into no activities. In school, he was reticent and shy and said he "didn't care for girls."

The precipitating stress in the soldier's current illness seemed to have been the birth of his first child one month before. Expressing a dislike for children, he said, "Babies make me nervous." Treatment in a military setting was not indicated and the man was separated from the service. A. T. K.

P. React. Depr. M:49:D:21 +4 28947'613– 2:12:6
B. Psth., Path. Emot.
Drug Add.
Suicidal

The patient was admitted to the hospital after a suicidal attempt. He had been out of work for a long time and had brooded over the fact that he was forced to be dependent upon his brother. About eight hours before admission he decided to end it all, poured out a handful of phenobarbital tablets, and took them. His brother came home and found him apparently drunk, but had him brought to the hospital when the patient told him what had occurred.

The patient had been a poor scholar in school and a frequent truant. He stopped at age 16 to travel with a carnival and since that time, when he was employed, he had mostly followed carnivals and worked in casinos or roadhouses, operating various gambling devices. He had been married 28 years before admission. That marriage ended in divorce after 17 years. He married again and was once more divorced about four months before admission. When he was working he made at times a good salary. Always an easygoing, irresponsible, jolly man who spent money rapidly and foolishly when he had it, he used poor judgment in choosing his associates and at various times had done a great deal of drinking. He had tended to resort to morphine and marijuana when in trouble.

In the hospital he was at first obviously under the influence of the narcotic. He gave this as his reason for taking it: "For the past few months I've been unemployed and dependent upon my brother for support. I have never before been dependent upon anyone. When my brother goes to work I have nothing to do but sit at home and brood over the fact that there is nothing for me to do. I have become more and more depressed." After recovering from the poisoning, he seemed to be his usual self. He was well oriented and there were no gross disturbances of sensorium or intellect. He appeared to be depressed but answered questions adequately and to the point, speaking spontaneously. He complained of some pain in his shoulder but recovered rapidly from such complaints. He had no insight at all into the inadequacies of his personality and he was not disposed to consider himself ill. He felt, probably with some justification, that if he could get work he would forget many of the things that were weighing upon him.

Ps. Sz., Paranoid	M:36:S	'29–41 (61)	2:3:18
Alcoholism			

This patient, a factory inspector of automotive parts, was admitted to the hospital in a grossly psychotic state with auditory and visual hallucinations and paranoid reactions. He appeared to be preoccupied with sexual matters. Soon after admission he put his head through a window and exhibited catatonic and negativistic behavior.

Information about this man's early life was meager. His parents had been inconsistent in their discipline; otherwise his home life was, as far as is known, not unusual. After graduating from high school he attended college for two years. On his job he was considered a steady and diligent employee. A shy person, he had feelings of inadequacy, apparently related to conflicts about masturbation. He also had guilt feelings about an embezzlement and was sensitive about not having achieved his economic goals. He was a solitary drinker and drank to excess. He was ill at ease with women and had not married.

After a brief series of electroshock treatments the patient changed markedly in appearance and behavior. The MMPI and other tests were administered at this time. After exploration of his feelings about masturbation and inadequacy, he abandoned his remaining delusions. Since the patient showed no desire to discuss homosexuality, this area was covered only superficially. W. M. H.

B. Psth., Asocial	F:36:M:7	+2	'294–6 (66)	4:3:13
P. Hys.		—270	'9–6723 (63)	4:5:16
Drug Add.				

Eleven months before admission to the hospital the patient had appeared before the parole board of the women's prison where she was serving a term and had been refused parole in spite of her alleged good conduct record. After that event she felt that "life was not worth living anymore." She lost her appetite and vomited whenever forced to eat. She changed from a friendly, cheerful, cooperative prisoner to a sullen, morose, and uncooperative one. She was restless, slept poorly, and did not respond to sedatives. On the day of her transfer to the psychiatric unit, she told the prison superintendent that she "wouldn't be alive the next day."

Her past health had been fairly good. At the age of 14, she suffered a severe facial laceration in an automobile accident and underwent extensive plastic surgery. Later she had several major operations for an abscessed kidney. At that hospital admission she was considered "psychoneurotic or malingering" (see the earlier MMPI obtained while she was on the surgical ward). There were no psychotic upsets. She attended high school for three years and was moderately successful but quit at age 17 to run away and marry a man who turned out to be a thief. She traveled with him for five years wherever his "business" took him. At the end of that time she divorced him after a severe quarrel. She thereafter made a living as a "shoplifter." When she was 28 she began to smoke opium and when that became difficult to get she changed to morphine. She was a drug addict for five years and was finally convicted for unlawfully procuring narcotics. After that she was arrested many times and on the last occasion was sentenced to five years in prison. After serving fifteen months of this term she applied for the pardon.

She appeared to be average in intelligence and was clear in sensorium and intellect. She was able to get along well with people and was cheerful and thoughtful in the ward activities. She was somewhat nervous and irritable at first but this disappeared shortly. She had mild outbursts of temper throughout the interviews. It was felt that at least part of her symptoms had been due to malingering. She was voluble but there was no flight of ideas. She always tended to lead the conversation away from subjects disagreeable to her. At one point she became somewhat unmanageable and was put in the disturbed section with her privileges taken away, whereupon she promptly began to behave again. The symptoms seemed to have a hysterical basis if they were more than malingering. In any case the pattern was not considered to be a virulent one. She was returned to the reformatory after study with suggestions as to how she should be handled, mostly based on the assumption that she was not a borderline psychotic or basically a character neurosis.

B. Pri. Child. M:17:S:13 +2 '<u>29</u>46–(51) 2:7:8
B. Psth., Asocial

The patient was admitted on a court order after he had aided an escapee from the city jail. The escapee, who had not known the patient very well, had asked the boy for clothing, and although two friends had tried to dissuade him, the patient had delivered the clothing and had driven the escapee and a girl friend to a summer cottage in his parents' car. All three were apprehended, and the father had requested that the boy be studied psychiatrically because he was poorly adjusted and antisocial.

The past physical history was noncontributory. The patient had had difficulty from early life in getting along with his parents. A disobedient boy, he had been sent to a private school because he was unruly in public school. Later he had returned to public school where he had made friends among reform school parolees and other undesirable companions. He had refused to participate in group athletics and had done poorly in so many other ways that he was finally transferred to a trade school. Although he had enjoyed his work, his performance level was poor. Before the present trouble he had been arrested once for speeding and driving without a license, and another time he had been arrested for helping to ruin tires on thirteen autos by using an ice pick.

In the hospital the patient was superficially cooperative, friendly, and socially acceptable, but there was an underlying insecurity about his inability to make friends. He confessed that he considered himself inadequate in athletics, personality, and scholastic ability. On several occasions he showed an inability to differentiate right from wrong. The temper tantrums evidenced at home were not indulged in during hospitalization. During his stay in the hospital there was no bizarre or abnormal behavior, and he was obviously not deeply concerned about his situation. Occasionally he was annoying to others, and he found it amusing if they resented his behavior. When he got into trouble, he had been on the point of being admitted to the navy, and on discharge it was recommended that the court permit him to join the navy.

Ps. Paranoid F:46:D:54 +3 '3–2 8:0:23
Mutilative

The psychosis with which this patient was admitted had been so slow in developing that it could not be dated. It had first been noticed at least eleven years before when the patient considered people who looked at her house to be agents of her divorced husband sent to spy upon her. When a member of the family did anything she did not approve of she would say, "You are not my dear daughter [or mother or father], you are someone else." The given member of the family would leave the room and re-enter, and the patient would then recognize him properly. This misidentification gradually progressed over the years. Finally the patient tried to drive her friends out of the house because they appeared to be total strangers to her. She also began to eat poorly because she feared the food was poisoned. She said she was unusually susceptible to the effects of electric rays. During the past year she had complained of lesions on her leg, which she said were inflicted on her while she slept, possibly by an X-ray machine that one of the neighbors owned. In the past few weeks the patient had slept with her bedroom door barred.

There were no past episodes of severe illness or psychological upsets. She was a high school graduate and had gone to a university for a while, failing at the first one she attended, then changing to a smaller school where she completed two years satisfactorily. She separated from her husband, who had abused her, and then worked to support her parents and children. She was a clerical worker and housemaid, never able to stay long in any one position. The patient developed a strong homosexual attachment to a woman for whom she worked. At one time she left her home and children in order to live for a while with this homosexual partner. The father of the patient was an unstable person who had squandered a small fortune on prospecting ventures. The mother was a nervous, dominating person who covered her inner nature by being very sweet and apparently yielding.

The consultants from the skin service believed that the ulcers with which the patient was afflicted were self-induced. Great difficulty was experienced in obtaining her true mental content. She very successfully covered up everything that she really was thinking. She said that the wounds on her leg were produced by an external agent and that she definitely knew the cause but would not tell it. The reason she gave for refusing to answer questions or cooperate in telling what she thought, was that she was protecting someone else. Except for the delusional content no abnormalities of behavior or mentation were observed. Ordinarily sweet and obliging, if really pushed she would show anger or burst into tears. She was finally transferred to a state hospital.

Ps. Toxic	M:45:M:19	+2	'3–6X (49)	11:1:21
		–5	'18 673–9X (51)	12:0:25

The patient had an acute attack of precordial pain, abdominal distress with tachycardia, dyspnea, and cyanosis four days before admission. He lapsed into a state of confusion with hallucinations and became unmanageable in spite of various medications, and his wife was unable at one time to keep him from getting dressed for work in the middle of the night. He was known to have been a fairly heavy drinker, but there was no evidence that he had taken unusual amounts of alcohol preceding the present attack.

For the past nine years he had had a kidney infection which had not responded well to treatment. Following a hospitalization a year before admission, when he received treatment for the infected kidney, he began to change in personality, becoming quiet and losing his interest in home, work, and social activities. He got worse after the death of his mother and acutely worse with the present illness. An easygoing person, he had mixed well with other people. He was a fairly steady worker but had been fired from a job he had held for six years just a few days before the onset of the present pattern of symptoms.

In the hospital the physical and neurological examinations showed nothing that would explain the illness. The patient was greatly confused and disoriented as to time, place, and person. He experienced continual hallucinations, complaining of seeing snakes and of feeling that the walls were falling in on him. He had no insight into his condition and was restless and sleepless. At times he was destructive, tearing up bed clothing. By the fourth day after admission he had returned to his usual personality although he kept to himself and was very quiet. He rapidly improved still more and became a good mixer with other patients on the ward. No certain conclusion could be reached regarding the etiology of the episode. There was no definite evidence that he had had excessive amounts of alcohol or that he was suffering from a toxic condition. He was completely recovered at the time of discharge.

Ps. Invol. Melan. F:53:M:9 +1 '31–468 5:2:10
P. Hys.

The admission complaints of this patient were centered around nervousness, irritability, insomnia, and depression. These dated chiefly from six months before admission when she suffered a severe attack of laryngitis with a breathing difficulty. The hoarseness and a cough continued for about six weeks. During this time she had several attacks of dyspnea which frightened her, and she experienced continuing insomnia. Crying spells developed and she was indifferent to her work and lax about her ordinary duties. She became absent-minded, leaving lights on and forgetting what she was doing. She was also indecisive and increasingly asocial. If she continued to feel this way, she said, she would kill herself. A sister had become insane and she feared that she might also. There were occasional short periods in which she would be fairly well and happy.

Inquiry into the patient's past history showed that the present illness was not as acute as it had first appeared. Her health had been fairly good, but she had undergone several operations and had been considered "nervous." She had never been pregnant although she had used no control measures. For a number of years her friends had noticed that her personality had been gradually changing to one less affable, more quiet and depressed. She was above average in intelligence and had been a relatively energetic and happy individual. She had been a good mixer, friendly, thoughtful, and kind, always at ease socially. In sexual matters she was somewhat prudish.

The patient was chiefly concerned about her inability to sleep. She cried and talked almost continually about this. She attributed all her problems to the throat disorder and believed that she never could get well. She denied that any factor was affecting her except the illness and the insomnia. Significant mood swings occurred during her hospital stay. At times she would be laughing happily and within a few minutes shedding tears copiously. She could furnish no reasons for these shifts although she cooperated well in examinations. She appeared to be willing to accept reassurance that she was physically well, insisting, however, that if only she could sleep she would get well rapidly. Heavy medication was given to help her sleep, and any decrease resulted in sleeplessness. In spite of warnings to the husband that his wife was a suicide risk, he removed her against advice and placed her in a private rest home. She was relatively unimproved at the time of discharge.

P. Hys. F:18:S:11 0 '31–47(68) 7:3:9

This girl's "nervous spells" consisted of somatic symptoms such as cold sweats and paresthesias, flushing of her face and neck, and the like. The first of these "spells" occurred about eighteen months before admission and was characterized by cold sweat on the palms of her hands, flushing of her face, neck, and chest, and tachycardia and palpitation. Later her arms and legs became rigid during a spell. She could tell when a spell would begin; usually it followed an argument with the family and lasted about five minutes. Conscious throughout the attacks she never was incontinent or injured herself.

Before the present difficulty, the girl's health had been good. There was a doubtful history of a "heart attack" two years earlier. An eighth-grade graduate from a rural school, she had left school to work on her parents' farm. Low average in intelligence, she was shy, friendly, cooperative, and cheerful. She liked to get things done in a hurry and was nervous when hindered. She had little interest in her future, showing no ambition or tendency to plan. The patient had never been out with a boy and claimed not to be concerned with sex. There was conflict in the family, apparently because the father was very strict.

In the hospital she was intact in sensorium and intellect and in general mental content. Not only did she express interest in her condition but she remembered minute details of her past illnesses. Although she was friendly and apparently talked freely she seemed to suppress her attitudes toward her home. Her condition was "due to nervousness" and there was nothing wrong with her physically, she thought. She was neat and normal in behavior on the ward. There were no delusions, mannerisms, or discernible abnormalities in her behavior. At discharge she showed enthusiasm over plans for a job away from home. It was felt that getting out of the home atmosphere in such a job was a good program and that she would probably have no further trouble.

B. Simple Adult Maladj. F:38:M:26 +14 '31–87962 8:0:11

B. Simple Adult Maladj. F:40:M:19 +2 '13–47869 7:4:7

The present admission was the second for this patient. The complaints were mildly hypochondriacal and appeared against a background of marital maladjustment. She had overreacted to her mother-in-law's pessimistic demeanor and to her husband's unemployment. She experienced occasional headaches and "blue spells." Some of the symptoms were found to be related to an acute hemorrhoid condition, treatment for which helped to determine admission to the hospital. The patient was only mildly disturbed psychologically and except for a long history of mild hypochondriasis, had seemed to be fairly well adjusted until the first hospitalization.

On admission the patient showed moderate concern about the headaches but said she did not want "to be a neurotic and kick about things." Discontented about her home situation, she said that the happiest time in her life was three years before when she took a trip away from home. Although mildly concerned about the scheduled operation for the hemorrhoidal condition, she appeared to accept that normally. Her heart pounded, she said, when she was asked to repeat digits in the psychological examination. She spoke of her "biggest difficulty" as being a "quick temper." The operation was performed without any particularly contributory events and gradually she became somewhat better. She continued to show considerable concern over family problems, and it was apparent that she did not meet these entirely adequately. At discharge she was greatly improved but basically not much different.

P. Hys. M:24:M:23 +10 '31–987 2:0:15

Three months before admission the patient had accidentally swallowed a mouthful of ethyl gasoline while cleaning a feed line in his car and had immediately experienced vertigo and vomiting. This persisted until the following morning, and there was also difficulty in breathing and dysphagia. In attacks that lasted about thirty minutes, his hand became numb with tingling up to the elbow. In the next months he experienced four of these attacks and received various medical and chiropractic treatments. At the time of admission to the hospital the patient was free of all symptoms with the exception of occasional periods of palpitation.

Six years before the present admission he had been a patient in a general hospital with pain in his right foot; but the physical examination at that time was negative, and it was felt that the condition was functional in nature. The patient had attended a country school through the eighth grade, stopping at age 14. Married at 17, for the past two years he had been on a W.P.A. job. Shy and retiring, but not particularly secretive or sensitive, he was described as a cheerful and optimistic person who "looked on the bright side of things in spite of financial difficulties" and who got along well with people. Although he had difficulty finding steady employment, he was said to be a hard worker. He and his wife appeared to be compatible.

When first seen in the outpatient department the patient was markedly tense, greatly concerned about his physical condition, and apprehensive that an attack might terminate fatally. Tenseness was still evident on admission, but there was no marked depression or euphoria, and he had a kind of verbal insight into his condition. At no time did his behavior show any evidence of abnormality. He was neat in appearance. He made a satisfactory adjustment on the ward, and he had no seizures while in the hospital, although he said that he occasionally felt palpitations. On several occasions he reiterated the belief that he was incapable of hard manual labor, and he also mentioned his intense dislike of work on W.P.A. projects. At the time of discharge he had made arrangements to work in another type of job, and the staff felt that with a good adjustment in that job he would probably have no further trouble.

P. Hys. M:38:M:26 +6 3′12– 7:2:14
P. React. Depr.

The patient experienced pain and weakness in his upper left arm and was irritable and depressed. His story was that he had been well until about eight months before admission, when one morning he was struck on the shoulder and left forearm by falling ice. For the severe pain that ensued he was given a hypodermic and was told to lie down. The morning following the accident he suffered a dizzy spell, was unable to sit up, and "everything turned black." Six months later he was examined by a physician for the insurance company which was to pay compensation for the accident. At the end of the examination the patient felt weak, had chills, and thought he was going to faint. He began to be depressed soon after this. Since the accident the patient had become cross with his children and had avoided his friends.

After finishing the eighth grade this man was employed as a semiskilled carpenter and at times as a mechanic. At the time of the accident he was working as a janitor. He had never had trouble doing his work well and was known as industrious. Independent by nature, he disliked seeking help from others. Associates thought of him as usually stable emotionally.

There were numerous neurological and physical findings but these seemed unrelated to any organic pathology. They shifted with suggestion and were different from one examination to another. Self-critical because he felt he was not living up to his obligations, and was not now taking care of himself, he wanted help so that he could resume work. The soreness and weakness of his left arm, he said, made it impossible for him to do anything. He was dissatisfied with what help he had received from friends, the insurance company, and others. Firmly convinced that his complaints were based upon organic disorders caused by the accident, he did nevertheless recognize the psychological nature of his irritability and depression. When discussing his troubles he became tearful and made little effort to associate with other patients. He repeatedly questioned the examiner about the compensation he might be awarded as a result of his accident. Since the whole psychotherapeutic approach was inhibited by the unsettled compensation situation, he was finally discharged with the suggestion that further study would be profitable only after the amount of compensation was fixed.

P. Hypo. F:53:M:12 +4 31′246–9 8:3:17

This woman had shown no particular personality problem, but she had been studied in a number of clinics because of what appeared to be arthritic symptoms, and mild emotional instability had been noted. It seemed desirable to evaluate this factor before she was given further exclusively somatic medication. She was also suffering from fairly severe insomnia and was somewhat anxious and apprehensive.

The past medical history included a number of major operative procedures, although the patient said that she had always had good health. She stopped high school in the third year—when she fell in love, the patient's father gave her the choice of marrying or continuing in school without seeing the man, and she chose matrimony. Apparently she had been an active and energetic person, social and outgoing. She seemed to have been somewhat of a gossip and a busybody. Generally speaking, however, she had been an adequate person. She worked after her marriage even though it was not financially necessary. After seventeen years of married life she left her husband, having remained with him that long because her mother had opposed separation or divorce. Her mother had recently died. For a while the patient operated a rest home, but when this failed she was forced to go on relief. A contributing factor in her inability to support herself was her rheumatism.

In the hospital no definite psychological pathology was revealed. She enjoyed helping others around the ward, was entirely cooperative, and entered into activities. She complained, however, of insomnia and of urinary frequency. A neurotic pattern, while not obvious, appeared as a definite substrata which usually she successfully hid. Apparently she was not suffering from very severe anxiety. She readily accepted suggestions that her insomnia, frequency, and emotional upsets were attributable to her difficult life situation, with apparently therapeutic results. After discharge she was to be followed as an outpatient.

P. Mixed F:21:M:12 +3 3′1̲2̲47–6 8:4:17

This young woman had begun to complain of abdominal pain during the latter part of a pregnancy three years earlier. Associated fatigue and nervousness were present, and she was hospitalized for a month. During a second pregnancy the symptoms reappeared in an aggravated form and she again went to a hospital. In the second hospitalization the attacks were associated with syncope. The syncope usually lasted for about ten minutes and she could be easily aroused during that time. Despite the fact that she underwent an appendectomy and a bilateral salpingectomy, the pain continued and she became increasingly irritable, often mistreating her children.

Leaving school in order to marry, the patient had finished the eighth grade. While she had lived with her parents it had been necessary for her to do heavy manual labor. She found outdoor life attractive, and she loved to hunt, fish, and go trapping with her husband. She was practical and energetic. A reticent person, she had few opportunities to make friends. Toward her husband she appeared to be submissive; while the couple seemed to be relatively happy, the patient did not enjoy sexual intercourse.

In the hospital she appeared as a short, dysplastic, slightly obese person. There was a marked hypertrichosis. She was concerned about the abdominal pain and the constant fatigue, and she ardently believed that no relief could be obtained without further surgical intervention. On these points she could not accept reassurance and, in fact, often showed clear displeasure at not being given physical treatment. In the psychological examinations she was inadequate and evasive. Tests showed her to be dull normal in intelligence. On the ward she was generally sullen, changeable in mood, and reluctant to enter into activities. It became apparent that she may have married her husband, who was twelve years her senior, in order to escape a home life that she had detested; actually she had merely exchanged this for an equally distasteful situation, since she hated keeping up a farm home. At discharge, she was symptomatically somewhat better, but the basic condition appeared not to have been altered.

P. Mixed	M:20:S:47	+3	312'478–9(51)	7:4:21
Ps. Sz., Simple				
Mental Deficiency				

The patient's chief symptoms were palpitation, dizziness, shortness of breath, and generalized weakness. A month before admission to the hospital, while working on a farm, he noted, "at times when I wasn't doing anything, my heart would start to jump around." Later he had an attack of faintness, shortness of breath, dizziness, and palpitation, during which he fell on the street but remained conscious. Similar attacks followed rapidly. Repeated studies showed no heart pathology. It was impossible to determine accurately the sequence of events and symptoms, since neither the patient nor his father, nor any other informant was intelligent enough to recall them clearly. It was established that he had been 4-F in the draft and his explanation of this was a "dropped heart, normal in shape and position."

The young man was described as having been cheerful and active before the onset of symptoms. Quiet and seclusive, however, he took little part in the activities that occupied most of his contemporaries. He spent most of his time reading and drawing. His father called him a hard worker. School had been difficult for the patient, and he was not at all interested in it. His I.Q. was 80.

In the hospital the youth showed marked worry about the chances of "passing out" during one of the attacks. This fear was related to uncertainty about the "hereafter" and his lack of definite religious beliefs. Lazy and passive, he showed no other interest in his problems, the examination, or ward activities and was content to lie in bed. He was finally persuaded to get up and be more active, but even then he lounged against the doorway or the wall. In occupational therapy he was given a simple project but in one week had not completed it. He developed no insight. The stubborn persistence of the symptom picture was not a hopeful sign, and although he was somewhat better at discharge, and had been partly reassured, it was felt he might need steady hospitalization.

B. Psth., Mixed	F:28:S:47	+5	31248'7–	3:9:17
P. Hys.				
Suicidal				

This patient, a university graduate student, was admitted because of restlessness and dissatisfaction of an undefinable nature. Asked in a class to make a case study of her own life, she had begun with great resistance, and when it was half finished she had come to the teacher and had poured out a great variety of conflicting material relating to sexual overactivity, emotional orgies, and attempts at suicide. A feeling of increased tension which she interpreted as sexual excitement appeared, making it difficult for her to eat, sleep, or concentrate.

As a college student in her early twenties she had received psychiatric help. In the first of two dramatic attempts at suicide she had drunk iodine in the office of a woman physician, and in the second she had slashed her wrist with glass. All her life she had had many bodily complaints, and in her early childhood deformed legs had necessitated the wearing of casts for many months. Her eating and sleeping habits had always been irregular. Her home life was unhappy, and while she was in high school she had done many odd jobs to avoid being at home. Later she had studied dramatics, at which she was very successful. After working with several stock companies, she found herself frustrated by the fact that her dramatic ability was appropriate for character parts, which she was too young for, and she decided to go back to college. She was sexually active from a very early age. At about age 10 she had begun to be attracted to other girls, and she became convinced that she was a homosexual. She was introduced to homosexual practices by an older actress. When this affair was terminated she became attached to a cult of homosexual women and finally was "married" by a "priest" of the cult to another woman whose ring she wore at the time of admission. The patient had been brought to the point of the suicidal attempts by her feeling of failure in the attempt to make an adequate heterosexual adjustment. She had a particular aversion toward girls who appeared "mannish," and she herself seemed very feminine in both body build and dress. She was a talented person and in many ways was social, friendly, and outgoing.

In the hospital her general demeanor was entirely normal. She expressed depressive attitudes about her inadequacies and feelings of inferiority. She had a great need for reassurance and sympathy, and she spent many hours discussing her problems with the therapist. (It was not directly established that she was homoerotic by nature.) She became somewhat more comfortable as she acquired insight into her early rejection of her family and into the entire pattern of development which had convinced her that she was "queer." She left the hospital to teach dramatics, a job at which she was very successful. After a year or so, she went into literary work and wrote several moderately successful plays.

Ps. Toxic F:42:M:78 +2 3′12487–(45) 3:3:15
B. Psth., Path. Emot.
Drug Add.

B. Psth., Path. Emot. F:43:M:29 +1 3′214–9(51) 7:4:16

The chief presenting problem of this patient was addiction to barbiturates. She had begun to use the barbiturates twelve years earlier to relieve migraine headaches. At that time she was also experiencing difficulties with her first husband who was a chronic alcoholic. For the year and a half preceding this admission (first MMPI) the patient's appetite had been poor, and she had steadily lost weight. During the last twelve years many physical symptoms appeared. As her physician became aware of her drug addiction, she lied continuously to mislead him. She neglected housework and often told her husband that she had worked all day when actually she had been idle. She became extremely weak, nervous, and tremulous. Her sexual desires became excessive.

The early years of the patient's life were uneventful. A telephone operator, she continued in her job for five years after marriage. This first marriage was ended by the death of the husband. Her second husband proved to be a much better marital partner. Before the onset of the hypochondriacal complaints the patient was described as having been a cheerful, cooperative, and pleasant person of average intelligence. She had always found it necessary to keep herself occupied with housework and other activities to avoid emotional difficulties.

When admitted to the ward she was nervous, euphoric, and disoriented. The barbiturates were withdrawn, but large doses of paraldehyde were administered occasionally to induce sleep. She was given electroshock and insulin shock treatments. These aided in clearing up her confusional state and brought her out of the psychotic behavior. Immediately, she was eager to leave the hospital and return home, asserting that now everything was fine, and that she would never again take drugs. These remarks were glib and not convincing. She appeared to have many conflicts but was unable to verbalize them. There were numerous psychotherapeutic interviews; but although she appeared much improved and gained 25 pounds, it was realized at discharge that she had not changed basically. A shallow and rigid personality was still her dominant characteristic, and there was little basis for a good prognosis. She was discharged only to be readmitted with a similar pattern a year later. The addiction in this case was relatively mild, and she was less confused. She was again discharged without a good prognosis and warned that this was a sort of last trial before more prolonged hospitalization in a state institution.

P. Mixed	F:19:S:113	+2	312′48769–(57)	7:4:25
P. Hypo.		+51	′3124–678(41)	5:2:17
		+53	′31429–(47)	5:2:23

The presenting complaints of this patient were nervousness and a variety of vague somatic pains and sensations. These were highlighted by tachycardia and a peculiar feeling of fullness in the stomach. The symptoms showed up when she was working "too hard," and she had initially been diagnosed by a physician as having rheumatic fever. In the course of the past year she consulted other physicians, used various medicines, and spent much time in bed under the care of a protective mother on whom she was dependent.

The patient's general health was normal until age 10 when she suffered a severe attack of pneumonia. Since that time she had had occasional dyspnea, and she dated all her difficulties from that illness. For years she used laxatives almost daily and once had a gastric disorder, diagnosed as ulcers, from which she recovered. At 16 she quit school because of "ulcers." Her grades had been average. She did not return to school but worked at various jobs, always avoiding heavy work. Her only specific ambition had been to "get married some day." Her intelligence was average, and she was regarded as cheerful and somewhat shy. She liked to "tear around" and enjoyed other people. Since age 15 these activities had steadily decreased as the hypochondriacal tendencies had increased. Her sisters regarded her as "neurotic."

Preoccupied with her somatic difficulties, the patient's emotions and attitudes were colored by an obvious desire for sympathy. She lacked interests and was called sensitive by the staff. Gradually she became more interested in activities and adapted fairly well to the hospital routine. During the latter days of her stay the somatic complaints diminished, and she gained in self-confidence. Her insight, however, was limited. The last month she was permitted to work part of each day in a private home but showed no genuine interest in this job. When finally discharged, she had made no definite plans for the future and did not appear to have changed much basically. The protection offered by her mother was considered an adverse factor in her adjustment.

P. Hys. F:21:M:36 0 31248769′–(47) 3:5:14
P. Hypo.

For ten months the patient had experienced intermittent attacks of heart pain, nervousness, headaches, and other peculiar sensations. These symptoms had begun three weeks after the birth of a child and had developed suddenly. Her doctor was concerned and feared the symptoms indicated a severe heart disability.

While attending school the patient had held jobs and was thought to be a competent girl. After graduating from high school she enlisted as a WAVE. Several months later she became pregnant and was dishonorably discharged. Subsequently, after his divorce, she married the man responsible for the pregnancy. Her husband's slowness in providing a home caused her anxiety, and she worried about their future. He was immature and dependent upon his father and mother, with whom they lived and where the patient felt unwelcome. Following the birth of the child, the question of its paternity was discussed throughout the small town in which they lived. Her greatest enjoyment had always been dancing. She was considered by many as immature in judgment.

In the hospital she showed signs of anxiety and the symptoms continued for several days. She was slow to face the facts of the sources of her anxiety, and she continued to depend upon her own mother and father for important decisions. The prognosis would have been good if sufficient time could have been spent in helping her to meet her problems squarely and also in manipulating the environment to relieve some of the pressures.

P. Mixed	F:38:S:124	+22	312'49–6	8:3:9
		+124	1'234–6	9:0:15
P. Mixed	F:39:S:91			

This woman, who was admitted to the hospital six times (four times before the present admission, first MMPI), complained of low back pain extending down the right lower extremity and nervousness. The particular pattern of complaints in any one admission varied according to the date. Besides the six admissions to this hospital she spent time in other hospitals. An adequate description of the complaints or of the treatment and surgical operations is impossible in a short account. For the low back pains she underwent a laminectomy, but no prolapsed disc could be discovered. At the time of admission a second laminectomy was being considered by the neurosurgery service. Numerous other complicated procedures had been used, and she had at various times worn braces and casts. She had been operated on for "appendicitis" and for a "floating right kidney." Apparently fairly well until about the age of 35, in the next years she accumulated one of the thickest records in the hospital.

The patient's personality was described as having been relatively good before the illness and on the whole she always appeared intact even during the worst of her complaints. Of average intelligence, she had worked as a maid and had proved satisfactory in her jobs, but she had never been able to establish social contacts. Her friends included no men. With a poor background, she had been unable to develop social skills. One difficulty was that she spoke brokenly because German was the only language used in her home and in her community. Originally a Roman Catholic, she had changed faith after leaving home and had become a Unitarian. Unassuming and passive, she was without well-developed interests and was almost totally lacking in enthusiasm.

In the hospital the patient appeared, superficially, as a stable person. It was true that she centered conversation and attention almost wholly upon her physical symptoms. Frequently she cried from the severity of the pain she said she was experiencing; she would not leave her bed at such times and showed every sign of anguish. Not only was she friendly to the personnel and the other patients, but she submitted readily to any form of treatment recommended. She mentioned daily that she "would do anything to get well," to earn her own living again. It was probable that the superficial appearance of normality, together with the absence of signs of nervousness or instability, explained the fact that so many surgical procedures were carried out in spite of some evidence that the complaints had a neurotic basis.

Realizing that this woman was causing a great deal of expense to the state, a long-time psychotherapeutic regime was instituted. Treatment included painful faradic stimuli applied to the regions of pain, as well as extensive reassurance and strong urging to become active. She was permitted, as far as possible, to express her feelings of frustration, and she was encouraged to gain insight into what was a problem with her, namely, a desire for a husband and a home. Since she was unattractive, and without ability to get along socially, it appeared unlikely that she would become acquainted with a suitable man. Cathartic types of psychotherapy had meager success because the patient was almost inarticulate and spent many minutes completely silent. Occupational therapy and social service, as well as nursing, were all mobilized. In the course of several months she gradually left the bed and improved to the point where she could go to a rest home. While she was at all times carefully checked physically, she was given no opportunity to indulge her physical symptoms. In general the staff and all who had contact with her spoke casually of these ills and said, if the patient became insistent, she should talk with a specially selected doctor. He did not always examine her but was at all times entirely reassuring, and never indicated that anything was severely wrong. After a year and a half of this intensive regime, the patient had become largely self-supporting again and appeared to have given up the pattern of somatic complaints.

P. Hypo.	F:60:W:73	+3	31'24 968–(47)	4:5:18
P. React. Depr.		–3	13'2489–(51)	5:1:21
P. Hys.				
Deteriorated				

Nervousness, epigastric distress, and numerous other somatic complaints were the chief problems presented by this patient. Although "nervous and high-strung" since adolescence, the first of the present symptom patterns appeared following the menopause. The symptoms occurred episodically and could be relieved by sedation. At the time her son left home to attend college her symptoms became much worse. She then showed extreme meticulousness concerning her diet and developed constipation and insomnia. Forced to quit her job, she was unable even to do housework. In the years that followed she had numerous medical examinations and treatments with several hospital admissions.

Until her marriage at the age of 38 the patient had been a "career" woman. Born and educated in a small town, she was trained to be a dress designer and left home to follow this career. She worked in many cities, earned high wages, and was well liked by her employers. After marriage she settled down, but when her husband died she went to live with a sister who was a schoolteacher. She worked as a saleswoman in a small department store until the present illness became too acute for her. Above average in intelligence, she was active socially, made friends readily, and was described as neither aloof nor overly sensitive. However, she was always interested in herself and her activities with little genuine concern for others, except possibly her son. She was known as one who required considerable attention from others—at first from her mother, later from her husband, and finally from doctors, nurses, and friends.

The patient was markedly concerned with her somatic complaints. Her whole life now revolved about them, and all her conversation was ultimately brought to focus on them. She was nervous, trembled, cried, and sought attention, sympathy, and reassurance. Her insight was superficial. During several weeks of the hospitalization she apparently gained considerable relief, but closer study showed this to be partly illusory. A few minor hysterical episodes were noted. Dependent on the hospital routine, she objected strenuously to the suggestion of discharge; and since psychotherapy had been of little value and progress in gaining insight negligible, she almost had to be evicted. The core of her problem was her egocentricity. There was a possibility of some organic brain damage due to arteriosclerosis. On discharge there was little to be optimistic about, but it was hoped that she could make some sort of adjustment in the private rest home to which she was sent.

P. Mixed F:43:M:22 +1 31′26–9(51) 5:3:18
P. Hypo. —71 132′78–46(43) 6:3:16

Most of the patient's ills were of long duration. She had experienced headaches for 25 years, abdominal pain for 12 years (she had been diagnosed as having an ulcer one year before admission), and other less localized pain. The headaches usually persisted from one to two days and occasionally could be relieved by five anacin tablets if they were taken early enough. Nausea and vomiting frequently accompanied the headaches. No evidence of ulcer was established by X-ray and the diagnosis did not appear to be certain. For the past few years she had no longer been able to concentrate on her work and had withdrawn from her friends.

Her past health had been fair. She had managed her home satisfactorily and had displayed fair judgment and ability. Said to be stubborn and indecisive, she also had been, on the other hand, cheerful and a good mixer until the recent illness. About her sexual life she was vague, but apparently it was satisfactory. The marital adjustment and home conditions appeared to have been fair until recently, when financial insecurities arose.

The patient discussed her problem coherently but with obvious evasion. She did not talk freely about her personal affairs. She considered emotional factors to be without importance, and she flatly resisted all attempts to tie these in with her illness. She insisted that she was trying hard to cooperate in working through her problems, but that her "illness was real." She chatted and played games with the other patients and cooperated with the regular ward routine. Her attitude toward the doctor was characterized thus: "You are the doctor. You tell me what is wrong." She seemed to say, "I won't talk or give in, in this game." During her entire stay in the hospital no one was able to get through this attitude. She did not change much and was discharged; the staff felt little assurance that her future adjustment would improve.

P. React. Depr. F:43:M:4 +2 3′126–98 2:0:17

This patient's nervousness was expressed in trembling, ready excitability, and sensitiveness, all of which had been present for ten years. Insomnia also was persistent and she harbored feelings of guilt. Reporting that she had been "nervous" as long as she could remember, she first felt an extreme fear of committing "unpardonable sins and blasphemy against God" three years following her marriage (eight years before admission). This continued for three months and did not again appear until a year before admission. In the interim she was sensitive and cried readily.

Described as always sensitive, at an early age she had lost her appetite for days if she overheard an argument between her parents even though she might not be involved. When excited she "trembled all over." Religious trends were early apparent. When she was 8 years old, as a result of reading a Bible verse about eternal punishment, she worried about committing an "unpardonable sin." A conscientious and hard worker, she exercised good judgment. She had not been asocial but was limited in social expression. An example of her particular ethical-moral code was her belief that having sexual relations on Sunday was sinful.

Prominent in the patient's thinking was indecision about the advisability of hospitalization. She felt certain she had improved considerably before entering the hospital. She said little about her feelings of sin and was reluctant to discuss the subject. Her intelligence was average and she was emotionally labile. When her present illness was discussed she showed agitation. She attributed her difficulties to environmental pressures. In view of the fact that the patient had largely recovered from the present attack and that she had had in the past a succession of ups and downs, it was felt she would probably continue to get better after discharge but she was likely to have future troubles. The complete symptomatic picture was not clear because she had so nearly recovered at the time of admission. Few somatic complaints were revealed in the interviews although her history included a number of operations and repeated visits to various physicians.

P. Hypo. F:23:S:58 +10 31′2648–(66) 6:5:14
Schizoid

The admission complaints for this young woman centered around headaches, pain in her side, insomnia, fatigue, dizziness, and anorexia. Two years before admission the patient had had periods when, she said, "I felt as if I were doped." These lasted for several hours and recurred several times a month. At the same time she became dissatisfied with her job in a grocery store; also, a brother, whom the family regarded as "the pet," was called into the navy. As time went on other physical symptoms were added to the original pattern. Her home medical doctor suspected hyperthyroid and prescribed medications which gave no appreciable relief. Much of the time during this period she stayed in bed. Finally she was admitted to the general medical clinic of the hospital where extensive studies were made for systemic diseases, with negative findings.

Never as robust as other children, the patient had avoided strenuous activities and had suffered from "anemia." Her father was a tenant farmer and she had felt inferior because of the low social standing of the family in the community. Her father was frequently drunk. She made a "C" average in school and graduated from the eighth grade at 14. She did housework for five years, then clerked in a grocery store until the present illness appeared. She disliked the clerking job and felt unjustly treated by her employer. Described as always shy and retiring, she was dependent on others. Quiet entertainments such as reading and walking satisfied her. Although she often worked in the evening to earn extra money, she had no ambition for a higher level job than housework. She had never attempted to leave her home environment, although she had opportunities to do so.

Uppermost in the patient's mind were worry about her home condition and a shallow concern about her illness. She appeared to be only moderately depressed and was apathetic about future plans and ambitions. She remained convinced that she had an organic illness. Laconic in her answers during the examinations, she volunteered no additional information. Her appearance was neat and her manner pleasant. Physically she was inactive. During hospitalization she showed no marked improvement, although she did become a little more active. The complaints and the apathy seemed basically unchanged. Attempts were made to remove her from the home environment but these having failed, she was discharged as unimproved.

P. Hypo.	F:25:S:79	+30	31267'894–	7:4:17
P. Hys.		+58	31'27684–X	11:2:23
		+72	31'26784–X	12:3:25

The patient's chief complaints centered around weakness, depression, general lassitude, inability to walk, a tendency to cry, and numerous pains and aches which had gradually grown worse over a period of at least a year.

Although there had been few specific illnesses, the patient had never had good health, and she had had considerable medical attention, with several physicians recognizing her problems as chiefly functional. She had taken some training as a teacher but had not completed the course. She had worked as a clerk and had never demonstrated any steady ambition. A rather inadequate person, who under stresses had taken refuge in sickness, she was in general a socially outgoing person with a good many friends. The family background was very poor. The father had been a drunkard. At the time of admission the patient was contemplating marriage to a farm boy who came from a respected family, and she was troubled about the contrast between his family and her own. She was also bothered because she did not like the idea of farm life.

One of her most obvious characteristics in the hospital was a high degree of suggestibility. She was admitted in a wheel chair because she was "too weak to walk," and her heart was beating at such a rapid rate that she thought she was about to die. When she was told that she was well and able to walk, she got up with a little help and walked normally. For a while she insisted that she was too weak to do occupational therapy, but when she was told she was able to do it, she took it up and worked satisfactorily. Depressed and obviously afraid of the doctors, she was exceedingly reluctant to discuss her problems and always retreated into accounts of her physical symptoms. When pressed on pertinent points she said she was so weak that the interview would have to be continued later. Although she became active and eager to return home and to take up life in her community, the staff felt there had been no basic change. It was apparent that although she could make an institutional adjustment, she would not make an adequate adjustment to life situations.

P. Mixed F:22:S:56 +4 31′2684–9 9:4:22
Schizoid

Postprandial regurgitation, weakness, and numerous somatic disorders brought this patient to the hospital. The history included a variety of somatic complaints since early childhood. Typical of these were "stomach trouble, awful headaches, dizziness, fainting spells, drawing feelings in the shoulder and neck."

As indicated, the young woman had never been well, and she had had a long sequence of medical attentions. Recently she had become useless in her home and had abandoned household duties because of weakness, vomiting after meals (without loss of weight), and lassitude. Valedictorian of her high school class, the girl had been ambitious to train for missionary work. For three years after high school graduation, she had acted as a school librarian. She had always had rigid and unbending attitudes in religious matters. Her few friends attributed her high standing at school to an excellent memory but felt that she possessed little native intelligence. A daydreamer, she had been sensitive, conscientious, and a diligent worker, at the expense of completely neglecting outside activities. Described as unemotional, she had not cried at her mother's funeral, her friends remembered.

In the hospital the young woman appeared to be preoccupied with numerous somatic ailments, such as not being able to "keep food down" and "stomach pain." She felt that the psychiatric ward was the wrong place for her. Although she professed a deep interest in religion, her actual knowledge in that field was not extensive. Her intelligence was tested as average. Indifferent and unenthusiastic, she was abstracted in the examination, and her responses sounded shallow. Her ideas were usually poorly expressed and showed blocking, and it was difficult to comprehend her meaning. She was restless and uncomfortable. Her movements were slow and she leaned against the wall when walking. She was soft-spoken and passive. During her hospital stay, the patient changed little and attempts at hypnotherapy and other approaches proved unsuccessful. It was recommended, therefore, that she enter a state hospital on a voluntary basis. However, two weeks before discharge she became much more accessible and showed a slight amount of initiative. Her case was reconsidered and finally it was decided that she should return home, where she might make a borderline adjustment.

P. Hypo. F:39:S:60 +1 3′12687–9X(55) 11:4:14

The patient's illness began at least twelve years before admission, with the appearance of general weakness, backache, and vague abdominal complaints. When a physician told her she had arthritis, she quit her job, returned to her parents' farm, and restricted her activities. A few years later she became worse, and then she rarely went outdoors in the winter for fear the cold might increase the pain. In spite of many treatments for the arthritis, her symptoms did not change. These consisted chiefly of weakness, insomnia, anorexia, dizziness, palpitations, and generalized pain.

Apparently she had not been particularly hypochondriacal during her youth. At the end of the ninth grade she left school because "it was too hard" for her. She was considered a low average student. For a long while she had been employed at housework; then she took a machine operator's job in a mill and worked for five years without advancement. During the last few years, she said, this work had become too difficult for her. After the onset of the symptoms she did nothing except occasional light housework, and she was content to be dependent on relatives. A shy, quiet, and reserved person always, she had few interests. As far back as she could remember, she had become ill whenever she felt "unappreciated."

In the hospital the physical and neurological examinations failed to show objective evidences of arthritis to a degree justifying the patient's complaints. Her thoughts, however, were chiefly on the arthritis. There were no gross disturbances of sensorium or intellect with the exception of this pattern. Tests showed her to be low normal in intelligence. She showed no insight and was convinced that she had a special kind of arthritis. Seldom did she volunteer any information and she was definitely retarded in speech. Toward anyone who might question the validity of her complaints, she was suspicious. Although she was cooperative, she was always passively so. She took baths and did other routine tasks fearfully, certain that the arthritis would be aggravated. She dressed warmly and always protected herself from possible chill. The patient's rigidity on the subject of her complaints was so great that no approach was discovered by which she could be helped.

P. Hypo. F:31:M:23 +2 31′26874– 8:2:23
P. Hys.

This patient was admitted to the hospital with numerous somatic complaints; nervousness, irritability, and "blue spells" were also prominent. The present illness had become definite five or six years before admission, when she developed a sharp body-awareness. Refraining from mentioning the symptoms to her family, she carried on her household duties satisfactorily. The symptoms totaled more than twenty, ranging from "spells of laughing and crying at the same time" to "stuffiness in the nose." Her memory seemed poor when she felt "bad." In the last six months she had suffered steady lower abdominal pain and had sought medical aid for this but had been unable to benefit from the reassurance she received.

312748′6–9

During the patient's last two years in high school she had occasional spells of amblyopia. Other hysterical evidences were observed at that time. She seemed well adjusted socially, often organizing family picnics and managing and planning other activities. Her friends and her family viewed her as stable.

The patient presented her history in a spontaneous fashion. Her bodily complaints were vague and she did not accept the possibility that her problems were due to psychological factors. She dwelt on the lower abdominal pains and distress. She was pregnant at the time of admission and appeared not displeased at this. Although she expressed concern about the financial condition of her family, she said they would "get along somehow." She was the sort of person who "kept her troubles to herself," she said. She had little initiative and did not mingle with other patients. There seemed to be no deep depression. In view of the long history of borderline adjustment and the multiple complaints, little hope was held for real recovery. Psychotherapeutic aid consisted chiefly in attempting to help arrange family affairs to relieve the pressure on her. It was thought probable that as the pregnancy advanced the symptoms might be significantly relieved.

P. Mixed F:33:M:36 +1 312748′6–9 (39) 4:6:20
P. Psychas.

The patient had been partially deaf for about ten years before admission. This had been accompanied by tinnitus and a gradually developing fear and nervousness. Beginning with her first pregnancy, when the deafness appeared, she had experienced a fear of crowds and had lost confidence in herself. She had multiple domestic problems and a long list of physical complaints. She had a fear of insanity. At admission she wore a hearing aid which helped her considerably but she complained of extraneous sounds that aggravated her nervousness considerably.

Although she was extremely self-conscious at the time of admission, she had not clearly been so in the past. A college graduate, she had no outstanding physical or psychological difficulties in the college period. During the last few years she had shown a tendency to deride her husband for his mistakes and failures. She had not been interested in sports or hobbies but would occasionally attend a meeting if accompanied by her husband. The husband appeared to be inferior to her, and the marriage was not a happy one. They lived with his parents as unwanted guests, and this embarrassed the patient. She felt her husband was not "getting ahead" as fast as he should.

The patient was restless and showed a great deal of emotional tension, by wringing her hands almost continually, for example. Her stream of thought was logical. Frequently she managed to bring her complaints into the conversation whether it was related to them or not. She expressed the thought that she was insane and insisted that tests showing her to be intelligent were inaccurate. With continued hospitalization she began to relax, took a passive part in occupational therapy, and gradually increased her contacts with the staff and other patients. A careful study was made of her hearing problems and she was given help with the use of the hearing aid. On the day of discharge it was noted that her symptoms were still definitely present, although she was more cheerful and was looking forward to returning home. Since little could be done about the home situation, the prognosis was not favorable for a good adjustment.

P. Mixed Drug Add. F:34:M:17 +3 31′<u>27</u> <u>48</u> <u>69</u>– 4:4:22

The particular complaints that brought this patient into the hospital centered around pain, for which she was taking morphine. When her supply of the drug was depleted and she was not able to obtain more she voluntarily entered the hospital. The addiction had begun about three years earlier when she had had intense pain from abscesses in her ears. Hypodermic injections of a drug she did not identify were administered over a period of six to eight months. When the pain finally stopped, she decreased the injections but took more phenobarbital tablets. The abscesses returned and when in addition she began to experience "arthritic" stiffening of fingers and pain, her doctor again increased the doses of the drug. When an examination indicated no good basis for either the arthritic discomfort or the ear pain she tried to stop taking the drug but found it difficult and came to the hospital for help.

This patient had never been robust and had had many illnesses and treatments. At age 10 she suffered from an unknown illness that kept her in bed for three months. This illness followed a fright and was initiated by an aphonia. Following this she had a series of "pelvic abscesses" in which the main symptom was pain. When she was finally operated on for these and nothing was found, it was decided that the history of abscesses was "unreliable." In spite of this she later underwent abdominal surgery twice. In school she was apparently a good student in spite of her irregular attendance. After high school graduation she worked for six years as a telephone operator and eventually became the chief operator. She married a college graduate when she was 26 and lived happily with him on a farm. There were no sexual maladjustments. She was a neat, energetic, capable person.

A most cooperative patient, she showed no unusual behavior in the hospital. She was able to give up the drug with minimum symptoms and day by day she gained insight into her general personality problems. She was encouraged to stay longer for further re-education, but refused to do so and went home somewhat against advice. It was felt that there was no reason to expect that she would change radically in her home adjustment.

P. Mixed F:41:W:33 +2 '3127 64–9 (57) 3:3:20
Drug Add. —39 371'2468–9 3:2:20

Ten years before admission the patient's husband had suddenly died, leaving her to care for three children, all young, on a mother's pension. Because she could not leave the children to seek outside employment, the patient helped supplement the income by baking and selling pastries. Very depressed, she cried frequently, complained of dizziness, headache, and fatigue. For these complaints she had been seen in the psychiatric outpatient department as early as nine years before admission. One year before admission her sister-in-law, who had helped in the care of the children and who had been almost the sole confidante of the patient, had also died. After this the patient became more despondent and was finally forced to stop all work because of fatigue, nervousness, nausea, and vomiting. A few months before the present admission she had been admitted to the hospital for physical and laboratory studies. These all proved to be negative, and she was discharged with a diagnosis of neurasthenia. Somewhat later she was again seen in the outpatient department and was given a supply of phenobarbital; she began to concentrate the day's dosage in order to sleep at night. Two nights before admission the patient took three pills and sat waiting for her daughter to come home. When the daughter arrived the mother was asleep and could not be aroused. The following morning the patient awoke, asked for sleeping pills, and when she learned there were none in the house she sent the child for more. When the mother began taking them "by the handful," the children became alarmed and a physician was called.

The patient's past history, except for her problems in the past ten years, did not seem contributory. A quiet, pleasant person, she had always been industrious although not strong. She was average in intelligence. Content to stay at home with her children, she had few outside interests.

In the hospital the patient repeated over and over, "I don't want to live. Leave me alone." She repeated other morbid remarks also. After recovering from the drug intoxication she did not remember saying these things and she gave no indication of why she had taken the drugs. She was pleasant and cooperative but seemed interested in nothing but her children and how soon she could go home to them. There were no gross disturbances of sensorium or intellect. She entered into ward activities enthusiastically and at no time showed any abnormal behavior. The social service helped her plan more adequately for the future of the family.

P. Hypo. F:47:W:51 +19 31'27684–X 10:2:16

Among the patient's exceedingly varied complaints were tiredness, anorexia, difficulty in keeping warm, aches in her abdomen, numbness in her extremities, and weight loss. She had first noted the symptoms in a mild degree about three years before admission at the time of her second husband's death, to which she had greatly overreacted. Six months later when she went to live with a sister, she had lost seventy pounds, had become very irritable, and had refused to work on the basis that she was too weak. She gradually limited her diet until at the time of admission she was taking only fluids. She spent the greater part of her time in bed. First admitted to the gynecology service for studies regarding the possibility of malignancy of the corpus uteri, she was transferred to psychiatry because she was a severe feeding problem.

She had been in good health previously. An eighth-grade graduate, she had made a good scholastic record and had worked as a dry goods clerk until she had married at age 19. Even after her marriage she had continued to work and was a very successful fur saleswoman. When she was 23 her husband died of tuberculosis, and two years later she remarried. The death of her first husband, and later the death of a crippled child by that husband, had not affected her nearly as much as the death of her second husband. An ambitious, intelligent, impatient, selfish, energetic, sociable, narcissistic person, she preferred active competition to the relatively calm life of a housewife. She had always been finicky about food. Although she was highly paid, she had been unable to save money, spending it for personal adornment and for pleasure. Apparently she was a shallow person with labile emotions.

The physical studies failed to show any pathology, but she was greatly disturbed about her physical condition, describing her somatic complaints in great detail. She thought that her irritability and conduct in her sister's home should be excused on the basis of her physical illness. "They can't expect a poor sick girl like me to do things right," she commented. She was troubled about the possibility of going to a state hospital: "You can't send a person to the state hospital if they're not crazy, can you, doctor? I'm not crazy, am I, doctor? I know just exactly what you intend to do. You can't fool me. You might as well come right out and tell me." There were no other obvious delusions, and her sensorium and intellect were clear. She was reserved with the examiner, apparently feeling that anything she said might be used as evidence for committing her to a state hospital, and she resisted any suggestion that her somatic complaints were linked with psychological factors. She was unusually careful about her food, but when she was faced with the prospect of tube feeding she made no more trouble about eating. There was no improvement in the hospital, and after some social adjustments had been made, she was discharged to try to live with her sister for a while.

P. Mixed	F:44:M:81	+31	31276′84–X (55)	10:9:16
P. Mixed	F:45:M:98	+28	213784′6–9 (53)	9:12:18

When the patient was first admitted to the medical service of the hospital for severe bronchial asthma of two weeks' duration, there was cyanosis of the lips and finger tips and other evidences of the disorder, but therapy for the asthma was difficult because she had mild cardiac damage. With such therapy as could be undertaken she improved, but when she complained of not sleeping well and became irritable and restless, she was transferred to the psychiatric service. The asthma attacks had begun with an upper respiratory infection nine years before the present episode, and they had gradually become more severe, particularly after the death of her only son. At that time hospitalization had been necessary.

Her previous physical health had been good, and there was no history of a neuropsychiatric disorder before. A high school graduate, she had married immediately after graduation and had never worked outside of her home. Her home life as a child and as an adult had been very congenial. A quiet retiring person with a limited social life, she was somewhat secretive and emotionally unstable, but before the present illness she had apparently led a fairly average life. She had been active in church activities.

In addition to the asthmatic problem the patient was exceedingly troubled about her son's illness and death. Although she was somewhat retarded, she was well oriented and intact in sensorium and intellect. She was depressed, irritable, and indifferent. She had partial insight in that she felt that her emotional problems contributed to some extent to her asthmatic attacks, and with help toward greater insight she began to do well without medication for her asthma. During her six weeks' stay on the psychiatric service, she had only a few minor attacks and one severe attack. On discharge she was greatly improved and was grateful for what had been done for her. If the environment was controlled so that she would experience a minimum of strain, the prognosis was considered good.

P. React. Depr. F:43:M:37 +20 312'78–9 2:6:11

This patient feared insanity. She complained of irritability, restlessness, feelings of tension, insomnia, and emotional depression. She was anorexic. Two years earlier she had suffered from an attack of "flu" and afterward had become emotionally disturbed, with tension, restlessness, insomnia, and loss of appetite. This depression responded promptly to two days of hospitalization, but she remained bedridden for a long time. A good period followed but shortly before admission she had again become depressed. There were multiple somatic difficulties and general weakness. The fear of insanity was expressed in the statement, "I can never be any better. I should do away with myself and not be a burden on my family."

She had always shown good common sense, had learned easily, and had been an unusually competent manager. She accepted responsibility and did her work seriously; in fact, she was noted for expecting from herself a high level of accomplishment. She met people easily and made a moderate number of warm social contacts. Regarding all signs of emotional display as weakness, she was careful at all times to keep herself under control. She had never been keenly interested in housework or feminine pursuits and had always wished she were a man. The reactive factors in the present symptoms were related chiefly to the marital and the filial situations. Her husband was an alcoholic and otherwise irresponsible. In addition her daughter showed irresponsibility and had made what her mother considered a poor marriage.

In the hospital the patient's complaints centered around a backache, and in addition, she objected to hospital routine, was dissatisfied with her room, and showed resentment toward everything and everybody. She appeared depressed. Willing to accept the suggestion that her family troubles had brought on some of the symptoms, she nevertheless felt certain that she had a somatic disorder. She held her body rigid and insisted that she was too weak to walk; she also protested that she had no appetite. Resentful toward the examiner, her greeting to him each morning was, "What are you going to bawl me out for now?" As time went on she gained weight, seemed more cheerful and less tense. She was encouraged to make more definite plans and to clarify for herself her thoughts about the home situation. At discharge it was felt she would make a satisfactory adjustment.

P. Hys. F:18:S:63 +20 312′784–9 5:2:13

The patient was admitted to the hospital because of a continual tremor of the right arm, which was exaggerated whenever she attempted to perform voluntary movements and which disappeared during sleep. The tremor, of ten days' duration, had appeared following a violent quarrel between two of her brothers. She had had several previous attacks of the same type, of brief duration.

At age 9, after the patient had been seduced by a neighbor boy who infected her with gonorrhea, she had been sent for two years to a school for girls under the guardianship of the state. Two years before admission she claimed to have been assaulted by a patient from an institution near her sister's farm, but the exact truth of that episode could not be determined. About that time she became very attached to an older woman who gave her clothes and with whom she exchanged many caresses. The patient was a physically attractive, apparently normal girl who had led a moderately adequate social life and who was of average intelligence.

No physical or neurological findings were pertinent. Other than the tremor, which she could not explain, she had no complaints, but she showed a great deal of emotional lability and frequently was unable to talk because of excessive blocking. When not being interviewed about her troubles, she appeared entirely normal and was active in ward activities and social interchange. After some preliminary investigation, deep suggestive therapy was instituted and she was told that she would have a dream in which the cause of her difficulty would be apparent. The dream occurred on the night that it was suggested and its contents were the quarrel between her brothers, the feelings of tension at home, and pains relating to the menstrual period. After some little time she had a night in which she tossed violently in bed and could not be quieted. There were clonic movements of the extremities and facial grimaces. Under deep suggestive therapy she stated that these were the result of her attempt to avoid masturbation. After these problems had been gone over with her she was discharged free of symptoms with a fairly good prognosis.

$312\underline{78}4'6–9$

The patient was married soon after her discharge from the hospital and was seen in another state about two years later. At that time she had one child and said that she had been free from symptoms and entirely well since leaving the hospital.

P. Hypo.	F:17:S:49	+25	$312\underline{78}4'6–9$	3:5:15
P. React. Depr.		+46	$3\underline{21}'76\underline{48}–9$	5:3:14
P. Hys.				
P. Mixed	F:24:M:33	?	283764'1–9 (63)	5:8:7

Depression, anxiety, and emotional instability were the complaints of this young woman on admission. Nine months earlier she had contracted an upper respiratory infection with characteristic symptoms, which later more or less subsided except for a continuing cough. At this time the patient developed abdominal pain. First experienced while she was in school, this pain had a sudden onset and was "sharp and knifelike." She was excused to go to the rest room where she "fainted" and was unconscious for fifteen or twenty minutes. The pain was sharp and continuous for two weeks, then gradually assumed a dull character with intermittent exacerbations persisting to the date of admission. There was also anuria for two and a half days, following which she experienced burning on micturition, dysmenorrhea, and a ten-pound weight loss.

Described by herself as having always been "weak and frail," the patient had never been able to play with other children because of fatigue. Her childhood diseases included poliomyelitis and nephritis. She had skipped the second and fourth grades and had completed two years of high school at the age of 17. Of normal intelligence, she made the honor roll occasionally and enjoyed school, taking an active part in all events. She liked sports, sewing, and reading, had many friends of both sexes, and apparently led a normal social life. She had not shown undue interest in health as far as others could tell, although she was described as having been a "finicky" child and she became easily upset if spoken to harshly.

At the time of admission to the hospital no pertinent physical findings could be elicited although extensive studies were made. She was preoccupied with the traumatic experience of pain and fainting. She appeared intact in mentation and orientation and was emotionally somewhat labile, particularly so when discussion was turned toward personal matters. She had almost no insight at first. She was neat in appearance and made a good adjustment on the ward. By the time of discharge she had verbal insight into her condition and the symptoms had completely disappeared. Because of her immaturity and the many unresolved difficulties, it was felt likely that there would be a recurrence of the pattern.

Seven years later she was readmitted with the same complaint pattern. She dated these symptoms from the first admission when, she said, she had felt that life was not worth living. Married a year after the first admission, she now had two children. The marriage had seemed successful at first, but the relationship deteriorated and the husband accused her of being sexually frigid and unresponsive. She in turn accused him of mistreatment and jealousy. She became preoccupied with sexual matters and said that she "had things to tell." There were innumerable physical complaints. Her illness and emotional troubles were uppermost in her mind. Even more clearly than when first seen, she was an immature and unstable person, occupied with numerous sexual conflicts. She was inclined to project her maladjustment onto her husband whose treatment of her was "brutal and inconsiderate." She demanded special treatment in the hospital and repeatedly said that she "could not discuss things" until she had "just the right doctor." Eventually she described sexual behavior with an older brother-in-law. She repressed her guilt over this; but when the brother-in-law began to repeat the behavior with her daughter, the symptoms suddenly increased in severity. She also described her inability to experience satisfactory sexual relations with her husband and expressed marked guilt that she preferred stimulation of the clitoris to sexual intercourse. With reassurance about these matters and after a thorough discussion of them, she was much relieved and the hostility toward her husband decreased. She was again discharged, this time with marked improvement but with the prognosis still uncertain.

P. Mixed F:47:M:28 +4 312'7849– 5:2:13

On admission to the hospital this patient complained of nervousness, insomnia, and headache. Well until six months earlier when her husband was called to duty in the National Guard, she then became ill and gradually the complaints increased in severity. A factor in her illness was the presence in the home of a 79-year-old psychotic mother-in-law, who was most difficult to care for. The patient could hire no one to help her because people in the small community were afraid of the mother-in-law.

As a child the patient had hoped to become a schoolteacher, but even then she had felt that she was "too nervous" for this type of work. Following graduation from high school she became a clerk until her marriage. An outgoing, sociable individual, she was active in lodge and church work. After her marriage she occasionally worked as a saleswoman or demonstrated household articles. She had always been high-strung and had considered herself frail. Her marriage appeared to be a good one, and there was one son who was 25 at the time the patient entered the hospital. Her medical history included a succession of surgical procedures.

In the hospital the patient presented multiple somatic complaints. She occasionally wept during interviews and was obviously depressed. She recognized that her present upset as well as the two previous ones were in some way psychogenic. She slept poorly and held herself tense; there was a definite tremor. As days passed she adjusted well to ward life and was a cooperative patient. She had the preconceived idea that a period of rest was all that was necessary for her to recover, and she was, therefore, courteously but positively resistive to therapeutic suggestion. She showed a desire to be advised to discontinue her social activities and to simplify her home life. This was one example of her polite but definite attempt to determine her own treatment and the general conduct of her hospitalization. She was not, however, a difficult patient in the usual sense of the word. She improved remarkably during hospitalization and at discharge was fairly well. Naturally, in view of the repeated depressions, it seemed likely that she would develop another one in the future.

P. Hypo. F:45:M:48 —34 3<u>12</u>786′4–9 8:2:15

The symptoms of this patient had appeared during the three months preceding admission, when she had become weaker, had had vague illnesses characterized chiefly by diarrhea, and had had a slight intermittent fever. She had become bedridden and had developed a number of other somatic complaints that finally came to involve almost all her bodily systems. This pattern had actually been present in a milder degree for a number of years, during which she had visited many clinics and a diagnosis of psychoneurosis had been made more than once. There had been, however, no clear psychotic upsets.

In the middle of the second year of high school she left to work as a clerk in a store. However, for ten years before admission she had been unable to work because of her physical complaints. During much of this time a mother's pension supported her, but when it was discontinued she had to be supported by her parents and by her children. Energetic and active when she liked things, her enthusiasm always broke down under adversity. As a child she had been stubborn and had had temper tantrums. Her marriage, which had occurred when she was 23, was an unhappy one. Her husband, who appeared to have been a shiftless person, had once been convicted of forgery. Eventually he left the patient and had not been heard of since. There were three children, two boys living and well at the time of the patient's admission. She had tried hard to give her boys a "good bringing-up."

In the hospital she voiced numerous complaints and worried that she might have a serious organic disorder. There were no real breaks with reality and she appeared intact intellectually. She was anxious, talked willingly, and answered questions loquaciously. Her conversation always centered around her somatic symptoms. She claimed to be unable to get out of bed because of weakness, and the slightest exertion accentuated her discomfort. Querulous and fretful, she showed no response to reassurance. Gradually she became somewhat better, gained weight, and finally moved around the ward, although she never became at all spontaneous in her activities. Slowly she began to show interest in leaving the hospital. The illness appeared to be deep-seated and there was not much probability that she would make an adequate adjustment. She finally returned home to try to live with her mother and an unmarried son, with follow-up interviews in the outpatient department for psychological support.

P. Hys. F:21:S:55 +4 3127′9486– 5:4:16
+24 3′21 796–4 1:4:9

This young woman came to the hospital with a two-year history of attacks of a peculiar nature. In the first one she suddenly fell to the floor, bit her tongue and wrist, and made numerous violent and purposeless movements. Similar attacks followed, frequently lasting as long as an hour and a half. In the latter part of this period the patient would be noncommunicative and resistive. She also complained of dysmenorrhea; the first attack followed a hysterectomy. There were other symptoms, a number of which appeared to be allergic in type.

Before the present illness the patient had been active socially, had had many friends, and had been considered a good worker. In the last three years she had become somewhat self-conscious, possibly because of extensive pelvic surgery which had kept her from social activity. She was employed as a stenographer. No particular event could be discovered which correlated with the onset of the symptoms. The convulsive attacks were not the earliest symptoms, but they followed a pattern of gradually increasing somatic complaints.

The examinations revealed no neurological findings that indicated organic involvement of the nervous system, and it was felt that the attacks were almost certainly hysterical in nature. When moved to the psychiatric ward, she was resentful and at first refused cooperation with nurses or doctors. Except for this she was complacent and apparently not much affected emotionally by her condition or problems. Seizures occurred if she was crossed. She became much better without special therapy and when finally discharged appeared to have a fair chance of making a good adjustment.

P. Hypo. F:44:S:74 ? 3128476′–9(49) 7:5:19
Paranoid

The patient had had multiple complaints of aches and pains since childhood. Particularly she had complained of weakness and inability to work. Actually her physical health had been fair. During one period she was treated for tuberculosis, but this had been arrested six years before admission. She had had at least three major operations, and there had been two short psychotic episodes in which she had experienced bizarre hallucinations and paranoid delusions.

She was dull normal intellectually but had completed the eighth grade at age 14. She worked on her parents' farm until she was 20 and then gradually assumed the role of a chronic invalid who did very little housework and merely did needle work in a dilatory fashion. She was rejected by her family and had always been shy and sensitive. She was unaggressive, dependent, and insecure. Apparently there was complete sexual suppression.

In the hospital the physical and neurological examinations were negative in spite of the numerous physical complaints. The patient was primarily concerned with these somatic disturbances, which she would describe in great detail. She showed marked antipathy toward members of her family and said that she was disturbed by their use of alcohol which she herself had strong convictions against. She felt that she was hated by her entire family. (This seemed, under the circumstances, not to be a delusion.) She wanted aid in getting away from the family and she wanted to be "cured physically" so that she could do productive work on her own. When discussing her family she would forget her physical complaints and would show evidences of adequate affect. Electroshock treatment was begun after other attempts to help her had seemed ineffectual. She did not respond much to these treatments either, but she did make a better adjustment in the hospital. As the time came for her to be discharged she returned to her old hypochondriacal routine. She left the hospital to live with her brother for a while as a trial, and it was decided that if she could not adjust she should go to a state hospital.

P. Hys. — M:33:M:7 — +2 — 312'8674- — 9:3:25
Alcoholism

On admission the patient complained of nervousness and of hand tremors which had begun three months earlier, three weeks after he had obtained a job as a truck driver. The tremors had rapidly become so severe that he had been forced to give up the job. On the day of admission he was unable to write his name. He dated his general nervousness from eight years before, when he had been treated for a goiter. Since then he had had spells of nervousness, irritability, and sleeplessness. Some of these periods lasted two or three weeks.

This man had always lived on farms. After completing the eighth grade, he was too restless to remain longer in school. His work history was not steady; he had held numerous jobs, all at the unskilled or semiskilled level. He was considered cheerful, cooperative, and easy to get along with. Disliking and avoiding responsibility, he showed restlessness whenever it was forced on him. For a year he had drunk heavily, and once he had served a thirty-day jail sentence for intoxication. His marriage had been a forced one. There were two children and the family was frequently on relief.

In the hospital the physical examinations revealed no pertinent findings. The psychological findings also were few. The patient's intelligence was below average. He was quiet and seemingly cooperative, but his resistance to staying in the hospital, it was believed, resulted in a partial suppression of some of the symptoms. The hand tremors disappeared soon after admission and he began to talk of going home. Finally he was allowed to leave before completion of a really adequate study. There seemed to be no reason to expect a significant change in this patient's behavior in the future.

P. Anxiety State — F:42:M:54 — +2 — 312'86749-(71) — 4:3:21

P. Mixed — F:42:M:82 — +2 — 3781269'4-(55) — 3:3:21

This woman's complaints, nervousness, weakness, crying spells, and general anxiety, had been present for about six months. In general her health had been good before the onset of the present illness, although until a year before admission she had been diagnosed as having a toxic thyroid. Neither treatment nor two operations had relieved the symptoms of this disorder, tremor and tachycardia. After the operations she had shown clearly hysterical symptoms.

At the end of the eighth grade, when she was 12, the patient left school. Then she worked on a farm at a man's job. After her marriage she continued to do much of the work and also managed the farm. Active in P.T.A. and church groups, she appeared at ease with others. She often gave parties for the youngsters in her vicinity, with whom she was popular, and she derived much pleasure in preparing for them. Her husband was described as a "weak" individual but their marital adjustment appeared to be reasonably good.

In the hospital although the patient talked freely and appeared to be cheerful and cooperative, she was not at all amenable to a realistic discussion of her problems and of the future. She showed some clearly hysterical avoidance reactions, refusing to read the newspapers, for example, because they distressed her. All her troubles she attributed to the thyroid condition. Her I.Q. was found to be about 120. At first she had frequent crying spells but these gradually disappeared. The present illness had apparently been caused by the restriction of her activities, due to the goiter, which contrasted with her previously happy and active life. At discharge it was thought that she would make a good adjustment. One year later she was readmitted with a new exacerbation of the symptom pattern. During this second hospitalization she looked at her problems more realistically and finally decided that she should leave her husband. Specific help was given to her in finding a new home and a job, and by the time of discharge she was again apparently well. This time it appeared even more likely that she would hold her own since she had made realistic plans.

P. Hypo.	F:33:M:58	+17	31286′79–	9:4:18
		+59	13268′79–	12:3:18
P. Hypo.	F:41:M:32	+1	13′2689–(49)	4:0:11

The primary complaints of this patient were lower abdominal pain, urinary urgency and frequency, vomiting, nausea, and dyspepsia. She dated the symptoms from a difficult labor which had resulted in the stillbirth of a premature infant. The patient had been examined in the outpatient clinic a number of times after this, but no adequate somatic explanation for the persistent pain had been found. A physician had recommended surgery for the removal of her "female organs," but this had not been performed.

The patient's childhood had been relatively uneventful. After completing the eighth grade at age 13, she worked on the family farm until she was married at 19. This husband died after two years, leaving her with a child. A year and a half later she married her present husband, a war veteran who was disabled psychologically and was considered a "queer" individual by the community. As the patient became aware of his strangeness, she became reluctant to appear in public with him. They had five children, all of whom appeared to be well adjusted. The patient had always been an energetic, happy person, ready to make the best of any situation. While she had never shown marked ambition, she had exercised good judgment and had met her problems in a direct and aggressive manner. Known to be somewhat egocentric, she did not, however, disregard the rights or feelings of others.

In the hospital she discussed her ills in detail, and she complained bitterly of the abdominal pain and of gas associated with belching and crampy pains. In addition she wished to remain in bed because of weakness. Emotionally she appeared depressed. She paid little attention to her personal appearance and took no interest in ward life. Although fairly cooperative in the examinations, she expressed resentment at any suggestion that there was a psychological background for her problems. In spite of gaining some insight into her condition she clung to the belief that her pains had an organic basis. The pains, however, did decrease in intensity. Not markedly better at the time of discharge, she returned to the hospital seven years later in almost the same condition. The course of the second episode followed closely that of the first.

P. Hypo. M:19:S:58 +1 31′2876–9 (47) 6:3:24
Schizoid

The presenting complaints of this patient were a feeling of fullness in his head and easy fatigability. Five months before admission he awoke one morning with what he called "fullness in the head." Three days before this he had become so fatigued at work that he had fallen asleep over his shovel, and during the following few days he had been more tired than usual. He sought medical attention and was treated, but without relief. Forced to quit work, he was finally admitted to the hospital.

At school the patient had had little trouble in learning but much difficulty in getting along with his classmates. Too shy to be a leader, he had always remained in the background and had made few friends. He dreaded talking in front of the class and refused to play baseball on the school team because he feared appearing before a crowd. At 16 he left school to work on a farm and remained there until the present symptoms appeared. Girls had not interested him and he had never gone out on a date. His ambition had always been to buy a farm with his brother and to run it in partnership. His interests outside of farming were few. He liked to sit alone and read fiction or just daydream.

In the hospital he expressed a desire to get well and go back to work. He said he felt strong enough to work in spite of his headaches and the feeling of fullness in his head. These would be all right, he thought, "if I don't work as hard as I did before." He wanted to stay out of the army and believed his work would exempt him. During the interview he was complacent but intense. He twisted his handkerchief, blushed, sweat, and avoided looking at the examiner.

Improvement was made slowly in the symptomatology but the patient remained shy and retiring. Although cooperative, he rarely took part in the affairs of the ward. He complained of intermittent and shifting abdominal pain. At his discharge instructions were given to his family to increase his social contacts. Although he was much better and he was able to go back to light work, it was felt that he might develop a more serious disorder later.

B. Simple Adult Maladj. F:27:M:45 +10 31′29 46–8 7:1:14
Paranoid
Suicidal

This patient was admitted to the hospital on a court order because of an emotional outburst in which she struck her husband and threatened suicide. She also had many bodily complaints. A year before admission four members of her husband's family had come to live with them, and about the same time the patient had become pregnant with her third child. Since then she had been emotionally very volatile and bitter toward her husband. No matter how fierce the rages, she had been able to keep her control in the presence of strangers until the last few weeks. At first she was depressed only periodically, but then this became her prevailing mood and she felt her situation was hopeless. She made impulsive suicidal gestures. She experienced continual pains in her head and over her heart and paresthesias, nausea, and vomiting, and she took heavy doses of sodium amytal.

The patient was of an average intellectual and social level. Her parents had been easygoing and unwisely lenient with their children. Her mother was known as a neurotic and this was supposed to "run in her family." The patient was thought to have poor judgment and to be inordinately proud and ambitious. She blamed her husband for everything that happened, even though her own work was spasmodic and ineffectual. Stubborn and self-centered, she belittled those about her and demanded her own way. She also boasted of an ungovernable temper. She was suspicious of others and clung to unreasonable grudges.

An attractive woman in appearance, the patient was sulky, sarcastic, and haughty in attitude and manner, and she antagonized other patients and ridiculed the staff. "I'm not crazy but I will be if I'm locked up here with these screwballs," she said. Her contact with reality was poor. No definite paranoid trends were noted, although she believed that her family and the welfare board were unjustly siding with her husband. "But just because I can't get along with my husband doesn't mean I'm crazy. Now that I'm here I can't get custody of the children if I do want a divorce." Minimizing her faults, she denied many of the facts furnished by others. She admitted many physical complaints but did not demand attention for them, since she attributed them to her general run-down condition. With time her manner became less egocentric and suspicious but she still was irate over the fact that the court had ordered her to be held. Her more paranoid reactions did not change until she realized that she was likely to prejudice her examiners, whereupon her manner became much more guarded. It was decided that she could try a home adjustment again but there was little expectation that she would be able to make the grade.

P. Hypo.	F:35:D:111	+9	31'297–	4:5:14
P. React. Depr.		+63	3'79148–6	6:3:14

The principal symptoms in this patient's illness were nervousness, depression, fear of insanity, an amnesic episode, and various somatic ills. The initial symptoms had appeared two months before admission when she had had to leave a temporary position because of nausea, dizziness, and a lump in her throat. The fear of insanity appeared when she noted that her memory for events of the past year was somewhat impaired. She first discovered the memory loss following a series of electroshock treatments, and concurrently a more marked depression with suicide thoughts developed.

Fairly well until about age 20, the patient then began to have severe back and side pains which came and went and forced her to leave a number of jobs. During the subsequent years she had many attacks of pain and other symptoms, and she underwent several major operations in a fruitless effort to find relief. Of average intelligence and with fair judgment in managing her affairs, she had completed the sophomore year of high school and had been a very good student. She was interested in sports, music, and reading. Apparently at ease with people, she was friendly, kind, and thoughtful. During her illnesses she showed a marked dependence on her sister and her mother. She was considered to be religious but not extremely so. She was said to be very stubborn occasionally. A competent stenographer, she had an occupational history which showed enormous irregularity because of her many illnesses. In general there was a tendency for the acute symptoms to be related to events in her environment. For example, after her father, a deaf-mute, was accidentally killed when she was 14, she showed a severe reaction. Her first definite illness, however, occurred about a year following her mother's marriage to a man the patient disliked. The patient's own marriage at age 28 was unsuccessful and ended in divorce. This was trying for the patient since she had desired and hoped for a reconciliation. During her illnesses her family devoted much attention to her.

When admitted to the hospital she was mainly concerned with her symptomatic picture. Rather distant during interviews, she made evasive answers, and at times tears welled up in her eyes although she did not actually cry. She admitted to being depressed and complained bitterly of headaches and dizziness. She said she knew that her trouble was "mental," but this appeared to be shallow insight at best. She got along well with other patients and was cooperative, although she expressed a dislike for the hospital. She made fair progress and most of the symptoms disappeared, but she never admitted that she felt good. When discharged she was at least back to her usual level of behavior.

Ps. M-D., Depr. F:54:M:23 +1 3'<u>14</u>2<u>679</u>-(51) 6:1:15
P. Hys.

The presenting complaints of this patient were nervousness, excitability, and irritability. These symptoms had appeared about nine months earlier when the family had moved into a large, gloomy house on a small farm.

Thin and sickly as a child, the patient had undergone a number of extensive surgical operations. She had also had previous depressions and during one of these she had been admitted to a state hospital. She described herself as bashful, timid, and terrified of the dark when she was a child. She had many friends and had always been happy until the onset of her first depression. She thought of herself as homeloving and wanting a secure and stable home more than anything. At 17 she had wanted to marry but her father had refused to give his permission and she was not married until she was 28. Her marriage and home life were happy.

The patient was of low normal intelligence and was well oriented. She exhibited emotional shifts during each interview but without any real outbreaks of emotion, and she was voluble and cooperative. She recognized that something was wrong with her but was unable to describe what she thought about it. She expressed worries about conditions at home. A few days after admission she no longer appeared depressed. This quick recovery indicated that reactive factors might be important. At discharge she seemed well and was eager to return home. It was felt probable that she would have other attacks.

P. React. Depr. F:35:M:19 +1 31'42<u>679</u>-(41) 6:6:11
B. Psth., Asocial
Suicidal

The patient was forced to enter the hospital by her family because of suicide attempts and because she was pressing for a divorce. She said that for fifteen years she had been dissatisfied with her husband's restrictions of her social activity. During the past two years she had become more depressed and also tired and irritable; her husband reported that she spent many hours gazing into space. One month she visited relatives in another state. There she associated with a man she knew little about. The two engaged in sexual intercourse several times and exchanged letters when she returned home. She asked her husband's permission to return to visit the man; he refused and she became depressed and made three unsuccessful suicide attempts. She subsequently refused to sleep with her husband and was very "cold" in everyday relations with him.

Her general health had always been poor, requiring almost continuous medical attention for multiple complaints. She completed the eighth grade and left school to do housework. Hoping to achieve a higher social level, she attended social and community functions. Recently, however, her social activities had been limited to close friends and relatives, and she began to indulge moderately in alcoholic beverages. Her husband was 41 and had asthma. There were six children. Of average intelligence, she was described as cheerful and happy before the development of the present problem.

31'42789–

In the hospital she was preoccupied with thoughts of divorce and concern about the future of her children and herself. At times she appeared somewhat depressed but was usually cheerful and happy. She had objected strenuously to being placed in a psychopathic ward, but once there she was quiet and cooperative. There was no clear explanation of her sudden change in the past two years, for although the marriage had never been successful she had previously made a fair adjustment. It was possible that the situation represented a mild manic episode. Psychotherapeutic measures involved chiefly aid in resolving her problems. Little real progress was made but she did have foresight and felt a responsibility toward her children and her home. Some hope was held, therefore, that with continued outpatient treatment she might make a satisfactory recovery.

P. Hypo. F:45:D:63 +5 31'42789– 3:7:16
P. Hys.

The somatic complaints of this woman included dull back pain (for twenty years), headaches, weakness, and fatigue. Not long before admission, the patient had experienced what she called "ptomaine poisoning." Following a meal she felt a full, aching pain over her entire thorax, her shoulders, and her neck, and since then she had had infrequent but regular spells of dizziness, usually associated with emotional upsets. She also complained of amnesic episodes in which "things went black" and in which, she said, "I did not know where I was or what I was doing." She developed a peculiar to and fro gait which disappeared if someone walked with her.

There was a history of three major operations and a peptic ulcer at age 25. No obvious symptoms had followed these episodes. She had an abnormal appetite and she said she was "always hungry, even after a heavy meal."

The patient had wanted to be a nurse, and she had done well in school but had not continued beyond the eighth grade. Before her marriage she had had a boy friend with whom she had had sexual intercourse. After the breakup of this "romance," she hated the boy and wanted to kill him. At 29 she married a war veteran who was still married during the first month of their courtship. He was extreme in his sexual demands and when she refused him he became irritable and sometimes struck her. He was lazy and shiftless and did not take care of their farm. The family lived in poverty. After three years the patient sued for a divorce, charging mental cruelty. There were two children. Next she lived with a brother until a sister moved in and "won my brother's affection." Four months before admission her brother had told her to leave his farm. She had since supported herself and her two children on $35 a month. Of a pleasant disposition, she was shy but made friends readily. She had average intelligence. She made a special point of disliking people with "dirty minds." She was sensitive about discussing her sexual troubles.

In the hospital the patient's thoughts, especially when she was depressed, centered around her early sex life, the failure of her marriage, and the puzzling behavior of her favorite brother. Accepting the possibility that her past history might have contributed to her somatic complaints, she nevertheless believed there was a real physical ailment. She was changeable in mood and reluctant to discuss her psychological problem. When depressed, she cried and remained in bed, but at other times she was very cheerful. Gradually she became more accessible, was helped by sedatives and reassurance, and gained a measure of insight into the source of her problems. However, the economic situation appeared to be insurmountable, and this precluded the possibility of a good adjustment. She was considerably better at discharge.

P. Hypo. F:43:D:107 +17 31427896′– 4:7:16
Ps. M-D., Manic
B. Psth., Mixed

"Sinking spells," with palpitations, frontal headaches, insomnia, and tenseness, were the chief presenting complaints of this patient. She had enjoyed good health until five years before admission when she had had her first "nervous breakdown." She was then the manager of a store and also operated a restaurant. At this period she was very successful. However, a few weeks after the opening of the restaurant, one night she suddenly experienced vertigo and became "panicky." This was followed by despair, loneliness, malaise, and insomnia. With psychiatric aid she recovered. About two years later her fiancé committed suicide and this brought on another bout of symptoms, from which she again recovered. From the original breakdown until the time of admission she experienced a series of ups and downs, and she gradually was reduced to working as a clerk. While in the latter job she fainted, was taken to the hospital, and was admitted to the psychiatric ward. She had divorced her husband before the onset of the present illness. During one period her earnings had more than doubled his.

Always a driving, ambitious individual, the patient's interests were uniquely centered in her work and she admired only financially and socially successful people. She enjoyed knowing and being recognized by "celebrities." For her work she sacrificed home and children whenever there was a choice. She felt that she compensated for the neglect of her children by providing them with material things. Up to the present illness she had been cheerful and optimistic and proud of her reputation for honesty and business success. Her social concepts were conventional. Throughout her marriage she had experienced frigidity.

In the hospital she had numerous somatic complaints, and one wondered how much these were a demand for attention rather than real physical discomforts. She was concerned about her loss of eminence and authority and considered herself a failure. She did not despair, however; she believed that if she could overcome the present illness she could regain her former status. Confinement in the mental ward was to her a "stigma." Her general appearance showed a slight degree of anxiety but her prevalent expression was euphoric. It was only when the patient was not occupied that her anxiety became apparent. Her clothing reflected poor taste and she was often careless in her dress. In the hospital she attempted on numerous occasions to display her authority by making brusque and insulting remarks to the nurses. Her case provided a great deal of difficulty from a diagnostic standpoint. Much of her behavior was hypomanic, when, for example, she led parties or other social activities on the ward. At other times obvious anxiety and depression made her appear a very different person. She derived benefit from sedation and other routine hospitalization procedures but was relatively resistant to psychotherapeutic approaches, her usual response being that she could handle her life if she could just get over her illness. She was improved when discharged but was not considered well.

P. Hypo. F:37:M:19 +8 '3142<u>8</u>-6 7:5:22

The patient had complained of headaches, weakness, pain in the abdomen and numerous other somatic symptoms for several months. A week before admission she had become acutely ill and had been admitted to the medical service, where a diagnosis of upper respiratory infection was made. When she recovered from this she still had multiple complaints for which the staff members were unable to find an organic basis, and recognizing a neurotic element, they referred her to the psychiatric unit.

The patient had never been very well. There were numerous surgical procedures in her past medical history. She was an eighth-grade graduate and thereafter until her marriage had worked in her father's business. Her family had regarded her as a sickly individual and had sheltered her from the outside world. She was unstable emotionally, having outbursts of crying whenever she was crossed. She was always envious of others, wanting to have things that they had, and this was a source of difficulty, because her husband could not provide her with everything. The patient had always sought refuge in physical complaints when faced with difficulties at home.

While the patient was in the psychiatric unit she acted normally. Her I.Q. was 84, and her behavior was indicative of a person of dull normal intelligence. It was difficult to get ideas across to her in examinations, and she showed little ability to grasp the abstract. She looked upon the hospitalization as a period of rest before she went home and at no time did she complain of any bodily difficulties; she said she had never felt better in her life. Although the diagnostic summary noted that she was obviously a psychoneurotic, judging from her history and the reports from the medical clinic, her behavior in the ward made it impossible to make a specific diagnosis.

P. Hypo.	M:22:S:23	−14	31′4782–	5:2:25
Ps. Sz., Paranoid	M:30:S:82	+1	4′3178296–(49)	6:5:25
		+79	4′893 16 27–(49)	5:5:23

The young man's complaints, headache, tinnitus, and scalp tenderness, had first appeared three years before admission to the hospital. Working at a job requiring heavy physical exertion, he apparently had been unable to keep up with the other boys of his own age and, consequently, had been teased. Subsequently he developed back pain and poor appetite, left the job, and returned home. In spite of rest and various treatments by the family physician, he became anemic in the course of the next months. Because of this, he said, his friends lost respect for him and began to shun him. This he thought was particularly true of his girl friends. Gradually he shifted from physical activity to intellectual studiousness. For a while he concentrated on his schoolwork and on playing the trumpet, but as he suffered more and more from severe attacks of headaches, he stopped studying and practicing, and remained idle at home until his admission to the hospital. He brought with him a carefully prepared list of his complaints.

Before the onset of the present illness the patient had been a fairly well-liked boy, not strong physically, but respected because of his excellent mental assets. Said to be kind, unselfish, and never suspicious, he desired, however, always to be the leader and when he could not assume this role, he usually made excuses not to participate. Rather shy, he tended to develop ideas that people were ridiculing him for one reason or another.

In the hospital he continually worried about his health and about whether or not he would be able to return to school and become a journalist. Repeatedly he asked, "When will I be able to go back to school?" He had many vague and indefinite aches and pains, and over and over he said, "Why do I have to have these headaches?" "These headaches are real to me and are severe, even though people might not think so." Well oriented, he showed no evidence of an intellectual limitation. There was obvious anxiety and depression. He discussed his headaches as possibly "functional." He talked slowly, choosing his words carefully, apparently trying to describe with extreme accuracy and detail all his bodily complaints. He was open and accessible to therapy and examination. As time went on he learned to differentiate two types of headaches. The first he ascribed to a spinal puncture he had received, the second was a "functional" headache. Gradually both types disappeared. Still later he became free of all complaints and decided that he felt well enough to return to his home and his work. The therapeutic approach had consisted chiefly of careful reassurance about his physical disorders and attempts to find a more adequate concept of their genesis. His positive response to treatment, as well as his many assets, spoke for a favorable prognosis, even though it was predicted that there might be return of the complaints if he met difficult situations.

Eight years later he was readmitted. This admission was requested by the authorities because he had broken into a home with the intent to steal. For several months he had been overactive, especially at night clubs, and had drawn attention to himself by annoying women. He had bought a home and had completely furnished it for his marriage although he was not even engaged. The earlier pattern of physical complaints had disappeared. He was discharged to the court with the recommendation that commitment to a state hospital be considered.

P. Hys.	F:24:M:114	+2	314′892–(47)	5:9:13
P. Hypo.		+77	′3–29(61)	8:13:13

When the patient first came to the clinic she complained of a great many physical symptoms: she had difficulty in accepting the fact that she did not have cancer; she had a feeling of "paralyzing in the head," accompanied by nausea; and she suffered from "nerves." She also had periods of considerable crying, although these were not reflected on the D scale of the MMPI. The patient was under considerable pressure in her second marriage. She had successively married two neurotic men. Each of these marriages had run a similar course. Along with this she had experienced frigidity, although she did report successful sexual relations with her first husband during the early days of their marriage. The patient had more than the usual interest in religion; she had the feeling that much of what she did was dictated directly by God. She wrote a great deal of sentimental poetry which was essentially pessimistic in outlook. An amusing side light was a list of some hundred character traits which the patient had constructed and intended to apply to any future men in her life. The patient began the first interview by saying she had thought that she had cancer. However, she had been told by her physician that she did not. She was very disappointed since she hoped that she might soon die.

The mother and the older sister of the patient were the domineering members in the family. While the father worked, he was not the main "breadwinner." The mother supplemented the family income by operating a store. The patient had apparently had the feeling for a long while that her father was not as strong a personality as she wanted, and she had always felt let down by his inability to combat the aggressiveness of his wife and older daughter. The patient described herself as passive like her father. During her childhood there had been a great deal of competition with her older sister. From every indication the older sister had always won, although there was no evidence that she was the intellectual equal of the patient. At about the age of 3 the patient had discovered that she could get attention and affection from her mother and sister if she were ill. The mother placed a great deal of emphasis on exterior appearances, constantly asking, "What will the neighbors think?" "What will the church members think?" She used this as a disciplinary measure for her children, especially for the patient. Here again, the father was no help.

Following the initial two or three sessions, which were largely devoted to an anamnesis (it would have been impossible to have stopped this process), the therapist became directive. This was done first by encouraging the patient to talk about specific matters in her early life and to try to see possible connections between her need to be ill and her role in the family. From here her attention was directed to finding out how this neurotic adjustment might have affected her marriage as well as her uncertainty about whether she wanted to become a professional woman or a housewife. During therapy she obtained a divorce from her second husband and decided to join the WAC. After 55 to 60 days the physical symptoms disappeared entirely and returned for only a brief moment at the time when the therapeutic relationship was being terminated. The second MMPI was shown to the patient during the final session and was compared with the first. The therapist felt that this technique was helpful in reinforcing the changes which had occurred in the patient's personality and radically improved social adjustment. At first she had withdrawn by avoiding people. By the time therapy was concluded, she had made a number of new acquaintances, was renewing past relations, and was having a fairly good time. A. S.

P. Hys. F:21:M:27 +2 31′4$\underline{89}$76– 9:2:21

Four months before this young woman was admitted to the hospital she had what was called "flu." The symptoms were those of an ordinary cold and she spent a week in bed. Next she developed a cough and lost her voice. Since then she had been unable to speak above a whisper, and for the first month she could not even whisper. A few minutes after admission to the hospital she suddenly began to talk in a high-pitched, faint voice, her first speech since the onset of the symptoms.

The patient's marriage of four years' duration was an unhappy one. The husband, a poor provider and an alcoholic, was irritable and cross and at times beat her. In the past she had been well except for a major operation for an "abscessed ovary" and occasional choking sensations brought on by emotional upsets. Her school record was poor. Although socially she was fairly well adjusted, she played a passive role. Incapable of entertaining herself, she always required company. She disliked work and usually avoided it whenever possible. She was readily depressed and her temper was short. She took almost no responsibility in any situation.

None of the physical findings in the hospital was related to the aphonia. Although verbally concerned about the loss of her voice, the patient did not appear to be genuinely troubled by it. On the day of admission when she so dramatically recovered her voice, she not only had no insight into the possible basis for the aphonia but was resistant to the possibility there was a psychological problem. Later she placed the entire blame for her difficulties on her husband and refused to accept any of the responsibility. Discharged as free of the admission symptoms, she had been so resistive to psychotherapy that it seemed probable she would continue in the same pattern and eventually develop other similar symptoms.

Ps. M-D., Mixed Suicidal M:41:M:20 +1 31'628 79–(69) 4:4:14

Ps. M-D., Mixed Suicidal M:42:M:58 +4 841'39267–(71) 5:10:24

The reasons for this patient's hospitalization were general hyperactivity and erratic overproductivity. Three weeks before admission his behavior became characterized by increased psychomotor activity, distractibility, irritability, excessive talking and writing, and fear that his behavior might jeopardize his professional position as a physician. This particular admission was one of a series that had begun six years before with a severe depression in which he had made an unsuccessful suicidal attempt. Following that time he had had alternating manic and depressive spells between long periods of normal behavior.

Of superior intellect, the patient had taken a serious point of view toward life from an early age. He had absorbed his parents' strict standards and had become a perfectionist, demanding only the best from himself and from others. He was possessed by a tremendous drive to be successful, and money and other material symbols were of first importance to him. His belief that he had unusual finesse in handling people did not equate with the facts, for he was not well liked by most people and was known as an exhibitionist.

Throughout this man's hospital stay he presented a problem in management for everyone concerned with him. Irritable and demanding, he slept poorly and snatched at every outlet for his abundant energies. He continually insisted that the place was "badly run" and that he was "going to leave." Finally he quieted down enough to be placed in the care of his wife. It was felt that he would recover from the present episode but would probably experience future attacks. As it turned out, two years later he was readmitted with much the same pattern, but in addition with considerable personality deterioration.

B. Psth., Path. Sexuality P. Psychas. M:54:M:19 +7 31'6472– 4:0:19

This patient entered the hospital voluntarily for psychiatric study after the discovery of a shortage in the funds which he had handled in his job as a clerk. He denied recollection of taking more than $2 although the sum missing amounted to $30. He believed that he had been mentally clouded for the last two months. After he was suspended from his job he filed a report in which he admitted certain minor indiscretions but denied the major theft, although he said that he may have acted without knowing what he was doing.

There was a history of an ulcer, and about four years before admission he had suffered an attack of "sciatic pain" in his right leg. Under stress the patient had always been fearful and apprehensive. He was known as a good worker and had been a clerk with the same concern for many years before the suspension. In his own financial affairs he exercised poor judgment. Despite an adequate income he was always in debt, and at the time of admission he owed $900, chiefly in medical expenses. Whenever he was alone he would become despondent and would often go for a long walk "to get away from myself." He had always worried a great deal about his health and his debts and had been troubled all his life with "unclean desires" concerning teen-age girls. Ten years earlier he had been accused of "watching and fondling" a 10-year-old girl, but, he said, "she was the hanging-on kind and gave me every opportunity." He had had other similar minor experiences. His wife was irritable and emotional, but he disclaimed any sexual frustration in their marital relationship. They had four children.

In the hospital the patient spent a great deal of time thinking about his recent financial difficulties. He felt that he might have been mentally confused by his sexual obsessions. It had been his habit in the past to retreat into sexual fantasies whenever his affairs came to a crisis. At times he cried when asked for details about his difficulties, and he expressed the thought that his mind had been clouded by his poor health and the sexual fantasies. By test his intelligence was in the upper average range. In personality he appeared to be similar to schizophrenic and neurotic patients. He provided a very severe problem diagnostically and prognostically. He had marked compulsive and obsessive thoughts and he was certainly not a simple problem of asocial personality. It was thought possible that he was homoerotic. At discharge it was recommended that he retire from work and that he continue outpatient contacts.

Ps. Sz., Paranoid F:28:S:44 +5 316 478'29- 3:6:10

Since the birth of an illegitimate child to this young woman three years before admission, her personal adjustment had become increasingly difficult. Her multiple physical complaints, which were increasing in number, were due to working too hard, she said. She shifted from one job to another, was malcontent, irritable, and unappreciative of any aid offered her. In the past few weeks she had been "too tired, weak, and distressed" even to attempt to work. Several years before admission she had got "messages from birds" and "priests preached sermons about me."

Coming from an unusually unhappy home, the patient claimed to have been mistreated by her parents. After considerable trouble with her studies she left school at the age of 18. Four years later she entered a convent, "because I was so unhappy," but she left there after only a year, explaining that she was physically unable to continue. In a few months she became pregnant, and for a while lived with the father of the child although she did not marry him. After the birth of the baby the patient had little to do with it, and at the time of admission it was being adopted by a relative.

In the hospital all the patient's spontaneous talk referred to her physical complaints, although she would also say, "I am depressed, worried, and have difficulty in concentration." She complained that "people never tried to help me." Her folks had always been mean to her and had hated her, she said. Evasive, she never talked directly to the point. For example, when she was asked how she was getting along she answered, "Do you think I need glasses, or is it my nose?" Irritated whenever she was pressed to answer any questions, she frequently commented, "No one can do anything for me anyway." She made a few friends in the ward and on the whole became slightly better, but at the time of discharge she was given a poor prognosis, and it was recommended that she accept a job, obtained for her by the social service, which would allow her to do easy work as a trial.

P. Hys. F:23:S:28 +4 31'<u>798</u>2- 5:6:18

This young woman was referred by her home doctor as a case of chronic encephalitis with possible brain tumor and rheumatic endocarditis. She was an achondroplastic dwarf. Her most obvious symptoms were her inability to speak above a whisper and her inability to walk. She also complained of backache, crampy abdominal pain, precordial pain, drowsiness, anorexia, and personality changes during the past year. About five months before admission the patient had begun to experience restlessness accompanied by an elevated temperature. This had continued in varying patterns with definite evidences of an infective process until about a month before admission she had begun to have days of such drowsiness that she could not be aroused even to urinate or to eat. A little earlier she had begun to lose her voice.

Her health had never been good and at one period she had been treated in a hospital for crippled children for marked bowing of both legs. A high school and business college graduate, the patient had hunted for a job and had been discouraged over not finding one. She had looked forward to a well-paying job so that she could do things for her parents. She had never had boy friends and said she preferred a career. Disregarding her physical handicaps, she engaged in such activities as swimming and skating. It was her code to be uncomplaining and cheerful. Her intelligence was average.

In the hospital the physical examinations showed some positive findings, but they were not consistent with the extent of her symptoms, and it was doubted that she had suffered encephalitic brain damage. With regard to the hospital procedures, she was indifferent and acquiescent. There was no sign of irritation or discouragement. She enjoyed describing her symptoms and declared that her only concern was the "heart disease." She was amused that her voice returned as soon as she was convinced by a specialist that its loss "was due to imagination." She showed no tendency to self-criticism and gave as her reason for not finding employment, "lots of others wanted the same position." She did not seem to recognize that her dwarfism could be a factor in her failure. To explanations of procedures or to other remarks, she usually answered, "Yes, doctor," without any evidence of a genuine appreciation. Once in the hospital she had a period of drowsiness when she could not be aroused by ordinary means. Electrical stimulation was then used, whereupon she became irritable, saying, "I'm tired of hospitals and being sick. Why do you try to wake me? You said I'd be out of here in two weeks and I'm still here." She was told that if she continued to improve she would be discharged in another week. In general, an effort was made to modify her standards for achievement and to help her accept a modest job where her appearance would be less of a handicap. This effort was only moderately successful, although it was felt that she would probably ultimately adjust fairly well.

P. Mixed F:31:D:40 +7 31'82476–(49) 6:4:24

Twice daily during the two weeks before admission and occasionally before that, the patient had had spells when she felt a lump in her throat and had great difficulty in breathing. Her face became flushed and her heart pounded, sometimes seeming to stop. The attacks lasted from a half hour to two hours.

Until six years before admission she had been in good health, but at that time she had begun to tire easily. A physician, believing that her thyroid was enlarged, had then put her on iodine for several weeks. She had had an eighth grade education, quitting school at age 15 to do housework; at the time of admission she was a waitress. Four years before, she had been divorced and had since lived at a hotel. She got along well with people, liked dancing and the company of the opposite sex. About a year before admission she had become pregnant and had had an abortion at the insistence of the man. Her anxiety had steadily mounted in intensity since the abortion and the failure of her plans to marry.

In the hospital the patient's thoughts were chiefly concerned with her past troubles. There were no delusions, hallucinations, or paranoid trends. She was well oriented, her memory was good for past events, and she was intact in intellect, but she was unstable and cried and sobbed easily. At first she said that the thyroid difficulty was her reason for coming to the hospital, but she came to understand that she had a functional problem. Socially quiet and shy, she never volunteered information but was cooperative and helpful in examinations, and responded readily to suggestive therapy. She was encouraged to make definite plans about meeting the frustrations of her life, and stress was put on the attitude she should take toward the events of her past life. She was discharged greatly improved, and it was felt that the prognosis was good.

Ps. M-D., Mixed F:54:M:91 +1 '31 84–X 12:3:25
+33 3'4186–X 11:24:1

During the month preceding her admission to the hospital the patient had exhibited signs of increased psychomotor activity. Restless, irritable, and demanding, she showed some elation, tended to be expansive, and spend money carelessly. Her behavior was frequently embarrassing to her husband. For a period of many years she had consulted numerous physicians for a variety of somatic complaints. No organic basis for the complaints could be discovered. Ten years before the present episode she had become depressed and had spent several months in a hospital. Subsequently she had experienced a number of minor attacks of depression but had been hospitalized only once more.

A normal school graduate, the patient taught kindergarten until her marriage. Her social adjustment was good, and she had diversified intellectual interests. A friendly and adequate person, she had not been accepted as well in recent years as she had been previously because some of her friends had recognized and reacted against increasing temperamental peculiarities.

In the hospital she was observed to be moderately obese and to have an elevated blood pressure with some signs of hypertensive change in the eye grounds. There was also a hypertrophic arthritis, which had resulted in an ankylosis in the right ankle. At the time of admission she showed a moderate degree of excitement. Her thoughts flowed rapidly and she was circumstantial and distractible. Constantly active, she was unable to apply her energies in an efficient manner. She was fully oriented and there were no hallucinations or other gross disturbances of intellect or sensorium. She considered the hospitalization altogether unnecessary, although she was "willing to put up with it." Gradually the symptoms abated although she continued to complain of physical discomfort. Many conflicts arose with other patients, but on the whole she was a friendly, well-poised person. At the time of discharge she was much improved; in general, the illness had at no time seemed extreme.

P. React. Depr.	F:22:S:57	+1	31876'249–	2:8:13
P. Hys.		+55	'648317–	4:1:18
Suicidal				

This young woman entered the hospital with the desire to free herself from "excessive" masturbation. She was bothered also by tenseness and depression. She had practiced masturbation ever since she could remember and had introduced foreign bodies into the urethra. These practices had been encouraged by a long period spent in bed with arthritis. She had made no previous attempt to control the masturbation. Subject to moods of depression on "blue days," she would then be preoccupied with thoughts of suicide; she had ineffectually used drugs and carbon monoxide more than once and at one time had tried to drown herself.

The patient was and always had been obese. Of good intelligence, she had a wide range of interests, including clothing design, music, and nature studies. During her childhood she had read extensively despite parental opposition. She liked mechanics and abhorred anything she regarded as "sissy." She was ambitious to be educated for office work and was only inhibited by her illness. Emotionally labile, she had always shown a marked need for affection and approval. Although physically unattractive, she had a direct manner and a sincerity which brought her many friends. She was experienced heterosexually and from an early age had been preoccupied with sex.

In the hospital she was placed in a ward where public exposure restricted the masturbation. There was an immediate decline in this practice and it continued throughout the hospital period. In one acute bout of depression she had thoughts of suicide. She was given a reducing diet and a full schedule of activities. As she engaged more and more in these activities she became freer in social contacts and appeared to be making a better adjustment. Definite plans were made to provide intellectual and recreational outlets for her in the period following discharge, and since she seemed to have not only superior motivation but perseverance, it appeared that she would continue to improve.

P. Mixed F:38:S:27 –3 31'92–4 4:3:14

Ps. M-D., Depr. F:40:S:41 +83 21376'8– 4:6:11
P. Mixed

The patient's admission complaints of weakness, weight loss, gastric distress, and attacks of tachycardia had gradually developed over a period of a year, following an attack of "flu." After the illness she had not returned to her usual state of good health. In the early stages of her illness, there had been an occasional partial loss of consciousness. Among the physical changes was a sixty-pound weight loss, and on admission she weighed only ninety pounds. In a long hospitalization preceding the present admission (first MMPI) she had received a complete physical study which had failed to reveal any disorder related to the symptoms.

A high school graduate of average intelligence, the patient had worked for two years as a clerk before going to business school. After a few months she discontinued the course and returned to clerking. When she developed "anemia," she was forced to stop work for six months, but she then returned to the job until a generalized weakness following a cholecystectomy made it impossible for her to work for a period of four years. When her health was sufficiently improved she took a position as a bookkeeper and maintained a fairly satisfactory work record until the present illness. As a child she had been known as a tomboy. An active, energetic person, she got along well with people except in her relations with men, where she was socially inept. She was unusually closely attached to her home. She was known as a hypochondriac and for many years was said to have annoyed her friends with detailed descriptions of her illnesses. Her mother, a selfish, hard, domineering person, had always encouraged the patient in her hypochondriasis and her attachment to her home. Her father, an average man, suspected that some of the patient's illness had a psychological basis, but the mother resisted the idea and felt that the patient was seriously ill.

On the ward the patient took a great deal of satisfaction in discussing her symptoms extensively. Placebo hypodermics were effective in temporarily relieving her pains. Her answers to questions were spontaneous, relevant, and coherent, but she insisted on remaining in bed because of her "weakness." When forced to get up she suffered a "fainting attack." Indirectly she complained almost continually about the hospital and the personnel. She gained considerable verbal insight into her problem, and at discharge she seemed considerably improved, but about two years later she was readmitted with almost the same symptoms. Two electric convulsive shocks produced an unfavorable response, and her general behavior was such that it was necessary to transfer her to the disturbed ward. Because of the development of depressive symptoms and the behavior disturbances she was transferred to a state hospital.

P. Hys. F:44:D:30 +3 31'06728 4 8:6:16

This patient's symptoms were choking spells, generalized nervous tension, and pain in her chest. Of several years' duration, these had not become severe until six months before admission. The choking spells were brief and were not associated with other phenomena. Many days she had as many as seven attacks. The most recent additional difficulty was depression.

Never robust, the patient began at age 13 to have fainting spells accompanied by generalized weakness. A diagnosis of heart trouble was made and a restricted life was recommended. Several major surgical operations were performed during the next years and at one time she was hospitalized with complaints resembling those of the present illness. Before her first marriage, she had worked as a domestic. She married at 20, was divorced four years later, and remarried quickly, this time to a 27-year-old widower with children of his own. This man died after two years and in a short time she married a 45-year-old man. After eight years of abuse from this third husband, she divorced him. The family, consisting of the patient, a married daughter and her husband, and two other children, lived in a three-room house owned by the patient. Her life was an active one and apparently she had formed warm social contacts. She had always tended to exaggerate any physical complaints. Whenever crossed, she showed a temper. This made a problem for relief agencies that worked with the family.

The patient was a powerfully built woman and appeared to be in excellent physical condition. Sure that her illness was organically caused, she objected to her hospitalization. She believed her trouble was "a bad heart." In spite of this she made a satisfactory adjustment. In the hospital she had occasional smothering spells, at first severe but later milder as a result of reassurance and explanation. Throughout her hospitalization she continued to have the spells but they did not interfere with her activities, and she was not distressed by them. At discharge she felt quite at ease even though the symptoms persisted in mild form. A good adjustment was predicted.

B. Psth., Mixed F:36:M:17 +5 319'74628– 5:5:12
Alcoholism

The complaints for which this patient entered the hospital were nausea, vomiting, epigastric distress, and anorexia. These symptoms had become so pronounced three months before that the patient had difficulty in retaining food. Her local physician, finding no organic basis for the condition, referred her to the hospital. However, before she actually entered, the symptoms had diminished. For the past three years she had experienced frontal headaches two to three times daily, tingling in her hands and feet, and tenderness in the pelvic region.

Although very intelligent, the patient apparently lacked good judgment, especially in matters concerned with sex. At 14 she had "quite a reputation with boys," became pregnant, and married at 15. After six months she divorced her first husband and married again at 18 following another pregnancy. She was promiscuous and increasingly alcoholic. At one time she threatened to kill her second husband with a bread knife, although in many ways they were well mated. A number of times she attempted suicide and once drank lysol. She showed poor judgment in choosing her associates and, likewise, in other areas of her life. She was usually cheerful and was described as emotionally stable by persons who knew her casually. Interestingly, she was religious and prayed every night.

In the hospital the patient was mainly concerned with the hospital admission itself. "I don't like it here because there is nothing wrong with my mind. I am sure my husband took me here so that he could get rid of me. He is probably getting drunk and playing around with women. He has done his share of it. He started it." She experienced a complete remission of the symptoms but at times showed emotional instability. When crossed she developed headaches and abdominal tenderness. She related the morbid details of her past history to other patients whenever they were willing to listen. She attributed all her problems to things outside herself and was inaccessible for therapy other than general laboratory tests. She attributed all her symptoms to overwork and fatigue. This woman had spent several periods in psychiatric units before, and it was predicted that she would probably return for future treatment. At discharge there was little or no optimism regarding her future adjustment. Three years later she was admitted to the neurological service because of a head injury from a fall, probably while she was drunk. The interim history was a continuation of her previous behavior.

P. Mixed	F:34:M:102	+1	32′1–9647 (74)	3:3:10
P. Psychas.		+90	3′1<u>29</u>– (53)	3:1:13

The patient's chief complaints were emotional instability, fatigability, insomnia, headaches, irritability, depression, and anorexia. These symptoms had been insidious in onset. About three years before admission she had had a "nervous breakdown" following a difficult pregnancy and delivery. Shortly before this episode her husband had been inducted into the army. She had required repeated reassurance from her physician and had finally been sent to the hospital for psychiatric examination. When she realized the nature of the examination she became indignant and left without completing the study. The return of her husband from the service pleased her but no improvement followed. The fatigue, particularly, persisted.

She was described as moderately friendly and given to frequent discussion about other people's activities; her interests were chiefly in reading and handicrafts. She was orderly and excessively clean. She had always been thought of as high-strung and irritable. Ten years earlier she had engaged in frequent sexual relations with a man who later abandoned her. Depressed after this, she did not appear ever to have recovered from the experience. She claimed to love her present husband but sexual intercourse with him had been unpleasant and unsatisfactory.

Disturbed at being in a hospital, she was afraid that she might have to remain a long time. She presented a beautifully arranged history of her illness with only slight intervention and guidance by the interviewer. There were evidences of extreme nervousness but little insight into the psychological factors in her problem. She related incidents showing that she had always been a meticulous person. She was given electroshock therapy, which was followed for a while by untidiness, forgetfulness, and other evidences of organic deterioration. However, before her final discharge she improved, and while the basic pattern of symptoms remained, she was somewhat more cheerful. An effort was made to improve the sexual compatibility of the patient and her husband, but he did not cooperate and little progress was made. In contrast to the man with whom she had earlier had intimacies, her husband was ineffectual and indecisive. It became clear that she feared pregnancies but felt a conflict because during pregnancy she was relieved of sexual intercourse. The presence of a long-standing pattern of complaints and inadequacy, together with her failure to develop much real insight, lowered the probability of complete recovery. However, at discharge, she had made positive improvement.

P. Hypo.	F:45:S:48	0	321′47–9	8:4:21
P. Anxiety State	F:45:S:34	+30	213′7–9	8:3:12

This patient had a long history of abdominal pain, nausea, vomiting, fatigue, depression, and anorexia, but the symptoms had been increasing in intensity for several years before hospitalization. The patient had undergone a nephropexy ten years before admission without relief of the symptoms.

Never a strong person, the patient had experienced her first serious illness at the age of 5, shortly after the death of her mother, when she had "brain fever" associated with marked nervousness. An appendectomy at age 16 had been followed by extreme weakness, which had persisted for a number of years. The removal of an ovarian cyst when she was 20 was followed by the appearance of a fistula that required six operative procedures. Others observed that every stressful situation increased her complaints. A shy person, she had easily hurt feelings. She was known to be generous. She was a regular church attendant. At one time her chief ambition had been to become a nurse. Dull intellectually, she had a school history of several grade repetitions and had finally quit at the eighth-grade level.

When admitted to the hospital the patient was well oriented, cooperative, and intellectually intact, but she was nervous, shy, restless, and complaining. She remarked that she felt useless and in the way, and it was noted that sudden noises frightened her. In her opinion the pain was entirely organic, although she recognized that it was worse when she was upset or worried. After gradual improvement she was finally discharged to the care of her relatives. She was readmitted a year later with a similar pattern, except that this time there was impairment of visual acuity, diplopia, mild headaches, and an impairment of her deep and superficial sensitivity which was thought to be entirely hysterical in nature. Reassurance relieved these symptoms somewhat, and she was again discharged, but there was no reason to believe that she would be much different following this discharge than she had been previously.

P. Hys. F:19:S:55 +3 3′21478–9 9:2:22

For approximately the last two years this young woman had been subject to spells of "fainting." At first infrequent, they increased until as many as ten or twelve occurred in one day. Her mother described the attacks as a loss of consciousness and said that the patient would fall to the floor silently without hurting herself and would lay motionless with her muscles flaccid for a few minutes. At times after she came out of the attacks she was still unable to move or talk even though she knew everything that was happening around her. The patient could not offer any explanation of why she had the attacks, and her mother said that no one particular thing seemed to set them off. Recently the episodes had become so incapacitating that the patient had withdrawn from school.

The past medical history was negative, except that menstruation had, in the past six months, become irregular and scanty. In school the patient did poor work and had failed the fourth and the seventh grades. At the time of admission she was a freshman in high school and most of her classmates were younger. She had had few real dates—perhaps none—with boys of her own age, but on at least three occasions she had had sexual experiences with older men that stopped just short of intercourse. The home environment was poor. The father, a heavy drinker, had been out of the home since the patient was 5. The mother was strict in her religion and taught the children that their father was a very bad person. There was a stepfather with whom the patient had strained relations. He appeared to nurse a particular grudge and antipathy toward the girl. The patient was usually friendly toward others, but she was obviously oversensitive and would be upset for hours after an adverse remark that she felt applied to her. She was ambitious to finish high school.

In the hospital the girl seemed normal for the most part. She said that her spells were "an inconvenience," but she seemed not to be overly concerned with them. She was particularly bitter toward her stepfather. When she was crossed or hurt she cried, became morose, and went off by herself. These spells did not last long. Her affect and general behavior did not appear unusual. About five days after admission she had an attack in which she showed a new pattern. She screamed and lay very limp, but moved in response to commands. A few more of these attacks occurred later, but they were all minor. After preliminary blocking, she talked readily with the examiners and admitted a fear that she would not be able to finish school because her stepfather might not allow it and because she might be "too dumb." She was permitted to tell her story completely and was given reassurance and some information about sex. Plans were also made to place her in a vocational school instead of the regular high school.

Ps. M-D., Mixed F:37:M:72 +27 32'16 7948– 3:1:15

The presenting complaints of this patient were nervousness and depression, with multiple bodily aches and pains. There was an involved medical history extending back six years. During that time she had consulted numerous physicians and had attended several different medical clinics in the hope of obtaining relief from back pain and other ills. She also consulted fortunetellers, healers, and the like. After her marriage (one year before admission) the nervousness increased. No treatment relieved her for more than a few weeks.

Before the gradual onset of the present problems the patient had always been in good health. A university graduate, she had worked as a private secretary and had been considered efficient and capable. She had continued to work long after the onset of the present symptoms. The patient had always had a strict conscience and was markedly attached to her family. She was well liked and honest. Although in some ways she and her husband were well mated she was obviously ambivalent in her attitude toward him. They lived with the husband's mother, and this occasioned considerable friction.

In the hospital she was tense, restless, and agitated. She complained of insomnia and demanded a great deal of attention and sympathy. There were no marked aberrations of intellect or sensorium. Depressed, she said that she had considered suicide. For the first two weeks in the hospital she attempted to monopolize the time of the nurses and of the staff doctors. She wished to be treated as a very ill person. Treatment, on the contrary, was fairly stern, and while she was given physical reassurance, she was urged to take part in ward activities and was not permitted to indulge herself by playing the invalid. With this regime she improved considerably in behavior and was discharged to the care of her husband. It seemed unlikely, however, that her adjustment outside of the hospital would be good, because no real change could be effected in her, and she remained unshaken in the delusion that her chief problems were somatic in character.

P. Mixed Alcoholism Drug Add. M:53:M:18 +3 <u>32</u>17′46–9 (43) 3:5:19

Headaches, insomnia, a cough, morphine habituation, and general nervousness were among the complaints of this patient. For as long as he could remember he had had periodic attacks of headache lasting from four to five days, and they had gradually increased in frequency. The pain, described as being "viselike," usually made him feel dizzy, and he frequently vomited at the height of the pain. Thirty years before admission the patient had been given morphine for the relief of one of these headaches and he had continued taking it since then. Until five years before admission he had restricted his use of the drug to the periods of the headaches, once about every five to seven weeks, but at that time he had begun to experience more constant pain and had developed a "liver condition," for which morphine had been given every two hours for about six months. When he showed evidence of "losing his mind" he was taken off this drug, but since then he had taken morphine once or twice a week in rather large quantities. The liver disorder was apparently alcoholic in origin.

The patient had finished the fourth grade in school and had made a satisfactory living as a truck driver and filling station operator. At the time of admission he had not been working for five years. He was described as stubborn and stingy, although he had good common sense and was very self-reliant. A friendly and thoughtful person, he nevertheless tended to avoid social contacts except within his family. At one time he had been a bootlegger and had been apprehended and fined on that count. He hated crowds because they made him nervous.

In the hospital he was worried about his physical condition and about the financial status of his family. Very set in his ideas, he "knew better than the doctors and the nurses what was good for him," but he adapted fairly well to ward activities and gradually entered into the general social events. His conduct of his life, his alcoholism, his bootlegging, and his asocial attitude toward groups indicated a psychopathic personality; there were also obvious neurotic factors in his lifelong inadequacy and in the pattern of the physical complaints on which the morphine addiction was based.

P. Mixed F:30:M:48 +3 <u>32</u> <u>176</u>4′8–9 2:3:11

P. Mixed F:32:M:113 +58 2<u>78</u>31′46– 2:10:7

The presenting complaints of the patient were pain in the jaws, anorexia, nervousness, unhappiness, and insomnia. A pain in the right jaw had begun eight years earlier. Four years later pain had appeared in the left jaw. The patient saw innumerable chiropractors, dentists, and physicians, and received extensive and varied treatments. Other symptomatic patterns gradually made their appearance. As the insomnia developed she became increasingly irritable and withdrew from her home and community activities. Peculiar hallucinations were present. The patient said that she frequently saw "funny people" at night.

The patient had undergone a number of major operative procedures before the onset of the present illness. She had withdrawn from high school in the middle of the second year. Throughout her schooling her grades had been poor, and she had failed one subject in the first year of high school. For a while she worked in a store but after she underwent a pelvic operation, her activities had to be somewhat limited. Previously she had enjoyed dances and other social functions, and she had many friends. Apparently congenial with her husband at the time of admission, she had found it difficult to adjust in the early days of her marriage and had frequently visited her mother. After the birth of a child she became sexually frigid.

In the hospital the patient was worried about her symptoms; she said, "I wish I could go out and do as I used to do and not be tired all the time." She described dreams she had; for example, "My child was drowning and I grabbed for her but always just missed her." She also dreamed about her dead father and brother. It was at first difficult to work with the patient because of her reserve. She presented the appearance of being impatient and hypercritical. Considerable medical attention was given to her, and attempts were made to build her up physically and to correct the malocclusion of her teeth. Her basic personality was inflexible, however, and while she obtained considerable symptomatic relief during the hospital period, the long history of the complaints suggested an unfavorable prognosis.

P. Mixed F:47:M:23 +56 32 1786'4– 2:7:9
Epilepsy

The patient had been epileptic since age 16. Seven months before admission she began to be seclusive, to worry excessively about her husband, whom she accused of infidelity, and to feel insecure about the future. In addition she had a marked fear of being left alone, was unaccountably worried and irritable about family matters, and had generalized vague somatic complaints. Since the epileptic convulsions occurred only about once in twelve to eighteen months, they were not a great problem.

Until the seventh grade the patient had received good marks, but she had failed the eighth grade because of a lack of textbooks. After she left school she worked as a domestic until her early marriage. Before the appearance of the present complaints she had been active, social, and interested in her home, but her ambitions had been directed toward a higher economic status than her husband provided.

In the hospital the patient worried about her children and about financial difficulties. Sometimes she doubted that the children were really hers, and occasionally she wondered who she was. She had never cared to go away from home because of the possibility of a convulsion. She had hated to seek help from a relief agency; and she felt that the necessity of this had contributed to her problem. She was cooperative and believed that hospitalization would help her. There was no definite evidence of a disturbance of her sensorium or intellect. Her I.Q. was 136. She thought menopausal symptoms had added to her difficulties, and she had a fear of becoming pregnant again. She was in a considerably better frame of mind at the time of discharge, and apparently she had made good progress toward working through her problems. The MMPI was obtained in the outpatient clinic when she returned later with a recurrence of the admission pattern of symptoms.

B. Simple Adult Maladj. M:39:M:18 +11 324′176–9 3:0:16

Fifteen years before admission the patient had an attack of extreme restlessness in which he felt all his muscles quivering, although there was no visible trembling. A "nerve" medicine relieved him, and there was no recurrence until shortly before admission when the symptoms returned with increasing intensity, along with profuse sweating even when he was not engaged in physical activities.

The past medical history contained nothing of positive importance although certain episodes indicated that he had been somewhat hypochondriacal or hysterical. Schoolwork was so difficult for him that he required seven years to complete the fifth grade. After leaving school he had been an itinerant worker, with the exception of periods of service in both the army and the navy. During recent months he had been on relief. He had many complaints about his wife who was, according to him, inefficient and a poor housekeeper. Almost everyone who associated with the man found it difficult to get along with him, and his wife said that he had spells in which, without provocation, he yelled, hit her, and threatened to kill her and to commit suicide. After the attack he always tried to make up with her, but he never admitted that the trouble was his fault. Three years before admission the wife had tried to get a divorce on the grounds of nonsupport, but the patient had successfully contested the divorce. Since then the couple had separated on a number of occasions. There were five children.

In the hospital the patient worried about his domestic difficulties and complained of backache, sweating, and nervousness. Although he admitted that part of his trouble was due to his quick temper and his stubbornness, he claimed that his wife was at least equally to blame, since she was unreasonable and he was a very reasonable person. A small, quiet-spoken person, he was attentive and deferential in manner and constantly called attention to his physical difficulties. He got along fairly well with the other patients and behaved reasonably well, although he was somewhat irritated by the behavior of the younger patients. He was discharged to return to his home after social service study and recommendations had been made.

P. Anxiety State M:45:M:16 +3 '3246–9(21) 3:2:21
Alcoholism
Drug Add.

The patient had been a "social drinker" since he was 21 years old, but he had begun to drink more than usual about eighteen months before admission when he developed a contracture of the right hand, which gave him great concern. About the same time he became worried and tense about his job and his financial situation, and to relieve the strain, he began to drink about a pint of whiskey a day. An operation corrected the contracture of the hand, but he continued to drink and to be emotionally disturbed. Given seconal as a sedative, he began to take overdoses. Persecutory delusions about his fellow workers appeared, and a week before admission he suffered acute hallucinations.

A university graduate and a very capable person, the patient had held a responsible job up to the time of the present illness. He was adequate socially though his feelings were easily hurt. A stubborn person with strong prejudices, he had been emotionally stable before his illness but had had a tendency to worry. He felt that he was the "black sheep" of his family because his economic success had not been as great as that achieved by his brothers. Hard working, overly conscientious, and sensitive, he was very fond of his home and children. There was a poor sexual adjustment because of his wife's inadequacies, but in spite of this they were strongly attached to each other.

On admission to the psychiatric ward the hallucinations and delusions had disappeared. He was stable, aware of his surroundings, and apparently clear in sensorium and intellect; there were no peculiarities in behavior or activity; and he was optimistic about his work situation. Although he did not like the psychiatric unit, he was interested and cooperative during examinations and expressed a willingness to accept help. After a few days he became relaxed and cheerful, was apparently satisfied to stay in the hospital, and enjoyed the rest and the sedative tubs. At the time of discharge he was almost completely recovered from the present episode. The staff felt that the contracture of his hand and his financial worries had operated to set up an anxiety state, which had a largely situational basis. With total abstinence and some psychotherapy, it seemed probable that he would make a good adjustment.

Ps. Toxic F:40:M:38 +17 3'2 697–8(45) 6:7:13
Drug Add.
Schizoid

The patient had been nervous all her life, but she had adjusted satisfactorily until her husband went overseas with the armed forces. At that time she began to worry about the nature of his work, fearing that he was on submarine duty. Her brother, a physician, gave her some sedation for her nervousness. Later he noted behavior changes and treated her for a short time in the hospital, where she was diagnosed as having a reactive depression with paranoid and schizoid features. When her husband returned to the United States he took her out of the hospital, and she did fairly well for a while. Moving around from place to place as her husband was transferred made her restless and nervous, but when he was finally discharged from the service, she did not improve. She lost interest in things, became irritated by a decrease in her husband's income, and, according to her husband, began accusing him of infidelity with his office help. They had arguments about the considerable amount of sedatives she took. At the time of admission to the hospital she was still very confused from the heavy sedation given to her by her brother following an unmanageable period.

There were no particular episodes of physical or mental illness in her past history. She had been married for twenty years, and although she had always been nervous, before the present illness she had made an adequate adjustment with her husband, who was apparently considerate and helpful. There were no children.

In the hospital she was confused, disoriented, and agitated. Her rambling speech and poor articulation made it difficult to talk with her. When her sensorium cleared she was logical, but she was confused about events immediately preceding her hospital admission. Within a week the signs of bromide intoxication disappeared, but there was an underlying defensiveness that made psychological study difficult. She made a fairly adequate hospital adjustment, but she objected to some of the routine. Efforts were made to help her in the home adjustment, and she was encouraged to discuss her problems. At the time of discharge it seemed possible that she would do fairly well, although from a standpoint of psychotherapy no real progress had been made with her.

P. Mixed　　M:67:M:15　　+1　　3′27 1684–(51)　　6:4:20

P. Mixed　　M:67:M:27

The patient was admitted to the hospital because of nervousness, insomnia, and other indefinite complaints of a neurotic character. He had not been well for the past 35 years. Shortly before admission the symptoms became so severe that he lapsed into an almost inert depressive state. He was quiet, seclusive, and hypoactive, occasionally breaking into tears; he could not express his thoughts verbally. He was first admitted to the hospital specifically for electroshock therapy, but after receiving four treatments he refused to continue them. He left the hospital against advice only to be readmitted shortly thereafter at his own request.

He had received a considerable amount of medical treatment in the past 35 years. He had taken special "cures," had undergone a number of major operations, and had been hospitalized twice for severe agitated depression. An eighth-grade graduate, he had worked most of his life as a rural mail carrier and had been reasonably successful. He was well liked by his co-workers and by members of the community. Always quiet and reserved, he had tended to be withdrawn, especially with strangers. His interests were narrow and in general he was a rigid person. He had always seemed satisfied with life.

3'27169–

In the hospital the neurological and physical examinations were essentially normal. He was clear in sensorium and intellect. His behavior was conventional. His thought was mainly focused on his illness. He had multiple somatic complaints. Tears would well up in his eyes during interviews but he denied wanting to cry. "I don't want to be like this but it's my nerves. Only the Lord knows what's wrong with me." He was restless and agitated. It was difficult to get him to associate with the other patients. After shock therapy he did not improve on the first admission but after further shocks during the second admission he did get better. He was apprehensive when he left the hospital, but on the whole it seemed to be fairly likely that he would make a satisfactory adjustment.

P. Mixed	F:29:W:22	+15	3'27169–	2:3:7
		+19	3712'86–	2:4:8

About a year before admission to the hospital the patient had begun to develop a host of physical complaints in addition to nervousness and depression. The symptoms had been with her almost constantly. There were occasional vomiting and frequent complaints of paresthesias. Her arms and legs often felt so numb that she was unable to use them. On several occasions she had fallen to the floor in a faint, but always without harming herself. The attraction she felt at high windows was so great that she had difficulty restraining herself from jumping out, although she disclaimed a suicidal impulse. While she watched, her brother had once jumped from an open window but had suffered only slight injuries. The patient's symptoms may have begun with the discovery that this brother had syphilis, since thereafter she had constantly worried that her children and she might have contracted the disease from him. The patient's mother said that her daughter had never recovered from the accidental death of her husband three years before.

Chronic fatigue and weakness had been present since the birth of her first child. Gonorrhea, which she had had when she was 16, had apparently been treated properly. In education she had reached the second year of high school, and although she had enjoyed school and had been a good student, the death of her stepfather had made it necessary for her to leave school. She had begun having sexual relations with her future husband at about that time, presumably contracting gonorrhea from him, and she had married him when she was 19. Following his accidental death she had had to go on relief after trying to make a living in various ways. Popular as a schoolgirl, she had in later years gradually become quiet and brooding and had tended to remain at home. She had two children.

In the hospital the physical and neurological examinations gave an explanation for part of her symptoms, but they did not provide a complete understanding of her illness. She frequently cried, and when not crying she spent a great deal of time daydreaming. She said that she felt nervous and restless, and that she could constantly hear the ring of the telephone call which "told me my husband was dead." During conversations she temporarily changed from an apathetic to an affable, agreeable person. She was open and accessible, but she spent much of her time in bed. She believed that her problem of "nervousness" was largely caused by physical disorders. She gradually became somewhat better and was discharged to return home after arrangements were made for follow-up medical treatments.

P. Mixed F:38:W:30 +4 3271'864–9 (59) 5:7:11

This woman's present illness had begun with her marriage, twelve years before admission. From the beginning her husband had been overbearing, dominant, sullen, and subject to episodes of mania. Six years after her marriage, following the birth of a third child and two miscarriages within a short period, the patient began to feel depressed and extremely tense. She recovered uneventfully. Later her husband was committed to an institution and two days later he died, leaving the patient four months pregnant. Forced to sell her personal belongings and her farm, she moved into a small place. After that she had little income. She markedly decreased her food intake and was admitted to a hospital, finally, in a severely cachectic state. She was fed intravenously for a while and was then transferred to the psychiatric hospital.

After completing the seventh grade at age 14, the patient had stopped school. Always a quiet, retiring child and afraid of her mother, she had been so dependent on her family that they thought she could never leave home. However, she did break away and later was married. Apparently she had always felt inferior and had had little desire to get ahead.

The most obvious problem, when she was admitted, was the emaciation. Her children's welfare worried her, and she wanted to be with them. She had no obvious paranoid trends. She admitted having a sensation like "turtles crawling over my legs," and "a pulling sensation on the skin." She also heard voices but could not understand what they said. Well oriented, she recognized that she was depressed but did not know what she was afraid of or what she was depressed about. It was difficult to induce her to eat and she was apathetic. In a relatively short time she began to gain weight and to improve, and she then took an active interest in some of the activities of the ward. At the time of discharge she was distinctly better and seemed well on the way to recovery from the present attack.

P. Psychas. M:18:S '32768– (67) 2:2:16

This college student came in with complaints centering around his "worrying and fatigue."

The patient was aware that he was an adopted child and was curious about his real parentage. His adoptive father was a tense person; his mother had recently died after a long illness, leaving a good deal of friction between the patient and his father. The boy described himself as perfectionistic, extremely neat, and in many acts compulsive. He stuttered occasionally, a symptom present from an early age although he had practically overcome it.

He was disturbed about sexual questions and was extremely defensive. He left after only one interview but came back six months later to discuss the difficulty between himself and his father which was becoming more acute. The interview was held at a superficial level and the patient did not care to continue therapy. C. K. A.

Alcoholism F:46:M:23 +1 '3294<u>18</u>-(37) 6:5:13
B. Psth., Path. Emot.

About once a month for the four or five years before admission the patient had gone on periodic drinking sprees lasting four or five days. Between bouts she was a total abstainer. She was a solitary drinker and confined her drinking to her home. Once started she could not seem to stop, and she was ingenious in saving household funds with which to buy liquor. When the money was gone she got more from her husband by threatening to go down to his office in an inebriated condition. She said that an unsatisfactory home life with her husband and their 16-year-old daughter, whom the husband favored, was the cause of her drinking. She said that she had to stay home alone all the time while her husband was away on business. She accused him of infidelity and considered her daughter an irresponsible, disrespectful, and disobedient girl.

There was a suggestion in the past history that she had had nervous breakdowns at ages 14, 16, and 25, the last episode being accompanied by "heart trouble," which was cured. All these episodes were characterized by weight loss, anxiety, extreme restlessness, and oversensitivity. Nervous, sensitive, and spoiled as a child, the patient had dropped out of school because of the second nervous breakdown and had finished her schooling under a tutor. At age 18 she married a man who later became a financial success. They spent money rapidly and foolishly, suffering such severe financial reverses in the 1930 depression that the patient had to go to work in a department store, where she worked her way up to become head of a department. She was later discharged, supposedly because of her drinking. Well liked, she had many friends, but apparently she considered herself better than other people, and when she did not get her own way she pouted and "flew off the handle."

In the hospital her uppermost thoughts concerned her husband's neglect and his possible infidelity, along with her inability to discipline her daughter. Clear in sensorium and intellect, she was emotionally tense, nervous, and somewhat depressed. She attributed her alcoholism to things outside herself. Although causing no trouble in the hospital, she was somewhat haughty in her attitude and she remained aloof. She became overconfident after attempts were made to work out some of the problems between her and her husband, and feeling that everything was solved, she wished to be discharged at once. When the staff advised a longer stay, she was resentful. Clinically she presented an immature, restless, spoiled individual's responses to a life situation with which she was unable to deal effectively. In other ways she was essentially normal. No real progress was made with the basic problem, but since the patient had many personality assets and did believe that she needed some degree of help there was hope that a satisfactory solution to the situation would be found.

P. React. Depr. F:24:M:13 +3 '34–279 5:2:15
B. Psth., Path. Emot.
Suicidal

This young woman was sent to the hospital by a court order because of attempted suicide. For a year she had been quarreling with her husband and had twice left him. Each did much to cause jealousy in the other. During the separations she had lived with a girl friend, who said the patient had been restless and sad. The husband and wife both drank. The evening before admission the patient went to the café where her husband worked and asked him to take her out. When he refused she went home, turned on the gas, and lay down on the floor. She had contemplated this act for several weeks. However, she did not seal the cracks around the doors and the windows, and three hours later she was discovered still alive. Jailed at first, she was brought to the hospital when she persisted in saying she intended to kill herself.

Although the patient had graduated from a two-year business course, she had held only waitress jobs. For a considerable time she had been in a sanitarium because of tuberculosis. In spite of the obvious involvement of two vertebrae, she left the hospital believing that she had never had tuberculosis. The patient's husband stated his own principles when he said, "A new job every six months and a new car every two years is our ideal." They lived in inexpensive rooming houses, ate in restaurants, and spent all their evenings in beer parlors. To enjoy as much cheep amusement as possible and not to worry about the future appeared to be the goal of both the patient and her husband.

In the hospital the patient displayed anger for having been institutionalized. It was obvious that she was in complete possession of her faculties and there was no evidence of any psychotic or severely neurotic upset. Alternatingly sarcastic and sulky she at first refused to eat with the other patients or to associate with them in any way. When she realized that her stay in the hospital might be prolonged by such an attitude she adapted fairly well to the ward routine. Censuring herself for having behaved in such a way that she was sent to the hospital, she claimed that a reconciliation with her husband had been effected and that she had no further desire to kill herself. Both she and her husband were anxious for her release, and she was discharged to the care of her husband.

B. Psth., Mixed Alcoholism   M:39:M:21   +3   3'412768–9(71)   4:5:23

A chronic alcoholic for ten or fifteen years, this patient had gone on frequent heavy drinking sprees, and he had been discharged from his last job because of drinking. He, his third wife, and his three children by a previous marriage had moved to another town, where down payments on a house and car, plus other expenditures, had exhausted his resources. When he failed to find work he became despondent and resorted, as usual, to drink in order to escape his despondency. He was unable to stay with Alcoholics Anonymous. His wife got secretarial work, but he was only able to get short-time employment and this intensified his depression and anxiety. It was through the efforts of A.A. that he was admitted to the hospital.

About twenty years before admission, he had received treatment for gonorrhea and apparently there were no residual effects. As a child he had greatly resented his mother's domination, and he had begun drinking as early as age 15. The youngest of six siblings in an affluent home, he had been sent to a number of private schools, making a poor adjustment in each case, but he had finally managed to complete high school and to enroll at a university. His schoolwork had always been broken up by drinking spells, and the same habit had made it impossible for him to keep a job very long. A dependent person even when he was not drinking, he had had a difficult time making adequate adjustments, and despite all his resentment toward his parents, he felt very much lost after their death. With each of his wives he had attempted to establish a dependent relationship, but in his first marriage the partner was more inadequate than he.

In the hospital the neurological examination was essentially negative and his sensorium and intellect were clear, but he was restless and anxious. He felt relatively little concern about his drinking, but he described himself as insecure and depressed. His I.Q. was 127. There was no psychometric evidence of brain damage. Polite and cooperative, he answered questions logically and in detail, was eager to please, and appeared overeager to accept suggestions, but he showed no initiative in his approach to his pressing problems. During his stay in the hospital arrangements were made for him to begin working shortly after his discharge. It was felt that if he could hold this job and make a better connection with Alcoholics Anonymous, there was a small chance that he might avoid serious difficulties in the future, but the staff had little hope that he would persist in any long-range plans.

Ps. M-D., Depr.   F:38:M:82   +6   '34 1287–(43)   7:2:27

The present illness had begun about four months before admission when the patient had had a spell of uncontrolled crying. This was prolonged and left her exhausted. She continued doing her housework for a while but still experienced occasional mild depression. These periods became more frequent and she went to a physician who after a complete examination gave her some medication along with reassurance. She nevertheless continued to be depressed, and finally she had only an occasional good day. Although she had had vague somatic complaints previously, these now became far more definite and she developed general malaise, anorexia, insomnia, and intermittent diarrhea. She again went to a physician who put her in a general hospital for a time, transferring her to the psychiatric unit when she did not improve.

The past history was relatively noncontributory except that she had had seven pregnancies, all of which had been terminated by spontaneous abortion. There had also been some possibly menopausal symptoms during the present illness.

She was a college graduate and had taken a special interest in music and dramatics. She taught school until her marriage fourteen years before admission. For one year she had cared for her incapacitated mother. Recently her security had been threatened by an unfortunate business transaction of her husband's. Before the present illness she had been buoyant, affable, and even-tempered, although she had complained about the amount of work she had had to do after her mother moved into the home.

In the hospital she fluctuated between severe depression and occasional cheerfulness. She was given shock treatments; after the fourth one she appeared to be much worse and objected so feverishly to the treatments that they were discontinued. She then began to improve, associating with the other patients and doing fairly well. She seemed nearly back to normal at the time of discharge, and it was felt probable that she would continue to recover from the present episode. Other attacks could not be predicted with certainty although she probably had a latent disposition to develop a depression.

P. React. Depr. F:55:M:26 +3 3′4216 78–(55) 5:1:22
P. Hys.

P. React. Depr. F:55:M:54 +11 3′42178–(49) 4:1:22

This patient was admitted to the hospital because of nervousness that showed itself in body tremors, insomnia, depression, uncontrollable crying, obsessive worrying, listlessness, nausea, and other symptoms. The illness had appeared about a month before when her husband had been unexpectedly discharged from his position as president of a company. When she heard the news she had become nervous and had begun to tremble. In addition to the other symptoms that made their appearance in the course of the next month, she became careless in her personal habits and indifferent to social matters. She was so concerned about the "stigma" of her husband's failure that she felt everything else was unimportant in relation to the "calamity" which had befallen her family. Her husband said the situation was not nearly as bad as she believed it to be.

Her general health had previously been fairly good. There was a history of tremor of her hands and lips for the past five years. Unusual stress had always brought on attacks of nausea and vomiting. She had had a laparotomy for uterine bleeding. At one time she had been studied at a clinic because of a tremor in her head that was thought to be Parkinsonism, but it was finally diagnosed as functional, and later the symptom disappeared. She had always been labile emotionally. She was able to handle household affairs and to plan adequately but she was hyperreactive to emotional stimuli. Although she had always had a good sense of humor she had tended to be pessimistic. She had married instead of going to college as her father had wished her to do. Her husband was a hard worker, and they had been socially successful and active.

In the hospital she was concerned about her husband's predicament and the injustice of it. She was filled with fears for the future. Her sensorium and intellect were clear, but she was indifferent and depressed and felt hopeless. Although she was cooperative, it took her a little time to fit into ward activities and to make friends. As she gained confidence in herself and in her ability to cope with the home situation she became anxious to be discharged. The psychotherapy was chiefly concerned with a practical handling of her attitude toward the environmental stresses. It was felt that with her discharge she would probably improve further, but the prognosis was not considered good because of the long-standing nervous tendency. Actually she re-entered the hospital with a relapse after twelve days. Shock therapy was discontinued because it was followed by a period of extreme depression, but she gradually began to improve. A friendship with a fellow patient, whom she apparently considered the only one in the hospital within her economic and social level, appeared to help her. At the time of the second discharge she still regarded "the problem" as a catastrophe, but she was willing to face life on the outside. This time the prognosis was considered good.

Alcoholism M:48:M:24 +1 342'619-8 (63) 5:3:12

The patient was admitted to the hospital because of chronic alcoholism. A year before, he had joined Alcoholics Anonymous but he was so disturbed by "their attitude toward my former drinking" that it had been of very little help, and he quit after several meetings. On four different occasions after his trial with A.A. he went to a sanitarium for chronic alcoholics to sober up. About a month before the present admission he became so concerned about the unethical actions of a friend of his that he began to drink heavily in order to get up courage to speak to the man about it. He had not been able to work since this time. He had begun to drink shortly after World War I, but he claimed not to have had much difficulty in controlling it until about eight years before admission when he was diagnosed as being hyperthyroid and was admitted to a veterans' hospital, where he apparently experienced hallucinatory symptoms that lasted about five days. In the next two years he had been admitted twice to hospitals for chronic alcoholism. He always drank alone at home and never became abusive.

He had worked his way through college and after graduation had obtained a good position in which he was professionally very competent. He had many friends but tended not to become confidential with anyone. He was outwardly social and friendly but there was evidence of inner conflict and anxiety. He preferred to stay at home, rather than to take his family out socially. Small things upset him. Since he felt that it would be admitting his own inadequacy, he had never delegated any responsibility to his wife.

In the hospital he was greatly concerned about his condition and expressed the desire to stop drinking. He was intact in sensorium and intellect. Emotionally he was easily upset, somewhat nervous, irritable, and tremulous, but in general he was friendly and cooperative. He felt that the ward routine was of no value to him, and he let it be known that he felt superior to the average person, especially to the other patients. After a week or two, he became more calm, jovial, and talkative, and he admitted that the hospital had helped him some. When he finally demanded his discharge against the advice of the staff, there was no real evidence that he had gained any insight into his condition or how to stop drinking.

P. Mixed	F:37:M:32	+13	3'427 816–(47)	4:0:16
P. Mixed	F:39:M:25	+1	31'2478–(37)	6:1:13
		+24	23'47168–9(32)	2:6:11

A month before admission to the hospital this patient, who had previously seemed well adjusted, suddenly became confused and excited. For twelve hours she had cried and talked about past events. A physician advised her to visit her parents, and while she was there her mother noticed that at times she was incoherent. When she returned home she went to a hospital where she occasionally vomited and complained of severe headache. She was discharged from the hospital to the psychopathic unit. About eighteen months before admission she had given birth to triplets. This pregnancy had not been planned, the couple having successfully practiced birth control for twelve years. The triplets were premature, and their care had caused a great drain on the family financial reserve. A month after their birth the patient had a nephrectomy, which kept her in the hospital for a considerable time. Later she had to stay in the hospital because of a prolapse of the uterus. These difficulties, along with the expenses, created a great tension in the husband, whose irritability had apparently helped bring on the present attack.

The patient had graduated from high school at age 17 and had immediately married. She had been very dependent on her husband, and he had always done all the buying, including the patient's clothes. Until the present illness she had been at ease with others, friendly, kind, and thoughtful. She had a compulsion to be unobtrusive and feared standing out in any situation. The husband considered her high-strung.

In the hospital her sensorium and intellect were clear. She appeared nervous, but contented. She was logical and to the point in discourse, but she gave the impression that she was hiding information, particularly about her sexual relations. She denied having any difficulties that necessitated hospitalization or treatment. No frank delusions or hallucinations were elicited. She had a childish, frightened attitude toward sex. During her stay in the hospital there were no abnormalities in her behavior, and no bizarre mental content was discovered. It was felt that the present situation was probably a neurotic reaction to environmental pressures. She was discharged much improved, but with a poor prognosis unless the environment could be rearranged so that she would be better able to carry the burden of her home responsibilities.

P. React. Depr. M:33:M:17 +11 '34 286–9 8:3:24
P. Hys. +34 4'23 1876– 7:3:26

For the past six months the patient had complained of headaches and dizziness which occurred when he watched moving objects. He also felt despondent, was uninterested in his surroundings, and was unable to carry out his routine work. About six days before admission to the hospital the patient suddenly experienced such marked ataxia that he had to lie in bed or sit in a chair. The melancholia became deeper, and there was unprovoked crying.

The patient, an eighth-grade graduate, had made a very poor school record. Until the present illness he had worked as an auto mechanic. Although he was a good mechanic, he had moved from one garage to another at relatively short intervals. At about the onset of the present illness he had been forced out of a good job by a man whom he had befriended. He had always been a matter-of-fact, cheerful, social individual and had shown fairly good judgment. Sensitive, he was eager to have people like him, and it was said that he was generous to a fault. He had always taken his responsibilities seriously and was mainly interested in his work and in his home.

In the hospital the general physical and neurological examinations indicated nothing of significance. Poorly nourished and small in stature, the patient spent his first days lying in bed crying, a manifestation that gradually disappeared over a period of about four days. At that time he disclaimed any remaining depression, took an active interest in ward life, and appeared normal. He was discharged completely recovered so far as could be determined.

P. React. Depr. F:54:M:17 +3 '34 619 278–X 12:2:22

The patient was admitted to the hospital because of marked depression and weeping. The present episode, one of four or five in the past three years, began when a woman made unkind remarks about the patient's attitude toward a son who had been dead for seventeen years. Unable to stop crying, the woman had

had to leave her work, and for a few days she had been unable to return. Her depressions were always characterized by uncontrollable crying, and they seemed to come on more readily when she was fatigued. Of a cyclical nature, the depressions had always appeared during the Christmas season, which was associated with the death of her son. She had a deep feeling of remorse about this son because she had got a divorce from her first husband shortly before the boy's death. Thirteen years before the present admission she had married her second husband, an epileptic and an alcoholic with whom she had been very unhappy.

According to the patient, her health had always been poor, and in addition to considerable treatment for a cardiac disease, she had undergone a bilateral mastectomy for the cosmetic effect. Very friendly and overly talkative, the woman was emotionally unstable, and had always been subject to "blue" spells, but apparently between depressions she was an adequate person and very good in the management of household affairs. Her hobby was gardening, and she put a great deal of energy into it.

In the hospital her chief concern was expressed by her question, "What can I do about my troubles?" There were no severe disturbances of mentation, but she cried much of the time, and whenever she directed the conversation she invariably turned it toward stories relating to her son. There were no paranoid trends except that she blamed her present depression on situations that had occurred in routine day-by-day living. She was well oriented, appeared to be dull normal intellectually, and was excessively desirous of an audience. It was noticed that slight things changed her mood so radically that even when she was unhappy she could be made to laugh very easily. Her general attitude was exceedingly superficial. There was a considerable tendency toward circumstantiality. Her condition rapidly improved in the hospital, and when she was discharged she seemed to be her ordinary self, but it was felt that she would almost certainly have other attacks.

Ps. Invol. Melan. F:50:S:41 +2 3'46271–9(59) 7:0:21
Paranoid

The patient was admitted to the hospital with delusions that she had been violated sexually and with throbbing abdominal pain. The complaints dated from about ten months before, when her brother and two close friends had died within a relatively short period. The first occasion on which she claimed to have been raped occurred in a private home where she was living. The next attack happened in a doctor's office. The third "assailant" was a man who had come to see her at the home of a friend. After these delusional episodes she felt a throbbing pain in her abdomen, became preoccupied and withdrawn, and worried a great deal because she thought she was pregnant or had contracted a venereal disease. The reassurance of physicians did not convince her.

The patient had had a number of illnesses in the past although none of them were particularly contributory to the present problem. The only other nervous disorder had followed her mother's death about nine years before admission, when the patient had been upset for three or four months.

Of good intelligence, the patient was a graduate of a teachers' college and had spent most of her life teaching grade school. She had experienced periods of great enthusiasm and overactivity, during which she spent her money "like a drunken sailor" and undertook such enterprises as flying or piano lessons. After these periods she was frugal and often somewhat depressed. A love affair at 23 had not led to marriage because her parents did not approve of the man. A sensitive, shy, snobbish and rather haughty person, she had always found it difficult to talk with strangers, but with people she knew she was friendly and cooperative. A sister, described as "cute, smart, and always healthy," had been a dominating influence on the patient's life from her earliest years, and when the sister married the patient had been very upset.

The hospital neurological examination was negative, and the physical examination yielded no evidence of sexual assault. The patient gave the outward appearance of being high-strung and ill at ease, but she was conventional in behavior and normal in sensorium and intellect. Her haughtiness aroused antagonism in the other patients. Her response to psychotherapy was good from the first, and she was quick to accept the fact that she was not pregnant and that she did not have a venereal disease. She began to have good insight, recognizing that many of her ideas were delusional, and the abdominal pain she had originally complained of gradually disappeared. On discharge, she seemed to have recovered from the present episode, and it was felt that she would probably make a good adjustment, but from the past history it seemed likely that there might be recurrences.

Ps. M-D., Manic F:43:S:58 +8 '34 69–2 (41) 6:4:17

The patient, a teacher, had had a heavy teaching load for some time. She said that she had been "neurotic" for a year, and she felt that her mind was "fuzzy." She had had transient dysphagia some months before admission, but it had disappeared after a few weeks. Her interest in religion had been increasing at a rapid rate, and she had been easily upset. Two weeks before admission she began to write down, frantically, her ideas on religion, psychiatry, racial prejudice, and nursing education. She slept only a few hours each night and ate very irregularly. She "bombarded" her students with her ideas and sent out more than 700 letters to such people as Stalin and the Pope.

Six years earlier the patient had suffered a depression, and had been treated with electroshock therapy. Three years later another nervous and hyperactive episode occurred, from which the patient made a spontaneous recovery. An intelligent person, she was capable of holding excellent jobs except for personality difficulties. Apparently she had been unable to get along with employers and resented authority. She had always been nasty to eligible men, she said, "almost as if it were a deliberate attempt on my part." The patient's brother described her as a person "who never stuck to anything for long" and who was "always enthusiastic about some one thing, but only for a little while."

On admission to the hospital she would scarcely talk of anything except religion, psychiatric treatment, and brotherly love. The ideas were disconnected and came out so rapidly that it was confusing to listen to her. Well oriented, she apparently was not suffering from hallucinatory experiences. She quickly improved and then felt very ashamed of her ideas, recognizing them as a camouflage for "feelings inside me which are wicked." Discussing her disappointment at being a failure in life, she said that she could have been a fine mother and wife and did not understand why she had repeatedly driven away eligible men. The thought of living alone was distasteful to her and she felt intense guilt about masturbation. At discharge she was completely recovered from the present illness, but it was felt likely that she would have future trouble.

Ps. Sz., Mixed F:24:S:42 +1 34817 62'9–(49) 6:9:13
Suicidal

The patient was admitted from another psychopathic hospital in order to receive further psychiatric evaluation. About seven months before the present admission she had entered the other hospital because of pain, nervousness, dizzy spells, confusion, inability to concentrate, and other complaints. There was a long history of various somatic disorders, outstanding among which was "stomach trouble."

During her early childhood the patient had had eyelid tics, nightmares, and episodes of nausea and vomiting. At the age of 6 she had been frightened by an elderly man who made sexual advances to her. She graduated from high school and after special training became a stenographer. Her I.Q. was 114. Two years before admission, while in a depressed and lonely mood following a family argument, she was picked up by a casual acquaintance, and they had sexual intercourse. She confessed to her pastor but was apparently left with guilt feelings. She became pregnant from this experience and was sent to live with relatives where she had frequent attacks of vomiting and hiccups. After the child was born, she arranged for a church announcement of its illegitimacy and then returned to live with relatives who did not really want her. At about this time it was found that she had a gonococcal infection.

In the hospital she was mostly characterized by her self-depreciating remarks. She was convinced that nothing could be done for her and wanted to know when she could leave. She took an uncompromisingly hostile and argumentative attitude. She had no obvious delusional or hallucinatory experiences, although it was felt that there were hidden delusions of grandeur and persecution. In discussion she was at times disconnected, confused, and rambling. At times she was preoccupied, took no care with her appearance, was easily agitated and anxious, pulled at her hair, twisted her clothes, and breathed heavily. She hoarded objects with which she might attempt to commit suicide or to harm herself. Psychotherapeutic study revealed many hostilities and much abnormal content, but it brought about no improvement. She was transferred to a state hospital.

Ps. Sz., Cat.	F:17:S:520	+10	'3482697–(49)	6:7:17
		+275	68497'3–X(63)	3:24:12

This girl had first entered the hospital following a series of fainting spells. These had begun about five months earlier with an attack of sobbing and crying which had been precipitated by an unfortunate incident at a school program. In the middle of a violin solo by the patient a string became loose, and although she managed to finish her piece, it sounded badly played. She felt embarrassed, humiliated, and above all disappointed that she had not lived up to the expectations of her father, who was lying at home slowly dying of cancer. At the end of the performance she cried hysterically, fainted, and did not regain consciousness until hours later when she awoke to find herself in a sanitarium. Given electroconvulsive therapy she returned home in three weeks feeling fine.

A second spell occurred when she was at a movie with her boy friend and began to worry about whether she should have stayed home with her sick father. Returned to the sanitarium for more shock therapy, she again recovered quickly. At this time her father died and after her return home she began to worry about her father's death and also about her brother-in-law, who had made sexual advances to her since she was 12. The family's evasions about her recent illness caused her anxiety, and she began to feel, she said, that they were "following me around, avoiding my questions, and not trusting me." After several more attacks of fainting and amnesic spells she was brought to the hospital for more intensive study.

Although she had had to compete for parental affection with six sisters, the patient had been deeply attached to her father and had received considerable affection from him. Her mother was never able to be frank or honest with the children, and she was excitable and in constant need of reassurance and guidance from others. The patient was an average student, was popular, and had many friends. However, she was easily hurt and retaliated in roundabout ways. When she was about 7 she had developed many gastrointestinal complaints and since the age of 15 she had complained of repeated headaches.

On admission to the hospital the girl at first was guarded and resentful about being sent to a mental hospital again. However, she was able to give a concise, relevant history of herself and no significant abnormalities were detected in the initial mental examination. After a month in the hospital and directly following a disturbing visit to her home, she began to talk about her problems. She felt that she was unwanted, that her mother did not like her, and that she was responsible for her father's death. The sexual activities with her brother-in-law also worried her. She was seen regularly from three to five times a week for psychotherapy. Instead of fainting spells she now had episodes of violent impulsive behavior, during which she fought with anyone who tried to control her. Auditory and visual hallucinations developed and insulin therapy was used. (The second MMPI was given after these treatments.) Psychotherapy was continued and a gradual improvement took place although it was still many months before she ceased to hear her father's voice. Several episodes of self-injury also occurred during the months following the insulin treatments. Gradually she gained some insight into the family situation. The psychotherapeutic interviews were aimed at establishing a good relationship with her family. She returned home to stay after a trial period. The family said she got along very well. During the daughter's illness the mother was also seen for interviews. After discharge the patient returned for outpatient treatment. E. B.

Schizoid M:19:S '348791–2(34) 5:2:22

This young high school graduate came to the center for vocational counseling at the suggestion of his father, who wished to find out whether it would be better for the boy to continue school or to find a job in the fall. The father told us that his son had had a "nervous breakdown" two years before, had been hospitalized, and had been given psychotherapy. He was discharged and returned to school but the following summer had another psychotic episode. Shock therapy was used this time, and he returned late to a private school, where he took a reduced schedule and graduated, but with mediocre grades. The school did not consider him college material, and his problem was to determine his next step.

The client himself talked mainly about jobs, but his father requested that we test for college ability as well as vocational aptitude. Shy and ill at ease, the boy showed strong feelings of inferiority. Both his parents and an older brother had been good students, but he had always been just average in his studies.

College aptitude tests indicated he had an average language ability but was poor in mathematics and below average in reading skills. His interests were in recreation and group work. To aid him in gaining a sense of status and in getting training equivalent to others in his own group, a trial plan was worked out for college with special work on remedial reading. He was intensely interested in this plan but undertook it with considerable anxiety. Early in the program his anxiety was so acute that he became fearful of another nervous illness. A psychiatrist saw him for a few interviews; he was given reassurance and achieved some insight. The program was continued as planned. He completed one year of college with passing grades in all but one semester of chemistry. He was discouraged by this and a little tempted to give up college. At one interview during the summer he requested the counselor's aid in getting a job, but he returned a few weeks later to say that he had decided to try another year of college.

D. F. C.

B. Pri., Child. M:17:S:38 +1 3'491 68–(53) 7:4:18

About three years before admission the patient took his sister's car and ran away from home for no apparent reason. The next significant incident occurred a year before admission, at a time when the patient was hospitalized for the treatment of corneal ulcers. The boy overheard a doctor say that he was going to be blind, and after that time he was depressed. Within the next few months he was involved in two major auto accidents, and as a result his parents refused him permission to drive. About three weeks before admission he told a story of having twice been kidnapped by a gang of men who were "out to get" his father, but when the police investigated his wildly told story of having fought off and escaped from the men, the patient confessed that the story was false. His only explanation was that there were times when he did not know what he was doing.

He had been in the hospital during the preceding three summers, first with jaundice, then for an appendectomy, and finally with the corneal ulcers. The first two years of his life he had spent in a hospital with eczema. At the time of admission he was in a twelfth-grade sight-saving class, and he had always been protected because of his eyes. He was a daydreamer, and he was submissive at home where he did his work carelessly but without complaint. His personality was good, and he got along well with people. He wanted to go into the army until he was 21, and then he planned to go into business.

In the hospital he was well oriented and clear in sensorium. He realized that what he had done was wrong, but he could give no adequate explanation for his actions other than that they might have been induced by a blow he had received on the head in a recent automobile accident. His replies to questions were adequate, but it was difficult to draw him out, and there obviously were problems he would not discuss. He appeared entirely normal around the ward, and he was always friendly and cooperative. He expressed hostility toward his home situation and it was apparent that he did not want to return there. His own mother had died when he was a child and he had a very real hostility toward his stepmother. He regarded his father as a "weakling." The social service attempted to change the home situation, but the stepmother refused to consider any suggestion that the boy live elsewhere.

F:21:S '36–27(55) 1:3:19

This college freshman came to the clinic voluntarily to discuss her doubts about her ability to make an adequate moral adjustment. She reported that she had recently become engaged after a very brief courtship and had then broken it off, also after a very short time. There was an identification with an older sister who had had considerable marital difficulty, and the patient was concerned because she did not form close attachments with boys.

A very lively and vivacious girl, she was apparently able to make friends readily. She liked to be with people and had many artistic and cultural interests. Although not endowed with physical beauty, she made a reasonably attractive appearance.

A series of four interviews took place, during which her rejecting attitude toward her own femininity, her identification with her sister and her father, and the conflict caused by some very early sex play with her brother and her parents' relatively rigid attitude toward sex were brought into the open. Following this release experience she was able to work out some personally satisfying integrations involving compromises between her career drives and her desire for normal sexual experience. It was at the close of this short series of interviews that she took the MMPI. A contact with her a few months later indicated that she was still retaining the gains she had made during the interviews. E. S. B.

Ps. Paranoid M:22:S:5 +1 '36–718 2:2:14

The patient had been apparently normal until two years before admission when his personality had begun to change. There was a marked increase in his consumption of alcohol; he squandered money and became irritable, taciturn, and depressed. At the time, he was a college student, and when his scholastic standing fell he left school to become a traveling salesman. He developed the delusion that representatives of the firm he was employed by were watching him and spying upon him, and as a consequence he resigned. When he returned home his parents noted that he was sleepless, irritable, depressed, and physically "rundown." For a while he became a kind of tramp, going from town to town, and in letters home he told of a young lady who, he believed, was following him. When officials notified his parents that their son was penniless and half-starved, they arranged to have him sent home. There he was irritable, easily angered, and difficult to manage, getting up at all hours to go for a walk, and frequently speaking of being annoyed by the young woman he thought was following him. On one occasion he went to a restaurant and ordered a meal for the girl, believing that she was in town.

The patient was an ambitious, enterprising person with unusually high moral standards. He attended a university for three years, making an unsatisfactory record only in his third year. He was unusually careful about his personal appearance. Although he was sociable, he was stiffly formal and ultrapolite, never fitting into any group, and his tendency was to cultivate the friendship of people who had money or prestige. Money was his one goal in life, although in general he never discussed his ideas or plans with anyone.

In the hospital he had marked paranoid trends, which consisted mostly of delusions of reference. He admitted that the evidence on which he based his feelings that people were spying on him and that the girl was following him was flimsy. When actually confronted with a logical statement of his situation he would say that he was probably wrong, but these admissions had no depth, and his behavior continued unchanged. He was well oriented and appeared composed though slightly depressed. There was no evidence of hallucinatory experiences. He said that he came into the hospital merely to please his parents and he did not feel that there was any need for the mental study. Although he was pleasant toward the examiner, and in general seemed fairly normal while in the hospital, it was apparently an effort for him to maintain this front. During his few days in the hospital his condition did not change, and it was obvious that the strain of being pleasant was becoming too much for him. Because his paranoid ideas were so definitely localized at a specific period of time, it was felt that his illness was a transitory psychotic episode, and that the patient would be able to maintain his place in society without future trouble. The problems and suggestions for his care were gone over with the parents and he was discharged to their care.

P. Anxiety State   F:22:M:15   +2   3712'4986–(53)   6:7:17

Immediately following the birth of her first child three months before admission, the patient began to feel inadequate in caring for it. The sight of the baby was enough to bring on an attack of vertigo, nausea, vomiting, weakness, and crying. She felt no confidence in herself and was afraid she would do something to harm the baby. She also demanded much attention from her husband and family.

All her life the patient had shown hysterical symptoms, and she had experienced vomiting and anorexia with every menstrual period since the menarche. She had such severe abdominal pains that she had to spend several days in bed each month. She was described as having always been nervous, and she developed dyspnea and palpitation on slight exertion. She had been treated for cardiac complaints, and some years before the present admission a diagnosis of psychoneurosis, hypochondriasis, had been made in the outpatient department of the hospital.

She had left school while in the twelfth grade, apparently having done fairly well in her schoolwork. At the age of 21 she married a man her family did not approve of and she became pregnant shortly after marriage. The child was unwanted by the husband, who blamed her for it. The patient was said to be shy, quiet, and reserved but always interested in doing things for others.

In the hospital the patient was very concerned with the problem of what she would do if she had to care for her baby and herself. She worried all the time about the baby. She considered herself as being nervous and worrying too much but she did not know what to do about it. In appearance she was neat, quiet, and shy, entirely normal in behavior and stream of thought. There was no marked evidence of depression and the emotional accompaniments of her worrying did not appear to be very deep. She complained of painful breasts and of cramps and nausea during menstruation. It appeared that her mother had been overprotective of her and had given her too much attention for her neurotic complaints. She was discharged to her husband after improving symptomatically but the long-standing character of her neurotic pattern made it unlikely that she would be much different in the future.

P. React. Depr.	F:48:M:36	0	37128'46–(45)	7:9:20
Suicidal		–51	237'184–(49)	8:4:17

The patient had always been nervous and tense but six years before admission, following the removal of her uterus, tubes, and ovaries, the nervousness had become more marked. She began having short depressive episodes and in the six months before admission the depression had been almost constant. She withdrew from her usual activities, had ideas of suicide, and became irritable and hypersensitive. There had been one possible attempt at suicide when she took an overdose of insulin.

The past medical history was not particularly contributory. She had been recognized as a diabetic eleven years before admission. The laparotomy was undertaken because of a suspected fibroma of the uterus. Restricted and overprotected by her parents during her childhood, she had been required to do an excessive amount of homework. She said this was the reason she had left school when she was in the ninth grade at age 15. Her intelligence was high average. She worked for a while after leaving school and was a reliable and hard worker. Married at age 21, she had few interests after that outside of her own household. Economically and socially the conditions of the home were poor.

In the hospital the patient was concerned about her situation as well as the living conditions of her family and her husband's attitude. According to her, he had opposed education for their children and was a heavy drinker. She realized she was ill and that emotional factors were contributing to her problem. She was friendly and cooperative but on the defensive, and she became extremely upset and wept when speaking of her family situation. She worked well in the hospital routine and received four electroshock treatments that appeared to help her. By the time she was discharged she was looking forward to her duties as a housewife with more equanimity. Plans for a change in the living situation were being made when she left the hospital.

Alcoholism	F:33:M:57	+7	3721 486'–(41)	4:12:14
Suicidal		+53	312784'96–(49)	4:7:18

The patient had begun drinking at age 19 and had become progessively more addicted to alcohol. She had had several attacks of delirium tremens and had attempted suicide; she was hospitalized several times, in the workhouse several times, and in a state hospital for inebriates once. She was discharged from the latter hospital two months before admission but began drinking again as soon as she was released, and she was brought to the psychopathic unit after she had planned another suicide.

Her past physical health had been good. She had an exceedingly irregular background. Her father was a chronic alcoholic who had been frequently drunk and who had often beaten the patient's mother. After divorcing him, the mother married another alcoholic who later committed suicide. As a child the patient had been shunned by other children because they were afraid of getting the dermatitis she had. She married at 19 after leaving high school and then she and her husband drank together. They had a 10-year-old child. The husband was eight years older than she. He had been discharged from a post office job because of pilfering the mails, and later he was sent to prison for stealing. After this the patient continued as a "lone wolf" drinker. She was said to have been somewhat promiscuous sexually, especially after her husband's imprisonment.

In the hospital the patient's sensorium and intellect were intact. She was distraught and nervous at first. There were no obvious delusions or hallucinations although she had experienced these shortly before admission when under the influence of drugs. Rambling but coherent in discourse, she was open and cooperative. She was concerned about her future and was determined to commit suicide unless she could control her drinking. In time she became more calm, was sociable, and ate well. There was little change in her general attitude even after several electroshock treatments. She accepted ward discipline under protest, and although she said that she was anxious to control her alcoholism, she could never really cooperate with the staff.

P. Hypo.	F:57:D:72	+1	'376842-1 (53)	7:5:8
		−22	17328'4-	7:2:20

There was no definite onset for this woman's admitting complaints, nervousness and numerous somatic pains and aches. She dated these symptoms from a fall when she was 10 years of age. When she was nervous or had to hurry, she noticed, the complaints became worse. Gradually the difficulties became more disturbing to her and she sought hospital aid.

As a frail and delicate child, the patient had experienced hysterical fainting when she was only 10. Her childhood had not been at all happy. She was a graduate of a two-year teachers' college, and at the completion of this training she married. After twelve years of unhappy married life she divorced her husband and worked as a domestic to support herself and her son. Later she became a hospital employee. The medical history included numerous clinical examinations and a number of major operations. First seen in the outpatient department of the psychiatric clinic three years earlier, she had then been diagnosed as having psychoneurosis with moderate depression and hypochondriasis. Outstanding was her inability to make and stick by decisions.

In the hospital she was mainly preoccupied with the somatic complaints, which varied in emphasis from day to day. These were always on the surface and she would pay little attention to anything else. On several occasions she expressed a fear that she might lose her mind because her memory seemed to be failing. Her verbal insight into her problems was fairly good. The patient's appearance was neat, her attitude and manner appropriate, and she had no obvious anxiety or depression. The real difficulty appeared to be her inability to decide on a course of action. For example, she waited twelve years to divorce her husband in spite of adequate reasons for doing so long before. After the divorce she continued to see him and one of the problems that brought her into the hospital was her indecision about whether to return to him. This would be a bad move, she seemed to realize, but when they were together he could talk her into it. Every effort was put forth to help her make her own decision in the matter. This general line of endeavor was not successful, since her one real, persistent purpose was to persuade the staff members to make all decisions for her.

P. Hys. M:33:M:12 +5 '38–46 7:2:21

This patient complained of convulsive seizures which had first appeared about seven years before admission. At first they had occurred only once or twice a year, but they had gradually become more frequent, though less severe, until at the time of admission the patient was experiencing five or six a day, usually after physical exertion. The attacks, which lasted from ten minutes to two hours, began with a blurring of vision, followed by a "loss of consciousness," during which the patient became rigid and threshed about. Upon recovering consciousness he experienced numbness in his hands and felt weak for about an hour, and then he resumed his activities with an occasional "ordinary headache" as the only continuing symptom. On one occasion there was urinary incontinence. Medication had no effect upon the seizures. After an outpatient study and a careful neurological examination the neurologists decided that the symptoms were functional in pattern.

Before the onset of the seizures the patient had not been outstanding in any way. An eighth-grade graduate, he had made a fairly satisfactory school record, but he had not got along well with his fellow students or with his teachers because, he said, "I was always sort of a pest." After leaving school he had worked for his father on the farm. Following his marriage at age 26 he had continued to live with his parents until he rented a farm for himself a few years later. The farming venture was not especially successful and he went on W.P.A., but again the salary did not provide for the family necessities and he did odd jobs to increase his income. However, the many bills he had incurred were a source of great concern to him. He was described as having always been somewhat flighty, easily depressed, and easily consoled. Apparently his most outstanding trait had been a lack of perseverance.

In the hospital he was friendly and very cooperative, making a completely satisfactory adjustment to ward activities. After transference to the psychiatric unit, he experienced no seizures and no abnormalities could be noted in his behavior, with the possible exception of a peculiar indifference to his long history of seizures. He was concerned about the fact that he was in a "mental ward," protesting that there was nothing wrong with his "mind," and attempts to give him some insight were unsuccessful.

Ps. Sz., Hebe. M:23:S 3'8<u>16</u>24–9X(61) 11:5:16

This young man was admitted with a history of nervousness, confusion, apathy, and attempted violence against his mother. He admitted having had auditory and visual hallucinations and he used neologisms and mannerisms. Frequently he was in good contact and realized that something was wrong with him.

The patient was dominated by his mother. Until the age of 13, he had slept with her. She prevented him from going out with girls by her obvious disapproval. She also prevented his participation in high school athletics but encouraged his regular attendance in church and Sunday school. Always quiet, neat, and well dressed before, he became slovenly, irritable, and hostile toward his mother and his brothers after his discharge from the army. He enrolled at a university but made a poor record there.

After his admission to the hospital his condition became progressively worse. He was more manneristic, his affect was less appropriate, and hallucinations were more frequent. Electroshock therapy was recommended. W. M. H.

P. Hypo. F:27:W:129 +33 <u>38</u>16724'9– 7:15:10

Originally admitted to the medical service, the patient listed some of her ills as headaches, backache, constipation, dysuria, and blurring of vision. On that service for two months, she was difficult to manage. Finally she became delirious and had terrifying hallucinations; the basis for these could not be determined, although a toxic delirium was considered. Obviously strongly affected by news, good or bad, and by the people who visited her, she was finally admitted to the psychiatric unit of the hospital for study, and in that admission no real findings resulted. An organic basis for the patient's troubles could not be discovered, and when she was discharged the general feeling was that she was a neurotic. In the present admission a similar pattern of somatic complaints was present.

After grade school the young woman had spent several years in the Salvation Army. A naive person, she had been considered mentally retarded. Her tested I.Q. was about 90. She had always been friendly and eager to help others. Her personal habits had been fairly good. On the whole, however, it was plain that she had been an inadequate person. Married at age 17, she had four children, and the family lived in a dilapidated, dirty house. When her husband died the local welfare agency took over the management of the children. An attempt was made to take the children away from the mother and place them in better surroundings, but the patient resisted actively and successfully.

In the hospital the physical findings were not helpful. The neurological examination was essentially negative. The patient, however, complained steadily of pain and various other organic symptoms. Her conversation was full of her children and she said she was proud of them. She was anxious to remain in the hospital and wanted to bring the children to the city. She had a poor understanding of the factors influencing her hospitalization and was exceedingly resistant to attempts to help her either personally or socially. There were no gross disturbances of intellect or sensorium. She cooperated fairly well in the hospital routine and was friendly with the other patients, but she was obviously shallow and immature. No real progress could be made with the case except in terms of the social agency work and she was discharged after reasonably adequate plans had been made for her by that agency.

Ps. M-D., Manic F:33:M:79 +36 38419'276–X(57) 3:10:18

Ps. M-D., Manic F:33:M:25

The patient was admitted against her own wishes under pressure from her husband and her family physician because of a manic attack. About two weeks before admission she had undergone a marked personality change. At first she assumed an affected speech. Then she said that something had "snapped" in her head and she was able to answer all the questions she had always wondered about. She became overactive and shouted at her parents and her husband, saying that she was curing them of their neuroses. She became obsessed with the thought that her daughter did not say what she was thinking, and she shook the daughter violently in order to "let her true ideas out." Two days before admission she asked her husband if he intended to kill her. When he answered negatively, she cried and told him that for the first time she realized that she loved him.

The past physical health of the patient had been good. She had had no other mental upsets. As a child she had been under the influence of a domineering mother and grandmother, and she had apparently been precocious. She had gone through the second year of college but had stopped after an auto accident in which she received a minor injury. Later, after her marriage, she went back and eventually graduated. She had had many boy friends while in college and was active and apparently normal in every way. After her marriage she discovered that she had no sexual desire, and while she could take part in sexual intercourse the experience was unsatisfactory. During this time, she said, her husband had become abusive and had threatened to kill her. She described him as a "neurotic" individual who was very jealous of her.

In the hospital the patient was mainly concerned about her guilt. The guilt seemed to concern her daughter who was a diabetic. She spent much of her time trying to diagnose her own condition and to formulate methods of therapy. She was perturbed by the fact that the staff did not listen to her suggestions. Her sensorium and intellect were unimpaired. She was alternately euphoric and depressed. She professed much more insight than she actually seemed to have. There was an occasional flight of ideas but in general she was cooperative and willing to tell of her difficulties. She was given sixteen electroshock treatments and there was a temporary remission of the psychosis. However, later she again became overactive and manic. Additional electroshock treatment was begun and was accompanied by psychotherapeutic interviews in which some of the conflicts were brought out. She gradually improved and at the time of discharge she seemed considerably better. About five months later she was readmitted with manic symptoms similar to those in the first admission. The content of her thoughts was also much the same and this time she was treated with baths and sedation. In this admission she showed one pattern that was somewhat different in that she was very demanding and sorry for herself, which made her seem exceedingly egocentric. She again improved considerably until she was almost ready to return home. However, it was recommended that she be transferred to a state hospital for at least a short stay.

B. Pri., Child. M:17:S:186 +30 38′46172–(73) 6:8:22
Schizoid

This youth was referred by his high school principal, who refused to readmit the boy to school until he was seen by a psychiatrist. The reason for the principal's alarm was that the patient, who had been teased considerably for his effeminate appearance and manners, confessed to his gym coach that he had once had a homosexual experience.

Early in his life the boy had been extremely affectionate toward his father, but he later reversed this and was then close to his mother. The latter was a dominating, rigid, anxious, overreligious woman. Because of her overprotection the boy had had little contact with other children as he grew up. His father was also a rigid, religious person.

The boy was approximately forty pounds overweight. In the hospital he was extremely fluent, indeed verbose on pseudophilosophical and religious subjects. He had some tendency to consider himself as marked for an important mission, to bring salvation to his schoolmates and others. He impressed the therapist as an immature and insecure youth, unable to find masculine interests and to adjust with members of his own sex. His grasp on reality was tenuous at times and distorted by the persistence of infantile traits and ways of thinking. He told of hallucinatory experiences in which he saw a black shape, "death," although his mother had not been able to see it. Over the period of six months he was seen 24 times for psychotherapy on an outpatient basis; his mother was also seen during this time. The therapy attempted to interpret whatever feelings were aroused by the therapeutic relationship itself and to discuss with him any problems he brought. He improved considerably in his school adjustment, received better grades, got along better with other boys, and became somewhat interested in girls, although he was still far from fully accepting his heterosexual impulses. While at first he was interested in a mystic, esoteric cult, he later focused his interest on a local church, adopted its tenets wholeheartedly, and planned to go into church work as a vocation. Because he felt no further need for help and feared that it was contrary to his religion, he stopped the therapy.

E. B.

B. Simple Adult Maladj. F:17:S:27 +1 3'867924–(32) 3:3:13
P. Hys. +230 '389–6(42) 3:3:18
P. Psychas.

This girl came for help because of prolonged crying spells, lasting from six to eight hours, and intermittent periods of depression. These had begun to occur earlier in the school year (she was a college freshman); she had had similar periods during her high school years. At times she became nauseated but was unable to vomit. Selecting which dress to wear became difficult for her, and even after spending ten minutes or longer in deciding, she would be dissatisfied with her choice. Between the periods of depression there were days of elation when everything was "beautiful and serene."

The patient reported that she had had a fairly happy childhood until her parents were divorced. After that she began to experience periods of loneliness and depression, from which she sought escape by absorption in scholastic activities. During high school she was considered a social leader, but actually she felt very disturbed during those years. When she came to college she had hoped to find relief for her problem but instead found it emphasized.

During the therapy the client cried a great deal and was particularly sensitive on the subject of her parents' divorce. When the family property had been divided, a lake cottage where she had spent the happiest days of her childhood had been sold. In this cottage the parents had lived on most amicable terms, and the cottage symbolically represented all the security of the girl's early childhood. As she gained insight into the relationship of her problem to the sale of the cottage, she progressed quickly into insights in all the social areas. Six months following the termination of therapy she wrote to the therapist, "I go along without letting things bother me very much. Since I have seen you I have never been gay and happy for long periods of time, but I have never been as unhappy. I seem to be riding a middle course. I am more social and like to have kids over, which I never did before. I go out both with friends and my family more too."

A. S.

B. Psth., Path. Emot. F:36:D:44 +20 39'1428–6 6:6:9

Increased appetite, fatigue, and obesity made up the complaint pattern for this woman. The increasing appetite had been accompanied by headaches, irritability, and occasional vomiting and nausea after meals. In addition, she found it difficult to relax and frequently had anxiety dreams. She had gained weight rapidly in the early stages and was self-conscious about it.

The history showed that a "paralysis" of the patient's lower extremity, lasting a month, had followed the death of her mother. There had also been a period in which the patient complained of weakness in her leg from a minor injury. Many medical procedures had been performed, including a bilateral salpingectomy and a hysterectomy with a bilateral oophorectomy.

Although the patient had finished much of the work for a high school diploma she had never obtained one. She had worked as a waitress and at stenographic and clerical jobs until her admission to the hospital. Her first marriage had occurred under the pressure of a seven months' pregnancy. After the birth of the child she had divorced her husband, had remarried, and had soon sought a second divorce. As a child she had been considered a tomboy. Socially she was aggressive. Friends said that she had always overreacted to sorrow.

In the hospital the patient was chiefly concerned about her constipation and about being overweight. Extremely dissatisfied with the diet offered in the hospital, she said that she would prefer a box of caramels. She resented the locked doors. She said her dead mother's voice often called for her when she was asleep. Apparently she believed that she possessed unusual powers: "My mother and I had a real close bond between us which stretched across miles. She knew when I was sick and I knew when she was ill. She had a second sight and since she died I have developed it. I have the gift of being able to look through people and to judge them." She was convinced that people discussed her obesity, although in reality her overweight was only moderately obvious. There was considerable variation in her affect, and she cried and laughed by turns. At other times she behaved irritably and was inclined to be loquacious and boastful. She frequently turned the conversation to the topic of sex. There was no severe break with reality and no gross disturbance of sensorium or intellect. She never changed in her strong feeling that "there is nothing wrong with my personality" and that "there is no reason whatsoever for me to be in a psychiatric hospital." Although she did in general cooperate in the activities of the ward, she resisted efforts to help her. By the time of discharge she had improved somewhat in her general attitude and was making acceptable plans for the future.

B. Psth., Asocial M:22:D 39′4 287 16–(74) 2:8:6
Mutilative

This young man, who was serving a prison sentence for assault with intent to murder, mutilated his Achilles' tendon with a dirk knife. He was treated and placed in solitary confinement. According to the youth's statement, the assault for which he was sentenced and imprisoned grew out of a gun fight that followed a card game. The prisoner had intentionally shot his victim in the leg, he said, in order to avoid killing him. He had entered a plea of guilty.

The prisoner's criminal career began at the age of 17, just after he completed high school, when he was arrested on a charge of grand and petty larceny. Convicted and sentenced to one year in the state reformatory, he was given a conditional parole two months later in order to join the army. After eleven months of service as a paratrooper he was injured in the back and was given an honorable discharge. On his twentieth birthday he was arrested for petty thievery and served four months in a county jail. Two years later he was arrested on vagrancy and theft charges and served six months in a county jail.

The youth's early home life had been sketchy and confused. His father disappeared when he was 10 or 11 and had not been heard of since. The prisoner and his brothers and sisters were scattered in different homes and he had long since lost track of most of the members of his family. A year before the present imprisonment the youth had married but his wife was now suing him for divorce. His employment record was one of varied pursuits and included jobs as painter, salesman, cabinetmaker's helper, office clerk, and hospital attendant. He had also been employed by a bookmaker and had operated a poker table in a gambling casino. His I.Q. was 105.

The prison classification committee, in considering the youth's case, classed him as an unstable psychopath and recommended that he be placed in the isolation lockup where the least reformable men are kept. He was rated as "criminally mature" and the possibilities for his rehabilitation were deemed poor.

R. C. K.

Ps. M-D., Manic Paranoid F:29:M:11 +4 3'<u>94</u>681–7 (59) 2:5:10

For a year the young woman had noticed a gradual onset of lassitude, easy fatigability, diminishing appetite, and loss of weight. Sent to a general hospital for two months, she was so depressed there, she said, that "If I had not believed in God, I would have taken my life." She could offer no reason for this depression and the only treatment she received was rest. When she was discharged from the hospital she seemed to be much improved, but she did not fully recover for several months. She then began to swing in the other direction; she developed excessive energies and engaged in manifold activities. She was impatient and critical of her husband, and she had ideas of reference that people were accusing her of infidelity and of using narcotics. She was boastful and exaggerative, and when angered she overreacted with hysterical crying or fainting.

The past history gave no evidence of definite earlier upsets, although she had always been prone to hypochondriacal complaints. She was graduated from high school at age 18, having spent the first two years in a boarding school. Her record was good and she liked school. Until her marriage she worked as a waitress and clerk. Described as "high-strung and nervous," she did everything with intensity, was energetic and efficient. Versed in psychiatric terminology, she used this knowledge in rationalizing everything so as to create a favorable impression.

In the hospital the patient was restless but showed conventional behavior. Her stream of thought was logical and adequate except about her reason for entering the hospital. On this she was evasive. She attributed all her marital problems to her husband's drinking. There were no gross disturbances of sensorium or intellect. Although slightly antagonistic toward staff members, she was friendly with other patients. It seemed that she had actually begun to recover from the illness before admission, and she was her usual self during her brief stay in the hospital. At discharge it was expected that she might again become depressed before long, despite the evidence that some adjustment of the home situation and other environmental factors had been achieved.

P. React. Depr. F:21:S '3948672–(53) 4:3:14

This young woman was brought in for treatment, in fact practically forced to come, by members of her sorority. The patient had been depressed for several weeks, severely so the last few days. According to her own report she was subject to depressions at irregular intervals. Her family and friends said that she had been "using too much benzedrine and alcohol."

The girl's father was an ineffectual, neutral person who had battled with his domineering wife for ten years before they eventually separated. The patient was the youngest of three children. Her brother and sister sided with the mother, and the patient felt considerable guilt because of her preference for her father. She idealized her brother and apparently her depression had been precipitated by his marriage.

The patient revealed a good deal of concern and guilt about sexual matters and apparently could find a relaxed adjustment only with homosexual boys. It was fairly evident that her ambivalence concerning her father was of grave significance. She rapidly showed evidence of a rather sticky transference and therapy was slow. Her imminent departure forced the therapist to make an early attempt to deal with the transference situation and the last weeks of therapy were stormy. At discharge she had improved some but little progress had been made with the basic problems. C. K. A.

B. Psth., Asocial F:24:D:6 +1 '4–1683(61) 5:1:15

The patient had had two illegitimate children in the two years since her divorce and had been under the care of a welfare agency for most of the time. She had, for the past two months, suffered spells of depression and crying alternating with elation, nervousness, and irritability. A week before admission she had begun to withdraw from people and to develop extreme dependence. Her husband was attempting to persuade her to come back to live with him and to gain custody of the two children after their remarriage. Because he was so unstable and undependable the welfare agency asked for a study of the patient before giving its consent to this plan.

The patient was of dull normal intelligence and had had difficulty in school. She had married at age 18 and had appeared to be making a good adjustment until, after two years, she discovered that her husband was carrying on an open affair with another woman. The patient had been a shy, timid, retiring child, constantly afraid of people and of doing things. Her childhood had been unhappy because of overly strict and moralistic parents. During the early part of her married life she improved somewhat and worked at a number of jobs, chiefly as a domestic employee. She described her former husband as "charming and conceited." She had numerous love affairs after their divorce. After she had her first illegitimate child, the husband begged for a reconciliation. Apparently he was willing to accept that child but when the patient arrived in the city where he was employed, she was already pregnant for a second time, and he was unwilling to remarry her then.

In the hospital she was mainly concerned with her present illness, her nervousness, and her indecision, although she did not show any symptoms during the examination. She expressed hope and confidence in the future since her husband wanted her back again. There were no defects of sensorium or intellect. She was apparently normal in her stream of thought. There were no evidences of bizarre behavior. She was somewhat inaccessible and assumed that she was in the hospital chiefly for a rest and to quiet her nerves. She had mild guilt feelings about the two children. She appeared older than her 24 years but was relatively lacking in psychological maturity and affect. She was cheerful and normal in ward activities but completely unapproachable for psychotherapy. She was discharged unchanged with a poor prognosis.

Ps. Sz., Mixed Paranoid	M:21:S	'4–19(43)	4:2:10
Ps. Sz., Mixed	M:21:S	8927631'4–X(65) '483–269(42)	8:33:14 9:2:23
Ps. Sz., Mixed Alcoholism	M:23:S	'43816–(43)	8:4:24

This patient was admitted to the hospital for the third time because of excessive drinking and peculiar behavior. On his first admission (first MMPI) he presented early paranoid symptoms and had a number of delusions which were vague and unsystematized. He left the hospital against medical advice after three weeks. Two months later his parents requested readmission because of peculiar behavior, failure to work, and somatic complaints. At this time he was apathetic and emotionally reduced, and his conversation was circumstantial, irrelevant, and revealed distortions of thinking and delusional ideas. He became disturbed and resistive on the ward. A diagnosis of schizophrenic reaction, mixed type, was made. After a course of insulin shock therapy, and also group and individual psychotherapy, he improved rapidly and was discharged at the end of five months. On the third admission he did not show any gross symptoms of his psychosis and after some supportive treatment was again discharged to return to his home.

Of average intelligence, the patient had finished the tenth grade and had then held jobs in skilled trades until he joined the navy. His mother described the young man as always well behaved, mild-mannered, and ambitious. She said that he got along well with others, liked outdoor sports, and was active in church work. The patient stated that he was always rather shy and sensitive, never made close friends, and stayed by himself much of the time. He acknowledged habitual masturbation but denied guilt feelings about this.

Although this patient continued to have difficulty in adjusting, he still appeared to be in remission of his psychosis after thirteen months. W. M. H.

P. Hys. F:18:S:64 +1 '4–<u>79</u>2X(55) 10:2:17
Schizoid

This patient had gradually been withdrawing from social contacts over the last two years and in addition had developed a jerky motion of the thumb. The latter symptom had been present for about six months. She had also become careless in dress and personal cleanliness. Whereas previously she had been interested in people, she now had become shy and would not stay in a room where there was a group of people even if those present were friends or members of her own family. The jerking movement of the right thumb had been preceded by an involuntary jerking of the arm, which had been especially bad when she was excited. With the disappearance of the arm jerk the thumb symptom appeared.

In her past medical history there was an acute febrile condition at age six, during which she had been delirious. She was a high school graduate, finishing at age 17. She made a good record and was socially active in school. It was only in the last year or two that she had changed in this respect.

The physical examination on admission to the hospital was negative. There were, however, a number of reflex findings in the neurological examination and it was thought probable that she had had encephalitis at some time. Her mental content was chiefly related to her fear that she was mentally ill. She was well oriented and did well in examinations, which showed her to be about average in intellect. She was quiet and cooperative, possibly a little depressed when she was questioned about the jerking movements. During her stay in the hospital she did not appear to be unduly shy and she showed no obviously abnormal behavior. She displayed definite artistic ability and therapeutic efforts were directed in part toward developing this talent. The diagnosis was not clear; there were possibly some hysterical symptoms but the contribution of the encephalitis, which may have been chronic, could not be determined.

B. Psth., Asocial M:18:S:8 +1 '4–96 4:0:21

This youth was sent to the hospital on a court order after the police had picked him up for molesting four girls in a theater. For the past six months he had become even less discriminating than usual in his choice of companions. For a couple of months his family had been missing sums of money, amounting to $200. When he was finally caught he denied his guilt, even though the circumstances left no reasonable doubt. Arrested at the request of his parents, he said in jail, "I took it but I'll pay it back. What of it?" Non-negotiable bonds, kept in the same drawer with the money, had also disappeared, and he persistently denied knowledge of these.

A high school graduate, the youth talked a great deal about becoming a lawyer but never actually made any plans. He entered a junior college but attended no classes, simply loafed in places around town. Growing careless in his dress and appearance, he neglected to have his hair cut for months. He excused himself for all this behavior by saying, "I'll get a fiddle and save money." The day before admission he sat for hours lighting one match after another. His intelligence had been tested as average. The boy had never learned the value of money, since he had only had to ask for cash and it had always been given to him. He had never been one to respect authority or age. He worked, if at all, inconsistently and spasmodically. Quick with enthusiasm, he lost it just as rapidly. He shirked responsibilities and never performed any chores at home. He was clumsy with his hands. He had always tended to play with boys smaller than himself and to bully them. Immature and overbearing, he would, it was said, "take money away from a 3-year-old," and he was described as "shy and sneaking." At school he was always alone. He had no apparent interest in girls except for the incident in the theater which led to the hospitalization. He had sat next to the girls and had placed his hands on their legs.

The patient was a well-developed, somewhat obese boy who spent his time in the hospital slumped in a chair, avoiding a direct gaze. Defiant and evasive in attitude, he refused to discuss his difficulties and denied any need for help. He appeared to be without emotion and without social feeling. There was no evidence of any personality assets that could be mobilized to his advantage. It was recommended that he be placed in an environment where discipline and supervision would be rigid, and he was discharged to the care of a sister.

Ps. Sz., Simple M:15:S:44 +17 '4–96(43) 5:0:20
B. Psth., Path. Emot.

The patient, who had always been a spoiled, irritable, and demanding child, became, at about age 9, more sullen, intolerant, and negativistic. He would play the piano until early morning hours, keeping the family awake. He developed somatic complaints in order to stay out of school, and in his temper tantrums he threw dishes, broke furniture, was profane and abusive. On one occasion he threatened his mother with a knife. He underwent brief hospitalization and was diagnosed as a psychopathic personality. Discharged to his mother, he failed to show any improvement and the present admission was preliminary to removing him from his home.

His past general health had been good. There was one illness that may have been encephalitis at age 5. At the time of admission he was in the tenth grade; his schoolwork was average, and though he missed many days, he managed to make up the work. He was extremely effeminate and was rejected by others boys as a "sissy." Most of his time he spent at home playing the piano and drawing pictures or "just fooling around." In school he was shy, seclusive, and quiet, having no close friends. Usually when he engaged in any activity it was with girls rather than boys.

In the hospital his physical and neurological studies yielded nothing of significance. He was extensively examined for a possible glandular imbalance. This study was also negative. In manner he was evasive and distant, and in answering questions his favorite response was, "I don't know." Rather flat emotionally, he behaved in markedly feminine ways. Psychological studies strongly indicated a schizophrenic fantasy life. In general he impressed the staff as having regressed to a very childish level. There was no indication of any homosexual tendency, although his extremely feminine appearance and behavior might indicate the future development of that. While he was obviously not clearly psychotic, the prognosis was bad and the possibility of a future schizophrenia was considered high. Chronic encephalitis also was a real possibility.

B. Pri., Child. M:18:S:36 +1 '4–98 (49) 2:4:11

This patient had always been a problem of one kind or another. He had been difficult to train in bowel and bladder control and at age 4 had wandered away from home unaccountably. He had had many difficulties in school, beginning as far back as the second grade, where he had been shy and withdrawn. He finally finished three grades of school after numerous difficulties with truant officers and teachers. There was an early history of petty thievery. He frequently took the family car without permission, and he had been apprehended while breaking into a grocery store where he took cash and merchandise. Sent to a reform school, he was paroled and was again picked up in a stolen automobile. He said that he always acted on impulse and without thinking, wanting to impress his associates.

His past physical health had been good. There were no obvious mental breakdowns. His I.Q. was 108. His interests were chiefly mechanical, especially airplanes and automobiles. His family background was irregular, and he resented his father particularly. His mother was dominant. His father had been involved in embezzlement and it appeared that this had, at least in part, been motivated by financial obligations incurred by the boy and his mother.

In the hospital the patient appeared to be withdrawn and answered in short sentences. He seemed to be trying to make a contact with the examiner, but he could not release himself. There was obvious blunting and he was ill at ease, but no obviously disturbed behavior was noted. His stream of thought and general behavior seemed rational. He wanted to go to a trade school. Tests indicated he had average intelligence with good mechanical aptitude. He was discharged to the court with the recommendation that a good placement in a boarding home and school might lead to satisfactory behavior.

Ps. M-D., Mixed M:54:M:73 +39 412'7386–X (55) 10:4:26
Alcoholism
Ps. Toxic
Deteriorated

This man was admitted because of headaches and personality changes, noticed for three weeks, and fainting spells, present for two days. Nervous, nagging, and careless for the past two years, he had become unusually irritable during these last three weeks. He showed inefficiency at work and loss of memory, and he began to swear although he was a devout Catholic and had not previously used profanity. His speech was circumstantial and rambling and he complained of a number of somatic symptoms. Two days before admission the patient began to go through the following sequence every hour. His speech became retarded; he mumbled and seemed confused for 45 minutes; and then he became quiet, stared, tensed his muscles, stiffened, and thrashed about blindly. During the latter period he also gasped and perspired. A few minutes of relaxation followed, and then he awoke with a start and became rational for a short time. He was not incontinent and apparently not obviously disoriented.

There were no previous psychotic episodes although he had apparently had a mild hypochondriacal tendency. For ten years he had been a heavy drinker and he was still drinking a good deal. A high school graduate, he earned a good living as a cost accountant. Described as high-strung, ambitious, and driving, he was not particularly sociable and had been somewhat obstreperous and seclusive. He worried about little things, and he always insisted on having order in his home and in his office. Somewhat paranoid always, he believed that people kept him from advancing.

In the hospital there was some evidence of brain damage. There was a questionable ventricular enlargement and a possibility that nutritional factors had played a role in precipitating the psychosis. However, these findings were not convincingly the basis for the symptoms. The patient was disoriented, confused, and assaultive. His speech was circumstantial and chiefly concerned small complaints about the staff and his treatment; he showed a paranoid attitude toward the nurses. When interrupted he would become disturbed. He was worried, angry, and argumentative. There were no hallucinations but he had delusions about "wires" in his brain being "all filled up." After five shock treatments he became quiet, friendly, cooperative, and rational. It was found that he had a gastric fistula and he was transferred to surgery for repair of the stomach. The postoperative course was uneventful. At times he seemed depressed, but he was generally quiet and cooperative. The case was never clearly understood and the prognosis was doubtful. The attack seemed to be most nearly comparable to a manic-depressive episode, mixed form.

P. Hypo. F:39:M:11 0 '413–9 7:1:23

The patient had a long history of complaints, chiefly of pain in the face and multiple arthritic pain, for which she had been treated extensively with varying success, but apparently no one procedure had been of permanent value. Her gall bladder had been removed, and she had had two operations for appendicitis and several sinus operations. She had once been diagnosed as having an enlarged heart. She took iodine for her thyroid.

She was an eighth-grade graduate who had done very well scholastically, and although she had wanted to continue school the low income of the family had made this impossible. She had always been nervous and high-strung. Her intelligence level was dull normal. She engaged in little or no social activity, and her husband and she were only moderately well adjusted. She frequently complained of his low economic level, and her claim that the two children she had had shortly after her marriage had weakened her and had made her unable to work was a source of irritation to her husband.

In the hospital although the physical and neurological examinations disclosed findings consistent with facial neuralgia and arthritis, the evidence did not seem sufficient to explain the extent and intensity of her complaints. In addition to the physical symptoms, the patient was concerned about finances and about the fact that her children lacked the privileges other children had. She had no insight into the possible psychological factors in her illness, and the woman felt she did not need hospitalization. She claimed her health was better than it had been for the past few years, and she continually expressed the desire to go home so that she could care for her children. On the ward the patient was friendly and cooperative and appeared normal, but it seemed probable that after discharge she would continue in her attempts to get somatic treatment.

P. Hys.	F:30:M:125	+2	413872'69–(47)	6:2:22
		+120	'1$\underline{437}$9$\underline{28}$–(47)	7:3:20

The patient complained of being nervous in every way. She felt pains, perspired freely, and had severe headaches and palpitation. She believed she was about to have a heart attack and complained that her stomach was "knotting up." In fact, there were few physical symptoms in the textbooks about which she did not complain. In addition, she was afraid that her husband was being unfaithful, that her mother was persecuting her, that something disastrous was going to happen to her child, and that none of her friends liked her. She also felt that she had strong feelings of inferiority, and she had a constant dread of impending death. She talked rapidly and in a typically hysterical manner. She had permitted her physical appearance to deteriorate. She had had complete physical examinations by almost every doctor in the community and was regularly pronounced to be in wonderful health, all of which was frustrating to her.

The patient was an adopted only child. The mother was a strong, demanding, and highly successful businesswoman. The father seemed to have been less successful in business. He was kind in a passive, undemonstrative way, which was a source of considerable consternation to the patient since he did not protect her sufficiently from her mother's rigid discipline. Typical of her early home life was the fact that her mother listened to her practice the violin and rapped her fingers with a small iron rod when she made a mistake. She was given no sex education of the hygienic sort and was warned of dire consequences should she go out with boys. As a result she conceived of sex as a loathsome and sinful matter. On the eve of her first wedding she was informed by her mother that she was an adopted child, and in such a way as to be seriously deflating. Her first marriage apparently was an utter failure from the beginning. The court granted custody of her one child to her mother, who used the child as a substitute son. Of course, the mother actively interfered in both the first and the second marriages of the patient.

The first therapy sessions were devoted to an anamnesis without any direction by the therapist. During the next block of interviews, the therapist directed the patient to certain apparently traumatic experiences in her childhood. From there the therapy moved into a discussion of the role which the patient's neurotic actions were playing in her adaptation to her mother, her son, and her second husband. At some points the therapist used a great deal of interpretation. During this period the patient-therapist relationship was analyzed in terms of some of the patient's feelings. At this time she began to make rapid progress. She had temporary setbacks and explosions, but many insights. There was a constant diminution of her anxiety and her near antisocial behavior. Her fear of sex changed and she reported making, for the first time in her life, sexual approaches toward her husband. The relationship with her mother became one of less dependence and less frequent contacts, and she accepted her mother as an emotionally sick person. She became much less protective toward her child and, with considerable glee, enrolled him for his first year in school. This woman cannot be considered cured, however. The second MMPI shows many of the same tendencies as the earlier one, but the scores approximate more nearly the normal range. The patient is currently on what may be considered a furlough. She feels free to return in the event she notes a recurrence of her earlier neurotic ways of meeting problems. The most encouraging signs are that she is now engaged in acceptable social activities, is getting great pleasure out of driving her car, and dresses up "fit to kill." A. S.

P. Mixed B. Psth., Mixed	F:31:M:60	+10	416'9378–	3:7:14
P. Mixed B. Psth., Mixed	F:31:M:9	–22	46183'792–	3:8:15

The patient, who was admitted to the general hospital because of allergies that took the form of upper respiratory difficulty and severe asthma, was transferred to the psychiatric service as soon as it became apparent that psychological factors were important in the complete pattern of her illness. On occasion she had previously had symptoms of an upper respiratory infection, and although medications had given her temporary relief they had always lost their effectiveness. There had been a gradual increase in irritability and the patient had been easily upset by trifling incidents. Her fatigue and weakness were so extreme that it became impossible for her to do her housework, and she tended to stay in bed constantly.

There were many periods of hospitalization and other medical attention in her past history. Osteitis of the hip, complicated by what appeared to be hysterical spells, had been treated operatively, and she had undergone several laparotomies. When she was a sophomore in high school the patient had stopped school, and until her marriage she had been sporadically employed. Even as a child she had been stubborn, resentful of authority, and emotionally unstable. A person who took little interest in her work, she had often been a truant from school, and the late hours she kept at night had constantly been a source of anxiety to her parents. At one time the juvenile court had considered sending her to a reform school but had placed her on probation instead. After her marriage she was a hard worker, but more and more of her time was spent in hospitals.

In the hospital she attributed her asthma to her last pregnancy and to her run-down condition. Her admission to the psychiatric unit distressed her, and she thought that she did not belong among the patients in that ward. On occasion she was listless, and at other times exceedingly argumentative. She felt that her marital problems had contributed to her condition, and she admitted having taken an overdose of drugs at one time because life was so miserable for her. Although she always insisted that her basic difficulties were organic and that anyone who did not concur simply did not understand her, she admitted that at times she had encouraged asthmatic attacks in order to obtain attention. She frequently demanded special privileges, and it was almost impossible to get her to follow any therapeutic suggestions. Just before her discharge she had a profane temper outburst and had to be placed in the disturbed section. Although she was discharged to her husband and returned to her home, she was readmitted shortly after with a similar pattern of difficulties. In this admission a number of drugs were tried, and when a regime was found that seemed to give her some relief she was again discharged.

Ps. Senile	M:48:M:46	+13	418'236 79–X	10:9:22
Deteriorated		+45	1'42836–9	8:3:21

For a year before admission the patient had complained of impotence and headaches, and over a period of five years he had become increasingly careless in his dress and in his farm work. Friends told his wife that he had acted queerly on occasion and that he had mistreated the farm animals. Of more recent origin was a marked irritability. Just before admission he had been involved in an automobile accident, the details of which were unknown, and when he had attempted to escape from the scene of the accident he had been apprehended and sent to the workhouse. Several times before he had been arrested for reckless driving. His personal injury as the result of the accident was limited to a swelling on the back of his head, but it was at this time that he showed evidence of a gross disorder, with greatly increased psychomotor activity. He became surly and secretive; he spent money indiscriminately and refused to work.

Previously he had been known for his good judgment, and everyone had trusted him. His hobby was gardening. An unaggressive, congenial, and friendly person, he was said to have always been somewhat stubborn and secretive.

Occasionally he had been a heavy drinker. An eighth-grade graduate, he had worked as a caretaker on an estate for eight years, and until the onset of the present illness he had always been a very reliable employee.

Although the patient felt that he was not ill and demanded immediate discharge from the hospital, the neurological examination showed consistent, scattered findings that seemed to verify the assumption of organic deterioration of the cortex. The man denied that there had been any recent changes in his behavior, and he had glib explanations for everything he had done. For example, he said that he had not worked after the accident because there was nothing much to do. Either he was confused about the accident or he falsified his description of it. On a few occasions he became sad, crying for short intervals. He had mild suicidal tendencies. Although he was not loquacious, his stream of thought was orderly. In appearance he was tired and disheveled. He had no interest in ward activities, and it was suspected that at one time he worked on a window with the intent of escaping. There was no change in his condition with hospitalization. Because his wife did not want him committed to the state hospital, he was discharged to her care, but the staff felt that he would soon have to be sent to a state institution.

Ps. Paranoid F:40:M:51 +42 '4186-(61) 7:2:23

The present episode had its onset about six months before when the patient had begun to speculate about Communist involvement in current airplane crashes. Her suspicions became more acute and extensive, and she began to check on her husband's activities. Finally one day when he was an hour late getting home she developed the delusion that he was a member of the Communist party and that the party was threatening him and her. She was afraid he would kill her in her sleep, and she became increasingly upset and unable to sleep. This situation grew gradually worse until the time of admission.

There had been a previous psychotic episode about eleven years before admission when she had stabbed her husband in the chest with a butcher knife. At that time she was ill for about four months. She had gone to college for two years and then had done office work. She was a devout church member. On the surface she was a jolly, easygoing, "life of the party" sort of person. It was thought by her friends that she was, however, sensitive to criticism and easily hurt, needing sympathy and warm interest. She absorbed a good deal of acrimonious criticism from her husband without fighting back. Her chief day by day pleasures seemed to come from a very active social life. She was moderately obese and eating apparently was one of her methods for controlling her nervous tension.

At the time of admission she concealed most of her ideas and appeared to be completely normal. Within a week, however, her delusions broke through. She found special meanings in radio programs and normal remarks by the staff, and she was hostile toward the staff. In other ways, however, her thinking remained logical, and her sensorium and intellect were intact. She seemed to have a remarkable degree of insight into the possible background for her symptoms. Seven electroshock treatments made her euphoric and overactive. Later she became more stable, and by the time she was discharged she was nearly normal. During interviews, she explained her difficulty on the basis of feelings of insecurity and dependence that went back to her earliest years. She also presented a clear picture of her husband's almost pathological domination of her.

Ps. Toxic M:38:M:27 +9 4'2-6X 11:3:20
Alcoholism
B. Psth., Asocial
Suicidal

A month before admission this man had become restless, depressed, and irritable. These symptoms had appeared soon after he and his family were requested to move from the farm they lived on, which was owned by the patient's mother. For one month before admission the patient became intoxicated at least three times a week, and during the last week he drank continuously for three days. After this drinking spree the patient read the paper until noon, walked to the barn, and later was found hanging unconscious. Cut down by his mother, he regained consciousness, was confused, weak, and ataxic. For at least a month before admission he had been increasingly careless in dress and had shown a few other regressive symptoms.

After finishing the eighth grade, the patient had worked as a farmer and a paper hanger. Following his marriage at age 27 he and his wife moved to his mother's farm and remained there until they were asked to leave, just before the patient's admission. When very young he had begun drinking moonshine whiskey, which was produced on his father's farm in a still. The largest amount he drank per day was one quart; this had occurred in the past year. Ambitious, he had always taken pride in his work both as a farmer and as a paper hanger. He worked best for strangers. All his life he had been subject to episodes in which he became seclusive, moody, and self-condemnatory. During these spells he usually quit work temporarily.

The neurological examination yielded no particular findings. There was no more than minimal evidence of neuritis. The patient attributed his trouble to influenza. At another time he said that his nervous breakdown was due to "too much alcohol, just like the snakes." He was anxious to get back to work on the farm. "I'll never drink any more, not even one, because one is just as bad as ten." There were no defects in his sensorium or intellect. Apparently he remembered nothing of the period just preceding the suicidal attempt in the barn. He condemned himself for his drinking, yet admitted no need for help. He was careless in his dress and possibly had recent memory defects. In the hospital he gained weight and claimed he was better than he had been in many months. When he left plans were made for him to live with a sister-in-law and to find another job.

P. Mixed F:24:S:9 +4 '4213– 5:2:16

In the last three years the patient had lost 53 pounds, and in the month preceding admission she had almost completely lost her appetite and had had severe constipation. Five years before admission the patient had weighed 130 pounds. After good-natured chiding about being fat, she had begun dieting. She lost her appetite and dropped to 118 pounds. She never again regained her appetite. In the next few years she had constipation, which she attempted to counteract by constantly chewing a laxative gum. Her weight continued to decline until it was only 70 pounds. About a year before admission she had a temporary gain to 95 pounds, but in the last six months she had gone back down to 80 pounds. There was never any fatigue, nausea, or vomiting.

The past history of the patient was unusually clear of obvious contributory factors. The second of four girls in a family that appeared to have been very harmonious, the patient had spent one year at a university, where she had spent money so extravagantly, especially on clothes, that her parents were unable to finance additional education. At one period the patient drank rather excessively four or five nights a week. She was a moderate cigarette smoker. She disclaimed having had sexual experiences but seemed to have a normal heterosexual interest. She had been a popular girl, and her ambition was to have a dress shop of her own. Her relatives thought she was "a bit wild, but not bad."

In the hospital the neurological examination revealed no evidence of disease. The patient was emaciated, but apart from the anorexia she was in fair condition. Her mental state showed no outstanding abnormality, but there was a lack of "depth" in her emotional attitudes, and she was indifferent toward her condition. She attempted to flatter the examiner into relaxing the surveillance exercised over her eating by saying, "You have given me such a different outlook on life that I know I will get well if you will just let me out." It was discovered by careful watching that she put food in her mouth, chewed it, and then spit it into a paper handkerchief or napkin. Upon completion of her meal she had a pocketful of food which she disposed of in the toilet. She also hid food in the radiator, and when she could she sneaked portions onto other patient's plates. She was caught in innumerable lies, and it was suspected that she stole money from other patients. In spite of every effort to get calories into her, she lost twelve pounds while in the hospital. She was taken out by her parents, who decided to try her at home. She died several months after discharge. The diagnosis clearly seemed to be anorexia nervosa.

B. Pri., Child. M:15:S:37 +1 '421378–6(49) 2:1:15

About a year before admission the patient was caught writing obscene material in textbooks used in the high school. He was reprimanded and made to erase all the books. Later he spent a night in jail after being apprehended for peeping into a woman's window. At that time he admitted other peeping episodes. About three months before admission while he was waiting to take a bus he stepped behind a young woman, placed his hand beneath her dress above the knee and held it there for a second. He was again taken to court for this offense and it was suggested that his parents have him admitted to the hospital for psychiatric evaluation.

His physical health had been very good. There were no past neurotic or psychotic episodes. He had always been a shy, self-conscious person, given to considerable daydreaming. He was narrow in his interests, irritable, and quick to flare up. Always a poor student in school, he had got along fairly well until high school, when his work became much worse. His I.Q. was 127. A neighbor had described him to his mother as a "perfect gentleman."

In the hospital he was conventional in behavior. There were no disturbances of sensorium or intellect. Occasionally he seemed belligerent but got along fairly well and joined in group activities. With psychotherapy he gained some insight into his problems, and it developed that his fantasy life had been much concerned with sex. Apparently his behavior had been in part aroused by a complete lack of any sexual information outside of infrequent and inaccurate communications from other children. There was a definite possibility that he felt great insecurity because of his social ineptitude and was attempting to convince himself of his own masculinity. His mother was oversolicitous toward him, which also seemed to be a factor in his behavior. He was discharged with a good prognosis.

B. Psth., Mixed M:43:M:46 +6 4217'83–9(53) 5:4:18
Suicidal

One month before admission, this man, after "a few whiskeys," shot and wounded his mother, then attempted suicide. The shooting was unintentional, he insisted. Something happened to his head, he said, and he could not recall the shooting.

There were no previous psychotic episodes, but the man had been treated for morphine addiction ten years earlier. When he was in the sixth grade, he left school. Irresponsible and temperamental, he was described as also being egotistical and nervous. There had been early hypochondriacal trends. He was a steady worker and had stayed at the same job for 25 years. However, he had always drunk a good deal and had spent money foolishly. He was separated from his wife, who was ten years younger than he. They had eight children, all of whom lived with the wife. The patient's mother was nearly 80 years old.

The physical examination in the hospital showed a severe defect and scarring of the lower jaw, lip, and tongue, due to the gunshot wound. The neurological examination was essentially negative. Well oriented about time, place, and person, he apparently had a partial amnesia for the events surrounding the shooting. He said he had been depressed because of pain in his side for the last year. He had no obvious hallucinations or delusions. He should not be punished for what he had done, he felt, since there must have been "something wrong with me" at the time of the shooting. While in the hospital he played cards, read books, and was helpful and cooperative. His claim that he was out of his mind at the time of the shooting seemed to relieve him of any worry over the whole matter. The few drinks he had had before the shooting had been taken to relieve the pain, he said. He was discharged back to the court, with the report that there was no evidence for psychosis either at the time of the examination or at the time of the shooting.

P. Hypo.	F:29:M:56	+10	42 186'73–9	8:5:17

Following a miscarriage six months before admission, this young woman complained of weakness, numerous somatic aches and pains, and dyspnea. Various physicians had prescribed a number of treatments, none of which had helped. The weakness became so severe that she spent much time in bed. She also complained that her head "did not work right."

Throughout her life the patient had been under par in health. However, no particular illnesses had preceded the present one. Apparently, her symptoms in a milder form had been evident since early childhood. An average student, she had graduated from the eighth grade. Until her marriage she lived with her family. Always shy and sensitive, a retiring sort of person, she took little interest in things outside her home. Emotionally she was labile, readily depressed by trifles, elated over slight successes. All in all, she lived a circumscribed, stilted, colorless, uneventful life.

In the hospital the patient was primarily concerned about her health. At all times she strove to keep the conversation centered around her physical condition. She complained of weakness and difficulty in breathing and said she had no appetite and was "too sick to live long." However, she ate heartily. It was with difficulty that she was induced to leave her bed and move about. Paying little attention to her personal appearance, she dragged herself about the ward, head hanging, with all the outward signs of a pathetically weak individual. Little change was effected; she remained essentially unapproachable and continually fended off approaches to her problem by saying, "There is nothing to be done." She was given reassurance about her physical condition and her husband was carefully instructed about the possible therapeutic contributions he might make. She was discharged to return home for a trial.

Ps. M-D., Manic	M:72:M:9	+2	'423–(69)	9:8:16
		—2 yrs.	431'86972–(57)	3:7:15

This man, a minister, was sent to the hospital on a court order because of unusual behavior. In the last year he had become resentful of his family and especially spiteful toward his wife. On one occasion he had firmly ejected her from his room, though he never became assaultive. Previously his daily activities had been well planned, but now he became very irregular, took baths at midnight, and roamed aimlessly about looking for things he had made, written, or done. He was voluble and talked extensively about religion and books he was writing. He had grandiose ideas about winning prizes and conducting religious services. There was some regressive behavior with inappropriate giggling and wide mood swings. There were also moderate ideas of persecution. In another town, where he was supposed to act as a relief preacher, he had been rejected by the church board and returned home because of his overactivity and grandiose plans.

He had had three previous psychotic upsets, widely separated in the course of his life. All had been essentially similar to the present one and all had taken considerable time for recovery. A minister for 45 years, he had been a fraternity man in his college days and president of his graduating class. He had never had any home church but had always been a relief minister. His family had never been financially safe, always running close to the margin. Between the psychotic episodes he was easy to live with, friendly, affable, cooperative, full of energy. Much of his time he devoted to reading. He had always shown exaggerated responses to disappointments.

In the hospital he had grandiose ideas and mild delusions of persecution. The neurological examination was negative and there was no disturbance of his sensorium or intellect. He was well oriented and normal in behavior and conversation. In discourse he was coherent but circumstantial. His conversation was full of his past life, the books he hoped to publish, and the prizes he expected to win. Most of each day he spent reading, writing letters, and talking with other patients. The prognosis was felt to be good for this attack, as it had been for the past ones. He was transferred to a state hospital for a time, although it was thought possible that he was able to get along at home.

B. Simple Adult Maladj. F:17:S:29 +1 '423–69 (70) 5:1:17

About a year before admission the patient had been placed in a foster home, and although she had adjusted well at first her foster parents came to feel that they could not keep her because she was sneaky and undependable. They had to keep private papers and accounts locked up, and she spread stories about the family. She had made up many excuses for staying home from school. When she was tried in another foster home, a similar pattern appeared, which made it necessary to terminate that placement also.

The patient had had some difficulty in school but had managed to get through the ninth grade. After one week in the tenth grade she refused to go back to school. Her I.Q. was 104. She lacked a sense of responsibility. Both her parents were feeble-minded, and her mother was in an institution. Her father was anxious to keep the family together but was unable to cope with the situation.

In the hospital the patient was well oriented, her responses were adequate, and there were no obvious neurotic symptoms or bizarre behavior. She gave the impression of being superficial, and she had an artificial bearing. She was pleasant but guarded, and there were a few times when she was stubborn. Occasionally she remained by herself. When she was discharged it was felt that in proper surroundings where she would have a sense of security she might be able to adjust.

Ps. Invol. Melan. F:49:M:38 +1 '42367-(57) 8:4:15
Paranoid

The pattern of difficulties appearing in this woman included depression, suicidal tendencies, insomnia, irritability, and pain. The onset of these symptoms was gradual and ill defined as to date. Vague personality changes had first been noticed six years earlier. These were characterized by a gradual estrangement from her husband, irritability, and compulsive behavior. Acute symptoms began one month before admission, immediately following a vacation with a daughter, to whom she had confided guilt feelings about an affair with another man. On returning home she had a sudden severe depression and talked of "ending it all." She withdrew from her friends and was preoccupied within herself. Her attitude toward her husband became sympathetic and patronizing. She cried frequently.

At age 21 the patient had borne a son out of wedlock and about that time she had suffered a peculiar stroke in which there were temporary hemiplegia and blindness. This seemed to be a hysterical attack. Throughout her life ill-defined spells of depression had occurred, but she claimed to have always been able to control these. She blamed much of her nervousness on an automobile accident in which she had been injured slightly. She also had such severe attacks of lower abdominal pain that she went to bed for two or three weeks at a time.

After completing the eighth grade at age 14, the patient went to work as a housekeeper. After her marriage she resented having to live in a small town and was dissatisfied with the social and occupational level of her husband. The latter was known to "like women and liquor." The patient justified her own affairs with other men on the basis of her husband's behavior. Although she had always been nervous and high-strung, she had shown exceptional ability in handling money and in planning. Her irresponsibility was evidenced by the fact that she frequently left her children without care while she spent an evening out. She herself had many interests and abundant energy. About her intimate affairs she tended to be secretive. She had many friends, mostly in the "fast" set.

In the hospital she appeared as an attractive, narcissistic woman, hostile toward any inquiry into her personal life. On other subjects she was friendly and even affectionate. Apathetic and detached when examined, if an important finding was mentioned she was immediately alert and interested. At first she was extremely depressed and kept saying, "It is all too late." She had mild delusions of reference and a vague suspiciousness. A remarkable improvement in the depression took place in the course of five electroshock treatments. The postshock memory loss was severe. She became cheerful, even overactive, and apparently recovered almost completely from the present attack.

P. React. Depr. M:20:S 42'3678–9(69) 4:6:16

This college student complained of a lack of motivation, a tendency to sleep all the time, occasional depression, and feelings of jealousy.

He came from a home that was broken by the death of his mother when he was a year and a half old. His father apparently was a paranoid, inconsistent person. After the death of his first wife he married a woman who made a very passive stepmother. The patient's half-brother was apparently a child schizophrenic. The family was well-to-do. The boy was taking training in a professional school and was extremely capable.

Passivity and dependence were prominent in the interview relationship. A great deal of time was spent on the Oedipal material present in the content of his dreams. There was considerable intellectualization, but he also managed to work through much emotional material, particularly about his jealousy of his girl friend. At the end of 23 interviews over a five-month period he was taking more interest in his work, slept less, and in general appeared more interested and better motivated. He made plans to go on to psychoanalytic therapy. C. K. A.

Ps. Invol. Melan. F:55:S:9 +1 4'2367819– 7:4:18
P. Mixed

For a year and a half this patient had become increasingly anxious and worried. She had been troubled by indecision and insomnia, and she had lost considerable weight. She had been living with a cousin, a widower, and his 14-year-old daughter. Her jealousy of an attractive, aggressive housekeeper, who was on friendly terms with her cousin, had precipitated the housekeeper's departure and had caused many quarrels and the exchange of many vicious remarks between the cousins. The patient had exhausted her emotional strength in attempting to make herself indispensible, only to find herself rejected by both the cousin and his daughter. When she became unable to concentrate on her work she had taken a leave of absence. Although she improved little, she returned to the home later. The daughter then ran away because she could not stand the discord.

Rectal surgery necessitated hospitalization for the patient, and since she was not allowed to return to her cousin's home after her recovery, the patient had then begun boarding out. About a week before admission, the cousin had sold his home, precluding the possibility of her return to it. She had beseiged her friends with phone calls and requests for advice on such trivial matters as these: "Should I go for a walk in the park?" "Where should I store my fur coat?" She took everyone's advice but reversed her decisions many times. Just before admission she had made a dramatic scene in a lawyer's office in which she demanded to know if the cousin still loved her as much as she loved him.

There were no previous psychotic or neurotic upsets. Her health had been considered good. She had always taken life very seriously, had a good work record as a stenographer, and had been held up as a model for her younger sister. She was a graduate of a business college. While her income would have permitted her to prepare for retirement, she had made no such preparation, and she had always shown poor judgment in financial matters. Obstinate and selfish, she was always having minor quarrels with members of her family, although she was peculiarly and closely attached to it. She was overly religious, had always liked to talk about herself, had taken up with many cults, and at times had imagined that she talked to the dead. She had always felt that she had been cheated by not having a husband or children, but she never had been able to accept the attention of men.

In the hospital her talk concerned herself and her troubles wholly, and she had a tendency to be overly concerned about trivial matters. At times she was in a mild panic state, frequently saying, "I can't stand it to be shut up like this. It's just awful. I can't stand the restraint." She was exceedingly angry because she had been brought to the hospital. A difficult patient, she was constantly on the move and made many requests, such as wanting to call friends. Although she changed very little in the hospital, she became somewhat more manageable. No really severe behavior disturbance was observed at any time. She was finally discharged to the custody of her sister, who planned to take her to another state where she would have an opportunity to recover.

B. Psth., Asocial Alcoholism M:34:M:9 +1 4'237-(47) 4:2:16

The district court referred the patient to the psychiatric unit for evaluation after he had been charged with failure to support his wife and seven children. An irresponsible person, he had always been an inconsistent worker who had never adequately supported his family, and his small earnings were a constant source of friction between him and his wife. Openly neglectful of his family, he frequently left them to drink and engage in extramarital activities for several days, returning home with only a small fraction of his pay. He circumvented in every case the efforts of probation officers and others to force him to contribute to the support of his family; he completely ignored appointments with probation officers, and it was difficult for them even to find out where he was currently living. When he was picked up before being admitted to the hospital, he was unkempt and was said to have been acting strangely.

His past history could not be obtained with any degree of accuracy. Until the age of 15 he had been enuretic. A marked kyphosis contributed to his feelings of inferiority. As the youngest of four children, he had been a favorite with his parents. Until he married at age 21 he had worked on his father's farm. He had entered high school but had stopped because he did not like it.

At the time of admission he showed a considerable feeling of inferiority and a lack of self-confidence. He said that he had never been able to handle money: "It sort of slips through my fingers." He had never had any hobbies and had not indulged in sports. He showed clearly that he put his own needs and wants above those of others. His course in the hospital was relatively uneventful. At times he was indiscreet in his associations with other patients, particularly the younger women. He showed no real interest in anything. It was impossible to help him much, and he was discharged back to the court with recommendations for his management.

Ps. Sz., Paranoid F:23:S:40 +7 4′23781–9 8:4:24

About nine months before admission, while being treated in a dentist's office, the patient had first experienced a fear of death, coupled with palpitation and dyspnea. There had been four other attacks before the one that led to hospitalization. For ten days before the present admission the patient had repeatedly said that she was going to die, "because her false teeth were breaking the blood vessels in her gums," and in her opinion she deserved death for having mistreated her parents. At the same time she accused her parents of having tried to poison her. An intensively religious person, she said that Jesus had once come to her room and had talked with her. Most of her day was spent either in crying or in prayer.

Except for hypothyroidism and myxedema, which had been controlled by oral thyroid medication, the past medical and psychological history contributed nothing. The patient had attended school as far as the eighth grade, stopping because of poor health, and afterward she had held numerous positions, mostly as a housemaid, but had never continued longer than a few weeks on any one job. For at least eighteen months preceding admission she had been unemployed. She was apparently dull normal in intelligence. Content to stay at home, she had never expressed any plans or concern for the future, and when she argued with her father about her refusal or lack of desire to seek work, she became depressed and unhappy. She disliked being with persons of her own age, preferring to associate with older people. An ardent church member, she disliked dancing and picture shows. She was described as stubborn and independent.

In the hospital there was no evidence of myxedema. Mentally she was markedly concerned about her fear of death and her delusions of persecution. Marked religious trends were exhibited in such statements as this: "When I go, I want to be saved." She also said, "The thyroid is the master gland and works on the nerves. My dentures have pulled my face out of shape. There is no circulation in my gums." She was, however, well oriented and showed normal mentation in other ways. She had absolutely no insight into her problems. Run-down and unkempt in appearance, she had an unpleasant personality, and her attitude was uncooperative. Unsystematized and shifting ideas of reference and delusions of persecution were also revealed during the hospitalization. Although she could never explain what she meant by it, she frequently said, "I'm well because I have been saved." During the hospitalization there was very little change in her symptoms, and when she was discharged to the care of her sister, it was felt that there was little chance of her making a good adaptation.

P. Hypo.	F:28:S:66	+1	42381'796–(53)	7:5:25
Schizoid		−184	431728'69–(63)	7:5:20

For many years this young woman had felt tired, listless, and run-down. In school she had been active in spite of this and had participated in many activities, especially sports. She felt she had been put under an extra strain by being advanced a grade. Her symptoms progressed until at age 18 she visited a doctor who gave her medication for anemia. She took a job but was soon forced to drop it because of "feeling so tired" and also because she noticed a weakness in her hands. She left other jobs after equally short trials. About a year before admission she was admitted to a general hospital for a thorough examination. Given vitamin therapy she left the hospital feeling much improved although nothing specific had been found in the studies. Shortly, however, she began to complain that her family made her feel like a parasite because she did not work. Formerly very fastidious, she now became increasingly untidy in dress and personal hygiene, the family noticed. When they spoke of this, she became angry and nervous and cried. She was irregular at meals and developed greater apathy and hostility to her family. First seen in the outpatient department in psychiatry, she was later admitted to the inpatient department.

Considered a smart child in school, she graduated at age 16 and then took a trade school course in art for two years. She worked at lettering leather and wooden goods in her first job. Her relations with her schoolmates had been good, especially with other girls. A truthful, cheerful, and stable person, she had always previously fulfilled her responsibilities at home and in society. Her brother, who had not seen her for four years, found that her personality had changed markedly from what he remembered. It was noted, however, that she had always been somewhat shy and sensitive and given to worry over somatic complaints.

In the hospital the patient blamed her present difficulties on unsatisfactory home relations and claimed that the family regarded her as a burden and that they took out on her their irritations at others. She complained her mother neglected her in favor of her brothers. There was some evidence that she resented the female role. Her sensorium and intellect were normal but she was indifferent and apathetic during the examinations. Most of the time preoccupied with her somatic complaints, she had to be continually encouraged to go to meals and to occupational therapy. Insulin shock treatment did not change the pattern materially. With the aid of the social service she sought a job while still in the hospital, but at discharge she had not found anything satisfactory. Contact with the social service department was to be continued. In view of the degree of immaturity and the long-standing maladjustment, the prognosis was thought to be poor.

P. Anxiety State	F:21:S:455	+10	423871'96–(53)	6:8:20
		+390	84'23917–(68)	6:2:21

This woman came in stating that she was a homosexual and that she did not want to do anything about the problem of homosexuality, but the symptoms of anxiety over her condition were causing her a great deal of discomfort. She thought she was sleeping only two to four hours a night; she was unable to participate in social affairs because of tension; and she thought she would be unable to maintain a satisfactory record in her schoolwork despite the fact that she had been making a good record up to this time. The homosexual element had been brought to her consciousness shortly before the first interview. She had suspected the possibility for some time before but had more or less rejected the idea as much as she could. She had been asked to one of the college social functions by a male classmate and the possibility of having to submit to "petting" on the date threw her into a state of near panic, typified by insomnia, anorexia, and precordial tension. This was the "clincher" which convinced her that there was no longer any point in keeping up the pretense which was designed to conceal her "true status" from herself. Eventually it was found that she had never participated in any overt form of sexual activity—masturbatory, heterosexual, or homosexual.

The family picture described by the patient entailed many sources of conflict. The relationship between her mother and father was evidently strained since the father had spent the bulk of his time away from the home. In consequence, almost all the rearing of the two children had been left to the mother, who supported the children by teaching school. The mother's management of the patient, as described by the girl, was more by dominance than by real affection. In recent years the mother had aided the girl materially in terms of clothing, college tuition, and college maintenance, but had repeatedly attempted to control the girl's selection of a vocation, mode of dress, and type of companionship. The patient felt, with a great deal of bitterness, that the mother's material provisions were her way of assuaging her own guilt for neglecting her daughter. The girl said, "I don't want clothing. All I want is affection." Although the patient had informed her mother of her "homosexuality," her mother rejected the idea, saying the girl was being dramatic. Another source of conflict was a younger brother. The patient felt that her brother was the center of attention and that she had been pushed to the periphery of her mother's affection.

The patient quickly built up a strong dependency relationship with the therapist. She was seen on a once-per-week basis for a period of three months. This series ended with the girl apparently fairly well adjusted. She returned to her home and wrote several letters to the therapist which indicated increasingly mounting tension. By the time she returned to school for the fall session she was in a near panic condition. At this time she was seen in daily sessions; she made a quick adjustment and therapy was tentatively terminated at the end of a month. Two months later the anxiety conditions returned and she was again seen daily. This was continued for three months and then decreased to biweekly. She continued in school during the spring quarter and shortly before its termination worked her problem through very satisfactorily. During this last period the anxiety attacks occurred sporadically and there was one spell of vermiform paresthesia which lasted about a month.

Following the end of the school year she obtained employment away from home and then returned to school in the fall. During this period she continued to progress. Just before she took the final MMPI she left a note for the therapist with this comment, "I can hardly wait for classes to begin. This doing nothing doesn't agree with me any more. Now I know the only solution to a lot of the problem is what you do. Make the most of every little minute and go until you drop. I am getting strict with me in the beginning and there can't be any looking around. Hah! Don't I sound different?"

The second MMPI still showed some tension in the Pd and Sc scale, the latter being T-70. On the rest of the scale she had an average over-all drop of two sigma. In all probability this girl will continue to have an occasional upset, but it is also probable that she will return to equilibrium fairly quickly. A. S.

B. Psth., Path. Emot. F:20:S:14 +3 423'8967-(43) 4:3:20
Suicidal

On the morning of the day preceding admission to the hospital the patient wrote a suicide note, placed it where it would not be found for some hours, and then went to bed after taking ten sleeping tablets. About eight hours later the note was found and when the family was unable to arouse her, they called a physician, who gave her stimulants and had her admitted to the psychiatric service.

Her previous health had been good. She had got along well in school and after she had graduated from high school at age 17, she had held a number of jobs for short periods. At three separate times she had enrolled at a university but had failed each time, accumulating almost no credits. She had made three previous attempts at suicide—by hanging, wrist slashing, and cyanide—but during this time she had maintained a very active social life and had had numerous friends, many of whom were, however, maladjusted. She had had both homosexual and heterosexual experiences. She talked entertainingly, laughed readily and frequently, and seemed to have a great deal of energy and vitality; but she overreacted to minor disappointments or frustrations, complained excessively about restrictions, sulked and was facetious whenever anyone tried to hold her in line. Informants could give no real reasons for her suicidal activities or for her other recent behavior.

In the hospital she talked freely about her history and showed considerable insight into her difficulties in that she thought her problem was mainly that of emotional immaturity. Her suicide attempts were the result of a conviction that psychiatry could not help her. She was restless and nervous in manner and somewhat disheveled in appearance, and she seemed to be under emotional tension. Her moods fluctuated widely, from outbursts of tears to excessive laughter. She was very distressed both at having failed in her suicide attempt and at finding herself in the hospital, but she developed a strong attachment to the therapist, which should have led to therapeutic improvement. However, no emotional or other appeals encouraged a more active and mature consideration of her difficulties, and there was little basic change. She was very resistant to any discussion of her homoerotic experiences; she simply implied that they had derived from conflicts and that they were a contributory influence on her suicidal attempts. She was discharged to return to her parents with a poor prognosis, in part due to the fact that she had an exceedingly low frustration tolerance.

Alcoholism M:28:M:21 0 4'239–1 (47) 5:5:18
B. Psth., Asocial

The patient was brought to the hospital from the county workhouse where he had been held after a five-day drinking spree. He had gone to a bar for "a couple of beers"; once started he could not stop. After two days he "blanked out" and remembered nothing until he was picked up in a hotel lobby by a friend of the family. This incident was typical of others over the past ten years. There were intermittent periods of sobriety that lasted from as little as two weeks to six months. Once started on a drinking spree he always extended it to an extreme.

His physical health had been good except for gonorrhea, which had been thought cured but had reappeared three weeks before admission. He completed about eleven years of parochial school before stopping. Apparently he had no learning difficulties although he frequently got into trouble. He was active in athletics. Leaving school to bum around the country, he held and lost many jobs; he was never dependable. When he did work on a job he was exceedingly capable and frequently showed so much promise that he would be rapidly advanced. He was dismissed from the marine corps with a bad conduct discharge. His wife had left him after tolerating a number of drinking episodes. He joined Alcoholics Anonymous and stayed away from liquor for four months. His parents usually went out of their way to get him out of his scrapes. He wrote bad checks and then phoned home for money to make them up. Apparently he had never had more than the most superficial and short-term goals, being impatient for quick results. He made acquaintances easily but never had any real friends.

In the hospital he showed no gross disturbances of mental content. He was concerned about the unjustness of being in the hospital and was busy with "big" plans for the future. His sensorium and intellect were intact. His attitude was sullen and aggressive. He was treated for gonorrhea but psychotherapeutically nothing could be done for him. Intent on behaving well enough to be released, he was fairly cooperative in general activities on the ward. He carried on an obvious flirtation with a young married woman who was also a patient. He was discharged recovered from the present episode but with an obviously poor prognosis.

Alcoholism Deteriorated   M:41:M:22   +1   4'263–19(69)   4:4:12

The patient had been drinking since age 18 and had been a severe alcoholic during the last two years. He had seldom attempted to help himself but had entered a state hospital and stayed a few days. On another occasion he had tried Alcoholics Anonymous but had not stayed long with them. Taken to a private hospital in a severe state of intoxication, he was difficult to manage and was transferred to the psychiatric unit.

He had been in good health except for the numerous alcoholic episodes. Pampered and spoiled as a child, he finally completed a year or two of college education and for a while was successful as a salesman. He had always spent money freely but had made no attempt to work in recent years. He had numerous personality assets, was a very good talker, and when sober was able to get a job readily, but he was immature, self-centered, jealous, and quick-tempered. His marriage was incompatible largely because of his emotional instability. He had six children and had been married fifteen years.

In the hospital he was belligerent and antagonistic at first but gradually calmed down. Frightened about his inability to do even simple tests at first, he feared that he had damaged his brain. This fear was partially substantiated by findings in the psychometric studies. After his recovery from the immediate symptoms he was discharged to return to his wife. About three weeks later he was readmitted after another severe drinking spell. Again he was demanding and belligerent but after two days rapport was established and this time he claimed to be really interested in getting help. Again, however, after he had recovered from the preliminary symptoms, he developed resistance and restlessness, finally leaving against advice. He was later committed to a state hospital that specialized in the handling of alcoholic cases.

B. Psth., Asocial Mutilative   M:21:S   '4267–(49)   4:2:13

This 21-year-old prison inmate was referred to the psychopathic ward because of destruction of prison property and self-mutilation by severing his Achilles' tendon with a dirk knife. Becoming an aggressive leader of a destructive group of inmates soon after he entered prison, he violated the rules by agitating, attempting to escape, mutilating himself twice, making "chock" beer, and creating a disturbance in the building. After mutilating himself, the prisoner was punished for cursing and abusing a guard and crushing a wash basin and commode. Later he was treated for superficial lacerations of his right leg and was admitted to the psychopathic ward.

Until his father's death, when he was 15 years of age, the patient had lived with his parents. His father had made a living as a dock hand on a dredge boat. Soon after his mother remarried, the boy left home. He claimed to have completed the eighth grade in school, but his actual grade placement was 5.4. The only jobs the patient had held were "roughnecking," and these for only short periods of time. The youth's criminal career began when he was 12 years of age. Arrested for burglary and sent to the state training school for boys, he served four terms and then escaped. While being sought, he committed a series of crimes including three filling station robberies and the theft of an automobile. For these later offenses he was charged with robbery by assault and sentenced to serve 25 years.

Interviews and studies indicated that the patient showed no regard for group values, had no loyalties or identifications. His crimes, as well as his misbehaviors in prison, showed impulsiveness and lack of forethought and planning. As an inmate, he was a constant source of trouble. He knew he was in prison for a long time, and to "do my time the hard way" was his sole expressed ambition. Little hope was felt for this patient's future. R. C. K.

Alcoholism	M:57:M:33	+1	42'67 389–(61)	2:5:21
		+24	42'3768–(57)	2:5:21

The illness of this patient really dated back 27 years when at the age of 30 he had begun drinking. The cause of his drinking at that time had been "an affair with a woman." His wife at the time of admission was the woman of that affair, whom he had finally married a year before admission. He was a graduate in law and before the onset of the present illness in its severe form he had been very successful. He described himself as a "secret drinker." For the past six years he had been unable to work at his profession. He had sustained many accidents and injuries while drunk and according to a physician he had been in various hospitals, several times with delirium tremens, though the patient denied this.

Except for his alcoholism, the patient had been well. He had graduated from law school at the age of 22 and had been well liked. He had had many friends and had been active in a number of organizations; he was an outstanding star in baseball. Apparently he had worked exceedingly hard at anything he tried and this appeared to be a factor in his problem. His physician said that the patient was trying to get into the limelight in order to cover up his feelings of inferiority and insecurity.

In the hospital he was well composed and conventional in behavior, logical and to the point in discourse. His sensorium and intellect appeared intact. When asked why he was in the hospital he referred to his drinking but said, "I think I have enough will power to quit drinking any time I want to." He was very neat and generally normal in appearance and activity. He made little progress in the basic revision of personality factors contributing to his problem, and though he was apparently normal at the time of discharge and felt he would be able to take care of himself the prognosis was very poor.

Ps. Psth. M:28:M:30 —35 426′78139–(73) 4:10:11
Paranoid —42 4237′8169–(49) 4:10:10

This young man believed that his present illness had begun following the loss of his garage and some equipment in a fire two years before admission. His wife, however, dated the difficulty from a blackjack beating he had suffered at the hands of the police a year before admission. In any event during the last months he had become increasingly concerned about his interpretation of the Bible and about the impending destruction of the world. The "persecution of the common man by big business" also troubled him. Since he had begun to have these ideas, he said, his friends and relatives, including his wife, had considered him insane and had "turned against me." Following the beating he had lost his ambition and had left job after job in rapid succession. At one point he became so angered about the way county aid was administered to his family that he went to the relief office and stole his application blank. For this behavior he was jailed for three days. At his wife's request he entered the hospital voluntarily.

He reported that he had had difficulty in swallowing since childhood and that he had had gonorrhea four times. He said also that he had many times been beaten with blackjacks. Although of average intelligence, he had made a poor school record. At the age of 14, when in the seventh grade, he was sent to a boys' farm for alleged drunkenness and a troublesome attitude. Innocent of these charges, according to his claim, he was forced to plead guilty because of threats by the truant officer. After he was released he worked as a farm hand for two years, then was arrested as an accomplice in a car theft. Always known as a troublemaker, he nevertheless claimed to have many friends. According to his view he was a sensitive person who must avenge every wrong done to him. He blamed his repeated unfaithfulness to his wife on her lack of sexual desire.

In the hospital the young man was seclusive, restless, and irritable, and he talked freely of his ideas and the loss of his wife's love. Gradually he participated more and more in ward activities and showed less concern over his own trouble. During the hospital stay he said that all his conflicts had been solved and "my mind cleared up." Because the staff felt that no real change had been effected, commitment to a state hospital was recommended. After a hearing by the commission, commitment was refused and he was discharged to go home. The prognosis was, of course, considered bad.

B. Psth., Asocial F:16:S:15 +2 ′4268–97 5:4:10
Deterioration

Inability to adjust in various homes, general delinquency, and shiftlessness were the factors in the admission of this patient. Although it was difficult to date the onset of these problems, the patient apparently had not made a good adjustment at any age, and every placement had ended badly. She had an unusual interest in boys, she kept irregular hours, and she was irresponsible and careless, with the carelessness extending to her personal appearance and general cleanliness. Two boys who had admitted having sexual relations with her had been sentenced to a reformatory about a year before the patient's admission to the hospital. She had then become a concern for the welfare board, and the present admission was a culmination of their futile efforts to work with her.

The patient was a congenital luetic; she had had continual antiluetic therapy, but at the time of admission the syphilologist felt that no further treatment was necessary. During the past year the patient had been under observation for a low abdominal and pelvic pain, but no definite diagnosis had been made. Because of her poor adjustment, her school attendance had been sporadic, but she had finally achieved about ninth-grade training. Only on a few occasions had she worked, and then just for brief periods; her work as a domestic had never been satisfactory. She was completely unable to plan for the future, unwilling to postpone any present pleasure for future gain, and unable to stick to a decision. A desire for immediate excitement such as dancing or other social activities was her only motivation. Her family background was very poor; the only fairly responsible person, the mother of the patient, had committed suicide by slashing her throat with a razor. The father had had syphilis, transmitting it to his wife, who had passed it on to the child.

At admission the patient was a fairly large and attractive blond, who appeared more mature than her chronological age indicated. There were slightly positive pupillary reflex findings, indicating the possibility of syphilitic damage. Although the patient at first denied most of the historical data given by the social worker, she later admitted all of it. She felt that she had never been given a real chance, and although she recognized that it was inadvisable, she was eager to return to the home of her father. Exceedingly desirous to get out of the hospital, she said that she wanted to study cosmetology. Emotionally she was composed, but occasionally she showed resentment toward control. Her intelligence was a little above average, and her adjustment on the ward was satisfactory, but she was not amenable to psychological help, and most of the planning for her discharge was done at the social service level.

P. React. Depr. F:30:S +20 4268'7-1 (37) 2:11:9

An interest in vocational guidance was the reason given by this client for coming to the clinic. Describing herself as unhappy in her present position with a somewhat domineering employer, she said she disliked being at anyone's beck and call. There was too little responsibility and opportunity to advance, she thought, and she had a poor relationship with the others in the office. She was nagged by the feeling that while her superiors were doing "important things" she herself was making little, if any, contribution.

The client expressed her vocational problem as stemming in part from the fact that because she was not happy in her home life, she needed satisfaction from a career. Her Italian-born parents had lived a stormy life together, each fighting for the exclusive love and attention of their two children. The parents remained together only because of the children—the client herself and an older brother who, with his family, had come to live at the parents' home. She felt certain it would be impossible for her to leave home, and if she married she planned to take her mother with her. Although she had held a series of responsible positions during the twelve years following her graduation from high school, the client expressed some complaint about each. The fault always centered in the job or in the office atmosphere rather than in herself. The young woman apparently had few social contacts outside her work, and while she hoped to marry some day, she had thus far met no one in whom she was interested.

The client discussed her life apart from her work only with the greatest reluctance. With little or no insight into the possibility that her vocational discontent might be part of a broader dissatisfaction or general emotional problem, she resisted strenuously any such implication. In regard to the presenting problem itself, it was difficult for her to express any specific interests or to face the implications of changing jobs at this point in her life.

When nursing was mentioned, she claimed she did not have "enough stamina"; when fashion design was suggested, she replied that she "couldn't afford to take a financial gamble." She did ask about various college courses but rejected the possibility of even night school when she learned of the fees; when pressed further she decided that she would not really enjoy college work. The strongest interest she expressed was in writing. Thus, while she wished to change to a job in which she could "lose herself," she was unwilling to make any of the sacrifices necessary for one of her age. When the importance of a good total adjustment was brought up, the client simply said that she felt the other aspects of her life could not be helped. A different job was the only answer, she was convinced. Although arrangements were made for further interviews, the client seemed disinterested and did not keep the next appointment. M. V. B.

Ps. Paranoid M:32:S:5 +4 42713'98–X(55) 13:11:26
Alcoholism

During the night about 36 hours before admission the patient suddenly began "to hear" the voice of a girl friend reproaching and threatening him because he had refused to marry her. When this recurred the following night, he became excited and thought there were burglars in the house. That morning he had been assaultive and had believed that the people of the village were talking about him. He had broken furniture and had struggled wildly against restraint. He related the onset of his symptoms to mild drinking during the week before admission. A few weeks earlier he had had a similar episode which had lasted only two hours. Except for severe periodic drinking for a number of years, the patient's past health history was not significant.

A precocious boy with high intelligence, he entered college at the age of 13, later dropped out, but finally graduated at 21. After three years in the navy, he became a lieutenant. At the time of admission he was earning a good salary as a schoolteacher. Somewhat introverted, he usually preferred to sit back while others took the lead. This tendency was not, however, especially noticeable. A friendly person, he had shown no outstanding deviations of personality, with the possible exception of the alcoholism.

At the time of admission he was experiencing auditory hallucinations and delusions of reference. He said he heard the voice of a girl friend reproaching and threatening him. These threats worried him even though he could not see what they purported. He was convinced that his drinking was the only basis for this episode. Apparently he realized that he was experiencing hallucinatory and delusory ideas, yet he was not seriously concerned and he was reticent about the details of the content. He did not care to stay in the hospital and on the second day his symptoms abruptly disappeared. After that he considered them foolish. It was likely that the symptomatic improvement was only a defense system covering the illness.

P. Mixed F:31:D:3 +2 42'739816–(49) 4:2:14
B. Psth., Mixed
Alcoholism

Regularly about a week before her menstrual periods began, the patient became tense and depressed, went to a bar, and began a drinking spree that lasted for several days. This routine dated back about five years to the time when she was divorcing her first husband and had trouble holding her job because of fights with her employer. She was then working as a stenographer. She had always drunk some but never before excessively. The first real spree lasted ten days. At first the episodes did not trouble her, but as they became more severe and occurred with every menstrual period she was handicapped by them. She took jobs in various cities and tried to help herself by joining Alcoholics Anonymous, but none of the procedures she adopted did any good. She married again but stayed with the man for only a short time since he made no effort to support her and her child by her first marriage. She went to a private hospital and took a liquor cure but reverted after leaving the hospital. Later still she received electroshock treatment but that also failed to help her.

The patient was a business school graduate and was above average in intelligence and general capability. She had always worked except for the period when she was pregnant and for a short time after the birth of her baby. She was a well-liked and very adequate person; however, she was impulsive and immature, tended to be dependent, and had poor judgment.

In the hospital the physical and neurological examinations were essentially negative. She was somewhat depressed, partly because she felt that so many things had been tried and had failed to help her. She was not particularly social toward other patients and was unwilling to cooperate in carrying out a program of therapy that might involve inconvenience for her. There was no bizarre behavior. She was highly emotional and obviously had poor control of her temper. Her insight was inadequate. She was not in the hospital long enough for a complete study and was discharged to continue with a private psychiatrist. Later she entered a psychopathic hospital in another city. The prognosis was considered to be very poor.

P. Mixed F:35:M:100 +3 4'<u>276</u>381–9 (30) 6:6:24

Five months before admission to the hospital the patient became severely agitated and began to worry about her son's intelligence as he recovered from a childhood disease. The lad was considered bright by his father and by teachers, yet the patient was not reassured. She developed insomnia and was in a state of exhaustion. Furthermore, she was unable to discipline the child and manage her home, and she had conscious death wishes against her child and her husband. She became progressively worse and began to talk of "going away." Later, when she spoke of suicide, she was admitted to the psychiatric unit.

Always in good health, the patient had nevertheless been unusually susceptible to exhaustion for the last twenty years. Even as a young child she had always tired first among her playmates and had had to rest. Love and affection had been lacking in her early life, and she had felt that her mother was unintelligent because she had not finished grade school. She had liked her father because he was kind to her, but, she said, "I didn't like him too much. I don't think I had an Oedipus complex." In school she was bright but had "an inferiority complex." She fell in love at age 17, became pregnant, and had an abortion performed. This experience created feelings of guilt. In college her feelings of inferiority and insecurity became more marked, and she began to be uncomfortable with other persons; previously she had been sociable. The change continued until she became a shy, quiet, and sensitive person.

In the hospital the patient was well oriented but depressed. She claimed to feel no emotion, yet she cried and smiled at appropriate times. Peculiar feelings of numbness over her forehead and neck were present. Relatively intact in sensorium and intellect, she was aloof, but in a somewhat subtle manner, for she was cooperative and friendly in ward activities. Thirty-three insulin shock treatments were given, with little effect. She was somewhat resistant toward psychotherapeutic approaches. She expressed a fear of returning to her husband and son, and she seemed to really lack interest in going back to them. The patient's underlying bland indifference balked every attempt to help her, and when she was discharged the prognosis was not felt to be good, although it did not seem likely that she would have an obvious break with reality.

B. Psth., Mixed M:36:M:3 0 '427 6389-(47) 1:2:15
Paranoid
Alcoholism
Drug Add.

This patient entered the hospital with a number of complaints but said that none of them was the real reason for his coming. When asked to tell about his illness he said that the staff was "getting into something that had no bearing" on the present admission.

Apparently the patient had been a chronic alcoholic for the past seventeen years, having begun to get drunk at age 15 or 16. He had had a number of trying experiences because of his drinking, but he refused to discuss these in any detail. He was a graduate of a medical school. He hinted that he had got into difficulties in another state because of his alcoholism, presumably in connection with his practice of medicine. For the last ten years he had initiated alcoholic sprees by taking benzedrine, paraldehyde, aspirin, chloral hydrate, and the like for three or four days before he actually began to take alcohol. He had joined an Alcoholics Anonymous group, and he felt it had helped him a great deal—he had learned to talk in front of a group and had got along better with his wife and family. In spite of his participation in A.A., however, he had never stayed "dry" for longer than seven to nine months. Apparently the main reason for his present admission was that he had been using morphine for the past few weeks and was frightened that it might take hold. It seemed certain that he had been in a number of sanitariums, hospitals, and jails in the past.

The man's past personality could not be determined with any certainty since he was the only informant and he refused to give any real information about himself. The staff thought that many of the statements he made were not true. In the hospital he appeared nervous and agitated, constantly paced the floor, and was very restless. He had almost no insight into his general problems. His sensorium and intellect were clear, and he showed no withdrawal symptoms after being denied drugs for three days. Before anything like a complete study had been completed, he left the hospital.

Ps. Sz., Mixed M:21:S:7 +1 427'8361-9(57) 2:4:21
Paranoid
Suicidal

Since entering high school at age 14 the patient had become extremely self-conscious, withdrawn, and seclusive. His convictions that his legs were greatly bowed, that he had a disfiguring kink in the left corner of his mouth, and that his teeth were deformed made him feel that he was repulsive to others. Because he had been incontinent of urine in a class, he had refused to go back to school and at home he had withdrawn from his usual activities, spending his time day-dreaming and reading. He developed rituals designed to keep himself clean and free from infection, for example, taking long baths late at night and dressing in a ritualistic way. On one occasion he had attempted to kill his mother with a knife but had been restrained before he could do her harm. He frequently talked of suicide and had made one attempt to kill himself by gas.

With the exception of the present illness, the patient's past history had been normal. Until dropping out in his third year of high school, he had done well enough in school, and though he had never been a really adequate person he had been fairly well adjusted. Since the onset of his illness, he had been unreliable and his judgment had been so poor that his family had given him no responsibilities about the farm. As a child he had been prone to aggressive outbursts, and he had always been secretive, stubborn, and nonconforming.

In the hospital his concern was chiefly with his "deformities," which he requested be corrected surgically. No amount of reassurance relieved him of his delusions. He was about average in intelligence, but he had very limited knowledge and interests. He had no apparent hallucinatory experiences. He kept himself immaculate. His affect was dulled, and he made no effort to become acquainted with other patients, or to enter into ward activities. He spent most of his time in his room and was inaccessible. There was no change during his hospitalization, and he was ultimately transferred to a state hospital.

B. Psth., Asocial F:22:S:27 —1 4′28– 5:3:20

The patient was admitted to the hospital because she had had two illegitimate children within the preceding two years, and social agencies had become disturbed about the seemingly unending problem she presented for them. There was no distinct illness, but she had always had difficulty in conforming to social standards, and for several years she had had indiscriminate sexual relationships.

Her past medical and psychological history was essentially negative. She had been in several automobile accidents but had suffered no serious injuries. She had left school at age 17 after getting to the ninth grade. When she had first come to the attention of social agencies she had been given tests that indicated an I.Q. of 69, but on two other tests she had scored 81 and 92. Her main interests were dancing, attending the movies, and going to parties. She had unenthusiastically considered marriage on one occasion. At first she had been protected by her family, with whom she had had a fairly good relationship, but as her behavior became more and more deviant, she withdrew from the family, and bad feelings developed. At home she was stubborn and faultfinding, impulsive and deceitful. She had few close friends, and the community, looking upon her as a lewd person, had ostracized her from the social contacts her family's standing would ordinarily have given her.

In the hospital there was no evidence in the physical examination indicating a venereal disease. Mentally she showed no clear-cut disorder. She talked willingly of her past experiences and said she was satisfied to remain in the hospital. There was no marked affect. Her statement that she hoped to conform more closely to convention in the future was not made with certainty, and even when she said she wanted to keep her children, it did not sound as though she meant it. She was helpful about the ward and took part in hospital activities. A somewhat narcissistic tendency was indicated by the amount of time she spent in fixing her hair, and in the care she took of her clothes and her body generally. Since she believed she had no particular problem that concerned the staff, she was relatively unapproachable. There was little change with hospitalization, and she was discharged with a poor prognosis.

B. Pri., Child. F:12:S:7 +2 '428 136–(68) 9:2:21
B. Psth., Path. Emot.

The patient was referred to the hospital for psychiatric evaluation because of uncontrollable temper outbursts and inability to adjust in foster homes. Since the age of 4 the girl had had a crippling of the left arm and leg, evidenced by a weakness of the arm and by contractures of the foot and leg. As the result of considerable medical and surgical treatment she had developed a marked hatred and fear of hospitals, doctors, and nurses. "They were mean to me and I hate them all," she said. The patient had been unable to stay in a boarding home because of her emotional outbursts and her generally ugly disposition. She was in the fifth grade at the time of admission and was having difficulty in school also.

The child had repeated several grades; she was of dull normal intelligence. She got along fairly well with her classmates, and she said that she had always been happy except when she was in a hospital. Her home life had been relatively happy, but her mother had been sent to a state hospital two years before the child's admission and the children had been put in foster homes because the father was unable to support them.

In the hospital the patient went into such a severe temper tantrum that she was completely unmanageable for a while, and even after she became more composed she showed marked antagonism toward staff members. She was oriented, however, and her manner and psychological content were normal. She displayed a marked indifference to her problems, but in other ways she was emotionally stable. For the first two days of her hospitalization she remained sullen and uncooperative, but before she was discharged she became seemingly fairly happy. Her negativism was undiminished, and she was discharged to be transferred to a state home school for girls because of incorrigibility.

B. Psth., Asocial M:22:S '42896–13 (49) 2:15:7
Mutilative

This young prison inmate was referred for an interview and an MMPI after repeated self-mutilations. The first time, he split the skin on his right leg, placed lye inside the wound, and sealed the opening with adhesive tape, thus causing a burn that incapacitated him for six weeks. A few months later he cut the tendons on the back of his left hand with a razor blade. Four weeks after that he severed the Achilles' tendon of his left leg with half of a double-edged razor blade, and a year and a half later he severed the sternomastoid muscle in a similar manner. Altogether, the man has 34 mutilation scars on his right arm and 41 on his left arm; his Achilles' tendons have been cut five times in as many years.

The inmate's early childhood was spent with an aunt and his grandparents. His mother reported that he was called "Big Boy" but was embarrassed by it, and when he grew up he asked that his family call him John. Because the boy's mother and stepfather worked all the time, his discipline was left to a Negro maid, to his aunt, or to his grandparents. The prisoner said that he had completed the seventh grade. His placement on the Stanford Achievement Test was grade 5.2; his I.Q. was not available. His school attendance, as recorded by five different schools, was irregular and his grades were consistently low. One teacher noted that he was "slow to learn, but otherwise bright." Another teacher wrote, "He was very slow, never completed anything; was large for his class; did not like being called 'Big Boy'." Truancies were reported "once a week." At 14 he ran away from home and the following year he was sent to a military academy. There he was frequently disciplined for "stealing, lying, smoking, and going AWOL." Before the school year was over he ran away and did not return.

The youth's criminal career began at the age of 17 with several arrests for vagrancy, followed by commitment to prison for automobile theft. After serving four years he was released. Within two months he became intoxicated and stole an automobile, for which he was arrested, convicted, and again sentenced to prison, this time for two years.

This man has caused prison officials more trouble with petty disciplinary problems than any other inmate in the system. The prison psychiatrist reports that, although the prisoner has been in and out of the psychopathic ward, the man is sane and shows no loss of contact with reality. In company with another prisoner, he stabbed an inmate nurse in the psychopathic ward and later was caught passing a note threatening to kill a Negro porter working in the isolation section. The prisoner is known to use benzedrine. He is belligerent and thoroughly oriented in criminal behavior, and he sometimes exhibits a smart-aleck attitude. He says he is "through with working." Inside prison walls he mutilates; outside he can get along with "a little gambling and light thieving." It is felt that he will probably be an institutional case the rest of his life. R. C. K.

B. Psth., Asocial M:16:S:50 +2 4'29-6(43) 4:5:17

The patient was admitted to the hospital because of truancy and delinquency. He first became known to the juvenile court about two years before admission after a 26-day truancy. He was put on probation. The next school year another complaint of truancy was made against him and he was judged delinquent and sentenced to a home school for boys, with a stay on probation. He violated this probation by committing three burglaries and the probation was terminated. He ran away from the home school and went to another state; later, returning to his home state, he was picked up by the police and sent to a reform school. There he showed such a violent temper that he was sent to the hospital for study.

He had had excellent health and there were no episodes of nervousness or mental upset. His school grades had been good until the last two years. Apparently he learned without effort. His intelligence was bright normal. He had held numerous jobs after leaving school, staying a very short time at each of them, but he had always moved on his own volition since he was a good worker and was never discharged. The exact history of the last two years was impossible to obtain since he had traveled about so much. He was described as having been friendly but he was without lasting friends. He had no hobbies and no other persistent interest. He had been depressed when rejected by the army, and it was following this rejection that he had begun to commit his more serious crimes.

In the hospital he was intact in sensorium and intellect. His behavior at no time was bizarre. He was convinced that he had "learned his lesson" and that all his troubles were over because as soon as "they" let him free he would get a job, hold it, and behave himself. He appeared to be sincere and confident. On the ward his behavior was exemplary. He made a good impression on the entire staff. At the time of discharge it was felt that he had a somewhat better prognosis than that indicated by his history. On the other hand, in spite of the good impression he made, it was recognized that the prognosis was still only moderately good.

Alcoholism M:38:S:5 +1 '429 38–(45) 2:4:16
B. Psth., Mixed

The patient was admitted because of acute alcoholism. This had begun as early as age 17. The routine had consisted of getting drunk every Saturday night.

The patient had been in the navy for about ten years and after his discharge, the periods of drinking became more frequent. Individual bouts of intoxication sometimes lasted as long as three weeks. He tried Alcoholics Anonymous and got along fairly well for six months but then regressed. He was confined in a general hospital psychiatric ward for about a week on one occasion after he had been on a five-week spree, during which he had drunk a quart of whiskey a day. The present admission was precipitated by the possibility of delirium tremens. Except for the alcoholism the past history was not very complete. He had stopped school in the eighth grade and had worked at various jobs thereafter until he enlisted in the navy. He had always been friendly and had freely mixed with everyone, according to his own statement, but there were indications that others considered him seclusive. He looked to alcohol as a way for getting everything and for having a good time. He had few interests and apparently had never been particularly aggressive sexually.

On admission to the hospital there was no gross disturbance of sensorium or intellect. He was confused immediately after admission but the confusion cleared up within the first day. He apparently had some minimal intellectual defects. He seemed to think clearly, but he was somewhat depressed and it was difficult to get from him any information that one could rely on. He was composed and conventional in behavior. He felt no need for help and did nothing to cooperate in interviews except to rationalize his position. He developed no insight into his problems and while he was improved with reference to the minimal signs of neuritis at the time of discharge, he was considered to have a very poor prognosis.

B. Psth., Mixed F:17:S:21 +9 4'29 867- 3:7:9
Ps. Sz., Paranoid

The present admission of this patient was precipitated by unexplained absences from school, breaking of dormitory rules, and dishonesty. She had been seen in the child psychiatric clinic three years before admission because she had experienced frequent spells of faintness and weakness. At admission she had the feeling that "her feet were growing together, and her bones were caving in." She also had ideas of reference. Because of a syphilitic infection in some of the students at the high school she thought that she had some of the symptoms of what she called the "bad disease." She felt that people were looking at her and pointing her out.

She had made a temporary borderline adjustment in a foster home but had then begun to break hours, coming in very late without any excuse. She had also developed complaints of headache, dizziness, and tinnitus. At one time, she said, she had taken thirteen aspirin tablets. She admitted shoplifting, and just before admission she told some people that she was pregnant. Of average intelligence, she had done C work in school but at admission had abandoned her schoolwork completely. Before the development of puberty she was described as having been cheerful and easy to get along with, but with puberty she became moody, overly reactive to little things, and resentful toward restrictions. She was, however, interested in cooking and had won several prizes in 4-H activities. She herself said that she was "spoiled." She explained that she had always wanted luxuries and had felt insecure if she was not dressed as well as her associates or better. When seen in the earlier child psychiatry admission, she was a "hostile, insecure, adolescent girl with strong feelings of resentment toward authority and every adult person. She did not feel that she was wanted and was fearful of establishing close relations with others. Her defiance and sullenness seemed to be a protection against what others might do to her."

In the hospital the physical and neurological examinations were negative. She expressed resentment at being hospitalized and showed great reluctance to discuss any of her problems. She frequently made the statement, "It's not fair." There were mild paranoid trends which were not systematized; no gross disturbances of sensorium or intellect were elicited. She felt that she was justified in abandoning her classes because one of her instructors had told her that if she was not interested in the work she need not come to class. Preoccupied, resentful, withdrawn, negative, and sarcastic in conversation, she frequently refused to give requested information by saying defensively, "I don't know." She made a poor ward adjustment, taking no part in activities. When she was discharged she had changed very little. Most of the staff's efforts were directed toward adjusting her environment and planning for her future.

B. Psth., Path. Sexuality M:23:S:20 0 431<u>276</u>'8–(94) 4:5:11
P. Mixed

This patient was admitted from the medical service after he had told the staff there that he was an "invert" and had asked for psychiatric study. At the time of admission he had an anal fistula, for which he had been receiving treatment in the medical clinic. He was a dysplastic person with unusually large ears, a peculiarly shaped face, and a gangling body. At admission he regularly used rouge and powder. He talked wildly and insisted that he was a "homosexual."

The patient had an I.Q. of 110; he had gone through two years of high school before stopping to wander about the country. From his early childhood he had been feminine by nature and had liked to dress up in girls' clothes and to play with dolls; he had generally been treated like a girl by his mother. He claimed that he recognized the peculiarity of his sexual interests as early as age 6. He got into no particular trouble and was not too different from other children, however, until his middle teens when his father and social pressures began to force him to be more masculine. From that time on he became increasingly maladjusted. A friend, a dentist, induced him to try homosexual activities. This introduction was followed by many experiences with this friend and other men. He was on the whole an honest and fairly reliable person, in intent at any rate, and in spite of his homosexual activities always tried, he said, to be "honorable and respectable."

In the hospital he was both eager to receive treatment and reluctant to be changed in any basic way. He showed some religious trends and was disturbed about his misconduct. The fistula had been brought on by acts of sodomy and it did not heal because these tended to recur. He was frequently in a fairly severe anxiety state because of his ambivalence toward his condition. His attitude toward treatment and the future might be expressed in his statement, "I've tried to live as a homosexual and I hate myself for it, but I can't help it. I want to try to live some other way now." He was discharged and was followed for five or six years by outpatient contacts.

Gradually, one by one, he gave up his feminine ways and manner of dress. He was given vocational training as a hairdresser. Throughout the whole period, however, he was exceedingly hypochondriacal as well as frequently ill from definitely somatic disorders. He got chicken pox and mumps among other diseases, seemingly having a weak body which betrayed him at critical points when he was almost making a good adjustment. There were frequent backslidings into homosexual behavior. He made at least one active suicidal attempt, and in a number of other suicide threats a good deal of drama was involved. At the end of six years he was fairly well adjusted and was self-supporting for the first time in his life, working chiefly as a church janitor. For the most part he no longer needed psychiatric or medical support.

Ps. Sz., Simple M:25:S:7 +1 4'31867-(53) 6:2:24
B. Psth., Mixed

The county attorney's office referred this patient to the psychiatric unit for study because of peculiar behavior dating particularly from six years before admission, when he had developed a multitude of hypochondriacal complaints. He had a record of numerous contacts with the law for drunkenness, speeding, and sexual misbehavior. Five years earlier his family had noted a definite change in his personality. He became nervous, restless, and withdrawn from people. At times his conversation was rambling and queer, with occasional references indicating grandiose delusions. Four years before admission he had been in a psychopathic hospital for three months. After a series of insulin shocks he apparently improved and was discharged with a diagnosis of schizophrenia. Since then he had worked occasionally but had held no job for very long. He also drank excessively and exposed himself to women. He had most recently been accused of carnal knowledge of a child.

The patient had graduated from high school at age 17 and had then worked as a truck driver and subsequently at various similar jobs. His entire family was considered peculiar, and his home life had been anything but pleasant. He had shown deviant behavior from an early age.

In the hospital he was withdrawn and confused in his thinking, but his sensorium and intellect were intact. He had delusions, including the fixed idea that he had had sexual intercourse with a prominent actress and was the father of her child. There was a split between his affect and reality. He was cooperative and made some attempt to associate with other patients, but he preferred to lie in bed. He was euphoric at all times. On discharge he was transferred to a state hospital.

P. React. Depr.	**F:29:M:89**	**+13**	**43'2167–9**	**8:5:17**
		+70	**231'748–**	**7:1:10**

Worry about her health, depression, and a general loss of interest in daily life were the highlights of this patient's admission complaints. The symptoms had a fairly abrupt onset about a year and a half before admission when the patient fell from a bicycle and hurt her lower back. Following this she showed great concern about her health. Any disease that she heard or read about led her to consult a physician. Her marked body concern gradually increased and became associated with a general depression and an inability to carry on her usual activities. She even neglected her personal appearance, spending most of her time complaining about her physical difficulties.

Average in intelligence, the patient had been known as energetic and hard working. Cheerful and not given to mood swings, she had always enjoyed social contacts and had seemed self-reliant. A waitress until she studied beauty culture at age 24, she had since then been a beauty operator. Her first marriage, to a man who was cruel and drank, had occurred when she was 15 years old. This husband finally died after infecting the patient with gonorrhea. She was treated successfully for this disease. While she was still working as a waitress she remarried. Her second husband, who had been employed as a hospital orderly, also died after a few years. She then kept company with one man for a number of years but married another, a man with whom she had had a relatively short acquaintance. Her third husband was not, however, her real love, and she stated that she was all worn out trying to keep her husband and the other man apart.

The patient was an unattractive, dark-complexioned person, who appeared to be in good physical condition. She was preoccupied with her troubles, particularly her physical complaints. Somewhat depressed, she showed a mild motor retardation, being content just to sit. Her facial expression portrayed sorrow. She was negligent of her personal appearance. In time she appeared to be much happier and did fairly well until arrangements were made for her to leave the hospital. Obviously reluctant to face her life situation, she then experienced some return of her depression.

Ps. Sz., Simple	F:15:S:13	+1	436'28–7X (45)	11:12:23
Paranoid		+10	46'89237–(39)	9:10:19
Ps. Sz., Mixed	F:18:S:72	+2	2783'416–(39)	3:7:19

Since infancy the patient had shown aberrant behavior, with recent exacerbations characterized by fears, depression, and a feeling of unreality. From an early age she had feared loud noises and other children, and as she grew older she would have nothing to do with youngsters her own age, insisting that she preferred the company of adults.

Other children regarded her as peculiar and teased her unmercifully. At age 13 she became acutely depressed, was obsessed by a fear of death, and had a morbid interest in cemeteries. She had hallucinatory visions of her own funeral and she saw skeletons everywhere. A visit to relatives brought about a gradual recovery from this severe disturbance. When she returned to school she gave bizarre recitations in the classroom, which incited unsympathetic laughter and teasing. A psychiatrist diagnosed her as having incipient schizophrenia but allowed her to stay in school. One teacher, who gave her considerable attention, helped her to some extent. The patient described herself as having "sexual thrills" in the presence of this teacher, to whom she sent frequent love notes, writing that she wanted "to marry the teacher if her daddy would let her." Neglectful of her personal appearance, she resented her mother's attempts to keep her neat and well dressed. She began to talk with her teeth tightly clenched and to grimace grotesquely. She was suspicious and jealous of the neighbor's children, and she was afraid that they would talk about her. On several occasions she was mildly assaultive toward her mother.

After hospital study (first set of admission data) at age 15 she was finally diagnosed as having schizophrenia. Eleven electroshock treatments at a private hospital failed to improve her. The present admission occurred after an interval in which she had continued to show the same behavior peculiarities.

An immature, small, thin girl, she wore glasses and had a moderate degree of lumbar scoliosis. The skin of her back, shoulders, and upper chest were covered with acneaform eruptions. On admission she was concerned primarily with her fears, repeating constantly, "I feel like I'm going to die. I'm afraid I'm going to die. This place isn't good for me. I want to go home." She also rambled on about various people, saying, "Mother nags. I'm in love with the married man next door. I'm really in love with my teacher. I thrill and thrill over her. I want my daddy. Can't my daddy come back and take me home please?" She was well oriented and had a good memory. Her I.Q. was about 80. There was a marked scattering of ideas and little logical consistency. She disturbed the other patients with her almost constant weeping and her statements about dying, and she followed the nurses and other staff members about the halls, complaining that she was made worse by being in the hospital. When she was finally told very positively that she would have to stop disturbing others and enter into the ward routine, her behavior almost miraculously underwent a great change. She became cooperative and relatively pleasant. At the end of the series of insulin shock therapy, with a total of about twenty comas, she was not deeply changed and was still obviously schizophrenic. She was, however, more tractable and at the time of discharge her family and she seemed to be better adjusted. The family was given considerable instruction about her management at home, and an attempt was made to help them see that in overprotecting her they had been taking a very poor approach toward her illness. It seemed probable that she would be able to continue her life outside a hospital for a time but that eventually commitment to a state hospital would have to be considered.

P. React. Depr. F:45:M:53 +9 436′821–79 8:7:18
Suicidal

The patient was admitted in a nervous, depressed state. Ever since their marriage 25 years before, her husband had been a heavy drinker, and she had contemplated suicide several times because of his alcoholism and cruelty. When he came home drunk and abusive, he swore at her and the children, spat on her, and pushed her around, all of which she tolerated because of her need for his support of their children. She had once arranged for her husband to take a "cure," but he had torn up the papers and had refused to leave home, promising that he would voluntarily stop drinking. However, his behavior had remained unchanged, and five years before admission the patient had attempted suicide by taking poison and sleeping tablets. Several months before she entered the hospital the patient's husband had knocked her down, bruising her, but she had continued to take his abuse until the night before admission when he was particularly threatening. Hysterical and depressed, she had telephoned the sheriff, saying that she would commit suicide if she was not taken away from her husband.

With the exception of two major operations, an appendectomy and a hysterectomy, the patient's previous health had been fairly good. At the time of admission she was experiencing some menopausal symptoms. The woman was of below average intelligence, and the family was of a low socio-economic level. She had failed the seventh grade and had left school to do housework and to work on her parents' farm. She was married when she was 19. She had never taken part in community activities, and especially since her marriage she had been nervous and unhappy.

In the hospital she was depressed, and her main concern was how to forget her husband and his maltreatment. Whenever her husband or her problems were discussed she broke down and cried, but in other ways she was mentally intact. She had good insight into everything except her reasons for not having left her husband previously. She was plain, but neat and cooperative. She quickly improved in the hospital, losing both her somatic complaints and her depression. Pleasant and cooperative with other patients and the staff, she adjusted well on the ward. When preparations had been made for her to go home, with at least some of her problems alleviated, she experienced a brief setback in contemplating the prospect.

Ps. M-D., Mixed F:33:M:23 +18 4'3726–9 5:1:19

Ps. M-D., Mixed F:33:M:15

Ten months before coming to the hospital the patient had first shown an uneasiness in which depressive elements were obvious. Because of her religious beliefs, she had felt great concern about taking quinine after missing a menstrual period, presumably with the intention of bringing about an artificial abortion, and she had gradually become more agitated and had lost her efficiency around her home. There were periods when she was somewhat better, but at one point the symptoms were so acute that she was placed in a sanitarium for a few days. The present admission followed another flare-up of the symptoms.

The past history was not particularly helpful. She had attended country and small town schools until age 16, when she had reached the eleventh grade. After a short business college course, she had worked as a telephone operator until her marriage at age 22 to a man eight years older than she. Intelligent and capable, she had mixed readily with others, had entered into local activities, and had shown no unusual emotional or nervous instability. Her husband felt that their marriage had been happy, but the woman's sister said the patient had been disappointed because she had not married a man she had been in love with before meeting her husband. The couple had three children, and a fourth pregnancy had ended in spontaneous abortion. The patient was reluctant to become pregnant again but because of her religious beliefs used no method of contraception not approved by the church. Some days after taking the quinine, when she thought herself pregnant just before the present illness, she had begun to menstruate.

In the hospital she readily told of her anxiety that she might have caused an abortion by taking the quinine, and although she recognized that her worry was probably unnecessary, she could not free herself of it. She was extremely tense and unable to sleep, but she did not think she should be in the hospital, and she was worried about financing her hospitalization, insisting several times on leaving. There were no obvious disorders of intellect or stream of thought, her conversation was intelligent and coherent, she dressed well, and she cooperated normally. For the first week her condition remained much the same, but during the second week she suddenly began to sleep well and became much more cheerful and composed. She was then released, but five days later she was readmitted in the same agitated state as for the first admission, and this time she was so preoccupied that she was unable to cooperate around the ward, her appearance was haggard, she slept poorly, and she engaged in aimless activities. Her husband finally gave in to her insistence that she be allowed to go home, and when she was discharged against advice in the fourth week of this hospitalization, the prognosis was poor. The nature of her illness was not clear.

Ps. Paranoid M:42:M:21 +6 '43728-9(55) 4:3:23

The onset of this patient's illness was insidious. He had never got along well with his wife, whom he had unwillingly married after she became pregnant. They separated a year after their marriage and remained apart for a while, and then lived together again until the wife inherited a farm and some money from her aunt, when she again left him. This was two years before admission. They had had several fights after that time and the wife tried unsuccessfully to have the patient committed as insane. He started divorce proceedings, but they were talked into living together again with the stipulation that they both go to a psychiatrist. The patient had spells of crying and talking about God and about how everybody was against him. A week before admission he became excited and wanted his wife to put her money in a joint account. He said that if the sheriff came out, he would shoot him. The psychiatrist to whom the patient had gone wrote the local doctor saying that the patient had paranoid trends; a hearing was arranged and the patient was ordered into the psychiatric unit for observation.

The patient had been in good health. He had at one time been treated for "high acidity." He was an eighth-grade graduate at age 16 and had always worked on farms. He liked to read the Bible and said that people who went to church were hypocrites, since reading the Bible was adequate. He was easy to get along with but had been nervous and high-strung all his life. He had periods of severe rage, but though he was always a suspicious person, he had never shown any really bizarre behavior. There were evidences that his marital maladjustment in general was in part due to his wife, who was sexually overactive and possibly had had affairs with other men.

In the hospital he had definitely suspicious thoughts about his wife, his family, and the deputy sheriff, and he believed they were organized against him. He was clear in sensorium and general intellectual reactions. He was cooperative but lacked insight and thought that he had been brought to the hospital to keep him out of the way. No bizarre behavior was noted though he was circumstantial in discourse. He wanted to start proceedings against the deputy for the treatment he had received. He also thought that his father's will had not been probated correctly and that something should be done about it. His behavior was never obviously delusional; there was a degree of rationality in nearly everything he did. It was obvious that if the patient was to be helped, the treatment would have to be a long-continued one. Neither he nor anyone in his family really appreciated the extent of his illness, and it seemed unlikely that much could be done for him.

B. Psth., Path. Emot. F:28:S:29 +1 4'379-(51) 7:2:21
Paranoid

A few days before admission the patient and her roommate had returned from a hitchhiking trip to find a note in their room from their landlady saying that the patient could no longer remain. The patient became angry, wanted to know why her girl friend could remain when she had to leave, and accused her friend of plotting with the landlady to get rid of her. In her anger she assaulted her friend and attempted to assault the landlady. Her father took her away the next day, removing her forcibly because she struggled violently and screamed. At home she continued to be unmanageable, in turn screaming, struggling, and crying. By the time of admission she had become less maniacal, although she was said to have fainted unconvincingly during the court hearing preceding admission.

The past history was not especially contributory until about a year before admission, when the patient was seen by a psychiatrist because of a depressed mood in which she threatened suicide; her family, however, had not taken the threat seriously. She recovered shortly from this acute episode. She explained the depression by saying she was an old maid, a misfit, and without friends. From her earliest years she had wanted to be a boy because boys did as they pleased, met people, got married, and lived as they wanted to; she had always been jealous of her brothers, especially when they married. She had never had many friends. As a child, she had stayed home and read much of the time. In constant rebellion against her father, she had been severely beaten many times for slight variations from his standards. Her tendency to extreme shyness had been enhanced during her late teens by the fact that she had been forced to wear old-fashioned clothes, and by the fact that the family had moved about so frequently that she had never been long in one place or one school. She had graduated from a teachers' college and had taught school for several years, but because of laziness and indecisiveness her record was poor. Although she always felt that if she could work where people understood her she would do all right, she had left a series of positions because she had been unable to get along with her employer or her associates. The patient had always been a selfish person, and with the possible exception of the girl friend she had lived with, she had never shown any responsibility toward anyone and had taken no interest in anyone. This friend was a homosexual partner in a relationship in which the patient was the passive participant.

In the hospital the patient was greatly concerned about the possibility of losing her friend and of being sent to a state hospital. She continued to "love" her girl friend, but she also wanted to see her punished for the trouble she had caused. The patient was depressed at her inability to adjust and to make something of herself. She had marked paranoid trends, chiefly directed toward her family, her friend, and the hospital staff. She was indignant at being in the hospital, and she denied the need for treatment. She felt that she was homosexual only because of circumstances, and the staff felt that this was a good explanation. During interviews her mood varied from vindictiveness and suspicion to friendliness and affability. She made frequent caustic remarks about others, and she always blamed other people and circumstances, rather than herself, for her troubles. She adapted fairly well to the hospital routine and showed some anxiety and indecision about the future. After social service preparation and the completion of plans for a job placement she was discharged with a poor prognosis and the advice that if she could not adjust she should go to a state hospital on her next admission.

Ps. Paranoid F:36:M:36 +3 '438–9(49) 8:1:26

The patient dated her present illness from about five years before when, she said, "I first began to feel run-down and sickly." At that time she believed that she was in need of medical attention but her husband did not agree. For two years she was "pepless" and found it difficult to do ordinary tasks. When a pregnancy was terminated by a uteran hemorrhage a partial hysterectomy was performed. During numerous visits to the doctor's office she developed an infatuation for him. She claimed that he flirted and made advances and that she knew by his actions he was in love with her. The physician was a widower, and the patient said that she first realized he did not love her when he remarried. At the time of admission she recognized the whole episode to be a "misunderstanding" on her part, yet insisted there had been "misconduct" on the part of the doctor. The physician's story was that the patient bothered him by coming to his office time after time with no particular complaint. One day after his remarriage the patient waylaid him in the presence of other people, accusing him of "breaking up" her own home and of marrying a "whore." Later she apologized for this scene. The physician notified the police of the situation and called the patient's husband but nothing was done.

The patient's past history was marked by numerous illnesses of one type or another and by "chronic sinusitis." Apparently she had had at least one nervous breakdown, although details were not available, and she had received extensive treatment for a "nervous stomach."

At the end of the eighth grade she had left school and had worked for a while. Then she married and later enrolled in a course in beauty culture but failed the state board examinations. In handling money and in managing the affairs of her home she exerted poor judgment. She was described as having been happy, carefree, and not given to excessive worry. With the development of the present illness, there was a gradual change in her personality, and she began to neglect her home and to spend money foolishly.

In the hospital she repeated in great detail the story of her present illness. In answer to the accusation that she had waited for the physician in public places, she said, "I could wait there if I wanted to, couldn't I?" In the hospital there were no abnormalities in her behavior except for the content of her discourse. She was cheerful and in general cooperative, although she had no awareness that she was ill in any sense of the word. Overtalkative and easily excited, she tired and annoyed other patients at times. She had definite hypochondriacal trends. She made no real change in the hospital and was discharged for a trial at home, with the recommendation that if she could not adjust she should go to a state hospital.

B. Psth., Asocial Mutilative — M:21:S — 43'829 761–(59) — 4:5:13

This youth was referred to the psychopathic ward for observation because of self-mutilation and an attempt to escape from prison. He had severed the Achilles' tendon of his left heel with a double-edged razor blade. Previously he had escaped from the prison farm, had attempted to escape two additional times, and had mutilated himself by cutting his right Achilles' tendon.

When the prisoner was 6 years of age, his parents separated and he lived with his mother until he was 15, when he ran away from home. He continued to attend school and graduated from high school. From that time on he held irregular jobs as a common laborer. The same year he left home he was arrested for the first time, for purse snatching. A year later he was apprehended again for the same offense. When sentenced to the state prison the first time, for burglary, he was an immature, unstable, irresponsible lad of 17. He served eleven months, maintained a good record, and was given a reprieve. He immediately joined the army but while on leave before going overseas he was caught in the act of robbing a private residence and was returned to prison as a conditional pardon violator. The conviction was for eight years. During this prison stay he began to show difficulty in making adjustments.

Observation of the youth showed him to be well oriented in criminal behavior and completely lacking in remorse for the grief he had repeatedly caused his mother. No delusions or hallucinations were present. He distinguished right from wrong, spoke with an easy flow of language, in fact was an excellent talker and adept at rationalization. The prison psychiatrist's statement said that the inmate was "a clever psychopath with traces of schizophrenia and hysteria, unable to adjust to prison, or to get along with the guards." The psychiatrist predicted that the youth "will be a problem while in prison" and added "nor will he be able to get along in the free world." R. C. K.

Ps. Psth. F:32:S:225 +1 4387126'9–(47) 7:7:17
Paranoid

When the patient was in her early twenties she had had a nervous breakdown, characterized by lassitude, fatigue, and inability to do any work. Even before this she had had disagreements with her teachers in college and had shown uncontrolled emotionalism and frank rebellion. She recovered from this breakdown and managed to get along, although she remained unstable and was always on the verge of another collapse. As physical symptoms developed she began to pay calls to physicians all over the city and was treated for this and that ill. A psychiatrist said at this time, "She shows a picture of severe neurotic involvement with psychasthenic features and a marked paranoid element." In one private hospital she received electroshock therapy, with little effect. The years passed in this fashion until, two months before admission, she "choked" while eating an orange and thereafter claimed to be unable to swallow solid food. She quarreled more violently than usual with her mother and, during the arguments, was profane and loud, a change from her usual behavior. She also became more than usually obsessed with the idea that she was going crazy.

The patient's past history was partly indicated by these episodes, but long before the events detailed, she had had many borderline physical difficulties. Above average in intellect, she had attended college for a number of years but had never done well because of her neurotic behavior. She became engaged, but after a visit to her fiancé's home she broke off the engagement, saying that the man's mother was "nuts." Except for helping her father she had never held a job. A perfectionist always, she apparently reached for goals above her ability to attain. In actual production she was never really successful at anything. She was cyclothymic in emotional tone and was generally resistive to almost everyone around her.

In the hospital the patient's main thought was the prediction that she was going crazy. She said, "My poor bean isn't what it used to be." She was intact in sensorium and intellect, and her behavior seemed superficially normal. She made an obvious attempt to be cheerful but was unconvincing. She recognized that her difficulties were psychological. Her replies to questions were normal and adequate. Although secretive in many ways, she gave the appearance of trying to be cooperative. She preferred to stay in bed but did follow the hospital routine when pushed. Her stay on the ward was characterized by ups and downs. There was some improvement but when she was finally discharged to go home the prognosis remained poor.

P. Mixed Schizoid F:22:S:76 +19 4398'7126– 3:11:15

About a year before admission the patient began to manifest great concern about her eyes. She felt pain and she thought she could not see as well as usual, but consultation with a number of physicians and frequent changes of glasses produced no definite improvement. Gradually she began to have spells in which she screamed, swore, struck others, and was destructive. She was in a sanitarium for four months but did not change. At times she was depressed, threatening suicide, and as her difficulty progressed she became very antagonistic toward her mother.

Never robust or strong, the patient had not had any severe physical illness, however. A high school graduate, she had got along well in school, but she was quiet, self-conscious, and underactive, and she had feelings of inadequacy. The girl was small in size, immature in appearance and behavior. She had always had a tendency to be readily depressed, and her relationship with her mother, a dominant, tense person, was an unhealthy one.

In the hospital she was greatly concerned and depressed about the condition of her eyes, which she felt was her only difficulty, and she wondered if she would "go mad" from the distress they caused her. There were no other delusions, no paranoid trends, and no obvious disturbances of intellect or sensorium. Her intelligence was dull normal. Although she talked readily, seemed cooperative, and adjusted fairly well in the hospital, it was impossible to establish good rapport with her. As time went on she made fewer references to her eyes and appeared to be somewhat improved, but she denied any possibility of improvement, saying that nothing could be done for her. Her mother's visits always brought out her worst behavior. It was impossible to determine whether her quick, nervous manner and choreiform movements, with tics and peculiar mannerisms, had a toxic or a functional basis. After arrangements were made for some changes in her home environment, the girl was discharged to be followed in the outpatient department.

B. Psth., Asocial F:21:M:14 +1 4′6–<u>132</u>(74) 0:3:8

When this young woman's husband left the country a year before admission, she began to neglect her housework and her children. Later, when her husband returned for a short leave, she regained interest in her affairs and behaved in a normal fashion. However, soon after he returned to duty, she again became lax. At this time she began to go out with other men, eventually every night. She took a job which left her almost no time or interest for her children. A sister, who had assumed partial care of the children, suddenly left, and when one night the children were found alone in the house they were put into the custody of the patient's mother-in-law. At this time the patient threw away her wedding ring and left the city. Shortly after, her husband arrived home and when he learned what had happened he found his wife and brought her in for diagnosis.

Three years earlier the young woman had slipped and struck the back of her head. She had been unconscious for five minutes and for months afterward she had suffered from weekly headaches over the right frontal region. Another accident had resulted in a miscarriage. Two years before admission she had had a mastoiditis and had been delirious for five days.

In school she had been an excellent student but had not finished high school because she became pregnant. A self-centered, deceptive person, she had always brought much trouble to her family. Until the present episode, however, she had fulfilled her home duties fairly well. In high school she had made no close girl friends and had been promiscuous with boys. Before her husband went into the army she had made a reasonably good adjustment as a wife and mother. Her first marriage had occurred when she was 16 in order to "give the baby a name." She had stayed with that husband only a few months and then had married her present husband.

In the hospital careful neurological studies revealed no evidence of a defect. Tests indicated an I.Q. of 116. Moody but otherwise normal in behavior, the patient did not seem to be troubled about her former actions and took them as a matter of course. Her adaptation to the hospital routine was good, although she was restless and frequently wanted to go home. She completely lacked any insight or awareness that she was ill, and psychotherapeutic approaches were ineffective. It was felt that she would probably adjust fairly well if she could live with her husband, but this possibility was remote, not only because of his army duties but because of his own instability.

B. Psth., Mixed F:16:S:39 +7 46′–<u>79</u> 5:3:14

According to a detailed social service report the patient had first come to the attention of authorities about a year before admission when she had been picked up by the police for sleeping in a used-car lot. Apparently not wanting to return home because the people with whom she had been living had moved to smaller quarters, she had been sleeping in used cars and in hotel rest rooms. The social agency had attempted to help her by a work-home placement, but the foster parents stated that she was negligent in personal cleanliness, irresponsible in her work, and irregular in hours. Her tendency to preoccupation led to her admission for psychiatric evaluation.

She had made satisfactory progress through the eighth grade, but her high school record was exceedingly unsatisfactory. She had been irregular in attendance, had been a disciplinary problem, and had taken little interest in her studies. After age 11 she spent considerable time away from home, maintaining herself by working as a domestic. Although she was a social individual and easily influenced, there was an ambivalence in her entire personality. She enjoyed such activities of "wild" young people as dancing and roller skating in cheap amusement halls, but she was aware that this type of recreation was improper, and she made a few unsuccessful attempts to associate with "better children." Because of marked socio-economic differences, however, she was usually unhappy and did not continue such relationships. Her family was poverty-stricken, with many children and very little money. The home was exceedingly dirty, and the nine children slept on the floor in one room.

On admission the patient was cooperative but seemed perplexed about being in the hospital and little concerned about her situation. She had better than average intelligence. At the times when she appeared preoccupied her answers to questions were brief and inadequate, but as rapport was established it became clear that the periods of apparent apathy were a front and that she was painfully aware of her poor family background. She realized that her conduct was inappropriate for her age, and she expressed some concern about her future. In time she came to recognize that she was easily influenced and in admitting her inability to stand up under rebuffs, she said that it was best for poor people like herself not to hope for too much. When her poor personal habits and slovenly appearance were pointed out to her, she accepted criticism and cooperated so that she made a better appearance. Apparently she wanted to make a readjustment, and arrangements were made for her to enter a vocational school. She was discharged to go to a residence home for girls while attending the school.

B. Simple Adult Maladj. M:49:S:34 +1 '46-9(65) 5:1:18
Ps. Sz., Simple

For seventeen years this patient had been a problem in his home community, and he was sent to the psychiatric unit by the court. Two months before admission he had been given a thirty-day jail sentence on the charge of "creating a nuisance" by following a young woman on a single occasion. Although there was no known instance of aggressive behavior, the patient had been in the habit of roaming the streets at night, appearing to wait for someone. When an unaccompanied woman passed he followed her home. On numerous occasions he had been seen peeping in windows. About eight years before admission he had stood trial in an alleged rape and probable paternity case, but he had been acquitted on a "no bill" verdict. The woman in the case, of rather questionable character, had been promiscuous with other men. It was the patient's opinion that the town marshal and local barkeeper were trying to get him out of town because he was against gambling and the selling of liquor. He said that the local "big shots" were paid to protect the local bar. When the possibility of commitment proceedings was brought up after he had served his thirty-day jail sentence, the patient requested evaluation by an outside clinic.

The patient had never had very good health, and several accidents had left him slightly incapacitated. After completing the eighth grade, he had worked at farming. Until the age of 25, when he gradually began to decline in ability, he had been known as a hard, ambitious worker. A shy, mild-mannered person with a tendency toward seclusiveness, he had never had close friends, men or women.

In the hospital he was composed, his behavior was conventional except for inappropriate laughter, and his stream of thought was adequate and logical. On personal matters he showed some hesitation and shyness. He was mildly concerned about his present situation and about the drinking and gambling in his home town. If anything was wrong with him the doctors would find it, he felt. There was no evidence of brain deterioration, and he was somewhat above average in measured intelligence. He changed little during his stay in the hospital. He was not really approachable, and he never gained any more insight than he had had at the time of admission. When he was discharged back to the court's custody it was with the general recommendation that he be shifted to another community if possible. From the standpoint of aggression it was felt that he was probably not dangerous.

P. Mixed M:32:D 462378′91–(84) 5:11:14
′43962–718(82) 6:7:18

This college student, a senior in history, was referred for help because he was not able to keep his grades up. He complained that even though he seemed to learn the material assigned in his courses he was unable to present it adequately in an examination.

The man was a veteran who had been discharged from the army with a psychoneurotic disability. He married while in the army but separated from his wife and finally divorced her. Before their separation his wife had joined the WAC and at the time he was being seen, she was also in one of the veterans' hospitals for psychotherapeutic treatment. He reported a great desire to make friends but apparently he tended to remain on the fringe of groups.

Even after the patient dropped out of school he continued to see the therapist, and he eventually worked through to an understanding of the ways in which he had avoided reality in order to build up preferred conceptions of himself as a highly talented, individualistic person. One very important set of emotional involvements he worked out was his attitude toward his former wife. It turned out that he had really not resolved his feelings toward her; after going through a period when he was on the verge of reopening their relationship, he finally decided to close it off. During this period also he shifted to a more realistic consideration of his occupational possibilities and plans. Indirect follow-up information indicated that he was holding his job and was continuing to operate effectively. The second MMPI was obtained late in the series of therapeutic interviews. E. S. B.

P. Mixed	F:25:M:44	+9	462738'19–(43)	5:2:16
		+36	3647 1829'–(39)	3:4:16
		+40	68 347129'–(37)	2:8:9

This young woman had been nervous since late adolescence. Tremors of her hands and feet, palpitation of her heart, and pressure sensations on her head were included in the pattern. Further troubles were intense anxiety, feelings of guilt about premarital promiscuity, insomnia, fear of crowds, and the like. She had become so nervous that she could not sit through an entire movie.

In general the patient's health had been good. She claimed to have had no difficulty in school but had led a rather "wild" life between the ages of 15 and 17. At this time she indulged in sexual intercourse with a number of boys, became pregnant, and left school to get married. She said that as a housewife she thereafter had remained faithful to her husband. She had three children. Always a sensitive and self-restrained person, she worried unduly about little things. For example, she was frequently embarrassed because her clothes were not as nice as those of other girls. Although she got along with people, she never joined social groups. Her father was a chronic alcoholic and her family life had been insecure and unpleasant. One of her sisters had become involved with the patient's husband, and the patient had heard about this just before the birth of her last child. The patient thought that she had bent over backward in "being good," for she had stopped drinking, smoking, and "tearing around" after her marriage. She was also very conscientious in her role as a mother. Her marriage had been reasonably happy until her husband's return from the service and his affair with her sister. He then became less affectionate and told her that she was too passionate and overemphasized sexual intercourse.

On admission to the hospital she was well oriented and had good contact at all times. Depressed and anxious, she worried excessively about her sexual looseness during her schooldays. Those experiences haunted her, she said, and "are always in the back of my mind." She thought her husband's present coolness might be due to these incidents and not to his war experiences as he insisted. Soon after she entered the hospital she became less tense but continued to complain of the physical symptoms. Three electroshock treatments were given and she appeared to respond favorably to these. Throughout her stay she continued to improve and was finally discharged to a boarding home for a period of recuperation.

Ps. Sz., Paranoid M:19:S:120 +1 4'6287-(67) 5.7:8

The onset of this youth's illness was insidious. A seclusive boy always, he had never made friends, could not get along with others of his age, and was irritable and demanding toward his mother. At 17 he left school to join the marines. He had completed his basic training and was in the final week of advanced training when he was placed in a mental hospital. After a month and a half he was discharged because "they thought something was the matter with my mind." After this he behaved in an even more peculiar manner and expressed bizarre ideas. Becoming a tramp, he begged for all his food, took no job, and spent his time sleeping, eating, reading, and seeing an occasional movie. More and more demanding of his mother and aunt, and more irritable, he frequently "shouted and screamed for hours." Although he never actually threatened his mother he demonstrated "Jap killing technique" on her with a long sharp knife. His last scheme had been to buy a horse (he already had purchased a saddle and gun) and ride west to purchase a large ranch and raise buffalo.

The youth's intelligence was good, especially in mechanical subjects. In school he had done well when he had attended and exerted any effort, but he had always shown poor judgment, particularly in handling money. Instead of participating in sports and in other recreation he would go off by himself to read. One of his interests was astrology, in which he firmly believed. He was described as being lazy and undependable.

In the hospital the patient was primarily concerned about when he could leave for the trip west. He had already made some initial purchases and he wanted to negotiate for the buffalo, cattle, and the like. When he had to miss the radio serial programs he had been following he was very exasperated. Tense, agitated, and excitable, he exploded angrily whenever his views were opposed. Lacking insight, he believed his troubles might be related to masturbation. At first he was thought to be dangerous, but gradually it came to be felt that this was not so, and he himself once admitted that his actions were a bluff and that actually he was afraid to fight. Toward other patients he exhibited an arrogant, inconsiderate attitude, yet he participated in group activities. A series of seventeen subshock insulin treatments brought no improvement. In interviews he expressed the certainty that everybody was against him and that he was left out of everything. The youth's aversion to hospital regulation and his desire to be "let alone" remained consistent through the entire hospitalization. Finally he was discharged to go to a state hospital.

Ps. Toxic M:43:M:15 +2 '4629-X(49) 15:10:15
Alcoholism

A month before admission the patient had taken a few drinks, contrary to his custom. Each morning during the next few weeks he promised his wife to stay away from alcohol; but each day he went to the local bar and returned home in a drunken stupor. There seemed to be no particular cause for this chain of events. Ten days before admission his wife told him to straighten out, or she would leave him. According to the patient, he spent the next few days in bars, sometimes not sleeping at night, and he was taken to the hospital by the police in a toxic delirium with evidence of neuritic irritation.

The patient had a residual paralysis of the right arm and hand as the result of poliomyelitis at age 8. Later he had developed chronic tuberculosis and had spent a year and a half in a sanitarium. Since that time he had had an artificial pneumothorax.

The patient was an eighth-grade graduate and had always been a somewhat irregular worker. About twice a year for ten years he had gone on two-week drinking bouts similar to the present one, but these sprees had recently been gradually increasing in frequency. His wife had supported him for the last fifteen years. When not drinking, he was a quiet, sensitive man, with good morals. He did not particularly enjoy social activities but was very interested in hunting and fishing. His irritability and his intolerance of the noise his children made around home were a source of conflict between the patient and his wife.

In the hospital the patient made a rapid recovery; his anxiety decreased markedly, the confusions and disorientation present at admission disappeared, as did the visual hallucinations, and he became very anxious about his wife, about the condition of his pneumothorax, and about his business. As he returned to his normal state there was evidence of considerable insecurity. He could give no reason for the drinking episodes, and he had no real desire for help or for personal understanding.

B. Psth., Mixed   M:26:M:25   +13   '462987–3(61)   5:6:12

This man was admitted to the hospital by a court order for investigation and treatment. He was charged with leaving his wife and children for long periods. He had served with the Royal Air Force as a transport driver in Burma. On being invalided out of the service, he could not settle down, had "bouts of blackness," and thought that people were against him.

Nothing was known about his early history.

He was diagnosed as being constitutionally inferior with psychopathic tendencies, and this diagnosis indicated no treatment. M. V.

B. Psth., Mixed   F:35:M:11   +11   4'63–   5:1:24
Drug Add.

When the patient was transferred from a general hospital on a voluntary basis, she complained of excessive nervousness and expressed a desire to overcome what she called a "morphine habit and alcoholism." Although she had apparently used morphine for sixteen years, there was a discrepancy between her version and that of another informant about when she first began to use it. For the last seven or eight years, there had been several hospital admissions and frequent arrests as the result of alcoholic "binges," during which she became abusive and used profane language. Among the clever devices she employed to get morphine from local physicians, by whom she was well known, was that of faking an attack of kidney stones, in which she pricked her finger to simulate blood in the urine. She had had at least two major surgical operations, one for a tumor of the uterus sixteen years before admission, and a cholecystectomy about twelve years before admission.

After graduating from a convent high school the patient had first worked in a department store and had then begun nurses' training. A premarital pregnancy at age 17 made it necessary for her to discontinue this training, but after her marriage her knowledge was sufficient to qualify her for practical nursing. In this capacity she had an excellent opportunity to steal morphine. As the youngest member of her family, she had always been spoiled, she said, and her nickname at one time had been "Stifflegs," because when she could not have her own way she stiffened out and became so obnoxious that her family always gave in to her. In general she was a cheerful, happy person, but she had a tendency toward moodiness and she was so eager for sympathy that she had developed the habit of crying on slight provocation. Although she had always been unable to handle money, she could get a new job easily, and her excess of energy was apparently one reason for her difficulties. Although her first child and her third one had died, a second was living and well. After eight years the patient had divorced her first husband and had married a man considerably older than she was. At the time of admission she was in love with a much younger man, but she insisted that she was very fond of her husband and that she wanted to continue her marriage because her husband was good to her.

There was no content disturbance on admission, and the patient was in excellent contact with reality. Her sensorium and general mentality were intact, but hers was obviously an immature personality. Chiefly because of her attempts to obtain morphine, she was unruly and uncooperative during her first few days in the hospital, and she cried and pouted like a child, but after this episode her surface attitude and manner were entirely acceptable. She had a superficial insight, and she insisted that everything was going to be all right because she had "learned her lesson." Although she wanted to be helpful on the ward, she also tried to get away with minor infractions of the rules, and she made little real progress while she was in the hospital. Her inability to profit by experience, her lack of appreciation of socially acceptable behavior, and her emotional instability were factors which made it appear unlikely that she would make an adequate adjustment.

Ps. Sz., Cat. F:19:S:36 +56 '463–2(57) 7:3:21

Four days before admission this young woman suddenly went into an acute psychotic state. This began in the mid-afternoon with such confusion that she was unable to continue work. She complained of sickness and was taken home, where she showed so much excitement that her mother thought she was drunk. Over and over she repeated that she had "told a lie" and consequently had decided to become a nun. (Three days before this incident the priest had telephoned the patient's father because of the bizarreness of her confession.) Heavy sedation was required to calm her, and her condition grew worse until she was brought to the hospital. At that time she experienced both auditory and visual hallucinations, grimaced, postured, and talked almost continually in a bizarre and incoherent manner. The patient's language was obscene and her actions at times assaultive.

There were no previous episodes of psychosis or obvious neurotic breakdowns in the patient's history. A person of average abilities, she had liked school and had graduated from high school when she was 19. After that she took a job as a waitress and performed satisfactorily. Described as a quiet and neat girl who "liked to tease," she had many friends. She was unusually modest, to the extent, in fact, that she refused to wear shorts and rarely went out with young men unless someone else was present. She spoke of men as "wolves." Her older brother often teased her and she felt that he was "against" her. In response to his teasing she often showed a hot temper. Always religious, she had seriously considered becoming a nun during the last few months. Her family life appeared to be normal, and there were no obvious contributory factors in that sphere.

In the hospital complete physical and neurophysiological studies disclosed no identifiable disturbances. She was grossly delusional and hallucinatory. Crosses, colored lights, and flies were prominent in her "visions." She misnamed members of the staff and talked obscenely about sexual matters. There was evidence of a strong sense of guilt, she was disoriented, her emotions were labile and her behavior unpredictable. Occasionally she reluctantly admitted that she had been sick but always felt that she was well at the time she made this admission. Various types of sedatives were given and she was forced to go to bed. After nine electroshock treatments she showed gradual improvement, became cooperative, dressed more attractively, and apparently tried to adapt to the hospital routine. Then she became puzzled about what had happened and she worried about it. At the time of discharge she was not entirely recovered but was greatly improved. It appeared probable that she would continue to have similar attacks but would recover and would be able to live a fairly normal life.

Ps. Paranoid F:44:M:57 +2 4′6<u>31</u>8–(57) 3:3:21

The court requested hospitalization for this woman after she had injured a neighbor child and had been charged with assault and battery. Three years earlier her husband had noted that she was misinterpreting events. At this time she became agitated and believed neighbors were spreading rumors that she was a "bad woman." She also showed increased irritability. Friends were sending her valentines that could be "taken two ways," she claimed, and she forced her husband to have postal authorities investigate. Her husband bought a home in a new locality but soon she became irritable and suspicious of her new neighbors. Set in her opinions, she flew into rages whenever anyone disagreed with her. Neighbors deliberately sent their children to annoy her, she insisted. It was this delusion that led to her assault on one of these children.

Her previous medical and psychological history was relatively noncontributory. Before the end of the first year of high school she left because she "lived too far from the school." Later, after six months at a business school, she went to work. In one job she had a peculiar experience. Apparently her employer paid her attentions, presented her with a check for $1000, and asked her to stay at a hotel with him for a week. According to her story, she refused and reported him to a social agency, but she herself was accused by the agency of "leading him along." Returning the money to him, she left the job. Of good intelligence, she was a steady worker. She was known as sensitive, secretive, and self-reliant. Other adjectives applied to her were stubborn, egotistical, and vain. She was interested in mysticism. Her greatest ambition was to be an author, but her lack of education prevented this, she felt. A responsible housewife, however, she got along fairly well until the onset of the present illness.

In the hospital she was deeply concerned about the fact that her neighbors had requested her arrest. She went into long and involved explanations of everything and showed a wealth of systematized delusional ideas. The appearance she gave was of composure and complacence, but also, in a subtle way, of indifference. Her intellect was good and she was well oriented. The only deviant symptoms that could be readily observed were the delusional systems and considerable circumstantiality in her discourse. She appeared to be cynical and haughty. Shock therapy brought no beneficial change and during her stay in the hospital she did not improve in any way. Toward the end she became defensive and denied her previous statements. This behavior was considered to be a cover-up procedure conscientiously assumed. In spite of the recommendation that she go to a state hospital, her husband took her home.

Ps. Invol. Melan.	F:50:M:87	+74	4'6328–(37)	8:2:19
Paranoid		+79	6'43 78–91(39)	2:3:17

This woman's immediate illness began one month before admission and coincided with the induction of a son into the service. The patient strongly disapproved of her son's decision to join the army, and there had also been disagreements between her husband and the son. Some months earlier her husband had left their home, and he was living alone. A long-standing incompatibility with her husband existed, but it was not until her son defied her wishes that she began secretly to acquire information so that she might obtain a divorce. She slept poorly, paced the floor, became depressed, and neglected her personal appearance. When brought to the hospital she was in a stuporous condition.

There were no previous nervous or mental upsets and no obviously contributory physical illnesses in the patient's history. As far as could be determined, she had a fairly routine childhood, attended high school, and married shortly after she finished. Her role was confined to that of a housewife and she had never held a job or supported herself. A woman of good social sense, she was interested in bridge and other recreational activities. There was no evidence of sexual maladjustment and the only deviant factor in her past personal history was her tendency to keep her troubles to herself.

It appeared when the patient was admitted to the hospital that she had received heavy sedation. She was resistive and uncooperative and for three days she remained mute and unresponsive. She ignored her surroundings, was negativistic, and would not feed herself. Then she began to ask to leave the hospital and she expressed a desire to see her husband. Her behavior changed; she began to respond and to cooperate but was still quiet and cried occasionally. Within the next weeks she kept busy with all sorts of tasks around the ward, apparently desiring to keep herself occupied, and she was eager to help other patients. She had self-depreciatory ideas. The worry about her son continued and she refused to believe that he was actually at sea. After eight electroshock treatments, there was a sudden change in her behavior; she began to dress more carefully and apparently returned to her normal mental outlook and condition. Although still concerned about her marital difficulties and her son's leaving she did not seem to be deeply depressed or otherwise emotional in discussing the problem. When she was discharged to return to her home, it was felt that she would probably make a fair adjustment.

B. Psth., Asocial F:38:D:12 +1 '4638–(59) 5:1:20
P. React. Depr.
Drug Add.

This woman came to the hospital from a state reformatory. There her record had been good until one month before admission when she had become nervous and depressed. For days she preferred to stay in her room and stare out the window. She frequently broke into tears, was careless in her dress, and refused to eat. Sometimes she felt an urge to move about, and after a long walk, she would be temporarily relieved of her symptoms.

The patient's childhood had been happy and apparently her home had been fairly good. She had made a satisfactory school record through the second year in high school. In her junior year she was sent to the reformatory for a few months for helping to distribute pornographic literature. While in the institution she became addicted to morphine. After this her life was a series of prison terms. The offenses centered around the drug addiction; for example, she was imprisoned four times for forging checks to obtain money for drugs. She was thought to have good learning ability and intelligence and good judgment except in relation to the drug addiction. Sewing and crocheting were her hobbies, and she read travel and biographical books as a pastime. She was friendly and cheerful in her associations with people. Her married life started out happily, but her husband was disappointed and despondent when he learned that she was a drug addict, and he divorced her while she was serving one of her terms in the reformatory. Sexually promiscuous then, she lived out of wedlock with a divorced man during her most recent interval out of prison.

In the hospital the patient's mental content was not bizarre. She dressed neatly and showed no peculiarities of activity or behavior. Expressing interest in any help that might be given to her, she declared that her life had been wasted and she blamed it on the morphine addiction. Why she took up the habit, she could not explain. When she talked of her forthcoming parole, she voiced the hope that she would be placed in a small town where friends could not influence her to take drugs. In talking to her, one had the impression of a person conscientiously trying to straighten out her life and make up for a poor past record. After less than three days in the hospital she said she felt much better and was less confused about her future. Her quick recovery surprised her. She gained no insight into her particular problem. She expressed deep concern about the health of her father, who was critically ill, and it was felt that this might have contributed to her depression. When she left the hospital she was to return to the reformatory.

Ps. Invol. Melan. F:51:M:16 +1 46381 27'9-(45) 6:4:20
Paranoid

This woman was admitted to the hospital on a police hold order because of an episode of agitation with depression, threats of suicide and assault, and paranoid ideas. The acute onset was two days before admission when the patient aroused her husband, slumped to the floor, and began to scream, cry for air, and say there was nothing left for her any longer. She continued to be agitated and when she was seen by a physician he found her confused, disorganized, threatening toward her husband, and experiencing delusions of persecution. The following night she locked herself in her room for hours and refused to see anyone. During the past year she had had frequent crying spells. She had also had various somatic complaints of a somewhat indefinite nature.

A high school graduate, she had next studied at a school of music. She taught music until she was married. After her marriage she moved to another city and again began teaching. She continued with this work until the present illness except for a few months while her mother was ill. Friends described her as a person who made a good first impression, but who was temperamental, overly sensitive, and easily hurt. She was a good conversationalist. Eager to get ahead as a teacher, she was ambitious for an advanced degree in music. Her home and personal possessions never satisfied her. She was also critical of others. She seemed to value money more than friendship and was self-centered. During the past year her tendency to be suspicious had intensified.

In the hospital the patient talked freely and exhibited considerable aggression toward her husband. Believing that she was unjustly hospitalized, she said this was her husband's method of proving her to be mentally unstable. He was saving his own face, she said, "because of his lying and cheating through the years." Her paranoid ideas extended to her home physician. She had "the goods" on her husband, she thought, and she believed that a divorce was her only solution. Much of the time, however, she felt that her situation was hopeless. She made a good adjustment to the hospital and took an active part in ward activities. She was encouraged to discuss her marital problems. At one time she decided "everything would be all right," but after talking to her husband, she made up her mind that it was hopeless again. She expressed no suicidal ideas and insisted that her previously expressed threats were "merely for effect." She came to recognize that her actions had been somewhat infantile, and she finally decided to make another try at her marriage. Her husband needed encouragement and praise rather than criticism from her, she concluded. At discharge she was improved, but the prognosis did not appear altogether good in view of the patient's long-standing basic trends.

B. Psth., Path. Emot. F:49:M:31 +2 46′3819– 6:4:10

The patient was admitted on a hold order issued by the probate court because of temper tantrums, neglect of her children, and general nuisance activities. On many occasions she had written to acquaintances and members of her family telling of her numerous domestic troubles, and twice she had suddenly left town without making arrangements for the care of her children. More recently she had taken a son with her to a dance and had stayed out until early morning, later telling her friends what a wonderful time she had had. She complained of forgetfulness, shortness of breath on exertion, and marked weakness.

An eighth-grade graduate, she had left school to work on her father's farm, often doing the work of a man. Preceding a cholecystectomy eleven years before admission, she had had fainting spells for a year. Before her illness she was known as an economical, hard-working housewife, who was sociable and apparently satisfied with her life in spite of the fact that the family was on relief. Four years before the patient's admission she had requested an insanity hearing for her husband, and although the husband had confirmed her testimony that he had been confined to a mental hospital for several months, neither the court nor the hospital had found any record of his commitment, and the commission had held that he was sane. At the hearing the patient had stated that her husband had spells when he was weak and helpless, that he drank heavily, and that he was very abusive at home, but only the fact that he had a very violent temper was clearly substantiated. The man was considered a good workman, and he had had no trouble with the welfare board. There were five children; several of them were feeble-minded, and at least one had been committed to a reform school.

The patient was a very obese person, and there was evidence of mild cardiac failure with some decompensation. She was under the impression that she had come to the hospital to rest and to get away from unpleasant conditions, and she was surprised to learn that she had been sent under a court order. She vigorously condemned her husband and said, "He doesn't believe in education or religion, both of which I believe in. Also he's very mean to the children. Once he almost choked one of the boys to death. I had him arrested on an insanity charge, but I made a mistake. I should have had him arrested on a cruelty charge." The patient's memory and mentation appeared to be intact, but she was of dull normal intelligence, and she readily found excuses for her behavior. She was pleasant and cooperative, however, and gained a considerable amount of insight into her problems. A diet, begun in the hospital, resulted in a weight loss which made her physically more comfortable. Though there was little basic change in her personality at the time of discharge, there was some improvement.

P. Psychas.	F:24:M:23	+19	4'638 2179–(41)	4:0:16
B. Psth., Asocial		–49	7'248631–9	7:3:12

Two years earlier, two weeks before the delivery of her second child, this young woman began to have fearful ideas which she could not describe. A few days after the birth of the child an aunt came to live with the family against the patient's wishes. The aunt was so peculiar in some ways that the patient feared she might go insane and harm the children. Two months later the patient began to have obsessions and to dream that she herself would go insane and kill the children. With the onset of these symptoms she became irritable and disinterested in her work, and she harbored guilt feelings over the obsessions. Her appetite diminished. Later she complained of sounds, such as frogs croaking, which persisted long after they were actually inaudible. Hospitalized briefly, she improved, but up and down periods followed and the symptoms remained until the time of admission.

Aside from these events in the preceding two years, the patient's past history made no pertinent contribution. She had left school when she was 15. Learning had always been difficult for her, particularly arithmetic and spelling. After leaving school she did odd jobs but did not keep any of them for long. She was married when she was 17. Her personality from her earliest years had been inadequate. Deficient in the ability to plan, she acted on impulse and was stubborn. Her intelligence was dull normal, and she could not handle money. Although she liked to be with people she was sensitive, difficult to get along with, often untruthful and deceptive when these devices helped her get what she wanted. Emotionally she had always been unstable and had indulged frequently in temper outbursts. She slighted her home duties and was not a good mother. She had known her first husband for only two weeks, and she married him "just to show the boy I loved." This marriage lasted less than a month, and she said she hated this man bitterly. A period when she had dates with many men followed, and finally she married again. Her first child was conceived before this marriage; in fact before she or her second husband had been granted divorces. By this marriage there were two children, neither had been wanted. The husband and wife quarreled almost continually and separated sporadically.

In the hospital the patient was mainly concerned with the thought that she would "go crazy." The intensity of her symptoms varied; often she showed verbal concern, but without anxiety. Although she apparently realized that something was wrong with her she never had any real insight into her problems. "Everything is due to hard work and not enough good times," she said. In general she was attractive in appearance and seemed outwardly to be normal and cooperative. On the ward she made a fairly good adjustment and improved. Some of the problems in her environment were cleared up, but it was felt that in the patient herself no real change had been made.

B. Psth., Mixed F:20:S:62 +14 463 8912'7– 9:4:23

This patient was sent to the psychiatric ward for study because of her inability to adapt herself to the life in an industrial school to which she had been committed as a delinquent child three years before admission. She had been a behavior problem several years before her commitment. The precipitating incident had been a school fight in which she was alleged to have inflicted physical injury on another pupil. At the detention school she had been unable to get along with the other girls, and when she was placed in work homes she worked poorly and developed numerous somatic complaints for which there was no organic basis. Her lack of response to any of the usual methods of handling girls at the school led to her hospitalization.

An eighth-grade graduate, the girl had had some difficulty in school, not because of lack of ability but because of frequent quarrels with other children. Since her family did not get along well with neighbors they moved frequently, making it necessary for the girl to change from one school to another. She had never been able to adapt herself to new situations. She apparently had been a stubborn, insecure child who was easily offended, and who, when frustrated, became depressed and withdrawn. The family was generally unstable, with a lurid history of various types of misbehavior.

In the hospital the patient complained of pain in her chest and back and said she had been unjustly committed to the industrial school, but she did not take either the physical symptoms or the idea of injustice very seriously. Although she was open and cooperative with examiners, no real contact was made with her. Because of an unusually low basal metabolic rate she was placed on thyroid medication. She adapted well to ward life and was helpful to the nurses, especially in the kitchen, but she was sensitive and easily offended. The physical symptoms disappeared readily on reassurance. In the psychiatric unit there was no real difficulty in handling the girl, and the staff was never able to decide whether it was because she was on her good behavior, or whether there were special problems connected with her residence at the industrial school. No clear diagnosis was reached, but everything indicated that this period was the only one in her life when she had got along satisfactorily with other people.

B. Psth., Mixed F:20:M:16 +2 4673'2189– 3:6:16

The juvenile court found the patient guilty of contributing to the delinquency of a 15-year-old girl, whom she had encouraged to stay away from home overnight without her parents' consent. Unemployed, both girls had made a practice of going to a local army post to meet soldiers, and the patient had taken various soldiers to her mother-in-law's house during the woman's absence. Frequently she had stayed with the soldiers until the early hours of the morning, becoming intoxicated and on numerous occasions having sexual relations with them. On the evening of her offense she had arranged a date with two soldiers for herself and the minor girl, and after several hours of drinking the two couples had gone to a hotel where they had each registered as man and wife. Early the following morning they had all returned to the army post, but the younger girl had refused to go home, and that evening the police had picked them up on the complaint of the minor's mother. Although the patient was not immediately charged with delinquency, it was suggested that she find employment. A complaint was signed the following weekend after she had gone to another state with a soldier instead of following the suggestion.

With the exception of an accident in which the patient and her parents had been trapped in a room full of gas from a leak in the main line, her past history was free of any contributory evidence. Both parents had died as the result of the accident, and the 3-year-old survivor was made a ward of her maternal uncle. She grew up in an atmosphere of delinquency, and at least one member of her family, a woman, had been engaged in "bootlegging and running a house of prostitution." The patient was described as a "flighty, irresponsible, impulsive, and oversexed" person who quarreled with everyone she came in contact with for any length of time. She believed that everything she did was right and that she should not be subject to criticism. Her main objective in life was to have "fun and to do the things I want to do." Described as a stubborn, unreliable, egotistical, and vain individual, she was also an inveterate prevaricator.

In the hospital the neurological examination was negative. The patient was not concerned about her present situation and insisted that it was her own business and that it was completely unimportant. She blamed everything on her previous environment and felt that people were overly critical of her. There was a marked restlessness and press of activity in her behavior, and she said that the hospital was a very dull place because there was nothing to do. In general her thoughts were logical and coherent, and she did not appear to be in the least depressed about what would follow her hospitalization. She devoted much of her time to her personal appearance, but she showed no comparable sustained interest in any other activity, and she had great difficulty in adapting to ward restrictions. She used an excess of cosmetics, and her hair was dyed. In prognosis the possibility of brain damage from the early near asphyxiation was considered, but in any case she was not susceptible to psychotherapeutic treatment, and she was transferred to the court for disposition.

Ps. Sz., Simple M:28:S:12 +4 467'839–(45) 4:8:12
B. Psth., Mixed
Suicidal

The patient was referred by the court because of indecent exposure, suicide threats, inability to seek or hold employment, despondency, and a disconcerting tendency to stare at people or into space. Although the man's behavior had always been somewhat abnormal, there appeared to have been a gradual change over at least four years. In that time he had been arrested several times for exhibitionism and vagrancy. Unkempt in appearance, he was temperamentally irritable, irresponsible, and depressed, often threatening suicide by drowning, cutting his throat, or taking pills. On one occasion he asked a neighbor to dig a grave for him.

As a boy the patient had suffered from osteomyelitis, following a fractured arm, that necessitated partial removal of some of his muscles. On two occasions he had contracted gonorrhea. Otherwise his medical history was noncontributory. At one time he had been suspended from school, possibly because of indecent exposure. He had never held a steady job, but he could give no apparent reason for the frequent job changes. One of the most irrational of these moves he explained by saying he had "felt like coming back home." He had never shown a marked interest in any subject or activity, nor had he ever seriously considered marriage and family life or any other kind of "settling down." He said he assumed indifference in social situations to cover up his shyness. About twice a month he went on "binges," and he claimed to have been promiscuous sexually. Specific evidence about his past life could not be obtained.

On admission to the hospital the patient's most notable characteristic was apathy toward any subject touched upon, with the exception of the loss of $400 in a celebration shortly before admission. The details of that story could not be elicited, but he was concerned about the loss. He felt he was not different from anyone else. His speech was slow, and he made vague references to things he refused to explain. He had an I.Q. of 107. There was no gross deterioration of intellect or sensorium. He did not change during his hospital stay. With the exception of constant apathy, shiftlessness, and mild depression, the symptoms that brought him into the hospital were not apparent. He was cooperative but tended to be flirtatious toward the female members of the staff. The prognosis was unfavorable, and he was returned to the court for disposition.

Ps. Paranoid F:31:M:32 +3 468'21 93- 5:15:13

Four years before admission the patient had given birth to her last child; throughout the pregnancy she had spent much of her time in bed, saying that she had "pus in the kidneys." Following the delivery she had had a swelling in her legs, and since then she had never been well, nor had she ceased to blame her husband for the unwanted child. She sought medical attention almost continually. Her local physician told her she might have a nervous breakdown, and the neighbors said that "her nerves would break." About three years before admission she woke up with an attack in which she could not breathe or speak, and she felt that a snake was coming up her throat. This panic lasted for several days. A diagnosis of chronic cholecystitis was made at one period, and she underwent a cholecystectomy. During the hospitalization for this operation she experienced hallucinations; in one of these she was told that if she did not take care of herself, her husband would outlive her, and that it was necessary for her to go to a hospital and stay there.

After that operation she had received various and extensive medications from numerous clinics. For the past two years she had been increasingly suspicious of her neighbors and of her husband, whom she accused of promiscuity. On one occasion she charged a neighbor of prowling about her house. She believed that the county commissioner and the county attorney were in colusion to prevent the separation from her husband which she had been demanding. Once when she went into her father's home she struck him such a blow on the head with a board that he needed surgical attention. She finally became unable to care for her home and children.

The woman left school in the eighth grade at age 16 and worked as a domestic until she was 17, when she married a man fifteen years older than she. Always moody and complaining, the patient had never been a good mixer and her interests had been narrow, but in general she had been able to take care of her family before the present illness. She had always had the attitude that she had been imposed upon and had been given a "raw deal."

On admission she was pleased to be in the hospital, frequently saying that she felt much better than when she was at home. She looked well, was friendly with the other patients, and took part in the ward routine. Except for a tendency to revert to her physical complaints, she showed no abnormalities of mentation. At times she refused to amplify on her statements. Her appearance was one of apathy and martyrdom. She said she had a feeling of impending disaster, stating, "I don't know what will happen if my husband's nerves break as mine did." Ideas of reference—about mind control, the infidelity of her husband, and plots against her—came out very gradually. Lacking insight, she blamed her condition on her husband, on the authorities, and on her physical disorders, and no amount of argument altered her conviction that she needed an operation. In general she improved, but very slowly. The only abnormal behavior she showed in the hospital occurred during a menstrual period when she stayed in bed most of the time and kept her eyes closed. She talked then of feeling the influence of other people's minds, and she seemed to be in a trancelike state. When she was discharged to the care of her brother, there had been no basic change in her condition.

Ps. Sz., Paranoid	M:36:M:15	0	<u>46</u>8'23–(51)	4:8:18

This man's symptoms, bizarre behavior, paranoid delusions, and hallucinations, had appeared gradually. He had first shown suspicion and jealousy of his wife shortly after their marriage ten years earlier. Openly accusing her of infidelity, he commented in public in a vulgar manner about her activities. Later he demanded frequent sexual relations under inappropriate circumstances. He became suspicious, locked up everything, kept a gun, and was unreasonable in dealing with his customers. Haranguing against members of a religious order, he argued illogically about "freedom of speech and freedom of religion." Gradually his suspicions of his wife diminished but the idea that he was being robbed persisted. In conversations he shouted and gesticulated wildly; there were periods of catatonic behavior. When he became threatening and violent toward his family and unable to work, he was admitted to the hospital on a court order.

At the age of 19 the patient had had a severe case of measles, but there were no psychotic or nervous episodes in his history. In the eighth grade he stopped school. At no time did he have any interests beyond his work and his family. Of average intelligence, he was a hard worker, was thought of as friendly and having a good disposition but easily irritated. The irritability had increased perceptibly each year.

On admission he was outwardly friendly but extremely defensive. His intellect appeared to be clear and he was well oriented. Most of the time he remained by himself, looking sullen and preoccupied, but on the whole he was cooperative. There was circumstantiality in his speech and he frequently talked to himself, although he denied having any hallucinations. There was no real doubt that he experienced paranoid delusions in the hospital but he would not admit these. Under the hospital routine he showed no violent behavior but his attitude did not change. During interviews or when under stress his marked hostility and resentment were evident. The patient was relatively inapproachable and eventually he was committed to a state hospital.

B. Psth., Asocial	F:17:S:39	+7	46'<u>829</u> <u>37</u>–	6:4:22
Mental Deficiency		+14	46'3897–	3:7:21
		?	'9–27	2:3:7

The patient was admitted to the hospital because of lying, extreme carelessness in her personal appearance, stealing, and threats to those in authority over her. About six years earlier a foster mother had made the first complaint about the patient's irresponsibility, lack of initiative, untidiness, and resentment of authority, traits which had made it necessary to place her in seven different foster homes. About a month before admission she had been apprehended in an attempted assault with a kitchen knife on a supervisor who had tried to discipline her when she had returned to the home in an intoxicated condition.

From the age of 3 she had been a ward of a children's aid society. Of dull normal intelligence and unstable, she had had to repeat a number of grades in school and had failed to complete the eighth grade. Although she was very pleasant when she had her own way, she was sullen and resentful when crossed. She was very suggestible and easily influenced. She had had only one close girl friend, but there were a number of boy friends with whom she was very intimate. Her father, reputed to be a drunkard and shiftless, had disappeared early in her life. Her mother had been committed to a state hospital with schizophrenia and complicating feeble-mindedness. Although she had two dull brothers, there were two other brothers and two sisters who were apparently well behaved and average in intelligence.

Although the patient adjusted well to the hospital routine and took part in all activities, she was irresponsible and untidy and showed almost no understanding of her problems or her situation. Since no good contact could be made with her psychotherapeutically, it was recommended that she be sent to a supervised residence school where special training was available.

Ps. Paranoid F:30:M:27 +1 4′683271–9 (84) 6:4:18

Ps. Paranoid F:31:M:8

This woman was brought to the hospital by the police. She had drilled holes in the floor of her apartment "to allow a snake to escape," and she had recently written the president's wife and the F.B.I. to enlist their aid in a search for her father. She also had numerous other delusions not directly related to her arrest.

Her past medical history included gonorrhea at an unknown date. She had also had an unusual number of physical complaints during her last pregnancy, which had been terminated five months before admission. The patient's childhood had been unhappy; her parents were divorced and her mother was said to be "queer." Except in situations where her delusional trends were involved, the patient had got along fairly well. She was apparently of limited intelligence; she did not reach the eighth grade until she was 18 years of age. A friendly person, she mixed well with persons other than her relatives. With them she had frequent outbursts of temper. At such times, delusional episodes often occurred. Her main difficulty with relatives occurred with the patient's mother and stepfather; her own sister, she felt, regarded her as inferior and "rather simple." The patient's husband was in the army and was usually away on foreign duty. Apparently the patient and her husband were compatible. There were two children.

In the hospital the patient was chiefly concerned about her parentage and her family history. She had numerous delusions. Her family wanted to kill her for searching into their past, and one of her relatives had cut her telephone wire, she believed. She had other ideas of this general sort, some of them bizarre. For example, she believed that her mother once blinded her by throwing skin over her eyes. Emotionally she appeared cheerful and alert, but she would cry on little provocation. She had no insight. Much of her time she spent in writing letters requesting help to search for her father, who had actually disappeared in her childhood. In ward contacts she was open, accessible, and cooperative. On the other hand, she was disagreeable about having been admitted on a court order. Soon she began to say that her delusional ideas were possibly untrue "since the doctors say so." However, it was felt that there was little genuine difference in her attitude, and since no real approach could be made to her, she was discharged to the care of her husband.

Six months later the patient was readmitted because she had continued to write letters demanding her "rights as a citizen." Some of these letters she sent to the president of the United States and to others in the government service. In contrast to the first admission, she was sullen, disagreeable, threatening, and irritable. Eventually she was transferred to a state hospital.

B. Psth., Path. Sexuality M:21:S:29 +5 46′83721–(89) 2:6:12
B. Psth., Mixed

The patient was admitted to the hospital on a court order. He was charged with grand larceny for having stolen many things of a peculiarly assorted nature, including a pair of pajamas, a bottle of cologne, several books, a toy frying pan, $25 worth of stamps, and a $5 bill. The patient's father had told the court that he believed his son was suffering from a long-standing mental defect, citing the fact that even as a child the patient had shown a lack of judgment and had had periods of depression and elation. The boy had read lurid, indecent literature and had treasured nude pictures, particularly of men. Five years before admission he had run away from home and had not been heard of for a considerable time. It was later established that during this interval he had engaged in a series of homosexual episodes and had been living with another man.

A very bright boy, the patient had done well in school when he had applied himself, and at an early age he had shown a talent for dancing, music, and drawing. In high school the boy had neglected physics and mathematics, showing a marked preference for such activities as dramatics and music. He had an I.Q. of about 120. As a youngster, he had liked to play with girls and to wear girls' clothing. Later he had impersonated females. He had an early interest in religion, mysticism, and ritual. While in high school he had got into his first serious difficulty with authorities by spending on himself money he had collected for Christmas baskets for the needy. From an early age he had had a tendency to lie and to be deceitful, and although he was extremely vain he had always had a remarkable ability to impress people. Repeatedly he had taken advantage of his charm to get himself out of various scrapes.

In the hospital he said that he believed his chief difficulties centered around his abnormal sexual desires. There was some evidence that he did not steal for material gain, and he could give no explanation for his thefts, claiming that they were done on the impulse of the moment. At the time he had stolen the articles which led to his arrest, he had been depressed because his girl friend had broken their engagement after discovering that he was homosexual. On some occasions he claimed that his only knowledge of having stolen articles was the discovery in his room of the paper in which the items had been wrapped. Critical of society in general, and of most people in particular, he claimed to have always been denied the pleasures that others had, and he felt he would have been better off had he been born a girl. He wondered if he were "completely evil," and if he would ever be able to "drive his evil thoughts out of his mind." He had contemplated suicide. The prospect of being sent to prison disturbed him and he said in that event he would commit suicide. However, he readily turned to the possibility of parole, and he was confident that he would not be given a prison sentence. He had no appreciation of the fact that many of his statements did not fit in with specific information obtained from other sources.

A small person who looked much younger than his age, he dressed neatly, and his mannerisms were effeminate and theatrical. On a masculinity-femininity test he was more feminine in general interests than the average woman. He claimed that his "perverted" acts with men had occurred under the influence of alcohol, and he believed that many of his homosexual friends were angry with him for having rejected their advances. His fear of venereal disease had made heterosexual relations impossible for him. It was felt that he was a danger to society, and he was returned to the custody of the court for its disposition.

F:22:S 4'68379–1 (41) 1:6:13

This college senior came in to discuss the factors which had led to unsuccessful love affairs.

She reported that she had been involved in a series of love affairs, all of which had been unsatisfactory. She was a good-looking brunette, vivacious and fluent and with considerable nervous energy. She was active in dramatics and other social activities.

A very short series of interviews involved an exploration of her attitudes toward herself as a woman and toward sex in general. These attitudes were related to parental influences and an attitude of competition with her sister. The problem was not brought to any very clear-cut resolution, although she did seem to get some symptomatic release. E. S. B.

B. Simple Adult Maladj. M:20:S:62 +1 46872'319–(69) 6:6:14

Three weeks before admission this young man was locked in jail as a result of the complaints of a woman and several girls. In the testimony it was claimed that he followed girls about the streets at night and made remarks in an attempt to gain their attention. It was also said that he "shadowed" a local detective for several months. This action he explained as part of an assignment for a detective's correspondence course. Picked up by the police, he was found in an insanity hearing to be free of psychosis, and he was sent to the psychiatric unit for observation.

In poor general health always, the patient had also suffered specifically from a curvature of the spine. He had had periods of severe emotional instability characterized by morbid anxiety and fear of going insane. Each time, after a few weeks in a rest home, he recovered. The youth's home background was poor. When he was 4 his father died and he was left with a psychotic mother. Shifted from one relative to another, the boy had never had a real home. In school he failed repeatedly, finally stopping in the middle of the ninth grade. He then worked at various odd jobs. Described as industrious, obedient, and economical, he was serious-minded and tried to make the best of his ability. Informants said that he gave the impression of feeling defensive against society, probably because of his deformity, and that he tended to be suspicious and questioning. Although he was definitely interested in girls they always avoided him.

In the hospital the young man's defensive and suspicious attitude was outstanding. This he exhibited toward all questions. Tests revealed an I.Q. of 87. Except for his reaction to personal questions he was cooperative and helpful and showed no significant emotional variations or instability. As time went on he became less suspicious and discussed his problems more freely. No real abnormalities of behavior were observed, and when he was ready for discharge he was placed in contact with the Big Brother movement. Plans were made for him to live in the city and work, and thus to try an entirely new and different environment.

B. Psth., Asocial	F:17:S:54	+20	46'89317-	5:7:11
		+51	6498'7-3	5:12:11

The patient was first brought to the attention of a social agency by a priest, who asked that an investigation of her be made. She had been absent from home for several days, and her parents knew nothing of her whereabouts. The investigation brought out the fact that she had been associating with older men, and at one time she was found in a room with a large number of men at four o'clock in the morning. She was sent to a guardian home after juvenile court action, and during her stay there she escaped at least once, but she was given an excellent record from this placement, and it was recommended that she be returned to her own home under court parole. Her parents gave no assistance in maintaining the parole restrictions, and she again indulged in irregular sexual conduct, frequently breaking parole. She was then referred to the psychiatric unit.

The patient had complained of dyspnea, hematuria, and weakness about a year before admission, but extensive study revealed no general organic difficulty as a basis for the symptoms. Three weeks before admission the patient had suddenly developed blindness, hemiparesis, and memory loss, which had gradually disappeared. There was no history of surgical treatments or traumatic incidents. The patient's schooling had been obtained in a convent school with the exception of one year in a public school, where she had done her best work, but she had left school when she was about 13 because of "nervousness." The patient said that she had not liked school. She had remained at home for a few months and had then obtained a job by misrepresenting her age. Later she and a girl friend ran away because her parents were "too strict" and would not let her dance or stay out late.

Always undependable, she showed no comprehension of social standards or ethics while in the hospital and felt that since a person lived only once he should have as much fun as possible. She had never had any remorse over her acts and had never felt that she had done anything wrong. Her family background was not unacceptable, although the mother was weak and easily dominated by her daughter. If one accepted the patient's story at face value, there seemed to have been no difficulties, but when the patient's stories were compared with those of other informants, much fabrication was revealed. On one occasion she had let it be known that she was going to be married, and a shower had been given for her, but although she had accepted the gifts there was no wedding and actually there had never been any boy friend who was serious about her. When the patient was confronted with the truth about an incident she would admit that she had been falsifying, but she would glibly continue to lie, modifying her story to fit the new situation. She objected strongly to hospitalization and felt that there was no need to give her all the attention she was receiving. When she was finally discharged to the care of her mother it was felt that she was almost certain to get into trouble again.

Ps. Sz., Paranoid F:29:S:54 +2 '469328–(43) 5:4:17

This patient was brought into the hospital on a court hold order issued on the complaint of her family. They contended that the patient, who had insisted on leaving home even though she was unable to look after herself, was nervous, irritable, and impossible to live with. The onset of the pattern was insidious. She had always lived in an unhappy environment. Seven years before admission two operations on her nose had left her so nervous that she had had to give up her job. After a period of severe headaches, when she also had ideas that people were talking about her having a venereal disease, she experienced a "nervous breakdown," for which she was given insulin shock therapy. After her discharge she thought that she had been given the wrong treatment, and that the medicines used on her were coming out of her pores and lining the bathtub with oily stuff every time she bathed. She finally took another job and eventually went overseas with the Red Cross. After a year she became "upset and nervous" and requested permission to return to the United States. She came back on a hospital ship and went to a hospital, where commitment was recommended, but her family refused to take action. Her sister and her mother considered her incapable and unmanageable.

She apparently had had good intelligence but had always been limited in interests. She impressed people as being tense and holding herself in. She was seclusive. She had always felt that she had the ability to do whatever she wanted to do, but that the rest of the family had tried to hold her back because they were jealous of her superior intelligence. Her family background was poor, marked by many arguments between her parents and difficulties with the police. She was deeply ashamed of her illiterate parents and her generally irresponsible family. Three of her brothers had jail records. Her father was described by the patient as cruel, dominating, and cold.

In the hospital the patient was well oriented. She talked freely about the shame she had always felt about her family, and she spoke with deep emotion when she insisted that they had prevented her from finding happiness. She evaded any discussion of her personal affairs, and it was difficult to establish contact with her, but a seclusiveness and inappropriate smiling indicated that there was a possibly extensive mental life that she would not discuss. After electroshock therapy she appeared to have improved considerably, but five days after this temporary improvement, she again became psychotic with complicated delusional systems, and she was transferred to a state hospital.

B. Psth., Asocial F:18:S:8 +1 4′6938–7(59) 6:3:17

This girl had been a problem to her parents over many years and the special concern of a social service agency for the past two years. The chief difficulties were truancy and running away. At one time she had been involved in a sexual episode and as a result she had been made a ward of the state. A year before admission she had left school and thereafter had held innumerable jobs, staying at each for only a few days or weeks. Often she disappeared for a week or more from her boarding home. She had many boy friends and often talked about marriage but it appeared that she was always the eager one and no actual marriage was known to have occurred.

The girl had been strictly raised. Her parents were fairly adequate, although her mother was said to have a violent temper. An attractive, seemingly mature girl, the patient showed poor judgment in almost every field of activity. She made few friends and held none for more than a short time. Although she admitted to sexual relations with at least one boy—with whom she was "in love"—she always took pride in the fact that she did not smoke or drink.

In the hospital the patient disliked the idea that people were "prying" into her affairs. Sure that she was unjustly blamed and that she had made only "one mistake" (the supposedly unique sex experience), she felt that if people would let her alone she would have no more trouble and would conscientiously try to "make a better place for myself in this world." She was cheerful and cooperative, except for her dislike of "prying," which made it difficult for any real progress psychotherapeutically. Her one constant defense was that she knew "what was wrong" with herself and if she was "let alone" all would be well. When she was discharged it was recommended that the next time she got into difficulty she should be put into a restricted environment for a time. If moderate limitations did not work it was recommended that more severe ones be imposed.

B. Psth., Path. Emot. M:33:M:16 +1 46'98–13(43) 7:4:13
Alcoholism

The patient was referred to the hospital by the court for a pre-sentencing investigation on the charge of child abandonment. A chronic alcoholic who had promised to reform at the time of his marriage, he had got drunk on his marriage night and had not gone with his wife on their honeymoon trip. In spite of this, the first years of the marriage were fairly happy, but his drinking gradually increased. When drunk he was abusive, aggressive, and irritable. His wife tried to separate from him four times, but each time she took him back because he promised to reform. When she finally decided to get a divorce he became violent, threatening to kill himself and his family. Shortly afterward he entered the home and attempted suicide after smashing up the place. He was arrested by the police and told to leave town, but he came back and assaulted his wife with a pipe. He had since been in jail.

The past history contained no obviously contributory factors. His childhood home life had been chaotic. He had been agreeable and likable when not under the influence of alcohol, but as time went on he had begun to have some of the alcoholic symptoms even when he was not drinking. A tendency to brag gradually came to be more and more characteristic of him. He had average intelligence.

In the hospital his thoughts centered around the injustice that the world had done him. He blamed his wife and his wife's relatives for his trouble, and he was full of requests and hopes for reconciliation with his wife and his children, but when he realized that the doctors were not going to help him achieve this desire he became depressed and sarcastic, although he had previously been pleasant and cooperative. His orientation and intellect were excellent, and there was no obvious evidence of deterioration. He was discharged to the custody of the court for sentence.

B. Psth., Mixed F:32:M:34 +1 4698'713–(55) 4:6:22
Paranoid
Alcoholism

This woman was admitted to the hospital because of alcoholism, extreme nervousness, neglect of her children, and paranoid delusions. Ten years earlier she had married against the wishes of the husband's parents. Discord resulted in separations, but the couple had repeatedly gone back together, until the husband was drafted into the army. He then sought the company of other women, and the patient so neglected the children that they were eventually placed in a boarding home by a court order. Some time later the children had been returned to the mother, but shortly before admission she went on a drinking spree and an investigation showed the children to be dirty and neglected and the home in disorder.

Her past health had been good, and there had been no previous mental or emotional disturbances. After her high school graduation she worked as a typist and clerk until her marriage. A popular girl, she had dated many men during her working days.

In the hospital she was unworried. She expressed feelings of persecution by her mother-in-law, but the ideas were not altogether unreasonable. She voiced suspicions of her friends and believed that someone had shot a gun at her. All she needed was a rest and a change of scenery, she felt sure. Aloof and suspicious at first, after a few days she became much more calm and friendly. With the staff, however, she remained impatient, and at times insisted they were wasting her time and theirs. Eager for a discharge, she cooperated, on the whole, fairly well. There were periods every few days when she apparently became depressed and withdrawn. These periods lasted about four hours. During the last two weeks of hospitalization she became scornful of the doctors and told other patients, "I can leave whenever I wish." There was little actual change and the prognosis was felt to be poor.

B. Psth., Asocial Mutilative — M:25:D — 47′2<u>39</u>–(55) 1:7:11

This prisoner mutilated himself by severing his left Achilles' tendon with a dirk knife. In addition three benzedrine inhalers were found in his possession, and he was involved in homosexual practices with other prison inmates.

Orphaned when very young, the boy made his home first with an aunt and then with a sister. At the latter home very little discipline was exercised over him. An older brother served a term in prison. At an early age the lad began to associate with a mischievous group of boys engaged in petty thefts. At the age of 13 he was first incarcerated, and he has spent practically all the remaining years of his life behind jail or prison bars. He claims to have completed the seventh grade in a state school for juvenile offenders and on a test given at prison he earned a grade placement of 6.6. The youth's first marriage lasted two months and he lived for seven months with another woman in a common-law relationship. His longest period of steady employment was six weeks as a truck driver; most of the time when out of prison he was "on the move."

The prisoner's arrest and commitment record shows thirteen sentences for burglary, theft, vagrancy, car theft, Dyer Act violation, violation of the national motor vehicle theft act, criminal assault, and being AWOL from the army. In a federal prison he participated in a race riot involving eleven whites and fifteen Negroes, and again at a medical center for federal prisoners he participated in a riot that involved his whole cell block.

The young man is a typically unstable and impetuous psychopath. There is no evidence for a neurological disorder or for psychosis. He is definitely belligerent, an agitator and a troublemaker. Easily discouraged in any undertaking, he shows no tenacity of purpose or desire to make good while in prison. Neither does he see any reason to try to get out of prison, for there are several detainers from various states awaiting his release. R. C. K.

Alcoholism Deteriorated	M:36:S:50	+1	4'72693–1 (67)	2:6:9
Alcoholism B. Psth., Path. Emot. Deteriorated	M:36:S:36	+1	4'2798–1 (65)	2:4:13

This man had first begun to drink heavily seventeen years before admission when he had lost a girl with whom he had been going for two years. The girl, a somewhat aggressive person, had forced him to have sexual relations with her twice a week. Her reason for breaking with him was that she felt he would never amount to anything. After the break he had wanted "to stay drunk for a year" and "to drink myself to death." Under family pressure he joined Alcoholics Anonymous but was not helped by them. He entered many different hospitals and rest homes to recover from the toxic effects of alcohol. He was admitted to the psychiatric unit from a general hospital, having been sent there after an unusually severe bout of drinking. Chronic otitis media, which had been present since high school days, had caused him to become partially deaf. In addition, he was very sensitive to the condition because of the odor.

In high school, which he had finished at age 18, he had had difficulties because of the deafness. His tested I.Q. was 115. After leaving school he worked at various jobs but held none for long. He had remained in the army only ninety days because of the chronic otitis media. People thought of him as being somewhat nervous and anxious, and he was said to be conscientious in many ways.

When admitted to the hospital he expressed concern about his illness and said that he really wanted to stop drinking. Friendly and cheerful, he talked freely but appeared to be nervous and tense. The psychometric examination revealed borderline evidence of brain damage. During his stay he lost some of the toxic symptoms and efforts were made to build up his self-confidence. Then, since he became eager to get out and "prove himself," he was allowed to go downtown several times. At the time of discharge he had obtained a job as a filling station attendant. Shortly after he left the hospital, he again began to drink and was fired from the job. Admitted to a veterans' hospital with delirium tremens, he stayed there for a while; after his discharge, he had another drinking spell, again he lost a job, and was readmitted to the psychiatric unit. Each hospitalization had almost the same pattern as the previous ones, and each time he left protesting that he would "remain dry."

B. Psth., Asocial	F:25:S:23	+3	472836'91–(45)	3:9:16
P. Psychas.		+25	2'9683–(49)	3:5:24
P. React. Depr.				

This girl came to the clinic because, she said, "I am thoroughly sick of myself as I am. I don't like myself. I am egotistical, self-centered. I can't make friends, or if I do, they can't stand me for long. I blow up. I call people down. Frankly, I don't care for myself one little bit." She had been feeling out of place in the college program and had projected the blame onto others, but a sequence of events had forced her to the realization that the source of the trouble lay within herself. She was considerably concerned also because she had been somewhat promiscuous sexually; she could not understand her actions in view of her accompanying guilt feelings.

The problem went back to the girl's early childhood. Her mother died when she was in the second grade and she went to live with an aunt. The economic level of this family was much higher than she had been accustomed to. She felt completely out of place. This was further enhanced by the attitude of her aunt's family, who repeatedly reinforced the idea that they were doing the client a distinct favor by keeping her. In all probability, the rejection of the girl by this family was stimulated by the presence of their own child. This child was about the same age as the client, but evidently of dull mentality. Inasmuch as the client was brilliant (I.Q. 150), there were unfortunate comparisons. The result of the rejection was apparently aggressive activity on the part of the client, particularly in the scholastic situation, which isolated her socially from her schoolmates. At this time she began to get some emotional outlet through stealing. Whenever she was under marked pressure she would go into one of the local stores and purloin something; then she would have a feeling of release. As she grew older the stealing activity disappeared, and her underlying tensions were released through sexual activity. She got through high school without ever having had the feeling of being wanted by any social group. She expressed this by saying she had felt like a "Pariah."

After high school she drifted from one job to another, never staying long in any one place. She would become disinterested, then careless; the carelessness would bring a reprimand, which in turn would provoke an outburst of anger, and then she would be dismissed. She finally joined the WAC, where she made a fairly adequate showing, but she found that willingness to participate in sexual affairs made her more desirable in the social situation. After the WAC came college, where her record was "spotty." She was frequently up before the student court for violation of the university code. Following graduation she took advanced work, and it was during this period that she began to realize the bulk of her problem lay within herself.

In therapy she was a most cooperative person: she was always prompt, always eager, always forcing herself to make insights. Sometimes she went at too rapid a rate, which upset her. She seemed to hold no animosity for the people who had rejected her during her childhood, considering this to be simply the ironic humor of fate. During this time she was also supporting her father, who was now an invalid. She performed this duty in an exemplary manner. She made a considerable reduction of her sexual activities but she never desisted entirely. As she put it, "I am a healthy animal. My body and I get into lots of arguments and sometimes I don't win." At the end of counseling the second MMPI was administered. It was felt that there was a possibility of a truly psychopathic element in this woman. This was talked over with her, and the suggestion was made that since the emotional pressure had disappeared she should make a definite effort to change her life.

The client was not seen for a year. Then she came back to the clinic under pressure and was seen for approximately fifteen hours of therapy. By this time she had almost entirely revamped her philosophy of life, and although a third MMPI was not taken, it was felt that the psychopathic element had been almost completely eliminated. Since that time she has undertaken further graduate study and, at the last report, was doing excellent work. A. S.

B. Pri., Child. M:14:S:44 +4 '47398–2(55) 4:0:23

The patient was admitted because of behavior problems including inattention to studies, truancy, pilfering, using his father's charge accounts, and general incorrigibility. The onset of this behavior had been gradual, but even at age 9 the patient was having difficulty in school, and two years before admission it was noted that he had no sense of responsibility in the management of funds or the handling of customers on a paper route. He was currently failing in two subjects, for which he blamed the teachers.

His past physical health had been good. He had attended six different schools in nine grades, but he had done fairly well until five years before admission. He had had no sustained interest at any time in any particular line of activity, although he showed sporadic interest in dancing, music, and art. His father felt that there was a failure of the deeper emotional responses, and that the boy had no conscience. He was described as selfish, irresponsible, and unable to appraise his own conduct. He loved attention and openly sought the limelight. Although he was easy to get along with, he was unresponsive to punitive measures.

In the hospital the patient was effeminate in mannerisms and speech, and he maintained a superior, sophisticated attitude. There were no gross disturbances of sensorium or intellect. He discussed his difficulties in a matter-of-fact, offhand way, readily blaming others for every irregularity. Although he was cooperative, he was highly defensive, and his manner of handling problems was to discuss volubly insignificant matters, or to assume a distant, abstracted look. He was superior in intellectual ability, he mixed well with the other patients, particularly the women, and he was happy when he was the center of attention. In interviews he was persistently resistant and demonstrated almost no ability to work with anyone. He changed very little while in the hospital, and it was not felt that he had made any real progress in insight. He was discharged as representing a problem in management rather than in therapy, but even with good management the prognosis seemed poor.

P. Hys. F:31:M:13 +4 47 6'2381–(47) 4:3:12
Suicidal

The patient said that her present illness had been precipitated nine days before admission when she and her husband attended a dance, where he became drunk and abusive. On their return home he struck the patient several times. The following morning she cried bitterly and then collapsed into a week-long spell during which she ate little, smoked many cigarettes, complained of severe headaches, and made several suicidal threats. When admitted to the hospital she immediately recovered her orientation and memory but said she had no recollection of the events since the day following the dance. She said that she had not had a happy moment since her marriage seven months before. Her husband had been excessively jealous, abusive, and frequently drunk. She got no satisfaction in sexual intercourse and had grown to dislike him in every respect.

Although the patient had had an unusual number of medical problems previously, none seemed especially pertinent to her present difficulty. Her schooling ended with the eighth grade. She had got along fairly well with people and had actively engaged in sports as a child. Ambitious to be a good housewife, she had apparently not expected much more of herself. She had had a happy childhood and had first been married to a man with whom she was very happy for seven years until she discovered that he was unfaithful to her. He admitted the infidelity and consented to a divorce, after which she married her present husband.

In the hospital she was a poorly developed, malnourished woman with a marked pallor. Otherwise, the physical and neurological examinations were relatively noncontributory. She seemed to be composed and well oriented. She was intact in sensorium and intellect except for the amnesia for the week preceding her admission. She described her husband as a "raving maniac" when drunk and said she wanted nothing more to do with him. Her chief concern was to get herself and her adopted daughter away from him. She recovered her memory for the lost week almost immediately after her admission and even before her husband had left the hospital. She rapidly adjusted and remained entirely normal, as far as one could see, during her whole stay in the hospital except for being considerably upset when her husband visited her. After she had made some fairly adequate plans for her behavior upon discharge, she left to go to live with her sister. She expected to obtain a divorce and to seek a third husband, with whom she hoped to have a better life. There was considerable doubt that all the facts in the patient's background had been brought out.

P. Anxiety State M:24:S 476′82193–(65) 5:3:13

The complaints of this youth, a university student, were never clearly delineated. He spoke vaguely of "nervous tension" and feelings of inadequacy which had been present for a long while but had in recent weeks become increasingly serious and disabling.

There was little in this young man's background that seemed pertinent to his difficulties. Born and raised on an isolated farm, he had few contacts with other children or adults during his early home life. His father, a rigid, demanding person, was the dominant figure in the boy's life. After high school graduation he entered college to prepare himself for teaching and later took a job in a small town school. Because of his feelings of inadequacy, he left this position after some months and returned to the university for further education.

In interviews with the therapist the youth appeared to be somewhat tense. He spoke with a loud voice but verbalized his difficulties well. One of his chief concerns was masturbation. Help for the youth consisted of group treatments over a period of two months. The sessions, not more than five in all, apparently brought relief, and the student discontinued treatment because he decided he felt "well enough to go on my own." C. K. A.

B. Simple Adult Maladj. F:18:S:33 +1 47682'93– 9:7:16

B. Simple Adult Maladj. F:18:S:12

The exceedingly irregular behavior of this woman in the small town in which she lived resulted in a court recommendation for hospital admission. Although it was difficult to identify the particular aberrations objected to, the patient was apparently very much disliked in the town, and she suffered from feelings of inferiority, in part because of the fact that she was illegitimate and of American Indian parentage. Unduly preoccupied with sex, the patient at one time had written a letter to the superintendent of schools claiming that a 72-year-old man had made repeated sexual attacks on her, and she had also claimed that she had fended off with a knife an uncle who had made an attack on her. She also told conflicting stories about an abortion which she claimed to have induced through the use of a knitting needle, but there was no good evidence to substantiate her stories.

The patient, who had an I.Q. of 89, had followed a very irregular course in school. She had always been set apart from the other school children because of her poor socio-economic connections and her Indian parentage. Apparently the patient had encouraged considerable adverse attention by dramatizations of herself, and she had begun to confuse her make-believe world and reality. She was slovenly, bathed infrequently, and objected strenuously when she did have to take a bath. She said in the hospital that she had never before been in a "real" bathtub, and this was entirely possible since her background was that of a marginal farming culture. In high school she had at times become so upset about her grades that she could not perform up to the level of her abilities. A grade school teacher described her as a "great liar and a good cheater," and she was so disliked by other pupils that she was always the last chosen for games or other group activities. She cried easily and without provocation, and from an early time she had had such an abnormal interest in the boys in her classes that she watched their every movement.

In the hospital she was apparently completely concerned with herself and her own problems. Well oriented, she showed no abnormalities of mental aptitude other than her defective intellect, but she was emotionally unstable, crying when she talked about her previous experiences, but laughing almost immediately with a change of subject. There was no evidence of insight. While she was in the hospital she made an effort to improve her appearance and personal habits, and with some attention to herself she became a not unattractive person. Her adjustment was very satisfactory, and she was discharged for a trial placement in a boarding home, where she remained for about three months and was then readmitted to the hospital on her own request. It was not established what the exact difficulties in the boarding home were, but she said, "If I don't get my own way, it's going to be too bad." She showed little appreciation for the help that had been given her, and apparently she had very little tolerance for any kind of frustration. She was discharged again to enter a working home.

M:26:S '478–13 (69) 0:5:14

A veteran majoring in police science, this college senior came on a referral from his psychology instructor. The client reported that his main concern was his apparent lack of emotional control. He cited as an example the fact that he seemed to cry very easily in certain kinds of social situations and that this might be a handicap in his field.

In most ways he seemed to be making an adequate adjustment. He was a very successful student and was apparently highly rated by his department. He seemed to be able to get along reasonably well with most people, although he was inclined to get into fights.

In several interviews he was able to relate his difficulties to his lack of security in some of his early relationships. He had been adopted by one family and his real sister by another. He had suffered several other blows during that period, which apparently resulted in an unwillingness to commit himself emotionally. With this as a starter he was able to relate this attitude to many of his present difficulties and found that he was able to exercise better control over his emotions as he became less afraid of them. E. S. B.

B. Pri., Child. F:13:S:35 +4 4'789–6 (59) 5:6:22

The patient, a ward of the state, was placed in her present foster home at the age of 5 months, and from the very first the child had been difficult to manage, a problem in feeding and in disposition. She was the illegitimate child of a feeble-minded mother, now in a school for the feeble-minded. The father was unknown. As she grew older, the behavior problems increased in severity, but she was seldom punished. When she was punished it had no effect on her behavior. In the past year, besides being disagreeable and disobedient, she had become assaultive and at times violent. She often abused the younger children in the family and willfully destroyed house fixtures. In explanation she said she was getting even with her parents for mistreating her. Reports from the social agency indicated that the foster parents treated her very well and had continued to keep her because they were sorry for her.

Her past physical health had been good, and there had been no obvious nervous breakdown. The patient was of average intelligence, but in the last year her schoolwork had been barely passing. She was always shy and ill at ease with strangers, but she got along well with her friends. A seclusive child, she refused to discuss anything with her parents and rejected their love and affection.

In the hospital the physical and neurological examinations were negative. Her mental content and behavior were normal. There was no queer or bizarre content or action, but she had no insight and did not recognize that she herself was the source of any of her problems. She was neat, and normal in mood, but she was indifferent throughout the interviews. In her hospital stay there was no problem in her behavior with the staff or other patients. Projective test evidences indicated a deep-seated anxiety and a few schizoid signs. She did not form any very useful rapport with staff members, and psychotherapy was felt, at best, to be a long-time proposition. It was advised that she be sent to a fairly strict boarding school. If that failed it was recommended that she be transferred to a residence reform school.

Alcoholism   M:27:M:19   +3   '479238-6(43)   0:2:23

The patient was admitted to the hospital because of alcoholic intoxication and delirium tremens. The specific period of intoxication leading to the admission had begun about a week before admission.

His past physical health had been reasonably good. About sixteen years before admission he had contracted gonorrhea and syphilis, for which he had apparently been treated adequately. He had been hospitalized for a previous episode of alcoholic neuritis. For about six months before admission he had complained of dizziness and difficulty with his vision.

He was an eleventh-grade graduate and had some additional business training. Between periods of drinking he was able to work and hold good jobs, but as his drinking increased in intensity his work level decreased. He was a genial person who considered himself a chronic worrier. When motivated he would show great energy output, especially in making financial plans. He was thought to have been sexually promiscuous before his marriage. His wife had tolerated his activities for many years but was threatening divorce at the time of the present admission. Apparently she had been devoted to him and the marriage was a good one except for the problem of alcoholism.

In the hospital the neurological examination showed a few signs of neuritis, but there were no definite evidences in either the neurological or psychological examinations indicating deterioration. He was depressed and worried that his wife would leave him and that he might not be able to get a job. He was obviously ashamed of his condition but had an almost complete lack of insight into his real difficulties and their severity. After a few days of depression and restlessness he began to enjoy the world and he seemed entirely normal. He was allowed to leave the hospital for trial periods and finally was discharged to go home, but the prognosis was considered bad as far as his drinking was concerned.

B. Pri., Child. M:14:S:25 +4 4'79 286–1 (51) 4:9:11

The patient had been stealing for five years. At the age of 9 he had begun by stealing from his mother, who had punished him by spanking him and restricting him to his room. Two years before admission he forged two checks, which he claimed were to cover shortages on his paper route, and he was put on probation. He took all this calmly and two months before admission was again brought before the juvenile court on a long series of charges including the stealing of various objects and window peeping.

His past physical health had been good except for measles at age 8, when he had a fever and was delirious. He had completed the ninth grade and was to go back into the tenth. His grades were mostly average and he was well liked by his teachers and classmates. He had worked at various jobs and had apparently been a reliable and normal boy until age 9. Because his father had died when he was 5 and his mother had had to get along on a very small relief stipend, the patient had bought much of his own clothing and had given his mother money. He was reserved but not shy or sensitive.

In the hospital he was not particularly worried about the situation he was faced with. There were no abnormalities of mentation or intellect. He was consciously at his ease and said he knew it was wrong to steal but could not help it. He said he did not plan to steal but just did it when the chance appeared. He was cooperative and polite. Most of his time was spent playing games with other patients. He read a good deal and caused no trouble. Although no psychotherapeutic measures seemed to have much effect on him, the staff felt there was a good chance that he would make a satisfactory adjustment if he could be placed in a home where he would be adequately supervised.

Ps. Sz., Paranoid M:25:S '479 38–(63) 4:3:17

This patient was hospitalized for "combat exhaustion" while in the navy. He was separated on points but made a poor adjustment to civil life and began to drink heavily. He enlisted in the army and shortly thereafter became psychotic. He was admitted to this hospital, on transfer from an army hospital, in a grossly psychotic state.

His behavior was apparently normal before his first enlistment in the navy at age 20, although he had been somewhat concerned about masturbation and homosexual ideas during his adolescence.

At the time of the examination he was making some spontaneous recovery after having had active hallucinations and paranoid delusions with considerable confusion and retrospective falsification. The patient was given insulin shock therapy, followed by intensive psychotherapy, over a period of five months. In individual psychotherapy it was brought out that during his early adolescence he had been approached by a hired man who was a homosexual and who talked a great deal about the F.B.I. Apparently, this was the basis for his delusions linking the F.B.I. with a ring of homosexuals. The patient's psychosis was precipitated by a homosexual experience. In psychotherapy he was considerably blocked, but after an amytal interview he was able to verbalize more freely. He gained considerable insight and showed that he was able to handle his conflicts satisfactorily. He was discharged from the hospital upon completion of the psychotherapy. A few weeks after discharge, apparently seeking reassurance, he returned voluntarily for a visit with the therapist and, at this time, gave the impression of making an adequate adjustment. The prognosis appeared to be fairly good. W. M. H.

B. Psth., Mixed M:21:M:26 +7 4'8–263(32) 2:6:10

This young man's complaints at admission were depression, listlessness, irritability, and a feeling that "everything was a mess" in his family life. Various physical symptoms had appeared five months before, coincident with the birth of his first child, when he had had marital difficulties and had felt he was no longer first in his wife's affection.

A relatively normal, healthy child until the age of 7, the patient at that time had scarlet fever, followed by a rheumatic heart disease. He was in bed for a year and was never again very robust. Kept at the side of a controlling mother, he was considered a "mama's boy" and the "booby" of the family. At the age of 14 he began to be a behavior problem, becoming involved in the activities of a local gang of boys, who stole and damaged property on one occasion. The patient left school after the eleventh grade against his parents' wishes and married at the age of 18, also against his mother's wishes. She felt that his wife was "low class and unrefined." Employed by his father as a laborer, the patient did not work steadily after his marriage and contracted a number of debts. He felt guilty because he had been seeing another woman during his wife's pregnancy, and also because he had frequently compelled his wife to perform perverted sex acts against her will. She threatened suicide because of his infidelity and he in turn threatened suicide if she left him. The situation was aggravated by the birth of their first child.

At the time of admission the patient seemed apathetic and had a slow, vague, uncomprehending manner. On the ward he was withdrawn and seclusive. He spoke of not being able to live without his wife's love, and of being extremely remorseful about his affair with the other woman. As far as could be determined he had merely followed the latter about and had never had intercourse with her. His dull, flat manner gave the impression of immaturity and borderline intelligence. A test showed he had an I.Q. of 100 with special difficulties in abstract thinking. After a week in the hospital he felt much better, was less worried, and was more friendly on the ward. His wife announced her decision to divorce him and he took this well and made plans to return home to his parents. On leaving the hospital with his mother he seemed fairly cheerful. This adjustment was apparently better suited to his limited ability to cope with problems than was marriage. E. B.

B. Psth., Asocial F:38:M:126 +6 4'8–69 5:2:21
Schizoid
Paranoid

This patient had been found guilty of bigamy. The complicated background for the bigamist offense was difficult to trace, partly because the patient had changed her name several times. About fifteen years before admission she had deserted a husband and two children in another state and had gone to visit a cousin. She told the cousin that she had divorced her first husband. She married again, and this time when she left home she did obtain a divorce. It was reported that she had tried to shoot her second husband. During her third marriage, the husband found that she was pregnant by another man. Because of her infidelities and alcoholism, he divorced her. It was at this time that she began to talk about her connections with important people and about her imaginary accomplishments. She lived with her fourth husband for several years and had one child by him, but frequent domestic quarrels resulted in a separation. Her story at that time was that she was "connected with G-men in Chicago." Without bothering with the formality of a divorce from her fourth husband, she changed her name and married still another man. The bigamy charge followed this marriage, and her stories were so bizarre that the court referred her for psychiatric evaluation.

No detailed past history was available for this patient and little information about her early personality pattern could be discovered, but it was established that various members of her immediate family had been detained in mental and penal institutions.

The patient was quiet and amenable to hospital rules, showed no oddities of activity, and engaged in games and activities with other patients without apparent abnormalities. A neat, attractive person, she usually wore a flower in her hair. There were no obvious mood changes, although she became momentarily irritable if addressed by her real name, and on one occasion when an attendant called her by her real name, she angrily replied, "Don't call me that name or I'll put a bullet through you when I get out of here." On a few occasions she was observed crying alone in her room. Her explanation was that she could not understand it all, that "things seem so fantastic, like something that has really happened but has not happened." Her I.Q. was 87. She steadily claimed that the bigamy charge was a frame-up, aimed at defrauding her and at obtaining possession of a million-dollar inheritance that would otherwise come to her. Along these lines she was obviously abnormal, and she also had complicated delusions about being a "G-girl," but she defended herself against any accusations of inaccuracy. The staff felt that the patient had no moral concept of right and wrong, and it was unlikely that her mental state would improve to any significant degree or that she would ever become a socially integrated person.

Ps. Paranoid F:51:M:28 +7 '48–7 (47) 9:2:22
Ps. Invol. Melan.

The patient's illness had had an insidious onset over the preceding seven or eight months. Her husband said that the first aberrancy he noted was a marked increase in her sexual drive. According to the patient, the symptoms became acute about three weeks before admission. In spite of her husband's denials she had come to feel that he was carrying on with a younger woman, and to support her accusation she had drawn more and more evidence from incidents about her. She said she had begun to "understand" little things that had "happened years before."

Fourteen years before admission she had had a similar episode but less severe. With the exception of a gall bladder operation, her general health had been good. Menstruation had ceased about five years before admission after deep X-ray therapy for dysmenorrhea and menorrhagia.

An eleventh-grade graduate, she had done well in school. She had taken considerable interest in a social group connected with her church and had recently been elected its president. Cheerful and easygoing, she had been especially good in working with children. She had been affectionate toward her own children, especially her sons, but even before her present illness she had been indifferent to sexual relationships. There were six children. In the household she had been the "boss," handling the money and the business affairs. She had a rigid sense of duty, with strong convictions about right and wrong.

On admission to the hospital she was well oriented and apparently intact intellectually, with no obvious deviant behavior. She was preoccupied with her husband's assumed activities, about which she cried easily and repeatedly. She interpreted past events in the light of newer "discoveries," until she built up a very intricate system. Her logic was good, but her basic assumptions obviously false. The diagnostic summary described her as a sensitive, rigid, and somewhat ambitious person whose paranoid ideas were extremely well organized and limited to a single subject. She frequently said that she did not need treatment, and that she could not see what the doctors could do for her. Even after four electroshock treatments her ideas remained fixed, but she was somewhat more comfortable.

B. Psth., Path. Sexuality M:16:S:47 +1 '48 12–(49) 5:7:22
Ps. Sz., Mixed

The patient's abnormal sexual behavior began about a month before admission when he exposed his genitalia to a teen-age girl. He made no further advances on that occasion and soon ran away, but during the following month similar incidents occurred three times. In each instance his advances were directed toward young women or girls, but his attempts at sexual relations were readily thwarted. When questioned by the police he admitted the incidents readily but maintained that he had not known what he was doing until completion of the action. He felt his difficulties might have begun during the summer when he was employed as a gasoline station attendant in a tourist camp. He spoke of disorderly, lewd conduct among the guests which disgusted him, and his disgust was complicated by a fear of his employer, a "fat, lazy man," who often struck him and who was a central figure in the frequent orgies.

Of average intelligence, the patient was in the second year of high school at the time of admission. He got along well in school and was interested in his studies. A somewhat introverted boy and given to excessive daydreaming, he had never made many friends of his own age, and his only achievements were in the Boy Scout movement where he was a junior leader. On several occasions he had been in juvenile court for petty larceny, but each time he had been paroled after promising to reform. His hobby was cooking. His family life had been chaotic, and an older sister had been a problem child for a while.

On admission he showed no obvious disturbance of mentation or sensorium. He did not think there was any reason for his being in the hospital. Normal in behavior and cooperative in attitude, he made a good ward adjustment, and there was no evidence of abnormal sexual behavior. It was difficult to establish rapport with him, however, and he did not talk freely at any time. No real insight was obtained into his problem. It was felt that he might be a sexual psychopath and might later develop a clear schizoid break. This diagnosis was, however, unsatisfactory. He was discharged to be placed in a foster home where there would be careful supervision.

Ps. Sz., Paranoid M:53:D '48 13 2679–X (69) 10:2:26

This man, a house-to-house salesman, was forcibly brought to the hospital after he was picked up for writing obscene letters to girls. The patient insisted that he was not ill, and he believed he was the second Messiah and that God talked directly to him. He also said that he must find a wife and have children. He had a long history of paranoid and withdrawing behavior and of vocational instability, and he had been hospitalized twice before.

Little was known about this patient's early home life except that his parents were oversolicitous. There was evidence that from a very early age the patient was troubled by inferiority feelings and religious preoccupation. His intelligence was estimated as average. After high school he had spent two years in an agricultural college. His marriage, to a woman who was known to be "peculiar," had been arranged by his parents and had ended in divorce. He had apparently had few friends and even fewer heterosexual contacts. His family relationships, however, seemed to be very strong.

This patient was put on an acute ward and specific treatment has not yet been planned. Despite his spontaneous recovery from previous psychotic episodes, the prognosis was not considered to be favorable. W. M. H.

B. Psth., Mixed F:15:S:27 +7 48<u>13</u>9'672–(55) 7:9:16

Since the age of 12 this girl had shown a progressive tendency to disregard authority. About a year and a half before admission she began to rebel against her parents' attempts to prevent her from associating with undesirable persons and from keeping late hours. She circumvented all restrictions and became overtly delinquent. On three occasions she ran away and stayed in hotels and trailers with girl and boy friends; she was consistently unreliable and untruthful. She was also known to have stolen from stores and from friends. Placed in a foster home, she remained there five weeks but could not adjust. Social agency workers found her to be resistant and difficult. In a children's center in another city the aberrant behavior continued and on at least one occasion, she had sexual intercourse with an adolescent boy. Finally she was admitted to the psychiatric unit for general observation and recommendations.

Two years earlier she had had "rheumatism" and at the age of 14 she had slept for four days and nights as a result of what was called "sun stroke." Otherwise, her early history was not particularly contributory. It was said that she "picked on other children" but "was not rebellious when disciplined." Until the fourth grade she did well in school but then her work changed. At the time of the hospital admission she was in the tenth grade. She blamed her troubles on her parents' refusal to allow her to have dates, which forced her to meet boys surreptitiously. Her interests were largely centered on "boys, romantic movies, parties, and things like that." Her six brothers and sisters, while they all left home at early ages, appeared to have been essentially normal in behavior. They had, however, resented the patient.

In the hospital the girl, a short, chubby adolescent, did not appear ill. There were no neurological abnormalities except that the Wassermann test was consistently positive, although the spinal fluid was negative. The patient was primarily concerned with utilizing her situation so as to obtain the most immediate pleasure for herself. She talked at length about her boy friends, movies, clothes, and how she had "gotten around" the restrictions of her parents. She expressed the idea that she had been admitted only to discover if she was pregnant, and she could think of no other reason why she was in the hospital. Unstable in mood, she was by turns happy and irritable, enthusiastic and sullen, depending on the amount of restriction imposed. Although always coherent and well oriented, she was evasive and often obviously untruthful. It was necessary to place her in a disturbed unit for a time because of her behavior with other patients, and while there she sulked and made no attempt to earn increased privileges. With male personnel she was alternately flirtatious, rebellious, and vulgar. She attempted to curry favor with anyone who interviewed her. A series of treatments for the syphilitic infection was given, but other approaches were on the whole unsuccessful. She was discharged to be transferred to a correctional school.

B. Psth., Path. Emot.	F:19:M:15	+7	4'817326-9 (59)	4:12:16
P. Hys.		—13	41'78 23-6	5:10:20

The onset of the patient's present illness had followed her marriage about two years before admission. She had fainting spells that lasted several minutes, and when she recovered consciousness, she attacked her husband or inanimate objects about her. During one of these spells, she was extremely destructive of clothes and furniture; sometimes she scratched herself. The attack would halt abruptly, and from five to fifteen minutes later the patient would appear normal though confused and sleepy. She claimed to have no memory of what happened during these periods. At first the spells occurred only during her menstrual periods, and after a bilateral salpingectomy she was free of them for a while. However, she then began to suffer from visual hallucinations that took the form of a woman in white robes holding a baby in her extended arms. The patient also saw "rings" of babies floating in the room. The hallucinations, which she realized were fantasy, continued until the time of admission.

The patient had undergone a bilateral salpingectomy, a left oophorectomy, and a subtotal resection of the right ovary, as a result of dysmenorrhea and menorrhagia. The salpingectomy, the patient said, had been performed without her knowledge.

She was a ninth-grade graduate at age 15 but then left school because of poor health and because her youngest sister had caught up with her. She had never been a good student and had stayed in school only because of pressure from her parents. She had been regarded even by her family as a problem child. She had never worked, except for a single month, and had always been lacking in responsibility and good judgment. She was unsuccessful in the management of her home. Determined and stubborn, she was friendly only as long as people adjusted themselves to her. Hysterical tendencies, which she used as an attention-getting device, had always been apparent. She had displayed a precocious sex interest at age 6 and some later delinquency, but since her marriage, she maintained, she had found no pleasure in sexual intercourse. She admitted having had premarital sexual intercourse with two men.

In the hospital she was egocentric and mildly hypochondriacal. Her primary interest was herself. There were no gross disturbances of sensorium or intellect. She was childlike, usually cheerful and happy, but this state could be upset by minor annoyances or disappointments. Her moods never lasted long. Although she was sloppy and messy in appearance, she was a reasonably good patient. Psychotherapeutically she gained a small degree of insight into her problems, but there was little on which a really effective psychotherapeutic approach could be based.

P. Mixed	M:14:S:45	+16	4'8193–(43)	5:5:22
B. Psth., Asocial		+24	'249 13–(37)	3:3:18

During the last year the patient had been guilty of many kinds of misbehavior. He had been a truant, had engaged in petty stealing and sexual misconduct, had carried a loaded revolver, had drunk alcoholic beverages, and had kept bad company. Community attention was directed to him by a petition alleging delinquency and filed by the superintendent of schools because of the patient's persistent truancy. He was placed on probation for that. Before, there had been a "scandal" in the town about his relationship with a young girl, who reported he had induced her to handle his genitalia. In addition, he and two other boys were known to be friendly with a middle-aged bachelor, reputedly a homosexual. The court had to take him in again when he, with some friends, discharged his father's pistol in a restaurant. This time he was referred to the psychopathic ward for study.

The previous history was essentially noncontributory, although he had had "stomach trouble, headaches, nervousness, sweating, and tremor." He had frequently been taken to a physician for these complaints. He had also had temper tantrums as a young child and had been eneuretic until age 12. The patient had a chaotic home and school history. He had lived with various persons, chiefly his grandparents. At school he did not do at all well. However, he had many friends, although recently he had been associating with boys much older than he and had belonged to no clubs or organizations.

In the hospital he was an alert, bright, interested, and cooperative patient. As he was examined, he was obviously attempting to play an adult role, and he appeared superficially open, frank, and self-controlled. He had an air of appraising the examiner and trying to keep one step ahead of him. He said he liked to make a good impression "so that they won't think bad of me." He discussed his delinquency in a matter-of-fact way and stated in the same manner that he was now aware that he had done wrong things and that he would change. He made several attempts to rationalize and project his responsibility, and he displayed very little anxiety. He was superior in intellect, with high mechanical interests and abilities. He showed a considerable disrespect for the rules and regulations of the hospital and he repeatedly committed infractions, even right after saying that he had learned his lesson from the last one. It was difficult to make any real contact with him, and he was only eager to get out. After considerable attention had been given to the plans for his immediate future, he was discharged with the recommendation that his mechanical interests be fostered.

Ps. Sz., Paranoid M:39:M:21 +3 48 267'3–9(65) 4:8:17

This man's change in personality had first been noted three years before admission when, following a civil service examination, he had become moody and despondent. The routine inquiries made by the civil service about his character seemed to be the source of his paranoid delusions. They were "spying" on him, he thought, and he decided his wife must be acting as informant. Whenever his wife left home he accused her of going to meet a civil service representative to plot against him. Later he conceived the notion that the house was "wired" and that microphones were hidden all over. He became withdrawn and preoccupied, refused to leave the house, voiced suspicions of his neighbors, and felt sure that his wife was unfaithful and that he was not the father of his children. Eventually the paranoid ideas included almost everyone he came in contact with.

The patient was a seventh-grade graduate, having left school because of "financial difficulties." Although somewhat above average in intelligence, he had always been a poor planner and had not been adequate in financial ways. In the civil service examination he took near the beginning of the present illness, he did very well. Regarded as secretive, shy, and sensitive, he never confided in anyone and had few personal friends. On the other hand he was self-reliant, honest, conscientious, and a respected member of the community.

The patient on admission was apathetic and seemed occasionally to be depressed. The most striking abnormality was manifest in his paranoid ideas. During his hospital stay he remained much the same. Cooperative and friendly part of the time, for brief periods he became tense and agitated and seemed to be confused. After such spells he seemed to be despondent but quickly returned to his usual appearance. The illness appeared to be a malignant type and he was transferred to a state hospital.

B. Psth., Asocial M:17:S:8 +1 4'8273–9(53) 6:10:23

Three years before admission the patient, at age 14, left school to take up the life of a tramp, wandering about the country as a transient worker. At times he would return home for unannounced visits and after brief stays would leave without warning. He drank a good deal and spoke unconcernedly about "getting girls in trouble." He had been arrested three times for drunkenness and had been apprehended once with other boys while stealing gasoline. When caught burglarizing the gasoline station he made no protest and did not attempt to escape. While in jail he managed once to get drunk. From there he was sent to the psychiatric unit for study.

His past history was not contributory, with the possible exception of severe scarlet fever at age 10. His older sister said that he had always been stubborn and troublesome. He had failed the second and fourth grades and had been in the sixth grade for the second year when he had left school. Without close friends, he had never felt any loyalty toward anyone or anything and had been incapable of taking responsibility of any kind. His home background was poor. The family was loosely held together, and the children all left home at early ages. The patient was the third of eight children, the rest of whom were not obviously maladjusted.

On admission the patient was well oriented and was aware of the general reason for his hospitalization, but there was no evidence of anxiety or guilt. He was dull normal in intelligence. Although he disliked the prospect of a reformatory term, he said that if he were put on probation he would probably break it. He cooperated fairly well in ward activities, but at no time did he show any capacity to form a relationship with anyone who might help him, and he was unable to take a responsible part in the consideration of his case. He was discharged back to the court.

B. Psth., Mixed Deteriorated   M:19:S:26   +4   '4827 63–X(61)   12:8:20

This youth came into the hospital because he was in trouble with the police. Nine months earlier he had stolen a valuable necklace and had been unable to give any motivation for his action. The necklace had then disappeared from his pocket, and he claimed it had been stolen from him. Placed on probation, he was told to see a psychiatrist twice a month. Six days before admission the youth stole a billfold from a lady sitting next to him in a theater. He had no need for the money and threw it away. At the request of the police, he found the money and willingly returned it. He was then referred to the hospital by the psychiatrist and the police.

The boy had been partially deaf since age 4 when he was struck on the head by a block of wood. He blamed the partial deafness for some of his behavior, since he had done poor work in school and had been teased by his playmates. At 11, a hearing aid was bought for him, and this helped him to do better schoolwork but left him still susceptible to the persecution of his schoolmates. He tried hard to make friends but always felt unsuccessful and uncomfortable. A surprising series of accidents befell him; among other things, he burned a leg and one arm was caught in a wringer. He was limited in his participation in sports, which he liked, because of the hearing aid. He claimed he had always been happy doing things with his hands, and he had earned his own pocket money by working for his father. At the end of the ninth grade he had enrolled in a trade school; he enjoyed that and was in training there at the time of the present difficulties. His parents believed that he tried too hard to be friendly and that some of his unpopularity resulted because he appeared to be "cocky." His tested intelligence was at the low limit of normal.

In the hospital the neurological examination indicated questionable signs of a brain injury. The psychological findings were consistent with such damage. Friendly, alert, and cooperative, he appeared somewhat childish for his age although he made a good appearance. His stream of thought was logical. He was afraid of what he might do if left alone—"Some crazy thing like stealing"—yet he was afraid to be with people because, he said, "I don't know what to say or how to act." He enjoyed the activities around the ward, and as time went on he seemed to be at ease. It was felt that he was overcompensating for inferiority feelings and attempts were made to plan more adequately for his supervision when he was discharged. In particular, he was to be tried in an environment away from home. He was finally sent to a state hospital for temporary hospitalization.

B. Psth., Asocial F:19:S:49 +2 48276'31– 7:10:23

This patient had been placed under the guardianship of a charitable institution at age 13 after the death of her mother, and since then she had made a poor adjustment in seven different homes. In each instance there was a fairly good initial adjustment, followed by minor thefts and deceitfulness. When she was accused of stealing she would first deny the theft, but if pressed she always finally admitted it. All the families she had lived with had found her untruthful, even about trivial matters. Except for short periods after she was reprimanded, her housework was carelessly done, and she persistently refused to obey orders. At age 14 she had become "boy crazy," and she admitted having had sexual intercourse. More recently she had been going out with various soldiers; she had apparently pursued in particular one who had a bad reputation. When he was sent overseas she went out with a friend of his, registered at a hotel with him, and had sexual intercourse. In explanation of her behavior, she said she was despondent over her friend's departure.

The girl had finished half the eleventh grade but had never made good grades. In the tenth and eleventh grades she had skipped school, on one occasion being truant for three consecutive weeks without the knowledge of her foster family because she always came home at the proper time. Although she had put in her application for work at a number of factories and stores, she had never shown any further initiative in getting work, and the month and a half she had worked as a waitress had been unpleasant to her. She enjoyed active sports. An immature person, she acted like a girl much younger than she actually was. She had few friends and had always been secretive and reluctant to discuss her problems. She resented any attempts to help her on the part of the society that was her guardian. When she was 8 years old her father had been given a penitentiary sentence for having carnal knowledge of the girl.

On admission for study and recommendation, she had no complaints and thought that there was nothing wrong with her. She resented being in the hospital. Although she was reticent and guarded in interviews, her orientation, memory, and thinking were all apparently normal, and she kept herself neat and well groomed. She was a little depressed, answered questions in a disinterested way, and instead of looking at the examiner, gazed out the window, smiling in a self-conscious way. For the first few days she refused to take part in ward activities, but she gradually changed. Her attitude toward the staff was antagonistic. Occasionally she cried but at no time did she actively cooperate in any of the studies the staff wished to make of her problems. Sometimes she said that she wanted to be sent to a reform school, and since almost everything except rigid supervision had been tried, it was recommended that she be sent to a home school for girls.

B. Psth., Path. Emot. M:22:M 4827'963-(65) 1:7:7
Schizoid

This private was referred to the psychiatrist by his commanding officer because of bizarre behavior and general vagueness of contact. He was completely irresponsible and complained of numerous hypochondriacal symptoms including headaches, "trouble swallowing," and exhaustion. His emotional depression was evident.

The son of immigrant Polish parents, the patient had been subjected to inconsistent handling by an oversolicitous father and mother. There was a lifelong history of pervasive maladjustment. He was closely tied to his parents in a hostile-dependent relationship. A poor student, he failed twice in school and was frequently truant. He constantly took new jobs and then left them. His current difficulty lay in the marital sphere. His wife, whom he had married after a ten-day courtship, had engaged in a series of extramarital affairs which she kept him informed about. He followed them with miserable but impotent intensity, going so far as to trace her and her lover to a hotel in a remote city and to report them to the hotel detective. However, he lacked the initiative, aggression, and self-esteem to take any definitive action in the matter.

The soldier was a physically slight individual. His army career consisted of a series of school assignments, all of which ended in failure because of his listlessness and lack of motivation. He was discharged from the service and no follow-up information was obtainable. A. T. K.

B. Psth., Path. Sexuality M:30:S:28 +26 48'291 367- 2:9:9
Alcoholism

The patient was a farm laborer. His room adjoined that of his employer's two daughters, aged 25 and 17, and he claimed that the elder daughter had led him to believe that she would welcome sexual advances; accordingly he had tried to enter her room late one night. When he had found the door locked, he had retired to his own room without forcing the door. On the complaint of his employer that the patient had attempted to enter the room he was picked up by the police and eventually sent to the hospital for study.

Most of what was learned about the man came from the patient himself. He had led a very erratic life; he had been illegitimately born in Italy, and his mother, who had answered a farmer's marriage advertisement, had brought him to the United States when he was 2 years old. The patient had gone as far as the eighth grade, where he discontinued his schooling after failing once. He had first become intoxicated at age 16 and had continued drinking, with bouts lasting from one to three days and occurring as frequently as once a week. An itinerant worker, he had been in jail on two occasions for disorderly conduct, and he readily admitted many sexual aberrations, including bestiality, masturbation, intercourse with a sister, and sodomy.

In the hospital he was entirely cooperative and well behaved, and showed no gross disturbances of intellect or mentation. He called himself "hot-blooded," and his comprehension of the social issue involved in the incident bringing him to the hospital was illustrated by his statement, "I won't ever break into a girl's room again. Next time I'll talk to them first." No real neurotic or identifiable anxiety was present, and he was accessible therapeutically. He was discharged to the court for disposition with the recommendation that if the patient was returned to society it should only be done with the strictest of supervision.

Ps. Sz., Cat. M:21:S:81 +30 48'2973– 3:1:16
Paranoid
Suicidal

The present illness of the patient had an insidious onset about six months earlier with the appearance of ideas of reference. He interpreted inconsequential remarks as meaning that he was unfit to associate with people because of a body odor indicating he was sexually "unnatural." Later he wrote a turbulent letter to his employers in which he referred to himself as a "dirty, rotten sexual pervert" and told of his introduction to sexual practices as a child, adding, "Sometimes I think I'm crazy." The patient had had good health until eight years before admission when he had developed a paralysis of all four extremities after anterior poliomyelitis. During his convalescence in the general hospital he lost his appetite, slept poorly, and was depressed. It was noted that he responded slowly and had a strong self-accusatory trend, with sexual colorings. Obviously hallucinatory, he thought he talked with God. He was considered suicidal. Feeding by tube was at times necessary because he talked of poisoning in his food and refused to eat. At this time it was suggested that he be committed to a state hospital, but during the proceedings he improved so much that he was not sent. After being fitted with orthopedic appliances he had been discharged from the general hospital; it was felt that a long hospitalization was not good for him because of his "mental condition."

By home study, he had completed the eighth grade. He had an I.Q. of 100. After extensive study by rehabilitation personnel it was recommended that he be trained to earn some money of his own, and it was noted that he had ideas of a peculiar type during this phase of his rehabilitation. He was a pleasant, friendly, and innately charming person, and many persons had tried to help him.

He spent much of his time in the hospital reading and listening to the radio. On the fourth day after admission he became acutely excited, tense, and fearful, talking at great length of his sinfulness. This condition lasted for about a week. Part of this time he was mute, lying with his eyes closed, his pulse and respiration rapid. Gradually he quieted down and began to work at occupational therapy, but a second episode with marked religious trends developed. He thought God had given him power to walk without crutches. He again developed mutism, refused food, and was incontinent. After several other periods of this type he was discharged to a state hospital.

B. Psth., Asocial	F:20:S:39	+1	4′83–(57)	5:4:23
		+30	4′839–(55)	5:3:25

This young woman was hospitalized on a court order because of social maladjustments including a preference for associating with Negro men. She had an illegitimate child by one of them. At age 15 the girl had begun to exhibit irresponsible behavior. In high school at that time, she was going with a Negro boy who was subsequently killed while hitching a ride. In reaction to this, she became hysterical and required sedation. Later, while in the "detention room" at school for truancy, she became acquainted with another Negro boy and had her first sexual experience. Not only did she refuse abortion when she later became pregnant but she maintained an attitude of calm indifference to her parents' concern. Next she ran away from home and was returned by the police. A psychiatrist, consulted by the family, refused to treat her. She became defiant and left home again. Next in the series of incidents leading to hospitalization was a "brawl" between a Negro friend of hers and a white man, apparently over the "sale" of the patient. The police intervened and took her and one of the men to jail. The illegitimate child was born shortly before the girl was brought to the hospital. When she refused to give up the baby, the psychiatric unit was asked to assess the problem.

Described by her parents as "headstrong, hard to discipline, and insistent on her own way," she was friendly and at ease with strangers but could never accept any kind of frustration. Toward anyone she thought responsible for frustrating her she became bitterly resentful. She was deceptive and frequently lied to get her own way. Although she spent most of her money for clothes, she was untidy and careless in appearance. The girl's parents were incompatible, and they had frequent quarrels, with threats of divorce and the like. The patient's I.Q. was tested at 115. In the hospital she was opinionated and haughty in attitude. While at first she was irritable and resentful over being hospitalized, she soon became happy and carefree and showed no concern about her problems. She stubbornly refused to give up the child and her attitute was one of "putting up" with everything until she was released. Little change was effected, and when the young woman was discharged it seemed probable she would have further trouble in the future.

Ps. Sz., Mixed F:27:S:10 +2 4837926'1-(45) 2:8:16
P. Hys.
B. Psth., Mixed
Suicidal

About three months before admission while visiting her fiancé, to whom she had been engaged for five years, the patient became pregnant but refused to marry the man, even when he insisted. (They had had intercourse on only two occasions, the second one initiating the pregnancy.) She returned home to resume her teaching job and although she wrote to her fiancé daily, often threatening suicide, she continued to go out with a local man in whom she was interested. She refused to tell her mother about her pregnancy. She developed palpitation, nervousness, forgetfulness, periods of depression, frontal headaches, and precordial pain. She was hospitalized in a general hospital after taking an overdose of quinine, apparently in an attempt to induce abortion.

The patient had always been nervous. An intelligent, cheerful, popular, and capable person, she had graduated from a four-year college course in three years. Her hobbies were golf and reading, and she had many personal friends. She admitted to sexual intercourse only with the one man.

In the hospital her main thought was how to obtain an abortion. Her idea that the pregnancy was an unfortunate accident remained fixed, and she considered the consequences only in the light of her future happiness. There was a blandness of affect inconsistent with the situation. She thought the pregnancy induced nervousness which in turn caused impairment of memory. She was neat, well dressed, alert, and cooperative in ward activities. Although she finally told her mother of the pregnancy in order to get her mother's consent to a therapeutic abortion, she decided to marry her fiancé before the abortion because he might not marry her afterward. When she left the hospital there was little change in her basic personality and no resolution of her real future problems since the staff had been unable to get her to be at all concerned with anything but her superficial problems.

B. Psth., Path. Sexuality M:17:S:21 +2 '486-(59) 7:8:13
Paranoid
Twin

This boy, who had been repeatedly identified as an exhibitionist, was sent to the clinic by the juvenile court. His method was to stand in front of an open window and cover the upper part of his body with a window curtain. The acts chiefly occurred in front of 9- and 10-year-old neighbor girls.

At the age of 7 the patient woke up one morning to find his right leg "paralyzed." The leg was movable at the hip and at the toes but not at the knee. There was no pain. He remained in bed for several days and the paralysis disappeared spontaneously. This episode was never explained. No other factor in his past medical history seemed contributory.

At the end of the tenth grade he left school to take a job, contrary to his father's wishes. He had never shown any interest in school and his grades were below average. No better at jobs than at school, he was mainly interested in neighborhood football and baseball games. Although he did not get into actual trouble in school or in the neighborhood, he was considered a "bad influence." Immature although independent, he was unable to make plans for the future or to appreciate what was happening to him. Tests indicated his I.Q. was about average, although there was a much higher score for performance than for verbal tests. A twin brother had a school and neighborhood record similar to the patient's. The family situation was not obviously bad.

In the hospital the patient found the routine monotonous. His main thoughts centered around getting discharged. Unconcerned about his troubles, he attributed his actions to "not being able to help it." The neighbors who had reported him "had it in for him," he believed, and the doctors were trying to "get something on him." Consequently he was defensive and evasive. When not under examination he appeared happy and was apparently even-tempered and well adjusted. At times he was loud and boisterous, especially in the presence of an attractive 17-year-old patient. No real contact could be made with him psychotherapeutically and he was discharged to go on probation.

Ps. Sz., Mixed Paranoid — M:22:S:16 — +17 — '486–9 — 3:3:20

A graduate student at a university, the patient had apparently been well adjusted until about six months before admission; then he had noticed that his lectures were unusually dull, he became unable to concentrate on them, and when he got home his notes made no sense. He felt that the professor and the rest of the class were conspiring against him to see how long he would put up with the poor lectures. When he went home for the Christmas holidays his family noticed that he was unusually quiet and that he kept by himself most of the time. A month before admission he became agitated and talked about a group of "Reds" who were out to "get him" at the university. On the list he made of them he included several friends, his roommate, and a few professors. It became increasingly impossible for him to continue his studies, and he developed ideas of reference. He got the idea that he should ask a girl in one of his classes, whom he did not know, to marry him. When she rejected the proposal, which he made at lunch after telephoning her for the date, he became depressed. There was a gradual development of more and more peculiar behavior and ideas.

An A student, the patient was fond of tennis and swimming, but he spent most of his spare time reading. Although he occasionally went out with girls, he had never before singled out any one girl. A somewhat aloof, serious-minded person, he had always been self-reliant and truthful.

On admission he was concerned with the thought that he had schizophrenia; he made a point of the fact that he regarded half of himself as a young boy 10 years of age and the other half a man. He did not want to be disturbed because he had so many things to think over. In his opinion several of his friends and some professors were conspiring to undermine his physical and moral strength. He also believed that his food and water were drugged. In general, however, he was well oriented and, as indicated in his idea about schizophrenia, he had a verbal insight into what was wrong with him. He spent all his time in his room alone, either lying in bed with his eyes closed and his hands folded on his chest, or sitting on a straight chair looking ahead. During the second week he began to show some improvement and took an interest in ward activities. After two weeks he was almost normal. His attitude and speech had become conventional, and he wanted to be released to go back to school. Although he admitted he had a few queer thoughts, he thought that he would be able to control them since he recognized them for what they were. It was suggested that he go home for two or three weeks and if he continued well, enter school the following quarter.

B. Psth., Path. Sexuality M:65:M:12 +3 4'86<u>17</u>–(49) 4:6:20

This man, a farmer, was ordered to the hospital for observation and study. A number of children frequently played in his yard, and one day they invited him to see a playhouse. Soon they all left except a 9-year-old girl. While talking to her he began to spank her softly and put his fingers on her genitals. Any further aggression he denied, and he said he did not disrobe her or expose himself. The incident did not alarm the child and there was no report of the matter until late in the evening when she told her mother. A physician was called and after examining the girl reported "signs of irritation." The child then claimed the patient had exposed himself. The child's mother hesitated but finally after a week she reported to the police and the patient was jailed. He could give no reason for his act. He was released on bail and returned home, but the neighbors demanded his return to jail, and it was then that he was sent to the psychiatric unit.

The patient had spent two years in an agricultural school, had worked at various jobs, and was considered reliable and capable. By most people he was regarded as an amiable person. Interviews with neighbors indicated that he had a reputation for lacking "sexual inhibition." His wife was frigid, he said, and he had been forced to extramarital relations in order to satisfy his excess libido. This resulted in the illegitimate pregnancy of a sister-in-law, a complaint by an acquaintance of an attack, and several "affairs" with women in the community. In the last few years, however, this activity had decreased.

In the hospital the patient was well composed and conventional in behavior. His stream of thought was logical and to the point. Of superior intellectual capacity, he showed no evidence of deterioration and was alert and cooperative. He rationalized everything he had done. His adjustment toward life was good, although he was mildly depressed. No real basis could be found for the man's aberrant behavior. It was felt that he might become worse as he grew older. His disposition was left to the discretion of the court.

B. Psth., Asocial F:15:S:26 +2 4862'<u>79</u>31-(51, 5:12:14
Suicidal

A month before admission to the hospital this girl had made a fourth attempt at suicide, this time by drinking formaldehyde. During the earlier part of the day she had been visiting with friends. Later she quarreled with her mother, who struck her. When her mother left the house, the patient contemplated suicide and procured a knife and a rope. At the last minute she changed her mind about the method and drank the formaldehyde. She was discovered by neighbors who heard her screams.

In her previous attempts to commit suicide the patient had used aspirin, iodine, and rat poison. Each time her purpose had been to join her dead lover. Although the girl had been exposed to numerous psychologically traumatic experiences, this series of suicidal attempts after the death of her lover were the only psychotic or obviously neurotic upsets in her history. The patient's schoolwork was marginal, not only because of her poor achievement but because of bad relations with her teachers. The social level of her family was low. The patient exhibited poor judgment and her interests were restricted, although she liked reading, dancing, and domestic work. Haughty and aloof except with a few friends, she was alone much of the time, but in spite of being at home so much, she was relatively self-reliant and independent of her family. She was known to have drunk excessively more than once. Her mother, who had divorced the patient's father and had later remarried, worked a good deal of the time, leaving her family at home alone.

On admission the girl was chiefly intent on presenting herself in a good light. She talked about the man she had loved and about her unhappy home life. Although she was free of obvious mental aberrations, she showed wide mood swings, ranging from spells of crying to spasms of laughter. She denied that she could be ill in any way, and in her view the suicidal attempts were unimportant. In fact she talked glibly of them. In the hospital she was so obstreperous a number of times that she was moved to the disturbed ward as a method of controlling her behavior. Her interpersonal relationships in the hospital were exceedingly superficial. It was decided that she should spend some time in a correctional home.

B. Pri., Child. M:16:S:26 +6 4869'1372-(51) 7:10:24
B. Psth., Path. Emot.

The patient's delinquency dated from the time he was 10 years of age when he had first engaged in petty thievery. This had consisted of taking small articles which he wanted but "couldn't afford." At age 8 he had acted as a lookout for an older boy during similar thefts. The patient said that he was not concerned about what he was doing as long as he got away with it. About two years before admission he had first become involved with the law when he broke into a house. He was placed on probation but broke it by stealing again. This kind of behavior continued until he was sent to the hospital for evaluation. He himself complained of marked nervousness, headaches, unhappiness, and depression. These he attributed to worry occasioned by his ostracism in his home town. In turn he had a feeling of resentment and distrust toward all individuals with whom he came in contact.

The patient had left school after completing the eighth grade. He had averaged below C in school and had not liked it. After leaving school he got odd jobs but did not stick to anything for long. He had always been something of a lone wolf, both at home and at school, tending usually to form a single very close friendship and finding it very hard to trust anyone else. His mother said that he was very stubborn. In his relations with his classmates, he was shy and sensitive. He did not have any known social relationships with girls. His family was apparently fairly well adjusted. The boy said of the father, "He would never do anything dishonest."

In the hospital the patient was an unhappy, sullen, and restless boy. He was defiant and suspicious toward the people who had brought him in and toward others who had tried to work with him. Shy and reluctant to elaborate on his story, he appeared emotionally unstable and showed a marked nervousness. He said that his contemporaries were not in the same trouble that he was only because they lacked courage or were not venturesome. He was slow to participate in activities of the group and appeared satisfied to be left alone. During interviews he maintained an attitude of indifference and negligent attention, with little apparent understanding of what was going on. Surprisingly he was reluctant to leave the hospital on the day of discharge. Little could be done with the boy himself, though efforts were directed toward preparing a way for him when he was discharged, and he was finally sent back to his parents and the county probation officer.

Ps. Sz., Simple F:30:S:48 +1 486'972–1 (61) 1:13:8

For the past year the patient had had a constant nodding of her head. This was aggravated when attention was drawn to it but disappeared when she engaged in a game or was otherwise distracted. The symptom had appeared while she was a patient in another mental hospital and it had become gradually worse. At times her whole body moved with her head. She spent some weeks in a second hospital, then was put in a convalescent home. There her conduct was poor—she played the radio loudly at all hours, for example—and finally the landlady requested that she leave.

Emotionally unstable, the patient had always been romantic and unrealistic, and her past history was full of illustrative incidents. Her father had died when she was small and her mother had been committed to a mental hospital. Throughout her childhood she had moved from one boarding home to another and had attended numerous private schools. At the age of 21 she had reached the eleventh grade. For three years she was the mistress of a 70-year-old man. Described as having always been nervous, she had many tics, staged temper tantrums regularly, and was selfish and demanding. The patient said that she only wanted to get rid of her "wiggle." Fearful of institutions, she wanted to "stay out of them," as she put it. She was pessimistic about her condition, and she appeared tense and depressed. The tic was her only difficulty, she felt, and she considered herself otherwise normal.

Her conduct in the hospital necessitated her removal for a short time to a disturbed ward. Most of the time she was content to lie in bed and daydream. She had made a scrapbook of a male movie star's pictures and was often seen kissing them. She was very untidy. Apparently she tried hard to impress everyone with her intelligence. Her moods changed rapidly; at one moment she would be happy and the next she would be crying bitterly. She was discharged to live in a boarding home. It was recommended that if this did not work out she should go to a state hospital.

Ps. M-D., Manic F:19:S:25 +1 '487–6(66) 4:2:25
B. Psth., Asocial

For seven years, dating from a severe case of pneumonia, this young woman's behavior had become more and more unusual. There were violent temper tantrums, accompanied by swearing, screaming, and throwing things, and set off by slight and seemingly inconsequential incidents. She took delight in shocking people with wild, lurid stories, and she tried to deceive people into believing she was married. During the past year the complaints had become worse, and in addition she had developed an enormous appetite for rich foods and a desire to sleep more than the usual amount.

The patient's health had never been good. Her childhood ills included rickets, endless colds, and attacks of vomiting accompanied by high fever. Until age 10, she was eneuretic. During the attack of pneumonia she was in a coma for two days. Although she had finished two years of high school without apparent difficulty she had been absent-minded and inattentive during the last year. She had been discharged from two jobs because of "nervousness." Of a pleasant disposition, she made friends easily, but she lost them just as quickly by her indiscriminate temper tantrums. She liked social activities and was especially attracted to men, with whom she flirted on every possible occasion. As far back as anyone could remember she had had periods of hyperactivity lasting a week. Low average in intelligence, she lacked good judgment and was immature. The family background was not unduly bad.

In the hospital she showed no worry about her condition and felt that "everything would be all right" when she went home. She said she had intentionally been acting queerly and could stop it whenever she wished. Well oriented, she was alert, friendly, and cooperative, and she showed no irritability or loss of temper during the first part of the hospitalization. Toward the end of her stay she became irritable. From the outset she showed resentment at questioning, and on personal matters she was unapproachable. "I don't want to be bossed," she said. "My mother spoiled me" was her own explanation for her problems. On the ward she was active, cheerful, and flirtatious. She received numerous letters, some from men in the service, and several of them asked her to marry them. Again and again she insisted that she "could behave" if she wanted to; it was true that she showed temper upsets on only two occasions, and both of these outbursts were mild. After her parents were carefully instructed about how they might handle her, she was discharged for a trial at home.

B. Psth., Path. Sexuality M:18:S:33 +4 487′2136– 4:7:21
Mental Deficiency

The patient was transferred to the hospital from the county jail for investigation because of mutual masturbation, fellatio, and homosexual activities. He admitted he had indulged in these practices since age 14 with strange men and three teen-age boy friends. He had met the older men while hitchhiking, and they had carried out their activities in a car on the outskirts of town. The boys had often dressed in girls' clothing and had then engaged in mutual masturbation and other practices, with the patient playing both active and passive roles. Their apprehension, at the home of one of the participants, was brought about by a boy who had become so angered at being excluded from the group that he had told his mother what was going on. She had informed the police.

The patient had left school in the ninth grade. The school had found him to have an I.Q. of about 75. After leaving school he had worked intermittently at a bakery and at housework. At home he did the cooking. Shy but friendly, he was usually cheerful, very stable, and truthful. In general he had tried to fulfill his responsibilities at home. He enjoyed cooking, swimming, horseback riding, bowling, and movies. He had been very uneasy in the presence of girls and had not had a date for two years. At about age 5 he had exhibited a type of fetishism in being fond of girls' clothes, and more recently he had shown the same tendency by taking his sister's clothes and objecting when asked to return them to her. Effeminate in his actions and speech, he also had a speech impediment so that he tended to lisp.

In the hospital he talked to some extent about having been brought in "because of sodomy" and about having been in jail for six weeks, but he spoke chiefly about the new understanding he had of his problems. He said he had "learned his lesson" and was sure he would never have similar difficulties again. He was well oriented, his memory was good, and there was no evidence of any defect of intellect. His insight into his problems and his future was exceedingly poor. His facial expression suggested stupidity, but he was cooperative and apparently eager to do well in all examinations. He especially liked to work in the hospital kitchen. He was happy in the hospital but after about two weeks was eager to go home. The I.Q. obtained in the hospital was in the low eighties. Environmental factors were thought to have contributed considerably to the pattern of his behavior, and careful placement was advised, with special consideration of both the home and the community to which he would go.

B. Psth., Path. Sexuality M:15:S:63 +7 487′236–9(71) 5:5:21

This boy had begun to indulge in overt homosexual acts when he was 11 years old. The first episode occurred with an older man who took him to a hotel room, gave him drinks, and practiced fellatio with him. These acts became more and more frequent and when he was 13 he was arrested for impersonating a woman. Occasionally he practiced mutual masturbation, often fellatio. He was sent to a reform school where he continued his practices. Placed on parole, he stopped for a few weeks, then resumed his former activities. When one of his "partners" stole his billfold and watch, the boy retaliated by taking the man's billfold and some of his clothes. Returned to the reform school, he continued his homosexual acts and was sent to the psychiatric hospital for recommendations.

There was considerable evidence that the boy had shown definite feminine trends since he was a small child. His grandparents, with whom he lived, had encouraged him in activities such as cooking and sewing. During his early life he had had few friends and had never been interested in active sports. He went through the ninth grade and did only moderately well. An illegitimate child, born to a girl who was 13 years old at the time, the patient was treated by his mother's parents like a real son. His mother lived in the home as a sister. The situation had been explained to him when he was 6 years of age.

In the hospital the youth was composed and willing to discuss his problems. His behavior showed definite feminine tendencies. He claimed that he would like to be helped if possible and that he wished to be freed of the homosexual habit, but he did not feel sure it was possible. His tested I.Q. was 109. His intellect and sensorium were entirely unaffected. Although he frequently expressed the desire "to do anything" that would help, the staff felt that this was a shallow statement. Actually when specific suggestions were made, the boy obviously shied away from anything difficult. Furthermore, he showed a preference for the men on the ward and was frequently seen holding hands with other young male patients. Whatever the origin of his problem might have been, the staff did not feel that any therapeutic efforts would likely change the patient much, and it was recommended that he be paroled and put in a social situation outside of the city, where temptation would be at a minimum and where someone might work with him and give him psychological support.

Ps. Sz., Mixed F:33:D:130 +13 4872361′9–X(57) 2:18:10
Suicidal +92 8426793′–(55) 1:13:8

The patient's acute illness had been precipitated by difficulties she encountered in an affair with a married man. When he began to lose interest in her, she became "hysterical" and panicky. Returning to her foster mother's home, she became more upset and felt that she hated this woman and must get away from her and hide. She ran out of the house dressed only in a slip and spent the night in a neighbor's cellar, where she was found in the morning and was taken to the hospital.

Because the patient's own mother was an alcoholic, she had been raised by foster parents, who were strict, religious people. The patient said, "My folks always gave me everything I wanted but I never felt wanted or needed; I always have felt lonely, alone, and frightened." When seen at the hospital the foster mother appeared to be a controlling and demanding woman, extremely hostile in a veiled way. At 20 the patient had run away from home, totally rejecting her background. After her first experience in sexual intercourse she thought of it continually and wanted intercourse with nearly every man she met. She had lived with her husband for two years before marrying him. They had a child and four years later were divorced, reportedly because of the husband's infidelity. The patient felt that she had never belonged to any one or to any group. She said she had learned to put on a "good front" and thus made friends easily and could be the life of the party; but she never had close friends. After she finished the twelfth grade in school she held many secretarial jobs. Tiring soon of each new job, she shifted from office to office.

On admission the patient was sloppy and seemed overwhelmed with shame and guilt. She was tearful at times, especially when expressing her feelings of fear and loneliness, although in general she appeared to be withdrawn, blocked, and confused rather than severely depressed. She had definite feelings of unreality and depersonalization, and she felt she was mentally ill and wanted treatment. Her course in the hospital was variable, but the general pattern of behavior which soon emerged was overt hostility to everyone in her environment, including the psychotherapist who saw her frequently during her hospitalization. After twelve electroshock treatments the patient said she felt exactly the same way about everything, but she admitted that, temporarily at least, her control and ability to adjust on the outside was improved. On the ward she covered some of her hostility with a moderately compliant exterior. She left the hospital, saying she might "blow up at any time."

During the following year she was hospitalized several times after a suicide attempt, and on another occasion after a spell of confusion and amnesia following an alcoholic interlude. Each time she improved with a brief hospitalization, but it was expected that she would continue to act out her conflicts and to react to frustration by further breakdowns. E. B.

B. Psth., Asocial   M:15:S:18   +2   48'726–(51)   7:7:23

Following a violation of parole this boy was sent to the hospital by a judge for the purpose of determining what should be done with him. Since age 11 he had frequently been involved in thefts and had played pranks such as breaking bottles on the highway and disrupting classes at school. At age 12 he had spent several months in a boys' reform school. Released, he had again stolen and with the money had lavished entertainment on himself and his friends.

The lad's home background was not outstandingly bad. There were seven children in the family, and it was said that the patient "is the only one who ever gets into trouble." A likable, boisterous boy, he seemed some years younger than his actual age. His intelligence was low normal. Although he made friends readily and appeared at ease with others, he tended to be domineering and demanding. He was usually cheerful and enthusiastic about things he himself chose to do. He had mechanical aptitudes and he showed interest and zeal in odd jobs that utilized these abilities.

In the hospital the boy felt no detectable concern or guilt about his troubles with the law. He gave no reason for the stealing, although he talked readily of it. Attentive and interested in the testing and the examinations, he nevertheless performed poorly. In general his behavior was "normal," and he was neat, natural, and open. On the ward other patients regarded him as somewhat of a nuisance because of his boisterousness and childish behavior. There was no evidence of unfulfilled needs in any emotional sphere. At discharge he was to return to the training school.

P. Mixed Schizoid F:32:S:35 +23 48′72936–(28) 6:10:21

The patient sought psychiatric help because she was worried that she might not be able to carry on with the job she had held for four years. She felt also she could no longer endure the burdens placed on her by an adolescent daughter who was a behavior problem. After one interview she seemed to collapse in a schizophrenic-like panic episode involving ideas of suicide, nightmares, tension and exhaustion, visual and auditory hallucinations of a persecutory nature, and a desire to escape reality.

The patient's father was an aggressive, domineering man who had never been very successful. Her mother was a sheltered, self-effacing woman, ruled harshly by her husband. From the time the patient was 13 her mother was apparently psychotic; she babbled to herself and was often out of contact with reality, but she was able to carry on her housework in a mechanical way. Until the patient was about 11 she was her father's favorite. At that time, as she became more self-assertive, her father became brutally punitive. Her conflict with her father culminated in a suicide attempt, after which she was sent to a mental hospital. She was reported to have had hallucinations of supernatural beings, but on that admission she took the commitment as an adventure and had no hallucinations or delusions and there was no evidence of psychosis. A diagnosis of hysteria was made, and she was sent to a boarding school where she did well.

After high school graduation she tried to work her way through college but became pregnant. A daughter was born and was raised first by the father's people, later by the patient, who waged a bitter court fight to regain the child's custody. At the time of the present admission the patient's daughter was living with her. At this time she felt very insecure and believed that her father and the child's grandmother were out to "get" her and had informed her employers and landlords that she was an unmarried mother. She worked as a receptionist.

The patient was vague about her sexual history. She felt that she attracted sadistic men and that no decent man would want to marry her.

A thin blonde, with a high-pitched, whiny voice, straggly hair, wrinkled clothing, and a worried, tense expression, the patient presented a pathetic appearance at the first interview. She was well oriented. Of superior intelligence, she tended to intellectualize and to utilize fantasy in a manner designed to intrigue the psychiatrist. Apparently she wished to startle her listener, to arouse pity, and to elicit reassurance. Her manner varied from oversweetness to suspiciousness and challenge. The "nervous collapse," occurring after the first interview, resembled a temper tantrum. Later she claimed that the hallucinations were only the product of her vivid imagination, cultivated because reality was so hard. Electroshock therapy was given, on an outpatient basis, with prompt improvement after one or two treatments. There were no more of the schizophrenic-like complaints. After two weeks of treatment she became so hostile to the relatives with whom she was living that they requested she be admitted as an inpatient. In the hospital she was less ingratiating and more critical of the hospital and the plans made for her. She continued to improve, however, and was ready for discharge in three weeks. By that time she felt able to carry on by herself. E. B.

B. Psth., Mixed F:16:S:42 +8 48′7391– 2:13:18

Eleven days before admission to the psychopathic unit the patient had borne an infant that had died shortly after birth. The pregnancy had been complicated by a pre-eclamptic state and puerperal infection. On the day of discharge from the general hospital the patient was trapped in an elevator between two floors and became extremely agitated and apprehensive. She then went to a home for unmarried mothers, where she experienced a severe hysterical reaction followed by "odd behavior."

The patient's pregnancy had forced her to terminate her schooling in the ninth grade. She had failed the first and third grades. Always a behavior problem, she was untruthful, got along poorly with her mother, and usually shirked responsibility in her home. She had had difficulties with her schoolwork, had shown defective judgment, and for many years had had an irresistible desire to go out with boys. She was easily frightened when she feared punishment, and she had feelings of inferiority. When the patient's father had died three years before, the mother had become somewhat disorganized and had found it difficult to carry on adequately with her three children.

The patient's pregnancy and the death of her child were apparently sources of unhappiness and disappointment to her, and she was much concerned about what the neighbors would think of her. She thought that the future held many problems, but she believed that some sort of job would solve her difficulty. One received the impression that she was making no effort to analyze her true emotional and psychological state. She believed that her hospitalization had been arranged to get her away from babies and their mothers. She made little effort to cooperate with the psychotherapeutic program and the other efforts made to help her. The girl took no real interest in her surroundings and initiated no conversations. Her intelligence was average, but she had a very poor fund of general knowledge. She remained listless, asocial, and hypochondriacal, and it was frequently necessary to use much persuasion to get her into group activities. When her requests were not immediately fulfilled, she became irritable, and when it came time for her discharge several times she flatly refused to go home or to go any place else. She said that she had no desire to make any effort to adjust in the new environment that the staff thought desirable for her.

P. Mixed F:16:S:49 +31 48 761'923–X(66) 2:19:5
B. Psth., Asocial

This girl was admitted on a court order for observation and recommendation; she had been a behavior problem at school and at home for four years. The pattern had begun with vomiting spells in school, for which she would ask to be excused. When a medical investigation indicated no reason for the vomiting the teachers were instructed to refuse to give her excuses. She then developed various somatic symptoms and began to play truant. Sent to a correctional home, she did fairly well there and lost considerable weight (she had always been obese). Next she went into a foster home and for another period showed good behavior. Later, however, she began to go out with an older man; she was again truant from school and sneaked out nights. The man was sent to the penitentiary on a charge of carnal knowledge, and the girl was again placed on probation. Then she developed an attachment for a relative of one of her foster parents and when this relationship was frustrated she had crying spells. She became more and more sensitive to remarks about her obesity and to gossip about her father, who was a drunkard. Welfare workers finally requested that a study of her be made, more because of the long-continued maladjustment than because of any particular misbehavior.

In the hospital she showed strong feelings of rejection by her parents; hostility was mingled with dependence. She was well oriented, friendly, and cooperative. Perceiving her own psychological maladjustment, she nevertheless blamed a good deal of her trouble on her teachers. She took a considerable interest in the activities of the ward and mixed well with the other patients. In interviews she was erratic but made progress in developing self-understanding. Because of the unexpected death of a close relative, she was suddenly discharged. Plans were made to continue contacts with the girl on an outpatient basis.

B. Psth., Asocial M:19:S:12 +1 48'7623–(49) 6:6:22

The youth, a parole violator, was admitted for study on a court order. He had been in difficulty with the law since he was 10, when he was picked up for petty thievery. Later he stole cars and had an irregular history of reform schools, breaking of parole, and the like. At one time he and another boy stole fifteen cars in a period of one week. In addition, they burglarized numerous houses. At the end of five weeks of this behavior he returned to the reform school voluntarily, confessed the car thefts, and was sent to the reformatory. Later, while out on parole, he became involved with a 16-year-old girl who became pregnant. This girl and the patient stole a car and lived together for some time. When the police found them the patient escaped. He finally consulted a lawyer who advised him to give himself up, which he did five or six days later.

His past medical history was noncontributory. The youth's I.Q. was 96. His school history was irregular, with poor grades because of truancy and other misbehavior. His first sexual experience had occurred at age 12, and after that he had indulged frequently. Described as a likable, friendly person who made an excellent first impression, he appeared frank and open, liked sports and movies, and in general seemed entirely normal. His family background was chaotic. His mother, with whom the patient had lived, was unstable and defensive about her son and never admitted that he had any undesirable characteristics.

In the hospital, although the young man faced a possible maximum term of forty years in prison, he appeared unconcerned and apparently did not worry. His own statement was that he had been thinking about what would happen to him "a little," but "if I thought much about it I'd go nuts." This latter prediction did not, however, appear to be deeply felt. His predominant emotional tone was one of shallow friendliness and indifference to his problem. He had no insight whatsoever into his antisocial behavior, attributing it all to factors outside himself or to a kind of indifferent fate. He fitted into the hospital routine well, except that he resented even the small amount of restriction to which he was subjected. No genuine personal contact could be established with him. He was discharged back to the court, and the outlook seemed to be poor.

B. Pri., Child. M:16:S:51 +8 487′6932– 3:7:13

For about the last four years this boy had shown signs of unrest. At age 14 he had run away and had spent several days in the woods near his home. Nine months before admission he had stolen his grandfather's car. Away from home for one week, he claimed to have been in another state, where he had maintained himself as a laborer. Next he had stolen some money from his grandmother and had traveled across the country. When he had heard that the authorities were looking for a man whose description, he thought, fitted him, he had written a threatening letter to the sheriff denouncing him for "putting the law on me," but on finding that his assumption was wrong and that he was unable to get a job, he had asked the travelers' aid bureau for transportation home.

Although he was not a disciplinary problem at school, on the playground he was boastful and left threatening notes about the things he intended to do to members of his class. For the last two years he had been infatuated with a girl classmate, and when she had not reciprocated his attachment he had threatened her. The school board, feeling that he was a bad influence, had expelled him. Other boys had been somewhat afraid of him at first, and they had been awed by his tall stories, but they had finally come to consider him harmless and to ridicule him for his stories. He had always had a feeling of insecurity, and he had few friends. Most of his time he spent by himself. Because his mother had died when he was 9 months old and his father had disappeared, he had lived with his grandparents, neither of whom was a very adequate person. The grandfather had been in a state hospital, and the grandmother, although hard working, was not stable.

In the hospital the boy presented no gross disturbance of mentation or sensorium. He said he had run away because life with his grandmother had become so unbearable that running away had seemed the only solution. He wanted to serve his sentence as quickly as possible so that he would then be free to handle his own problems. Ultimately he wanted to be an explorer and study old ruins. Although he adapted well to ward life and was at no time a problem, he resented having been sent to the hospital for study, and he spoke to other patients about his intention of breaking out. In extensive studies made of him, it was found that he had an I.Q. of 120, with high mechanical aptitude, but no real progress was made with him, and he seemed incapable of good interpersonal rapport. When he was discharged to the custody of the court on the completion of these studies, it was with the recommendation that if possible he be trained in a vocational school while living in a boarding home, but it was felt unlikely that the boy would take advantage of these opportunities.

B. Pri., Child. F:16:S:26 +1 '4879-6(61) 9:5:11

This girl had been placed in a detention home three years earlier, and in the beginning her adjustment there had been good. The picture had gradually changed, however, as competition with other girls and striving for attention became too great for her. She had a series of temper tantrums characterized by rigidity, enlarged eyes, abusive language, and a general defiance of authority. In addition she became violent, hitting and biting other girls and the matrons and destroying property. These spells lasted about a week. Various methods of punishment had been tried—isolation, ignoring her, exclusion from the honor roll. Between outbursts she was disobedient and plotted with other girls against the institution.

Originally referred to the detention home as a result of domestic difficulties and her own incorrigible behavior and disobedience, the girl had at first been placed in foster homes. She adjusted in none of these. She was frequently accused of stealing, was noisy and boisterous, and demanded constant attention.

'489–

She was, however, very religious. Although she denied all knowledge of sex, others disputed this. In school she was a quick and alert pupil, but her disobedience and her refusal to follow the routine prevented normal progress.

In the hospital she showed a great deal of concern about the future, particularly about the problem of whether she should return to her mother or try another home. Staff members felt that there was little genuine emotion behind her remarks. She would say casually, "If I can't do something about my anger I will never get any place." However, she consistently placed the blame for her misbehavior on external situations and declared that she had no control over what happened to her. Intellectually, she was at the dull normal level. On the ward she behaved well, her manners were good, and she was not overactive. She was somewhat demanding of attention. In general during the hospitalization nothing untoward was observed. At discharge arrangements were made to place the girl in another foster home on trial. There was little expectation that she would adjust well, however.

P. Mixed F:25:S '489–(47) 4:2:22

This girl came to the clinic at the suggestion of her mother to discuss job possibilities. A college graduate with professional training in library work, she had been unsuccessful on library jobs and at present was working as a sales clerk in a local department store.

In the first interview she was almost too well controlled about her past difficulties. She discussed her interest in art and her attempts at painting. She had little to say about her family and did not describe any difficulties except to remark that she and her mother lived in a very small apartment, which at times was hard on both of them. Inquiries about her library work brought out the information that she had seemed immature, nervous, lacking in poise, slow in reference work, and increasingly irregular in attendance. A conference with her mother revealed that she had been hospitalized once for a nervous illness, which had interrupted her library work. After the girl's discharge from the hospital at that time her psychiatrist had left the staff and there had been no follow-up of any kind.

Within the next year we saw her for a number of interviews and she shifted jobs several times. She saw no prospects of returning to professional work and turned to a short business course, but she did not complete it and continued at sales jobs. She showed increasing tension and excitability, which finally appeared to be real hypomania. Thirteen months after our first contact, and the administration of the MMPI, she had another severe psychotic spell, was hospitalized, and was treated by psychotherapy. Electroshock therapy was considered but was not used.

At the end of another year she had been discharged, had finished a course in secretarial training, and had been on a secretarial job for four months. Her mother reported that she seemed better than she had been for years. D. F. C.

B. Psth., Path. Sexuality M:26:S:8 +1 '489-(57) 9:3:20
Schizoid

Three days before admission this young man had visited a roadhouse with several friends. There he became drunk, left the party, and walked to his brother-in-law's farm. After arriving he went into the barn, had intercourse with a cow, and caused the death of three other cows by inserting a pitchfork handle into their vaginas. Taken into custody, he confessed but claimed he was so drunk he had no knowledge of his acts.

The past history for this man was obscure. After completion of the eighth grade he had worked at various jobs until he enlisted in the army. It was possible that while in the army he had contracted a venereal disease. After severe combat experience he had been discharged, only a week before the present episode. People thought of him as shy and retiring, and some regarded him as intellectually slow. Even before his army years, he had been promiscuous. He had planned to be married in a few months. Nothing was known of the girl.

On admission to the hospital the man seemed bewildered about what was happening to him but was composed and answered most questions quickly and logically, although sometimes he refused to answer or was evasive. Outwardly he showed no signs of nervousness or tension and, in general, was somewhat apathetic. He completely lacked real insight into his motivations. He mingled freely with the other patients. One day he mentioned to a nurse that he had proposed to his girl friend on the night of the trouble and had been refused. This he had never told to anyone else, and it explained in part the difficulty experienced in attempting to work with him. There was no evidence of a gross personality disturbance other than the episode just before admission. The patient was returned to the custody of the sheriff.

B. Psth., Asocial M:21:D 4891'367-(53) 2:11:11
Mutilative

This youth, in company with another prison inmate, had used a dirk knife to sever his Achilles' tendon. Except for this mutilation he had a good conduct record. Along with his companion he was transferred to the psychopathic ward for observation.

First arrested at the age of 14 as a runaway from home, he was returned to his parents by probation officers. In a few days he was picked up for possession of a stolen automobile; he was released after being held for thirty days. Next he appeared in court on a charge of car theft. He was then given four years' probation for violation of the Dyer Act. Placed in a county welfare home, he soon escaped but was apprehended for larceny of a motor vehicle and charged as a parole violator. Given a three-year sentence to an industrial school for boys, he attempted to escape from this institution but was caught and served out the sentence. Before his commitment to the state penitentiary (the present sentence), he was arrested for suspected violation of the Selective Service Act, and later he was picked up for being drunk and disorderly. For the latter he was given a two-month jail sentence. His present two-year sentence is for theft. He had entered a rooming house under the pretense of obtaining a room and later he had removed therefrom a radio valued at $125, which he had then sold to an unknown person for $5.

The records indicate that the inmate's parents had separated when he was a child. Both had remarried since. He was reared by his mother and his stepfather. His mother, now about 40, is a high school graduate and in good health. She was formerly the manager of a drive-in stand; her present occupation is unknown. At the time of the prisoner's last contact with his stepfather, he was making a "pretty good living." The patient has a brother, who is at the present time thought to be employed as a lineman. His sister's present address is unknown. She had been arrested at least once for "staying out too late nights."

The inmate's former wife had been married twice previously and had two children. They were divorced because they "quarreled all the time." He had left school at age 12 after completing the fourth grade. He said that he quit school when he ran away from home because of his stepfather.

The prison psychiatrist described him as having an "inadequate personality with a history of maladjustment in early life, and many disciplinary disturbances." His recent behavior is definitely that of a psychopath with low mentality. No hallucinations or delusions were detected. His power and judgment are faulty. He obviously will never adjust to any of the prison work units.

R. C. K.

B. Psth., Asocial F:21:S:37 +4 '4<u>89</u>2–(74) 9:4:18
Epilepsy

The patient was admitted to the hospital because of recurrent "fainting spells" and behavior disturbances characterized by irresponsibility, bad manners, an unkempt appearance, and drunkenness. When at age 16 she first began to experience the fainting spells, characterized by a loss of consciousness and falling, they more or less coincided with the menses, but they had since become more frequent. The patient denied any knowledge of the nature of the attacks, but she described an occasional aura-like sensation of "spinning around" preceding an attack, and after a seizure she found it necessary to "sleep it off." She said she had had no "spells" during the nine months before admission. After her discharge from the WAC with a diagnosis of idiopathic epilepsy, she enrolled in a university where her behavior aberrations brought her to the attention of the state Vocational Rehabilitation Agency, which referred her to the hospital for study.

Her past history included a severe blow on the head at age 12. The personality deviations had not set in until two years after the accident, and she was said to have been a delightful and charming child up to the age of 10 or 12 years. She had undergone an appendectomy and an operation for an ovarian cyst, and she had been troubled with dysmenorrhea and menorrhagia. After the patient had graduated from high school she had been a government clerk until joining the WAC.

Although in the hospital she was well oriented and intact in sensorium and intellect, she was apathetic about her illness and about the difficulties her behavior created, and she was inclined to falsify facts about her life and about her ward behavior. Her cooperation was superficial and seemingly insincere. Soon after admission she was observed in a typical epileptic seizure, and she was placed on medication. With regard to her irresponsibility and her antagonistic attitudes, she was unapproachable psychotherapeutically, and she demonstrated almost no ability to recognize her problem. It was felt that much of her behavior was unacceptable more to her parents than to society, and the extent of her misbehavior never became entirely clear. It was evident that her attempts to go to college, encouraged by her parents, were inconsistent with her intellectual level, which was little above average. It seemed that under the stress of being pressed to overachievement, and of having idiopathic epilepsy, she was resorting to infantile behavior.

B. Psth., Asocial M:38:S:15 +3 4′8923–(45) 5:10:11

Three months before admission the patient, who was a university student at the time, committed the first in a series of three robberies. He was caught during the third robbery when he drove into a police trap. He surrendered and pleaded guilty to his thefts of that evening and the earlier ones as well.

While in the navy he had been hospitalized for a fractured jaw and a severe head injury, which he said had resulted from an accident. Following his discharge from the navy he had osteomyelitis of the jaw; since in the medical records there was no history of any accident it appeared that the trauma had been incurred in a fight. A month after the first of his robberies he had again suffered a fracture of the jaw, which this time he blamed on a skating accident. He stayed in a hospital for a few days and then signed out against advice.

The patient was very high in college aptitude but had completed only the tenth grade before his admission to the university by special examination. He had successfully completed two quarters of engineering before the present problems arose. His mother said that he had occasionally been depressed and irritable but that she had noted nothing otherwise unusual in his behavior. In the navy he had been in extensive combat. His naval conduct rating was good, indicating that he had committed no misdemeanors that came to official attention.

In the hospital the physical and neurological examinations were essentially normal. The patient was entirely oriented and showed no abnormalities of sensorium, intellect, or mental content. He exhibited no unusual emotional reactions. Well adjusted to his environment, he cooperated fully and seemed to be psychologically intact except for a lack of deeper affect. He was much concerned about returning to school and continuing his education. In a way he had good insight; however, the staff did not feel that this insight was indicative of any effectual adjustment of his momentary tendencies to long-time goals. He was returned to the custody of the police with the recommendation that he be institutionalized, at least for a period. The prognosis was at best doubtful.

B. Psth., Asocial	F:19:S:31	+1	489'263 17–(55)	4:8:22
		+26	496'87–(49)	4:6:19

Apparently until the age of 17 the patient had been an exemplary girl. At that time her parents objected to the new friends she was making, considering them a bad influence on her. The girl then became secretive about her movements. She was sent to a convent school but felt inferior to the other girls and continued to see persons who were objectionable to her parents. She became pregnant after leaving the convent and was eventually picked up by the police at a hotel where she was rooming with a man. After the child was born the patient stayed with it for about six weeks; then she disappeared and was next caught forging her mother's name to checks. She was treated for gonorrhea during the time she was held by the police on this charge. There were other events similar to these. She was finally sent to the hospital for evaluation under a charge of falsification of identity.

Her past medical history disclosed that she had been sick at age 8 with what her mother called "rheumatism of the brain." This illness could not be clearly defined, but there apparently had been a hysterical factor in it. It was said, for example, that she could see only one object in her visual field at any one time. She was somewhat above average in intelligence. She was described as always having been impulsive. She had been the leader of a Girl Scout troop and had liked basketball and other sports.

In the hospital she was well oriented, coherent, and logical. She resented being brought in and blamed her mother for it. She could see no reason why her behavior should concern other people and apparently felt no sense of wrongdoing for any of her actions. Cheerful and friendly, she mixed well with the other patients. She was superficially concerned about what might happen to her, but at no time could any useful rapport be established. She was completely unreliable in what she said. She was discharged after preparation had been made for a period of probation and follow-up studies by the social service.

B. Psth., Path. Sexuality	M:64:M:6	+3	4'89̲37–(71)	1:3:12

Admitted on a court order for observation after he had been charged with taking indecent liberties with a child, the patient confessed that during the preceding year he had indulged in similar activities with six other small girls, chiefly by fingering their genitals and encouraging the children to handle his.

Apparently he had engaged in sexual misbehavior throughout his adult life; on the records there was a 45-year history of aberrant sexual behavior beginning with "window peeping." After four arrests on such charges, he had been committed to a state hospital for approximately a month. About ten years before admission he had again been caught window peeping and at that time had admitted sex play with a 10-year-old girl. Knowing he had syphilis, he had infected his first wife. He had also contracted gonorrhea.

A high school graduate, he had set up and successfully operated a small business. Socially he had always made a good impression, and he had engaged in many constructive and acceptable enterprises, including the Boy Scout and Y.M.C.A. movements. He had many hobbies and interests. Although his second wife had little sex drive after the menopause, their marriage was happy and compatible. They had no children.

On admission there was no positive evidence of an active venereal disease. Well composed, he was indifferent and complacent about his conduct and its consequences; he did not believe he had experienced any abnormal urges but rather that he had "fallen to the temptation of normal urges presented by God," and therefore he thought his case rested in God's hands. Although there was a possibility of early organic senile changes, he was intact and sound in intellect. He was also cooperative and overly anxious to behave correctly. Since no progress could be made with the problem of re-training and treating him, it was finally recommended that he be considered a sexual psychopath under the law governing such cases.

B. Pri., Child. F:14:S:73 +1 4′8937–(51) 5:6:18
B. Psth., Asocial

The patient's problems began a year before admission when she was seduced by a family friend whose children she was caring for. Under the threat of informing her boy friend of their intimacy, this man had sexual relations with her twice during the following month. Three months later she was found lying in a snow bank, and as a ruse to explain a possible pregnancy, she claimed she had been attacked by a stranger in an automobile but had managed to escape. During this period she became less tolerant of criticism. Later she also had sexual relations with a young man she had just been introduced to. Still later she was picked up by the police and was found to have syphilis, for which she was treated. Placed on parole in the custody of her parents, she broke parole a month before admission and was sexually intimate with one of her companions. Eventually she was again arrested by the police and was sent to the hospital.

There were no past psychological disturbances. She had lived with foster parents all her life, her real parents having died when she was 2 months old. In school she had completed the sixth grade; though she was of average intelligence she had had to repeat the second grade. After discovery of the syphilis she had not been permitted to return to school. She made friends easily, got along with others, and was self-confident, but she was careless with money and had a tendency to lose track of time. Quick-tempered, she did not hold a grudge. Her foster parents had taken her brother to live with them at the same time they had taken the patient. She had other siblings, but nothing was known of them except that one of her sisters had been apprehended for sexual misbehavior much like the patient's. The foster parents had treated the patient as their own child and had provided a comfortable home.

In the hospital she had a positive serological reaction for syphilis and treatment was given. There were no contributory physical or neurological findings. She was well oriented, mature beyond her years, and fearful that she might be sent to a reform school. She got along with other patients and with the staff. She was much interested in art and drawing, at which she showed great proficiency. On the surface she was emotionally stable, but she was indifferent toward her general behavior, and on the whole she was little concerned about what people thought of her. She was discharged to the court for disposition with a generally unfavorable prognosis.

Ps. M-D., Depr.	F:20:S:40	+11	489376'21-(47)	2:10:18
Schizoid		+36	'38149-(51)	1:5:10
Paranoid				

This young woman's illness began about two months before admission with complaints of fatigue and headaches. At that time she was living in a college dormitory because of strained relations at home. She finally became so weak and tired that she left school and returned to live with her parents. A little later she became agitated and irrational, talked of her "sins," and was depressed. Two days before admission she refused to come downstairs to dinner and showed extreme resentment when her father attempted to comfort her. Later she stuffed a bar of soap into her mouth and it took the combined efforts of three people to dislodge it. She was negativistic, closed her eyes, and refused to speak. At this time she was admitted to the psychiatric unit.

The patient's general health had never been good. Her physical ills included severe asthma, difficulties during menstrual periods, and dermatitis. Three years earlier she had been referred to a psychiatrist in an attempt to relieve her of allergies. For two years she had been under his care, but the allergies remained much the same. She had many depressed and moody spells as well as periods of overactivity. Although never a social success, she had not been entirely inactive socially, having been president of one or two student clubs. The year before admission had been a hectic one, however. Not only did she lose interest in social activities but she was so negligent in her schoolwork that she received incompletes and failures in all her courses. A perfectionist, she strove always to get to the "bottom of things." She was devout and belonged to a minor religious cult. Interested in people, she nevertheless had extreme difficulty in making close friends because of her aloofness and sensitivity. She was narcissistic and dependent. At the time of admission she was engaged to a man but was not concerned about when they would be married.

In the hospital she was negativistic at first—she stared at the interviewer and made no responses. After a few days she began to talk. Being in a mental hospital was a source of disturbance to her. She worried about "the hurt my father must be feeling." Full of profound thoughts, which she expressed freely, she tended to jump from one idea to another without elaborating any one. She was well oriented and mentally alert. Tests indicated an I.Q. of 118. After a week she was much better organized in her thinking but was bothered by severe asthmatic attacks and depressive spells. There were frequent relapses into mutism and manifest paranoid ideas. A month later she was given three electroshock treatments which seemed to help considerably. At the time of discharge she was much improved, and it was felt that she would probably continue to recover from the present attack, although the long-range prognosis was not good.

B. Simple Adult Maladj. F:18:S:57 +16 4'89̲6̲– 2:6:13

Ever since she was a little girl the patient had been a behavior problem. She had always been unable to get along with children of her own age, preferring the company of younger children. She was undependable and almost continually disobedient. After her mother's death two years before admission she had been placed in various boarding homes, but in each instance the foster parents became so disgusted with her that they refused to keep her. She often used physical complaints to keep from having to take examinations at school. She was careless with money, she neglected her personal appearance, and her behavior showed no restraint even when she was in public.

In high school, where she was a senior at the time of admission, she was inconsiderate of the feelings of others. She told many lies and had not been averse to stealing from her mother at times. She had considerable energy for such activities as hiking or horseback riding, but housework was so distasteful to her that she refused to do it. She had made no friendships with boys and only one of possible significance with a girl friend younger than she. Her mother had died suddenly, and her father, a considerate, patient, and helpful person, had tried to take care of his daughter. An older brother, an epileptic, had died when the patient was much younger.

The patient was an unprepossessing, ungainly girl with a somewhat masculine build. Her teeth were carious. She assumed that her hospitalization was prompted entirely by her frequent disobedient acts, and she accused her classmates in high school of being mean and unreasonable. She spoke of liking to spend money foolishly. She had an I.Q. in the average range, but she was emotionally immature. She frequently said, "I know it is wrong to do such things, but I seem unable to resist temptation." Although her answers to questions were relevant and coherent, she was reticent in discussing her personal problems. She got along fairly well on the ward, although her table manners were noticeably defective and she was impulsive, loud, and untidy. At times she had precipitate vomiting after meals. As she continued in the hospital her behavior improved somewhat, and she managed to absorb a few of the social amenities. On discharge she went to live with her aunt, but since her supervision would probably continue to be inadequate the outlook was precarious.

B. Psth., Path. Emot. F:24:S:51 +5 4'896–2 5:4:21

From the time the patient was 3 or 4 years old, her parents had noticed that she had a tendency toward instability and always liked to have her own way. When thwarted she would fly into tantrums; on one occasion she had broken the car windows with a flashlight during an argument. Another time she had come home tired, and because her father did not immediately answer a question she asked, she had thrown dirty water on him. On two occasions her mother had called the police to settle arguments; the second time the patient was referred to the hospital.

The patient had had an attack of poliomyelitis when she was 13 years of age; this disease had left a residual weakness of the thigh so that she had to wear a brace a good part of the time. Because of this handicap she had been refused admission to several business schools and had allegedly lost at least one job. A fair student, she had finished high school and after that had worked at various jobs. Her vocational ambitions were numerous; at one time she had wanted to be a doctor, later a medical technician, and more recently a secretary, but she had never been steady at work or study. Never self-sufficient, she had had to live with her parents. A cheerful person, she made friends easily. Her most obvious abnormal tendencies were directed toward her parents. Her father, an ineffectual person who had been unable to hold a steady job, was content to live with relatives and was completely dominated by his wife. The patient was an only child. The three frequently quarreled among themselves.

On admission the patient was not worried about her confinement, although she did show some concern about what her friends would think. She had fair insight. Cheerful although somewhat evasive in manner, she cooperated well in all ways and showed none of the behavior that had led to her admission. Arrangements were made for her to go to a business school at state expense, and it was recommended that she live away from home. The prognosis was considered to be good.

B. Pri., Child. F:14:S:12 —9 4896'271–X(57) 8:19:18
Twin

The patient's present illness was of long standing. She first began "running away" at age 11 when she was living at a county home school for girls. At that time she gave the excuse that the officials were too strict and she wanted to be with her twin sister. She was then sent to a private correctional school with her twin. Apparently her conduct there was satisfactory. Thirteen months before her present admission she was sent home to live with her mother and stepfather. She got along well for a while, but then her mother became more strict, she said, and refused to let her go out evenings as frequently as she wanted to. Her mother, she complained, also "tried to pick my friends for me" and made many false accusations about the girl's father. This led to friction and the patient began to stay away from home more and more. She met a number of boys who, she said, offered her marriage. At one time she was found living in the home of one of these boy friends.

The patient's past physical and psychological histories were otherwise relatively negative. Her intelligence was about average, and her school history was not helpful since it had been irregular because of factors beyond her control. During the past year she had become interested in boys older than herself and had stayed out late no matter what the consequences. She was not an aggressive person and appeared shy and self-conscious. She described herself as usually being happy and said that she was most relaxed when she was out with her friends. Her parents had been divorced when she was 6 years old. Her mother had worked as a bartender and waitress and had later remarried. Apparently the mother drank a considerable amount of alcohol and the patient had seen her drunk on many occasions.

In the hospital the patient was shy and self-conscious, fidgeted about, and seemed reluctant to answer questions. She blushed when asked about her conduct. She admitted that most of her difficulties arose from her uncontrollable desire to be with her friends; she blamed no one else for her problems but apparently was wholly unable to make a realistic attempt to change. She said that when she was released from the hospital she would go to live with her mother and thought she could get along with her. This statement was made in spite of much evidence to the contrary. She made friends with other patients and for the most part got along well with them, but the friendships were superficial and there was no evidence that the patient made any real attempt to behave better or to form deeper attachments. She broke hospital rules almost deliberately. She was discharged to go to a state correctional school.

B. Psth., Asocial M:25:S:8 +9 4<u>89</u>76'2-1 1:10:9

The patient had a long history of stealing dating from the age of 5, and as he grew older this tendency resulted in numerous incarcerations. Just before admission to the hospital he had broken a seven-month parole from a reformatory for men. At age 16 he had been convicted of car stealing, and shortly after his release from the reform school he had stolen another car. There were many similar incidents. Because of a history of numerous head injuries, he was sent to the hospital for investigation of possible brain damage as the basis for his "kleptomania."

At the age of 2 he had been unconscious for several days after landing on his head in a fall from a high chair. When he was 7 years old he had fallen from a tree, again hitting his head. At age 21 he had been unconscious for about eighteen hours with a persisting paralysis, as the result of a football injury. He also had a history of recurrent fainting spells, which were, however, not accompanied by convulsive seizures.

After graduation from high school the patient had attended a religious school for two years, but he had left when he got into some difficulty with the faculty. His ability was apparently superior and he had always shown good judgment. Both before and after his recent misbehavior he had been active in athletics. Since the beginning of his difficulties he had been very secretive, especially with his parents and had revealed only the things he wanted to. His self-assurance was very great, and he had a high opinion of his own abilities. He had a total disregard for the rules and regulations laid down by society; he said, "I feel I can have anything I wish to have. Why should anyone stop me?" On the other hand, he had always been meticulous in fulfilling his duties at home. Generally he had been cheerful and stable emotionally.

In the hospital the physical and neurological examinations were entirely negative. He was reluctant to talk, indifferent about his future, calm and composed. He spoke without emotion about his experiences and was indifferent to the fact that he would probably be sent back to the reformatory, but tears did come to his eyes when he realized that prison would separate him from his newly acquired fiancée. There was no such display of emotion when he spoke of the sacrifices his parents had made to protect him from the effects of his offenses. The patient recognized that he should not do the things he did, but he said that he was unable to restrain himself; he believed he acted as he did because there was something wrong with him. In other ways his attitude and his manner were relatively conventional, and he was cooperative, open, and normal on the ward. No evidence was produced to indicate that his aberrant behavior dated from the football accident, and it was felt that the patient had probably been markedly maladjusted over a period of many years.

B. Psth., Asocial M:20:S:10 +1 '49–1267 (41) 4:6:16

This youth's father signed a court order requesting that his son's psychiatric condition be studied in spite of the denial by the patient and his mother of any need for such investigation. The mother admitted the young man had lost weight, had shown irritability, and had begun to make threats against people, but he never carried out the threats or meant to do so, she claimed. She also admitted that he had been involved in drunken riots and had behaved aggressively toward people. She related this behavior to his army experience. Two years before admission he had been discharged from the army because of "nervousness," according to his mother's story. Several months later he was arrested for being involved in a drunken riot. Later he was again arrested for drinking and was put on probation for a year. At that time he began to go out with a girl of 19, against his father's wishes. The patient spent considerable time at the girl's home, often when her parents were not there. Later the couple obtained a marriage license and the girl lied about her age, which, it turned out, was only 14. The patient's mother then asked that the police get the marriage license back from the couple. The young man was arrested for contributing to the delinquency of a minor, but no action had been taken at the time he was hospitalized.

The youth's history was essentially noncontributory before his entrance into the army. There were no past psychological difficulties. In school he had had no trouble with his studies or conduct and had completed the eleventh grade. When he returned from the army and went back to school, he was soon expelled, supposedly because he could not get along with the teachers. Next he went from job to job, giving vague reasons for leaving each. Although he seemed to have no close friends (except his girl friend), he was not obviously asocial. During the course of the present illness he had been completely unreliable, falsifying and in general behaving with no reference to the consequences.

In the hospital the youth was well oriented but agitated. In intelligence he tested above average. He kept his aggression on the verbal level but was boastful and threatening. He was emotionally labile, though the variations in his affect were always minimal, and the affect seemed shallow. There was no deep-seated feeling, animosity or love, toward either of his parents. Indignant that his "character was being examined," he seemed fearful of the outcome and vehemently insisted that he was "completely normal in all ways." It was felt that his emphasis of this statement indicated overcompensation. As time went on, he calmed down to some extent but was always on the verge of an outburst. He was somewhat antisocial and assumed a haughty, self-righteous attitude on the ward. Throughout his hospitalization he continued to make demands for special treatment. No real rapport could be established with him and he was basically little changed on discharge. The pattern indicated a poor prognosis.

B. Psth., Asocial M:35:M:5 +1 4'9–26(47) 4:3:16

The patient was brought into court on a bigamy charge. His second wife, while planning to sue for divorce on charges of nonsupport, had found that her supposed husband had never been divorced from his first wife. The patient asserted that his first wife had informed him he was divorced, but the court sentenced him to serve an indefinite time in prison. The sentence was suspended on condition that he discontinue seeing his second wife, but immediately after his release, a probation officer found him at her home. The man was referred from the jail for psychiatric study.

The past medical history was essentially negative except for the fact that he had been rejected for military service because of a peptic ulcer and an exophthalmic goiter. He had been irregular in school attendance, but he had completed the eighth grade. Although he had held various jobs as a skilled workman, he had frequently been absent from work, had saved nothing, and had contributed very little to the support of either of his wives. He had a police record for delinquency, truancy, and petty larceny. Of average intelligence, he was described as moody, restless, glum, and inclined to tell falsehoods, often without an apparent reason. Outwardly, however, he appeared to be happy-go-lucky. He was a good conversationalist, interested in athletics, and an avid reader of comic books.

In the hospital he showed considerable anxiety about being in a psychiatric unit because he feared his sanity was in doubt. He was cooperative, at ease, well oriented, and intact in sensorium and intellect, but he had no insight into the social meaning of his behavior, and his explanation for his actions was inconsistent and full of falsifications. In appearance he was apprehensive, anxious, and aggressive, and in conversation he was overly voluble. His hospitalization was disturbing to the other patients. He associated with women patients against the doctors' orders and enjoyed telling his problems to anyone who would listen, but he insisted that he "had learned his lesson" and that if he got out of this mess he "would never get mixed up again." When he was discharged back to the custody of the court, the prognosis for his aberrant social behavior was considered poor.

B. Pri., Child. M:15:S:23 +1 '49–2817 (53) 1:1:11

Some time before admission the patient had returned to his own home after living for several months with a favorite uncle. He hated his home because of its poverty; in addition he was disturbed because his girl friend had been going out with other boys while he had been away. He soon lost interest in his studies and began missing classes. Two months before admission he and two friends were job hunting when a strange man invited him to a room to discuss a job. This man began rubbing the patient's genitals but when he made further advances the boy fled. Disgusted about this experience, the patient broke into a schoolhouse that night and stole some things. A week later he broke into a filling station and was caught.

The boy had been frequently ill as a child; particularly when he was very young he had frequent sore throats and colds. Because of the family's poverty his parents had sent him to live with relatives during several of his long bouts of illness. In general the boy's misbehavior had increased whenever he had had to live at home. He was a friendly person and at least in the last few years had had many friends. Superior in intelligence, he hoped to go to college. His father had been sent to jail for forgery about six months before the boy's admission to the hospital.

In the hospital he was intelligent and cooperative and no abnormal mental content or bizarre behavior was noted. There was a manifest conflict between feeling loyal toward his parents and being ashamed of them. He had a desire for money and wanted to be successful. He was worried about the possibility that he might be sent to a correctional institution. He seemed to come to understand his problems much better during his stay in the hospital and at the time of discharge, it was arranged that he should live with his grandmother. It was likely that he would make a good adjustment and have no further trouble.

Alcoholism	M:49:D:24	+4	4′9–6378 12	3:2:15
		+17	′491–673	3:3:17

For the past two years the patient had frequently exposed himself when he was drunk, had been involved in street brawls, and while under the influence of liquor had spoken to young girls and women with whom he was not acquainted. His usual drink was beer, sometimes supplemented with whiskey, and he drank with his friends as long as he had the money.

After he had finished the junior year of high school he had joined the army. He had begun drinking at age 18 after his term of enlistment expired. He had left home at 20, wandering all over the country doing odd jobs, finally joining the Canadian army for overseas duty. Later he had re-entered the United States army, where he had remained until about a year before admission. He had got along fairly well in the army but had never been promoted. He was not ambitious, was always active and boisterous, and never assumed any responsibilities or obligations. Married for a few months, he had been divorced by his wife for his unreliability and his excessive drinking.

In the hospital the neurological and physical examinations were noncontributory. He believed that he had been used as a scapegoat by the judge and that his conviction might have been brought about by "gossiping women." He boastfully talked of his drinking ability, his sexual experiences, and his fighting power. He was indifferent about his admission to the hospital, saying, "The food and beds are much better than in jail." Verbose and somewhat circumstantial, he was, however, friendly and cooperative, although he tried to take charge of the activities of the younger patients. When he was transferred back to the county jail, few recommendations were made since the modification of a pattern of such long standing seemed improbable.

B. Psth., Asocial	M:30:M:12	+3	49′–673	1:5:16

This man had pleaded guilty in district court to a charge of forgery, having cashed checks totaling $100. Through his father's influence he was transferred to the psychopathic ward for investigation.

The history included no episodes of a psychological or neurotic character. He had reached the twelfth grade and had done average schoolwork, but even as a small boy he had been a problem to his family. This misbehavior began with lying, petty thievery, and running away from home. As he grew older he began to charge merchandise to his father and to borrow money in his father's name. Never settling down to steady employment, he worked periodically at such jobs as auto racing, stunting, and parachute jumping. Three years before admission he served ninety days in jail for petty larceny. Numerous other times he had escaped jail sentences because of his father's influence. Although he earned good money at his spectacular feats at fairs and other shows, his associates stole or borrowed so much that he seldom had any left. He married and soon after a child was born, his wife left him. They were not, however, divorced. A year later he married again, committing bigamy. He lived with this wife for only a few weeks and, later, he admitted paternity of a child by a third woman to whom he was not married. The patient came from a respectable family of good financial means and social standing. His father had come to believe that his son must be suffering from some mental disorder and had, therefore, requested hospitalization.

On admission the patient showed no distortions of mental content. He was aware of the reason for his presence in the hospital. Claiming to have no objection to the investigation, he vividly described many of his brushes with the law. Of the social implications behind his acts he showed no recognition. Tests indicated he was somewhat above average in intelligence. His talk was glib and boastful, and much of his conversation was objectionable to other patients. At first adaptable and cooperative, he later became sullen at ward restrictions. He would, he felt, be able to conform to acceptable standards in the future. He was somewhat philosophical about the impending prison sentence. He was discharged back to the court with a report indicating a poor prognosis. The court paroled him at the recommendation of his father.

B. Psth., Asocial M:39:M:33 +6 4'9138– 9:2:24

Admitted on a court order, the patient was accused of cruelty and neglect toward his wife and family. For the past three and a half years the county welfare board had been concerned with the case because of repeated reports of physical violence by the patient toward his wife and children. Three years before admission he had been given a ninety-day sentence for beating his 2-year-old child over the head with a board. His wife admitted that he often struck her and their oldest girl, but she was so afraid of him that she would not report him. The situation dragged on, and eventually the patient lost his W.P.A. job and thereafter did little work because of "abdominal pain." One day when a social worker called at the home, the patient lost his temper and made unreasonable demands for relief. In the last few months the children had had numerous abrasions and contusions, but these were always assigned by the parents to natural causes.

The family physician described the patient as "vicious, unstable, and stupid." As a child he had engaged in petty thievery. Once convicted of burglary, he was sent to a reformatory. He left school at age 16 after getting to the sixth grade. His I.Q. was about 97. He was thought by some to be a good worker but hard to get along with. When angry he usually worked harder. He was occasionally cruel to animals. Persons of his general type apparently were numerous in his family history. His wife was found to have an I.Q. of 56 and was demonstrably incapable of managing her home and children. There were six children and the wife was pregnant at the time of the patient's admission. The family had lived in a succession of small houses and rooms, all "hardly fit for occupation," according to the welfare board.

In the hospital the patient said, "I feel fine. The pains in my stomach, on the left side, are gone. I have no worries." He thought that a minor operation performed on him had "remade" him and that he was a "changed man." When asked about his treatment of his wife and children, he said, "I love my wife and kids. I don't want to hurt them. When the kids don't mind they should be trimmed." He denied having ever been cruel. About the welfare board he said, "They've done well by us, but they don't always keep their promises." Composed, affable, and pleasant, he was entirely cooperative during this hospitalization. He felt he had "no mental trouble"; nevertheless he was willing to stay in the hospital for observation. He spent his time in reading, occupational therapy, and playing games. He had no physical complaints and frequently said that he was eager to go home and work. Social agencies were consulted and plans were made to straighten out the family situation. It was recommended that the wife be sterilized, and attempts were to be made to remove the children from the home.

B. Psth., Asocial M:38:D 492'3671-(51) 4:12:10
Mutilative
Drug Add.
Alcoholism

This prisoner was referred for observation because of self-mutilation, including the severing of his right Achilles' tendon, and suspected use of benzedrine.

His parents having separated when he was 7 and divorced when he was 8, he was reared by his mother and grandmother. His father had been an excessive drinker. Following the divorce his mother worked as a domestic to support herself and her two sons. He claimed to have completed the seventh grade. On a standardized test he earned a grade placement of 8.5 and showed an I.Q. of 88. The man's own story was that he started the "use of drugs at the age of 18 because of worry." A social agency reported that the family had been known to them for years; contact had begun with treatment for an insane brother. The prisoner's longest employment was for twenty months as a common laborer. His mother stated that he "didn't stay at one job long."

As to his criminal record, the prisoner said that when he was 14 years of age he began stealing cars, and because his maternal uncle was the juvenile judge, he was placed on probation seven or eight times. He estimated that he had been arrested fifty times, with jail sentences ranging from sixty to ninety days in six cities. The charges included vagrancy, drunkenness, fighting, disturbing the peace, petty larceny, and possession of narcotics. His arrest and commitment history contained 27 entries. At the age of 22, he received his first prison sentence, a one-year commitment to the federal prison. At 27 he was again sentenced to a federal prison. Seven years later he was found guilty of grand larceny and was given a five-year sentence. With six others, he escaped by "mugging a guard," but all the prisoners were caught four hours later. Two years afterward he escaped again by slipping away from a work squad.

Now serving a fourteen-year sentence for assault with intent to murder in connection with robbing a pawn shop, the man is considered dangerous and a constant source of trouble to prison authorities. In spite of repeated warnings, he loafs on the job; he has been placed in isolation for conspiring with another inmate to attack a common enemy; and he is frequently transferred to a new job for disciplinary reasons. In addition he has made home-brew in his cell and has been punished for loud talking in the mess hall and for refusing to work.

An escapee from another state penitentiary and wanted in still a third state, this defendant, officials strongly urge, should be given no consideration in respect to parole. It has been recommended that he serve his entire time and then be released to the authorities of one of the two other states.

The diagnosis is "a definite psychopath with hypomanic trends." He shows some effects of drug addiction and the excessive use of alcohol, but no impairment of his mental faculties. The conclusion is that a man of his age and long-established habits will in all probability continue to be a problem to himself and to society, whether in or out of prison. R. C. K.

B. Psth., Asocial M:30:D 4′9237–(55) 4:6:19
Mutilative

This prisoner was referred to the psychopathic ward because of his participation in two mutinies and his self-mutilation by cutting off the end of the little finger on his left hand.

An only child, he lived with his parents until he ran away from home at the age of 16. Although he attended school only until the end of the ninth grade, his grade placement score on tests was 11.0. His I.Q. was 92. The prisoner lived with a common-law wife for three years and had one son by this union. Later he married but his wife is now suing for a divorce. His only employment was with carnivals traveling over the country. The prisoner was discharged "not honorably" from the army. His first arrest, when he was 20, was for petty larceny, and he received a five-month jail sentence. Since then his records show sixteen convictions, for forgery, burglary, vagrancy, and violation of the Selective Service Act. The present incarceration is for forgery, a four-year sentence, and he has three detainers against him.

When interviewed, this man showed no mental conflict and no loss of contact with reality. He was frank in expressing his resentments toward the officials of the prison, and he blamed them vehemently for the "deplorable conditions on the farm, dirty sleeping quarters, and unsavory food." He said that the intimates drew lots to see who would mutilate himself in order to call attention to these conditions and, since he drew the agreed number, he immediately cut off the end of his finger. After his recovery from the mutilation, he was placed on another prison farm and reports are that he is getting along well. R. C. K.

Alcoholism M:51:M:13 +2 '49318–(45) 5:2:23

The patient had been a chronic alcoholic for at least ten years. His latest drinking spree began a month before admission. Each night he came home from work drunk, surly, and assaultive toward his family. His business lagged, his friends and family became more and more antagonistic to him, and he was finally persuaded to come to the hospital for treatment. His excuse for the latest difficulty was a vague, pleuritic pain, which he felt alcohol would relieve.

Except for the drinking habit, his past history was not particularly relevant. There was one previous institutionalization for alcoholism. He had been an excellent student, graduating from high school and from a school of pharmacy with a high average. After he had failed in various business ventures he had finally joined his father in the operation of a drugstore. When his father's death had made it necessary for him to run the store alone he had begun to drink heavily. A friendly, thoughtful, gregarious person, he had a good general disposition, but he was overly sensitive to criticism. During a drinking episode he became a very different person. His wife believed him to be "oversexed," but with the exception of the gradually developing drinking problem the family was not too badly adjusted.

In the hospital the patient was unconcerned about his problems, feeling that symptomatic treatment was sufficient to bring a full recovery. He completely lacked any insight into the true seriousness of his condition. There was no evidence of an alcoholic neuritis. He was nervous and high-strung, but he was completely cooperative and pleasant. Although he answered questions rationally, he was difficult to draw out. The general picture he presented was that of a normal businessman, and it was only in reference to the history that an illness could be discovered.

B. Psth., Asocial M:34:D 49'326–1 (61) 2:7:12
Mutilative

This inmate was referred to the psychopathic ward because of repeated violations of prison rules, refusal to work, and self-mutilation by cutting off the end of his left little finger with an ax.

As a child, the prisoner lived with his parents at home until his mother was committed to a state hospital, where she later died. A sister and a brother of the prisoner are now in a state hospital. He completed the fifth grade in school. The man had three marital failures. His arrest history began when he was 19 years of age; since then he has served at least thirteen jail sentences and has escaped twice. Sentenced to a military prison during the war, he escaped seven times. He served two previous terms in a state penitentiary for burglary and bigamy. At present he is serving three and a half years in the penitentiary for swindling by check and has two detainers against him. A constant source of trouble within the prison walls, he has spent more than six hundred hours in solitary confinement for insubordination.

The prison psychiatrist diagnosed this man's case as "a psychopathic personality without psychosis, with emotional instability, irresponsibility, and poor life adjustment." The summary further stated, "His main interest in life seems to be a greedy, egotistical, self-satisfying effort to gain power and material wealth. He is incapable of fair-minded relationships, but rather he sees his fellow men as only a means to an end, a tool to satisfy his own selfish striving. Intellectually, he is probably capable of knowing right from wrong, but emotionally he has no desire or wish to distinguish the two. He will be honest and fair-minded only so long as this brings benefits to himself; once these benefits cease, he will gain them in any possible way. This man will be a menace to society if released and is likely to be a problem prisoner if retained in prison." R. C. K.

B. Psth., Path. Emot. M:47:M:20 +2 '4936–(73) 2:1:15

The patient had a long history of periodic bouts of excessive drinking, each of which, once started, he had been unable to stop. It was difficult to get a really complete history for the man. He had apparently had periods of relative freedom from alcohol. The most recent of these lasted three and a half years, during which he was actively associated with Alcoholics Anonymous. He drifted away from the organization, feeling that too great demands were made upon him, returned to drinking, and neglected his practice as a physician. He was admitted on a court order requested by his sister.

He had had a number of previous hospitalizations and contacts with the police because of alcoholism, and he had at one time been involved with the authorities over a presumed addiction to morphine. He had worked his way through medical school and had been a successful physician. He had taken little part in social life because of his devotion to his practice. Usually an affable, friendly person, he was easily irritated when things went against him. There was good evidence that he had been irresponsible toward his obligations to his wife and family. This recently had extended in part to his patients. He had a basic dependency on his family, however; he expected them to help him out of his difficulties and always had a ready excuse for what he did.

Apparently not deteriorated mentally, he was well oriented in the hospital.

He was defensive and evasive but his insight was relatively good and there was no disorder in mentation. During his stay in the hospital he showed gradual improvement. However, while he was superficially cooperative and normal in his behavior, no real progress could be made psychotherapeutically, and when he was discharged, the prognosis was definitely poor.

Ps. M-D., Manic Schizoid F:33:D:85 +4 49'3816– 7:2:23

About two months before admission, while she was ill with a stomach disorder, the patient became nervous and run-down and left her job. She spoke of having been hypnotized by a psychiatrist, talked about religion and sex, and apparently began to experience auditory hallucinations.

She had had two previous nervous breakdowns separated by about three years. Both were similar to the present one and had required hospitalization. After her high school graduation she had led a somewhat disorganized life. She studied dramatics, art, business, and other things, but never followed through in any line of work. A brief marriage was terminated in divorce. The actual work she did was mostly as nursemaid and housemaid; occasionally she did secretarial work. She appeared to be an energetic, active person, whose main difficulty was a lack of emotional control.

In the hospital she was tremendously concerned about religion, mysticism, psychology, and various cults, and she talked rapidly and at great length about them. Her speech showed a flight of ideas and there was a definitely bizarre content. Her sensorium was clear and she was apparently not experiencing hallucinations. She was friendly and cooperative for the most part, although she was emotionally labile. In time she calmed down and finally was able to return to her community. She had little insight and apparently her usual behavior at its best did not markedly differ from the milder periods of her illness.

B. Psth., Asocial Mutilative Drug Add. M:28:S 4'96–71 (57) 1:6:12

This prison inmate, a big man (5 feet 9 inches tall, weighing 309 pounds), purposely severed his left Achilles' tendon. The mutilation was his first violation of prison rules.

Reared in a large city, the prisoner and his brother had been well known to the probation department. His arrests began at the age of 17, with traffic violations first, later forgery, attempted murder, theft, assault and battery, larceny, and burglary. His present sentence is fifteen years for robbery.

4'9678–132

The man is a "stable psychopath" and an admitted user of benzedrine. Aggressive, he frequently displays temperamental hostilities toward the guards. He is sluggish, slovenly dressed, dirty, and careless about his toilet habits. The man's chief regret, after severing his tendon, was that it impaired his skill as a boxer. He has responded not at all to overtures of the administration in his behalf, and those in charge feel little hope for anything but trouble from this man, either in or out of prison. R. C. K.

Ps. Sz., Simple	F:18:S:54	—1	4'9678–132	2:4:12
Suicidal		+5	94'867–31	1:3:11

An inmate of a girls' reform school for about two years because of sexual delinquency, the patient was brought to the hospital because of suicidal threats, irritability, and general emotional instability. She was usually quiet but she had crushes on other girls and told vulgar stories. She was described as being silly, her moods were unstable, and she was considered a "tattletale." Her school progress had been extremely irregular. At times she had been on the honor roll, but in recent months the behavior had deteriorated. When she lost the privilege of attending an honor roll party, she smashed a window with her fist, telling a roommate that she was going to end it all. Failure to be appointed a nurse's assistant produced a severe temper outburst in which she became defiant and disagreeable. She spoke of suicide and removed the screen from her window as though to jump, because she "wanted to get away from everything."

Her sexual delinquency began at age 14, when she admitted having sexual relations with two men. Placed on probation, she violated it and finally was sent to the reform school. Her I.Q. was 108. Because she had never liked school she had frequently been a truant, but she was interested in school sports. When she was in one of her better moods she was very cooperative and pleasant, but she had always been childish and immature. The patient's family had been a community liability for many years, but her older married brother wanted the patient discharged from the school and placed in his home.

In the hospital the patient said that her truancy was due to her association with girls who did not like school. The first time she had contemplated suicide she had gone on a hunger strike, and she explained it by saying, "I wanted to try out something. I wanted to see how long it would take a person to starve." The second suicidal impulse had made her take off the window screen. In explanation this time she said, "I wanted to get away from everything. I got sick and tired of everything. I was tired of being locked up." Moderately depressed and pessimistic about the future, she thought her situation was hopeless, but she was not inclined to do anything to remedy it. Hospitalization represented a form of punishment to her. Uncooperative in interviews, she was slow in answering questions, and her stay in the hospital was marked by impulsiveness, irritability, mood variability, discouragement, and self-depreciation, in addition to several temper outbursts and other obvious emotional upsets. It was finally decided that the usual psychotherapeutic methods and facilities were of little value in this case since the disorders had a deep basis in the girl's personality. Recommendations about her parole were made, and she was sent back to the school for disposition.

Ps. M-D., Manic Paranoid M:31:D:56 +5 49'68-72(39) 3:8:12

The patient was transferred to this hospital from a state hospital, where a diagnosis of paranoid condition with an underlying psychopathic personality had been made during a ten-day hospitalization. The patient had made threats against various people, had struck a boy, and had kept guns in his car. Finally he had been arrested after he speeded in town through red lights, ran up on the curb across from the police station, and kicked on the door of the station. Later he claimed this had been to test the integrity of the police officials, who, he felt, were too lax. At this time he talked irrationally, repeated such statements as "I am not the second coming of Christ," and expressed ideas of reference.

One of six children, the patient was the favorite of his mother. The latter was an extremely unstable and inconsistent person. The children never knew whether to expect "a spanking or a piece of cake" when they came home from school. Cruel punishments were used, and once the mother attempted to throw the baby into the furnace, but was restrained by the other children. Such traumatic incidents were not uncommon throughout the patient's childhood. The father was described as usually being a timid, nonauthoritarian person. If he did try to discipline the children the mother flew into a rage. There were bitter quarrels between the parents and occasionally the father beat his wife.

The patient had been an active, aggressive child. Placed for a while in an orphanage, he finished the eighth grade there and then ran away. On his own, he went "on the bum" for many years. Eventually he entered a small business and was very successful. His first marriage lasted five years. It had never been a happy one, and a second marriage was being dissolved at the time of the hospitalization. The patient had a record of a series of arrests on minor charges from drunken driving to slapping his wife. Always an active person, he ate four or five meals a day, drank heavily, exercised vigorously. He belonged to many clubs. His sexual relations with his second wife had been infrequent and he denied any extramarital intercourse. Before marriage he had engaged in intercourse regularly beginning at the age of 13.

On entry the patient was superior in manner, supercilious, defensive, and frequently hostile and indirectly sarcastic. His speech was overproductive, and his flight of ideas had a paranoid coloring. Rationalizing all his difficulties, he claimed he had been "railroaded" into the hospital. There was a conspiracy against him, he believed, and he was eager to get out to fight it. He had no insight and denied that he was sick in any way. On the tenth day he ran away while out on pass and was returned by the sheriff of a nearby town. He then changed for the worse. He talked incessantly, paced, and kicked at the door. After five electroshock treatments he quieted down. His manner was superficially cooperative but faintly sullen. A sister who visited him at this time said he was "his old self again." Later the patient ran away again and appeared at his sister's home. Since he seemed to maintain his improvement he was discharged as recovered. A few weeks later he visited the hospital on his way through town. He still showed no insight into his illness and spoke of his belief that people had not helped him "as much as they might have." E. B.

B. Psth., Asocial M:16:S:9 +1 4'<u>96</u> <u>83</u>–(45) 3:7:16

This youth was sent to the hospital by authorities of a boys' training school for a personality evaluation. A disciplinary problem at the school, where he had been returned after violation of parole, he was said to be bellicose. He engaged in frequent fights, which he seemed to provoke systematically, and showed no tendency to alter his behavior pattern in response to the usual punishment for such transgressions. His repeated combativeness toward other boys encouraged the feeling that the boy might be psychotic. There was real danger of a mass retaliation by the other boys which would lead to the injury of the patient.

The boy's background included a series of foster homes. A continual disciplinary problem, he was first charged with truancy at age 9 after the death of his father. At age 13 he stole a car. Later, while on probation from the reform school, he threatened to use a gun during an argument with his sister. Still later he was apprehended for petty larceny. In and out of trouble, he had been moved here and there and his schooling had been exceedingly irregular. The boy's I.Q. was 96.

In the hospital he was concerned with his desire to become a free and independent adult. Minimizing all his misdeeds, he interpreted his acts as self-preservation rather than as transgressions against society. He denied any need for help and felt that he was entirely normal. His emotional tone was appropriate and there was little evidence of marked emotional instability while he was in the hospital. His behavior was good, he was cooperative, and he showed no peculiarities. His attempts to dominate group activities were not offensive. There was psychometric evidence that indicated a possible organic impairment but the physical and neurological examinations did not answer the question of whether or not there was some brain damage. An electroencephalogram was "borderline normal." The psychiatric staff made few pertinent contributions to the case, and he was returned to the school with general recommendations for practical methods of handling him.

B. Psth., Asocial F:16:S:18 +3 4'968<u>37</u>–(63) 2:2:23

The patient was admitted to the hospital because of nervousness, insomnia, emotional instability, and headaches. About a year before admission she developed a definite dislike for school and her friends. She became irritable and restless, lost her interest in sports, hobbies, and other activities, was a truant from school, and stayed out late at night. Her parents' attempts to change this pattern were unsuccessful and during her temper spells she threw things at them and threatened to leave home permanently. Placed in a hospital for three weeks, she seemed improved but gradually reverted to her former behavior. She made friends with undesirable people and frequently stayed out all night with boy friends. As a consequence of one wild party, she and several other youngsters were placed on court probation.

She had completed the tenth grade with average marks. Learning had been easy for her, and she had done well in school until the onset of the present pattern. She had held several part-time jobs but had given them up because they bored her. Always a nervous and somewhat high-strung person, she had been active, energetic, and interested in many things. Apparently she had always wanted to be the life of the party. From the time of puberty the opposite sex had held a great attraction for her. Formerly open and truthful toward her parents, she had become secretive and deceptive after the appearance of the present pattern. In general her home was a good one.

On first impression in the hospital she was composed and conventional, but she was emotionally unstable, very easily angered, unreasonably attracted to men, and absolutely undiscriminating in her friendships. She had no insight into the fact that her behavior was at all unusual. Her main interest was to gain the attention of men. She was not extremely difficult to control in spite of her deceitfulness and resistance. It was recommended that her parents change their methods of attempting to handle her, and it was felt that the return of her older brother to the family might help somewhat, but her prognosis was very poor.

B. Psth., Asocial   M:21:S   '497-1(43)   4:3:11
Mutilative
Drug Add.

This young man was referred to the psychopathic unit because of self-mutilation while in the state prison. He severed his right Achilles' tendon with a dirk knife.

Until the age of 5 the boy lived with both parents; then, following their divorce, he made his home with his father. After completing the ninth grade in school he worked at odd jobs in a café and, for a short time, as a truck driver. When he was 16 he joined the navy. He was given an "undesirable discharge" at 17 because of a conviction by civil authorities while absent without leave from the service. In this conviction he was committed to the state prison on a 25-year sentence for robbery, burglary, and assault with intent to murder.

The present offense was the prisoner's first arrest. His "within the walls" record is poor. Twice he has attempted to escape; he was charged once with mutiny; and he has been punished for refusing to work, impudence to a guard, and self-mutilation. The prison physician reported that the prisoner uses benzedrine, and the warden said that the youth is a homosexual.

An excerpt from the warden's report follows: "This man has more intelligence than most men in prison. He is very nice looking and a leader among the inmates. I have spent considerable time trying to analyze this mutilation case, which involves two other inmates at the farm. The case appeared a very complicated one at the time. The subject told me that his mother had given the assistant warden $35 to get him a good job in the kitchen. He stated that anyone with $25 could buy a good job. I wrote his mother and told her I would like to see and talk to her. She came and told me that she had never given an employee any money and the most she had ever sent the boy at one time was $2. She further stated that she was a poor woman and did not have the money to send if she wanted to. She told me that when the subject was a small child he would come home and tell colorful stories that were not true. The mother stated that her son was mentally irresponsible. After being in lock-up for some time, he gave a lot of information which proved to be untrue. This was done in an effort to gain sympathy and consideration at the expense of other inmates. He was brought before the disciplinary committee. While he was being considered, he was told of the information that his mother had given and as a result he was very abusive to his mother. This man is definitely a sex problem. He was known to force homosexual relations upon other inmates at the point of a knife. My prediction is that this man will build in the future a notorious crime record." R. C. K.

B. Psth., Path. Sexuality M:21:S:25 +5 '497-6X(57) 12:5:19

The history of this patient as given by his sister included unusual behavior suggestive of fetishism. She said that he kept articles of women's clothing secreted in his room. These appeared to have been stolen. She also said that he had taken these articles to bed with him, utilizing them in the practice of masturbation.

He had held a number of jobs and had been dismissed from all of them for incompetence or unreliability after only short periods of employment. He had been three times convicted of theft at ages 15, 17, and 19 and had been sent to a reform school on each occasion. He had had a severe attack of pneumonia at age 10 and there was some indication that the present illness was related to that attack. He was a first-generation son of Italian immigrants. His schooling had been much interrupted by the terms at the reform schools and by the pneumonia. He felt that he had always been unable to complete his share of family duties and had been "a nuisance" to his mother. He accused himself of making no serious effort to be of help to his family. He was described by others as listless, without ambition, and easily led. His I.Q. was 88.

In the hospital the neurological data including an electroencephalogram were interpreted as normal. The patient expressed complete innocence about his sentences to the reform school. He was well oriented and was intact in sensorium and intellect. He was somewhat apathetic, and there was no evidence that he had any insight into his problems. He showed no outright schizoid or other bizarre behavior. No real rapport could be established with him. He developed some interest in his surroundings while in the hospital and learned a number of games, engaging fairly well in social activities. He had several periods of enuresis. At the time of discharge he was mildly euphoric in contrast to his mild depression at admission. Otherwise, there was no real change. Continued institutionalization was recommended, and he was transferred to a state hospital some time afterward.

P. React. Depr. F:18:S:38 +3 '49 7231–6(57) 2:6:12

The present illness of this patient apparently began three weeks before admission with an attack of influenza. The girl, a college student, fell behind in her schoolwork and began to worry about final examinations. Her fears were chiefly centered around thoughts of the disappointment her parents would feel if she made a poor record.

The previous history showed no outstanding contributory factors. An honor student in high school, she was a hard worker, both in and out of school. Until the illness she had been able to earn the money for all her college expenses. Of a pleasing personality, she had many friends and was interested in drama, music, and art. At home she was tense and nervous because of the behavior of her parents and the presence of an epileptic brother, whom she was afraid of. She was stubborn at times but was truthful and showed no neurotic trends. Her parents were both high-strung, her mother domineering and aggressive.

In the hospital the young woman voiced the conviction that she was selfish and stubborn. She was self-depreciatory and had ideas of reference. Her family had suffered ill treatment from her, she insisted. She also believed that she could not carry out the most ordinary activities in a normal, responsible, spontaneous way. Everyone was acutely aware of her shortcomings and she was being watched critically, she told the staff. Except for this pattern of thinking there were no disturbances of intellect or mentation. She was depressed, perplexed, and apathetic in manner. Her troubles were due to a "confusion of ideas," she felt. She showed considerable blocking, an inability to finish sentences, and a moderate amount of circumstantiality. She sighed frequently and cried a great deal. During the first week she said and did odd things, but she was always well behaved and cooperative. Gradually she began to talk with others and eventually was permitted to leave the hospital for days at a time. She had a second acute attack, but again she began to get well. At the time of discharge she appeared to be completely recovered. It was recommended that she live with one of her brothers in order to help free her from the situation at her parents' home.

Ps. M-D., Depr. F:32:M:54 +2 49'8-6(37) 8:3:18
Schizoid

Ps. M-D., Depr. F:32:M:45 +2 7842136'9-(32) 6:7:19
Suicidal

The patient was transferred to the psychiatric unit from a general hospital for study and treatment. The present illness had begun eleven years before, following an illegal abortion. At that time the patient had had a period of nervousness. This nervousness reappeared when her mother was committed to a state hospital. At still another time the patient herself was sent to a psychopathic hospital, where she was noisy and destructive. She was paroled from this hospital and during her parole secretly married a man who soon thereafter became a chronic alcoholic and caused her considerable concern. Her husband went into the army for a while and after coming out he, the patient's sister, and the patient set up housekeeping together. A month before admission the patient asked the other two to leave her alone, which they did. Thirteen days before admission the sister returned to the apartment to find the patient posturizing and carrying out bizarre activities. The entire apartment was bedecked with sheets, altars, effigies, crosses, and other objects peculiarly arranged in groups of three.

The patient's physical health had been good. A college graduate, she had been a librarian. As a child she had been shy and dependent though she had been popular. She was described as determined and vehement in her ideas.

In the hospital she was occupied with posturizing, and apparently most of her mental content centered on religion and racial equality. Her sensorium and intellect were intact. Her emotional tone varied from cheerfulness to obvious belligerence. She recognized that she was not acting like others but nevertheless felt that she was rational. She remained assaultive and uncooperative until about a week after admission when shock treatment was begun. She received six treatments and steadily improved. She became more her natural self, appearing immature and generally insecure and indecisive. She was discharged to the care of her husband and her sister. The prognosis was felt to be only fairly good. Two months later she was readmitted. She had made frequent ineffectual attempts at suicide as well as an effort to smother her husband with a pillow. Five more shock treatments again seemed to bring her back to normal.

Ps. Sz., Paranoid M:24:S:19 +5 '4983-(74) 3:5:9

Two years before admission the patient was discharged from the navy because of a personality disorder. He then entered a university, where he was a trial to his fraternity brothers because of his unusual frankness and individualistic behavior. He became acquainted with a girl student and, though some of his relationships with her were conventional, there was also unusual behavior. He once entered the sorority house demanding to see her. When she appeared, he argued with her, then struck and slapped her. He left when requested to do so but later returned, forcing his way in through a window. Friends persuaded him to enter the psychopathic unit voluntarily after this series of episodes.

He had had good health. There were no previous behavior upsets, except as indicated in the navy discharge. He had done average work in high school and was the favorite student of the teaching staff there. An active, serious, purposeful individual, he had always been well liked by everyone. He had been very shy toward girls and had had only two dates while in high school. He had always been meticulous and hard working.

In the hospital he was cooperative. His statements were coherent, his behavior essentially conventional. There were no obvious disturbances in mentation. He admitted that his behavior might be considered unusual by the average person but he defended himself, saying that his reasons though poorly expressed were adequate and justified him. At times he did consider the possibility of going to a psychopathic hospital for a longer stay but always rejected the idea ultimately, feeling that he knew what he was about. It developed that the boy's family had been characterized by a surprising number of peculiar persons, and his behavior was apparently explicable both in hereditary and environmental terms. The staff was somewhat at a loss in understanding what had occurred and in making a prognosis. An underlying paranoid trend was felt to exist though nothing clearly of that nature could be elicited.

Ps. M-D., Mixed	M:27:S:41	+3	49'87-1	1:8:10
Alcoholism		+31	9'476-1	5:3:13

The patient first became ill three years before admission when he developed symptoms of excitement. He was given hospital care, and after a short period he returned home to recuperate. His improvement was gradual, and it was doubtful that he ever completely returned to his normal level. Restlessness and irritability were present for about a year, followed by an obvious depression, which lasted several months, and by excessive drinking. Although he had difficulty concentrating, he continued his work. During the winter preceding admission his motor activity again became excessive. He was overly talkative and showed impaired judgment. The alcoholism persisted. Throughout this episode there were short periods of depression alternating with manic behavior, and during the three months before admission he was unusually aggressive, irritable, and bitter toward his family and others.

The past history was noncontributory. He had finished high school at age 16 and had gone on to a university, where he had done poor work. Although he finally had been admitted to law school, he had failed a number of courses and had had to be satisfied with completing the bachelor of science degree instead of the bachelor of laws. He rationalized his failure on the grounds that his parents had required too much outside work from him. In the development of the present illness he had persisted in his attempts to study law but had accomplished nothing. A well-mannered, agreeable person with abundant physical energy, he had always taken great pride in his achievements. His interest in women had always been superficial and transient.

In the hospital he spoke vaguely of a "nervous breakdown" and indirectly explained that this prevented him from completing his law course or engaging in profitable work. He was obviously deeply disappointed over his failure, and he was anxious to avoid full recognition of the fact that he would never be an attorney. He appeared satisfied to remain in the hospital and implied that it was the place for him to stay until he was thoroughly rested. No outright delusions, hallucinations, or other abnormalities of intellect or sensorium were elicited, but he was overtalkative and circumstantial. Most of the time he was euphoric, but at times he was irritable. His judgment was poor and he never really recognized that he was ill. His improvement was slight, and he was finally placed in a private sanitarium.

Ps. Sz., Mixed M:24:M:114 +11 49'8716-3(55) 5:2:16

This veteran had been hospitalized for mental illness while in the service. After his discharge he held many jobs, changing frequently and never staying long in one place. He settled down after his marriage and apparently made a satisfactory adjustment until just before his second child was born. According to his wife, the patient changed a great deal during her second pregnancy. One day he left home without any warning and did not return until after the birth of the child. He often spoke irrationally. Once while intoxicated he was arrested and placed in jail, where he started a fire in his cell; subsequently he was committed to a state hospital. The physical examinations there were negative, although he was in a state of acute excitement when first admitted. His symptoms gradually subsided and he was transferred to this hospital seven months later.

School had been difficult for the patient and he had repeated the first, fifth, and ninth grades. At 17 when he was in the ninth grade he left school to enter the army. While stationed on one of the Pacific islands he fell in love with a native girl and wanted to marry her and remain there. Because military regulations would not permit this and because his buddies disapproved of the idea, he became very unhappy. Not long after this he was hospitalized, received insulin therapy, and was discharged from the service. Early in the patient's marriage he had had some difficulty with his wife because he wanted to cut his own timber and build his house after the fashion of the natives on the Pacific island. In other ways also the patient gave evidence of his preoccupation with his "island romance."

On the admission ward he made a good adjustment and was then transferred to the privileged ward, where he was quiet and cooperative. There was one exacerbation in which he had periods of hyperactivity when he would strike his head against the wall and kick furniture, followed by periods of semicatatonic stupor. He made a spontaneous remission and eventually was released for a trial visit home.

C. W. S.

Ps. Sz., Simple F:20:S:36 +5 49'872–3X(63) 10:6:18

This young woman was admitted because of decreased efficiency, lack of spontaneity, and a self-inflicted dermatitis. The acute phase of the illness began seven or eight weeks earlier when one evening she came home from assisting with the housework at a neighbor's "wearing a silly look." She rapidly became passive and inactive, could no longer work, had difficulty dressing, and sat alone in the dark for hours.

The patient's past physical health had been exceptionally good. There were no severe episodes of nervousness. In the seventh grade she had left school to take over the family housework after her mother's death. Known as efficient and capable, she was also introverted and shy, did not meet people well, and made few friends. She had always been very dependent. On the other hand there was little obvious emotional expression. She had been apparently happy and content. She was devoutly religious and limited her friends to those of her faith.

In the hospital she was passive and withdrawn. Over her entire body she had a pustular dermatitis. While she expressed a passive desire to have this cleared up and could not account for its onset, there was evidence that she rubbed and scratched herself, keeping the dermatitis active. There were no disturbances of sensorium or intellect and she was well oriented. Although retarded in her responses, she was cooperative and pleasant. She admitted auditory hallucinations such as "God is speaking to me and telling me to lead a good life." She showed no paranoid trends. After some encouragement she participated in the activities of the ward but showed little spontaneity. Fourteen insulin subcoma shocks resulted in only a slight improvement. Still withdrawn, she required pushing and persuasion even to move. The prognosis was poor. When she was discharged to her family it was with the expectation that she would be able to continue as long as she was given family protection.

B. Psth., Asocial M:20:M:10 +1 '498 73–2(51) 7:0:23

This was a peculiar case in which the patient was sent to the hospital for a determination of his mental competence. The young man had been drafted two years before, shortly after undergoing a hernioplasty, and he had been eager to pass the navy qualifications. Before this he had worked steadily and had been temperate in habits and tastes. While in the navy he complained of "kidney trouble" and said he thought he needed another operation. Shortly after this his mother received a letter saying he was suffering from a "nervous disorder." He was transferred to a psychiatric center and was discharged from the service about nine months before the present admission after receiving electroshock treatments. He had been diagnosed as having dementia praecox and was allowed total disability. His behavior contrasted markedly with that before his enlistment. He now drank, smoked, kept late hours, and was unable to hold a job for any length of time. On one occasion he was accused of stealing from an aunt. He was also suspected of participation in another robbery, and some of the stolen articles were found on his person. He called this a result of "cleaning up the mess left by the robbers." The police picked him up for the robbery the day after he was married to a girl he had been engaged to for some time.

Before the present illness there was little of note in his history except that he had been enuretic until he was 12. A high school graduate, he had been industrious and had maintained a fair school record. He was described as having been quiet and shy but friendly. He had always been somewhat immature.

In the hospital the youth appeared to be entirely normal. Tests indicated an I.Q. of 117. There were no guilt feelings that could be detected and no obviously abnormal behavior. He felt he was a victim of circumstances and his attitude was insincere and evasive, though he attempted to appear friendly and cooperative. He behaved fairly well throughout his hospitalization. Occasionally he was sarcastic to other patients, but he did not actually antagonize anyone. He was returned to the custody of the authorities as not psychotic, although the staff had not gained an adequate understanding of the problem he presented.

B. Psth., Asocial M:16:S:44 +3 '49876–21 0:11:6

The patient, sent to the hospital by the juvenile court for observation, had been showing delinquent traits for approximately two years before his admission. On several occasions he had stolen articles, mostly things without great value although once he did steal a bicycle, and he had established friendships with other boys who were also delinquent. He was taken to the juvenile court when he came under the guidance of a social agency. Because of his intractability, efforts to help him were generally unavailing, and people quickly became discouraged in their attempts to work with him. He was seen several times by a psychiatrist, who advised that he be admitted to an inpatient psychiatric service.

The patient had had no previous psychological or physical difficulties that seemed pertinent. Until the onset of the present problems he had done fair work in school and had reached the tenth grade. He intended to continue his education. Since childhood he had been irresponsible and difficult with people, and he had shown considerable irritability. He had strongly antagonistic feelings toward his mother and his siblings. Shortly before his birth, his father had left home and nothing had been heard of him for a long while. After his father and mother were finally divorced, his mother remarried but she was again divorced shortly.

In the hospital the boy discussed his behavior in a reserved manner, never telling more than he thought was already known. He accounted for his behavior by saying that he was impulsive, a trait he did not think he could overcome. He made very shallow emotional responses, with no evidence of remorse or apprehension about what he had done, but he was somewhat worried about the possibility that he would be placed in a penal institution. Although he adapted fairly well to hospitalization he was always on the verge of getting into trouble. He exhibited no bizarre behavior and there was no evidence of a definite psychosis. Efforts to form a psychotherapeutic relationship with him were not successful. The prognosis was poor, and the suggestions for his future were concerned chiefly with his management in the training school to which he was sent.

P. Hys.	F:19:S:60	−14	498'763-(63)	3:2:21
		+62	9'8417-6(55)	3:5:12

This girl came to the clinic with a variety of complaints, none of any magnitude but together they seemed to add up to a comparatively mild anxiety. She felt out of place socially and complained of a lack of self-confidence, feelings of loneliness, and sensitivity to criticism. She felt pressure particularly in the social situation and made a thorough nuisance of herself in her college dormitory by forming deep emotional attachments to some of the other students. These relationships were apparently not homosexual in nature. The girl was finally motivated to come to the clinic by a psychology student who had administered the MMPI and had given her a cautious summary of the results. This happened just in time since her case had grown to such magnitude that it had come to the attention of the student court.

A main factor in this girl's early childhood was an impermanent home situation. Her father died when she was young and with her mother working, she was "farmed out" to various relatives, spending the bulk of her time with her grandmother, to whom she had little, if any, emotional attachment. Actually there was no parental figure in her life until adolescence. In speaking of her mother, the girl commented that she was a very charming and attractive person but somehow they did not seem to be related in a mother-daughter sense.

In adolescence the girl got her first mother-surrogate through a strong emotional attachment to a playground director. The woman was evidently very understanding and treated the girl with the utmost kindness for about a year. Then the relationship evidently began to cloy and the playground director "let her down" abruptly. This was followed by a series of crushes on almost any adult woman who showed the patient an iota of kindness. At this time she established some relationships with other children of the same age but these seemed to have been of a fairly superficial nature. Her adolescence was more or less a blind search for a satisfactory mother-substitute. Because of this she was naive in the conventional social graces and as a result undoubtedly antagonized many of her acquaintances. When she came to college she found herself almost completely isolated socially, and the series of emotional crushes resulting in her referral followed.

During therapy she developed a similar attachment for the counselor, being almost unwilling to act without his approval. Despite this, a nondirective approach was used almost exclusively, since it was felt that the girl had to be encouraged to develop self-autonomy as soon as possible. She worked through the therapy uneventfully, although she was reluctant to break off the relationship which had proved so satisfactory. A year later she was seen for three sessions by another psychologist, who felt that there was nothing seriously wrong with the girl but that she lacked an adequate knowledge of social graces, and he directed her in this area. From that point on she made a satisfactory, although still somewhat immature, social adjustment. A. S.

Ps. Sz., Hebe. M:21:S '6–29(57) 5:3:17
Paranoid

This college student was encouraged to come to the office by his family, who reported that he had been withdrawn, uncomfortable with others, and suspicious. He spent most of his time daydreaming and complaining of physical manifestations of approaching old age.

He was the only child of a dominating father, who had been discharged from the navy after shock treatment for depression, and a chronically tense, neurotic mother. She reported that the boy's early childhood had been characterized by compliant and inhibited behavior.

Unable to look at others, he had no friends and spent much of his time calculating the batting averages of professional ball players, but he never went to games because he felt that other spectators were looking at him and talking about him. He continually bit his nails during interviews, was eager to leave, and spoke hesitatingly if at all. He mentioned guilt over masturbation and hostility toward his father, and he frequently laughed inappropriately. He finally left the university and remained at home. C. K. A.

B. Psth., Path. Emot. F:62:M:21 +1 '6–7149X(66) 10:5:12
Mental Deficiency

The patient was sent to the hospital by the county welfare office, which had first heard of her as being probably insane. Further study indicated that she had always been a social problem. She had been inefficient and unable to keep her children in a decent manner. At various times her I.Q. had been listed at the borderline imbecile or moron level. The psychological reports pointed out, however, that this standing might be somewhat low because there were confusing elements in her behavior. Her physical health had always been good.

She had had eight children, the last when she was 47. Very little was known about her early life or personality. She had been much affected by the death of her father and had apparently worried about it for many months. She had always been moody and had cried a good deal of the time, sometimes showing her agitation by pacing the floor. During the past month she had been in three different boarding homes but the landladies had ejected her because she refused to clean up, talked about men and taverns, and was generally disturbing to the other occupants.

In the physical examination at the hospital her thyroid was found to be large; there was a history of hyperthyroidism that apparently extended back to her childhood. This was not considered to be a clinical problem, however. She was uncouth and peculiar in behavior. There were no gross disturbances of sensorium or intellect, no hallucinations or obvious delusions. She adjusted fairly well to the hospital routine but had to be supervised at all times. Sometimes she was loud and silly. The problem was felt to be one of low intellect combined with poor training in social relationships and responsibility.

Ps. Paranoid F:33:M:28 +11 '6–7893 7:2:11

About a week before admission the patient developed aggressive feelings toward her husband, was suspicious of him, and thought he was trying to harm her. At one time she made a physical assault on him. She also had a number of unsystematized, bizarre delusions and hallucinations, but her sensorium was more or less intact. She did not seem to have been taking drugs, and there were no obvious precipitating factors. Over the past seven or eight years, she had had several similar episodes, about one a year, each following the same pattern. It was thought that the attacks might be related to her frequent headaches. Usually the spells lasted a month but milder episodes were shorter.

The past history was not contributory. After some high school education she had begun to work in a factory. Her intelligence was good, she was a good manager and worker, and she got along well with people. She had one child, a boy of 9, in whom she was very interested. Two years after this child was born, the patient had again become pregnant. When she finally aborted, the husband showed so little interest in her welfare that it affected her attitude toward him. Thereafter she maintained a certain degree of coldness toward him, and they were not harmonious sexually.

The neurological and physical examinations on admission were negative. The patient had a variety of bizarre and fantastic delusions and both auditory and visual hallucinations in which there was a strong paranoid coloring. She misinterpreted things and had periods of double orientation. Although she claimed to be unhappy, she did not manifest any great emotion and described her strange delusions without much feeling. She talked rapidly with many irrelevant associations. At times she was irritable, objecting particularly to her detention in the hospital. Within a few days she appeared to have completely recovered, but she showed a surprising lack of insight into her illness. For the most part she now became a haughty, distant person who was essentially cooperative but who showed no tendency to unburden herself. She objected to the routine and felt there was no reason for her to be in the hospital. The staff was unable to determine an etiology for the episode, although the possibility of toxic factors remained; the only other reasonable suggestion seemed to be that she was characteristically paranoid.

P. React. Depr.	F:14:S:30	+10	61'83792–	5:9:11
Ps. M-D., Depr.		+26	'6149–73	9:1:13
Ps. Sz., Simple				
Ps. Sz., Simple	F:19:S:67	+1	2'64871–X	11:8:19

The patient's illness began when she was about 14 years old, following the death of two sisters, when she became depressed, could not eat or sleep, and cried frequently. She also had dreams in which her sisters talked to her. Hospitalized for a month with marked improvement, she had no further difficulty until two years before the present admission when she left high school following an attack of flu. After this she worked as a housemaid, taking jobs in many different homes but staying in each only briefly. She was moody, depressed, and uncooperative, and there was friction between her and her mother. Three months before admission she was admitted to a general hospital for treatment of gonorrhea. She was pregnant at that time. She was discharged after arrangements had been made for her to stay at a girls' club, but she continued to be so depressed that she entered the psychiatric unit in the present admission.

An honor student in school, she had taken little interest in extracurricular activities, and her moody, withdrawn behavior came between her and possible friends. Until age 17 she had never had dates, but for the past two years she had met boys at theaters and drugstores and had been somewhat promiscuous, even though she claimed not to find sexual relations particularly pleasant. She had never been in love with any of the boys she had gone out with. Her father was a quiet, unassuming person who had had some difficulty in supporting his family. Her mother was jealous because the father was very friendly with the patient; she also resented the fact that her husband did not support the family better. The patient had been very attached to her two sisters, one of whom had died at age 15 with a brain tumor and the other at age 11 with an acute nephritis.

In the hospital the physical examination indicated that an abnormality of the kidneys was highly probable but the symptoms were not acute. The patient's pregnancy was normal to the time of admission. She was indifferent and apathetic. Her mental depression and retardation seemed superficial, and she responded adequately to direct questions. Within a few days she was less depressed and began to participate in ward activities, making friends with other patients, especially with the men, to whom she made so many overt advances that she had to be reprimanded. Later she again became upset and depressed, particularly when asked about her future. About that time she developed a vaginal blood clot and had abdominal pains, fever, and hematuria. She went to bed and complained of being tired and weak, but she apparently enjoyed the attention she received and was happy to have someone take care of her. It was recommended that she be transferred to a state hospital, but in the interim she needed continued contacts with the obstetrical department.

B. Pri., Child.	F:14:S:14	+4	'6238–(55)	6:8:12

When this girl was 11 her parents began to notice that she cried readily and was easily disturbed. This pattern continued and she often "cried herself into a fit over nothing at all." Whereas she had formerly been energetic and had liked to play, she now withdrew and said that other children made her nervous. She lost interest in things and appeared to tire with a minimum of exercise. Unless a light was left on she refused to go to bed, although previously she had never been afraid. A fear of cows also developed. In addition she claimed to have difficulty in swallowing solid food.

The girl attended a rural school with an enrollment of only one other pupil. She attributed her repetition of two grades to the fact that she had gone to a town school for a while. Her achievement level was at the seventh grade. She found it difficult to concentrate and to assimilate new material but was well behaved in school. At home she helped her mother dutifully. Although considered shy she made friends easily and was regarded as trustworthy and truthful. Apparently she had not had any particular worries. Her social contacts were limited, and she had seen only one movie in her life. The patient's brother and sisters appeared to be normal.

On admission the physical examination indicated a diffuse symmetrical enlargement of the thyroid gland and other symptoms of hypothyroidism. She was a purile, timid, and somewhat farmerish-looking girl; she always had a dull expression on her face. She giggled frequently and wrung her hands much of the time. Vague and indifferent about everything, she voiced no complaints. Tests showed her I.Q. to be about 81. She gave short and incomplete answers to questions and showed no spontaneity. Although cooperative and quiet she took little interest in the ward activities. Because she was so shy, giggled so much, and made silly remarks, she was not well accepted. In occupational therapy she sat and watched others most of the time. She liked the other patients and the nurses, she said. She was put on thyroid medication, and she improved considerably, especially during her last week in the hospital. At discharge it was recommended that she leave school and take up a simple vocational activity.

B. Psth., Asocial M:17:S:13 +3 '624–913 (47) 2:4:11

The patient entered the hospital voluntarily at the suggestion of his probation officer. He had made an unsatisfactory adjustment in school and society when his family had moved to the city five years before admission. He became withdrawn and the few friends he made were younger than himself. For four years he had engaged in petty stealing and automobile thievery. Stealing a motorcycle led to his being sent to a training school for boys; he was put on probation but soon he stole two electric motors. This latter episode led to his hospitalization.

A senior in high school, he lacked a genuine interest in school activities. His main interest was in mechanics. He had never been given any real responsibilities by his parents, who supplied his material wants without question. His only real job experience had been as a janitor for two months at his father's place of business. Average in ability, he was shy, sensitive, immature, irritable, and impulsive. He seemed to have no guilt feelings about his behavior. His father worked long hours and his mother resented the fact that her husband did not accept more responsibility for the children. The patient had a brother who was also delinquent. When the boys got into trouble, they managed for a while to get attention from their parents;. whichever one was currently in trouble would get a lion's share of the attention.

In the hospital the boy was cheerful and cooperative and talked freely on a superficial level. Whenever his troubles were discussed, he became defensive and emphasized that he was not abnormal. He rationalized all his misdeeds. He had feelings of insecurity but these did not go deep enough to motivate him. He was not at first particularly anxious about his hospitalization; later he became restless but said it was better to be in the hospital than to face what the law might do to him. He was obviously more interested in himself than in anything else and was somewhat of a nuisance to the other patients because of his boisterous spirits and attempts to attract attention. No real rapport could be established with him and little could be done in the way of psychotherapy. A controlled environment was recommended, and it was suggested that some older person be made a consistent source of authority.

P. React. Depr.	F:56:D:22	+6	624'3819–(68)	4:5:11
		–83	2134'6879–(68)	3:2:14

The principal complaints for this patient were depression, vomiting, insomnia, and anorexia. Her illness had appeared after surgery for jaundice due to cancer. The operation, although successful, was immediately followed by persistent vomiting and a poor appetite, for which no organic basis was discovered. Then she showed extreme annoyance and depression over small disturbances. Particularly she felt that the operation had been mismanaged and that she had been roughly treated. At home after the operation she had a fairly good week, then abruptly the symptoms returned in full force.

Among the patient's known assets were good intelligence, friendliness, and cheerfulness. However, her good disposition persisted only when everything suited her, and she had always been readily disturbed. Both of her marriages had been stormy and had ended in divorce. Except for the emotional instability and frequent depression, there were no factors in the past history that seemed contributory.

On the ward the patient was well composed and her behavior conventional. Illogical in discussions, she tended to "run on" and to jump from one topic to another. She had no real insight into the fact that her troubles were petty and greatly exaggerated in her thinking. On the ward she was pleasant and friendly and mingled well with other patients. She improved considerably, although she gained little further insight and became homesick. At discharge it was felt that she would probably be able to follow a regular routine, and the prognosis was favorable.

Ps. Psth. Suicidal Mutilative	F:33:M:23	+6	6247'389–(43)	4:5:11
Ps. Psth.	F:36:D:72	+6	497823'61–(59)	2:7:10

The patient's complaints at the time she was first seen in this hospital were a compulsive desire to mutilate and kill herself and recurrent episodes of elation and depression. This was but one in a long series of hospitalizations beginning at the age of 18 after a suicide attempt. During the next fifteen years she had been in hospitals in four different states following suicide attempts or outbursts of violent behavior. On one occasion she had an impulse to break a large glass store window; she told the owner what she wanted to do and begged him to call the police. When he did not take her seriously she went ahead and smashed the window. In one admission acute alcoholism was a problem. She received electroshock and insulin treatments, with never more than a temporary improvement. At one time hallucinations and delusions were reported, and she made an attempt to murder a hospital attendant by forcing her head in a toilet bowl. The possibility of epilepsy was raised and the patient gave a history of convulsions. Later she denied this, however, and no conclusive evidence of a convulsive disorder was ever obtained.

The woman's parents were both alcoholics. When the patient was 6 they were divorced. She then lived with her mother, who married four more times. Her father remarried five times but the patient saw little of him until her present hospitalization, when he began to visit her. The two then behaved like sweethearts. The patient remembered being impulsive as a child, wanting to run in front of cars or jump from high places. Once she crushed a baby chick in her hand "to see it die." Above average in intelligence, she did adequate schoolwork but did not mix well socially. She felt she was inferior and had many moody spells. After leaving school she lived many places and held innumerable jobs, often as a waitress or dice girl in night clubs. At 17 she eloped and was married secretly. When she found she was pregnant she had an abortion at her mother's insistence. The marriage terminated in divorce shortly afterward. At 20 she married again; she claimed that this had been a happy marriage and that she had divorced this second husband only because she was unable to become pregnant again and "did not feel it fair to remain married." She remarried again shortly, however.

In this hospital the patient's behavior was characterized by daily disturbed episodes, during which she became excited, paced, shouted, pounded the walls, broke windows, and inflicted wounds on herself. When not in an excited spell she was pleasant, charming, fully cooperative, and seemingly distressed about her condition. However, attempts at psychotherapy were not found to be helpful, nor was she aided by ten electronarcosis treatments. The difficulty in handling her outbursts made her transfer to another hospital necessary. A lobotomy was finally performed and following this all her more disturbing symptoms disappeared. She was able to adjust relatively well for a year without hospitalization, living with her father and holding several minor jobs for short periods. During this time she divorced her third husband while he was overseas.

At the end of a year, one day on her way to inquire about a new job, she had a spell of amnesia lasting thirty minutes. Then she developed a severe headache and a recurrence of her impulses to destructive behavior, and she entered this hospital a second time. She had improved somewhat in her ability to control her impulsive outbursts; however, she continued to be a problem to herself and others, and she complained of the persistent headache. This was accompanied by obsessive thoughts such as the word *God* repeated over and over. It was felt that the first lobotomy had not been extensive enough and a second one was performed. She did not at this time manifest the usual post-lobotomy syndrome. The headache was relieved and she reported that her impulses were not so intense and uncontrollable. No further improvement was expected and she was discharged to her father.

E. B.

B. Psth., Asocial	F:30:M:27	+1	62487′3–(39)	6:11:4
P. Hypo.		—41	2467′831–	4:11:7

This woman was brought to the hospital by her husband, who requested that her behavior abnormalities be studied. For nine years she had been in love with her husband's brother. Every time he appeared she showed discontent with her home life, but as soon as he left this disappeared. The odd behavior associated with the discontent consisted of reading cheap literature, becoming irritable, developing hypochondriacal signs, threatening to kill her five children and herself, and probably engaging in extramarital relationships. She was pregnant at the time of admission, and it was thought probable that her husband was not the father.

The patient described herself as having always been "sickly." She apparently had had difficulties with her teeth and sinuses and had suffered from colds, headaches, and the like. She had always lived in small towns and at a low social level, from which she wished to escape. In high school, which she attended for two years, she earned good marks. Tests indicated an I.Q. of 120. Formerly she had read many good books, but recently she had preferred cheap love magazines. She had got along well with people earlier but lately she had become withdrawn socially. She also slighted her housework. Unyielding and stubborn, she demanded her own way from her husband, whom she regarded as her intellectual inferior. Actually, this seemed to be true. She was considered to have low ethical standards. Although she admitted to no sexual relations with her brother-in-law, she described him as a "better lover" than her husband and, according to her husband, once said that her brother-in-law could be with her any time he wished. The couple had five children. The husband was weak-willed and afraid of his brother, and once he even allowed himself to be ordered from his own home by his brother. He always took his problems to his wife's parents to ask their advice. The brother who was so prominent in the case appeared to be an irresponsible, unreliable, reckless person, who was unlikely to assume any responsibility for anyone.

Except for a five-month pregnancy the patient was physically and neurologically free of any organic signs that would help clarify the situation. Her wish, she said, was to do "what is best for the children and for my husband so the home won't be broken up." It would be hard for her to love her husband again, she claimed, yet she expressed a willingness to try. She was cooperative and intact psychologically in mentation and sensorium. Around the ward she was not so depressed that she could not seem to enjoy herself. During the latter part of her stay in the hospital she was eager to return home to her husband and children. The case was a difficult one to assess and the staff efforts were mainly directed toward a study of the environmental factors. Among other recommendations it was suggested that the husband's brother be kept at as great a distance as possible.

B. Psth., Path. Emot. Alcoholism Suicidal	M:21:M:7	+5	6'2748-1 (74)	3:6:11
B. Psth., Path. Emot. Alcoholism Suicidal	M:22:M:38	+2	72486'3-1 (63)	3:5:17

The patient was admitted to the hospital because of alcoholism, depression, restlessness, insomnia, and attempted suicide. The onset of the symptoms was insidious. He began drinking when in high school and then drank more heavily while in the army until he was medically discharged. He then enrolled in a university and went on many "alcoholic sprees." After his wife left him to visit her parents he began to drink almost continually. He attempted to divert himself from his depression by deliberately seeking gaiety and engaging in "wild" parties, but these did not seem to help him. While drunk he was hostile toward his mother. The day before admission his mother found him attempting to swallow eight phenobarbital tablets.

His past health was good. While in high school he had been interested in dramatics, oil painting, and writing narrative poetry. In the university he was studying business administration, made friends easily, and was well liked despite the fact that he was self-centered and aloof. He was subject to temper tantrums and always sought means of avoiding responsibility. He prided himself on his "lurid" sex life. His wife was an apparently well-adjusted and sensible person. Their married life had been satisfactory except for the patient's increasing alcoholism and his extramarital relationships.

In the hospital he was cooperative and courteous at all times. He appeared somewhat anxious and apprehensive and was disgusted at finding himself in a psychiatric ward. While he recognized that he was depressed, he had only superficial insight and thought his drinking was merely a rebellion against family ties. He was egotistical and spoke through clenched teeth with a dramatic air. He enjoyed being the center of attention. There was no abnormal behavior or obviously abnormal content. He seemed to make very good plans for the future and was certain that he would abstain from drinking, finish college, and begin to accept his adult responsibilities. On discharge he went back to his wife, but the prognosis was considered very bad.

About a year later he was readmitted with an interim history of the same behavior. He had been discouraged, bored with life, and irregular during the year. Apparently he had done relatively less drinking but just before this admission he again drank heavily and threatened suicide. This time he was eager to leave the hospital and said he would "go nuts" if he could not leave. Again he felt that he had solved his problems.

B. Simple Adult Maladj. M:52:S:17 +5 627'8139– 6:12:5
Alcoholism
P. Hypo.

This particular illness appeared a year before admission when the patient began to complain of severe headaches, which he said "were never absent," and for which he had gradually increased his nightly doses of sedatives. He was said to have changed in personality, becoming careless and indifferent and spending most of his time in bed. The patient had begun drinking heavily at age 15 and had continued through his life. There were at least three past admissions to state hospitals, chiefly because of alcoholism. He had had delirium tremens three times, with definite hallucinations. For a number of years, he said, he had experienced almost continual auditory hallucinations. Voices would say to him, for example, "Harry is an old booze hound." These "voices" were not markedly male or female, and he could never identify them. In the past few years he had been drinking somewhat less.

The patient terminated his schooling in the seventh grade at age 15. Unmarried, he said that he had had heterosexual experiences with many girls, most of them much younger than he. He had always had poor judgment and no foresight. On the other hand, he was well liked by a number of cronies who regularly came to his house to while away the hours. He preferred to live alone. An active and energetic worker before the present illness, he had also enjoyed outdoor activities. He was described as trustful and childlike in his attitudes toward religion and toward his superiors.

Except for minimal signs of neuritis, the neurological examination in the hospital proved to be negative. The patient had numerous somatic complaints, chiefly sensory in nature. The hallucinations were present and appeared benign. He had no ideas of reference or persecution. He showed some apprehension, fearing that he would not regain his health and that he might die. He was tested as dull normal in intelligence. In spite of his complaints that he did not sleep, hypnographic recordings showed him to be sleeping eight hours a night. He was given reassurance and physical therapy, and he recovered from the present pattern of complaints.

P. Mixed F:22:S:9 +1 628'7314–(74) 5:10:12
P. Hys. −39 8'2971634–(68) 4:5:11

The patient was admitted to the hospital because of persistent vomiting after meals, a forty-pound weight loss, and amenorrhea. The illness dated from about two years before when the patient was in high school. She had been going out with a classmate frequently but her family wanted her to marry another man. She therefore left home, began to work as a waitress, and fell in love with a Protestant boy. The patient and her family were Catholics and when her family learned of the new affair, they told her that she would no longer be welcome at home and would lose her religion if she went through with the marriage. She abandoned her job and went to a distant city, where she worked as a welder. While working on a ship, she nearly fell from a very high place. She continued to work that day but the next morning when she got up she vomited. The vomiting continued and she finally had to give up her job and return home.

Her past physical health had been good, and there were no previous mental or nervous upsets. She finished the seventh grade at age 13 and left school to work on her family's farm. Her family was hard working and thrifty. The patient apparently accepted their standards. Five years before the present illness the patient's mother had experienced a nervous breakdown and had been hospitalized; an important symptom in her mother's illness had been inability to eat.

In the hospital the patient was somewhat retarded, depressed, and fearful. Her mental content was normal, and her sensorium and intellect were intact. She seemed to have good insight but was reluctant to discuss the conflicts she was obviously concerned with. She finally became more free in talking about her problems and said that if her home situation could be straightened out, she thought her vomiting would stop. Apparently the desire to marry the Protestant boy was still her uppermost problem, and a consultation was arranged in which the patient and her family discussed the entire situation with a member of the staff. After this the patient markedly improved and returned home free of symptoms. The family had agreed to the marriage, and the patient planned to work for a while, gaining her weight back before the actual ceremony.

Ps. Sz., Paranoid M:26:S:16 +10 6287'4319–X(71) 10:11:18

This man had been "nervy" and had felt "different" from others since childhood. His feelings of inferiority and his persecutory ideas made employment impossible, and he entered the hospital as a voluntary patient.

He was the illegitimate child of a neurotic mother. He went to a grammar school but did not continue his education because of "chorea, chest trouble, and asthma." He was always shy and a bad mixer and did not get on with people. On leaving school he became an engineering apprentice and held several jobs for various lengths of time. He had been on the unemployment register for two years before entering the hospital.

Diagnosed as having schizophrenia, he underwent a course of modified insulin therapy and one electroshock. He left the hospital against medical advice.

M. V.

P. Mixed	**F:48:S:44**	**+4**	**6312'794–(41)**	**7:2:14**
Drug Add.		**+37**	**216'379–(45)**	**8:4:10**

The patient's trouble had begun sixteen years before admission when a romance of five years' duration had been terminated. The patient, a technician, had been seriously in love with a scientist she worked with, and they had had sexual relations. Their plans for marriage fell through when the man broke off the relationship because of religious differences. After this the patient began to drink heavily, and she suffered guilt feelings over the intimacies which she could not overcome. Gradually, because she felt tired, exhausted, irritable, unhappy, and miserable most of the time, she began to take benzedrine sulfate to relieve her feelings of sluggishness and lethargy. When her mother died a year before admission her condition became worse, and she was forced to give up her job because of numerous physical complaints. She began taking seconal and developed a mild addiction to it; her decision to come to the hospital was due to her fear that the drug might get the best of her.

A graduate in technology, the patient had been excellently recommended by all her employers. In school she had been actively interested in activities and sports and had been entirely adequate socially. She supported her mother and had put her brother through two years of college. A likable person, she had worked hard and had succeeded in nearly everything she had attempted. She considered herself self-conscious, however, and she had feelings of inferiority which she compensated for by hard work.

In the hospital the physical and neurological examinations were essentially negative. On admission she was in a state of acute barbiturate intoxication; she was disheveled in appearance and somewhat euphoric, and her sensorium was clouded. She could not give an adequate history and was mainly concerned with her anxiety and guilt. She professed gratitude at being allowed to enter the hospital. Within 24 hours most of her confusion cleared. She adjusted well to the routine and was cooperative and pleasant; no bizarre behavior was observed. She was able to discuss her problems, and she developed good insight. At the time of discharge she had come to look favorably upon the possibility of marriage, and she faced her problems generally with an acceptably realistic attitude. The feeling of inferiority was apparently an important factor in her entire life, and her fundamental problem was an obsessive-compulsive one with overlying depression and other symptoms. Providing she continued with the plans she had made, the prognosis was felt to be good.

Ps. Invol. Melan.	F:53:M:58	–5 yrs.	**6'31284–**	**8:6:16**
Ps. Invol. Melan.	**F:54:M:39**	**+1**	**2'37186–49(57)**	**6:7:11**

This patient's complaints centered around insomnia, forgetfulness, general nervousness, and pains on the top of her head. She was tense, worried excessively, believed that she was "slowed down mentally," and feared becoming insane. The symptoms had been worse for about two months. In that time she had become withdrawn and inactive.

Previously the patient's health had been fairly good. In her early thirties she had had an attack of "mucous colitis," which was characterized by nervousness, diarrhea, and insomnia. Her husband said that the pattern of this illness was similar in many respects to the present one. The menopause had begun about five years before admission, without any particular disturbance. She was hypertensive and there was some evidence of brain damage.

Above average in learning ability, she had been a teacher in a country school for six years before her marriage to a wealthy farmer. She was regarded as cheerful and optimistic, not excessively depressed by disappointments, well adjusted in her home and community. In general her past history contributed little of aid in understanding the present situation.

In the hospital the patient's main thoughts concerned her illness, her fear of insanity, and her various somatic complaints. She steadfastly pointed to her pains as evidence of an organic disorder. Her thinking capacity appeared to be greatly reduced, although her general knowledge was good. She believed herself to be irretrievably on the way to insanity. Although she did appear concerned and puzzled, she did not seem to be as depressed as further investigation proved her to be. She failed to improve at first, but following five electroshock treatments she recovered a good deal of animation and looked much less sick. She remained, however, ill at ease and irritable. The insomnia also persisted, and some of her somatic ideas. She was finally permitted to go home and travel with her husband. It was felt, however, that the long-time prognosis was not good, since probable vascular changes were contributory to the whole pattern. One year later she was readmitted with the same pattern of symptoms. She again received electroshock treatments and the discharge status was similar to that for the first admission.

Ps. Psth. F:33:M:63 +18 '6327 841–X (43) 10:1:25
Paranoid

The present illness of this patient dated from about five months before admission when her husband left for the army. She insisted on working while he was away, but the work she undertook was too hard for her and it upset her. She had financial troubles and she frequently went without food rather than use any of the money her husband had deposited in the bank for her. She withdrew from social contacts and her husband noted that her letters became more and more morose. He got an emergency leave and found his wife confused and refusing to read any printed matter. She believed that there were special references to her in various newspaper articles and that these references were placed there to depress her. The articles made her feel guilty because of her lack of contribution to the war effort. After threatening suicide she was taken to a private sanitarium, where she received electroshock treatments without improvement.

The patient had had no previous psychotic upsets and her physical health had been good. She was a high school graduate with an average record, and after her marriage she was an efficient housekeeper, taking great pride in her home. She was friendly and enjoyed social life. She read extensively and was well informed. Others called her "vain, egocentric," and described her husband as oversolicitous to a degree that made her dependent upon him for all decisions. She needed his sympathy for even the slightest distress to which she was subjected.

In the hospital the physical and neurological examinations were essentially negative. She was uncooperative and when asked a question would say, "If I can only talk to my husband, then everything will be all right." Her actions were childish. She threw articles at nurses and once smeared feces on the wall of her room. After two weeks her temper tantrums and other misbehavior had sufficiently abated so that she could be transferred to the open ward. There she was careful of her appearance and her attitude improved, but she had spells of depression when she would cry for long periods. She gained favors by coaxing and she tried to bribe the nurses with such statements as this: "I don't trust anyone else but I have faith in you and I know you'll help me." She gradually improved until she was fairly well but her childishness and active dependence upon her husband were still obvious. Commitment for a while to a hospital was suggested by the staff, but her husband arranged to care for her at home. At the time of discharge it was felt that her paranoid ideas were merely hidden under a surface appearance of unconcern.

Ps. Sz., Paranoid F:51:D:9 0 634'12–(34) 7:8:14

For three weeks before admission the patient had complained of a backache. This and a number of other physical complaints took her to a health service, where it was recognized that she had a general psychiatric disturbance, and she was referred to the psychiatric unit. She complained of having been bothered by "funny" people for six and a half years. She said they had first begun to annoy her while she was living in another state, where they stole her personal belongings and ridiculed her. She thought her husband was "cuckoo" because he allowed this to go on. She had spent some time in a state hospital but after her release had not been appreciably better. She changed her residence numerous times to get away from her persecutors. She thought that they tried to hypnotize her and to control her mind. She also believed they were poisoning her.

The patient had attended a number of normal schools and universities and had taught grade school for a considerable time. No information was available about her previous personality although it was discovered some time after her admission that she had had numerous hospitalizations, apparently with paranoid breakdowns. She had been married twice, first to a man she had had to support and then, after divorcing him, to a professional man. Later she also divorced her second husband.

In the hospital she appeared quiet, well mannered, conventional, and courteous. She was well oriented and willing to talk. There was no special disorder in her stream of thought. It was only when she spoke of the "funny" people who were following her that she showed any bizarre mental content. It was thought that she had auditory hallucinations, though one could never be sure. She said, "I am not imagining these things. It's all true. I don't care what anyone says, and I was sent to the state hospital so that they couldn't get at me. I've never had any mental trouble." She changed little during her stay and she was finally discharged to return to the state hospital.

Ps. Sz., Paranoid F:33:M:95 +3 '637814–(53) 4:2:12

The patient came to the hospital voluntarily because she "needed a rest." She was under the pressure of excessive religious fervor. About six months before admission, while sitting at home knitting, she had suddenly had the impression that "God most certainly exists" and that a brother she had been very fond of, who had drowned some time before, was in heaven and extremely happy. The patient would not admit that this was a vision but she was greatly overjoyed, knelt by the bed, and intermittently wept and prayed for some time. She had doubted the existence of a deity previously because of the unjustness of her brother's sudden death. Later, while having sexual intercourse with her husband, she had the impression that from the union would come a great savior of mankind. She immediately developed a much stronger interest in church work; she sold her wedding dress and engagement ring for money to give to a missionary group and attempted to make many other sacrifices of that kind. She refused to believe that she was not pregnant. Later she told a priest that she was atoning for the sins of the world, had frequent fights with the devil, and felt the world was coming to an end. Once she said that a miracle would coincide with the termination of her supposed pregnancy.

Except for seasonal asthmatic attacks, a vague history of arthritis, and a few other somatic complaints of a somewhat hysterical nature, the past history was noncontributory. The patient was an eighth-grade graduate but had not gone on because the school was so far from her home. As a girl she had had a very limited social life and infrequent dates. Usually her brother had acted as her escort. She had never worked except at home. Married for thirteen years, she had always been fond of children but had had none. A quiet person, she spent a great deal of her time reading or listening to the radio; she tended to accept everything commentators said as the ultimate truth. Since the onset of her illness she had become excessively emotional as well as religious.

In the hospital she was well oriented and intact in sensorium and intellect. She took considerable pleasure in interviews and was very dramatic. The thoughts uppermost in her mind were religious in nature. She pictured herself on one side of the road and the "anti-Christ" on the other, with the mass of humanity passing between them and having the choice of the two sides of the road. She cried openly when she mentioned her brother. At the time of the first interviews she still believed she was pregnant despite her regular menses. She felt obvious relief with being able to tell her troubles freely. During the time she was in the hospital she fluctuated between friendliness and seclusiveness. Since electroshock therapy appeared to make her worse, she was shifted to insulin shock and for a while showed marked improvement. Although she was much better at the time of discharge, the prognosis was considered poor.

B. Psth., Asocial Mutilative M:30:M '639–(64) 2:6:12

In this case the MMPI was given to the prisoner twelve years after a self-inflicted amputation of the middle finger of his left hand. Meanwhile he had been released from prison with the expiration of his sentence and recommitted on a five-year sentence for assault with intent to murder. Since his return he has made a good adjustment in prison and shows an emotional maturity that was noticeably absent before. If he is the kind of individual this MMPI indicates he may be, the change that has taken place in his personality growth represents a major transformation in human behavior. The prisoner had married a worthy and capable woman, and it was because of a remark made by one of his former buddies that he assaulted and is again in prison. The following case record of his earlier imprisonment also throws light on some of the situations contributing to the practice of mutilation which is so common in prisons.

The prisoner was first admitted to the penitentiary at the age of 18. According to the juvenile court of the town in which this man grew up, the section of the city his family lived in was considered the worst; and the court has had more hopeless cases from that neighborhood than from any other. The prisoner's father, a harsh, unrelenting man, punished the boy severely during his childhood instead of trying to understand him. When the prisoner was in his late teens, his father deserted the family. His maternal grandmother and two other maternal relatives were inmates of mental institutions. Early known to juvenile authorities, he was first arrested at the age of 7 as the result of a fight. It was said the boy had also tried to burn a house down. At the age of 9 he was considered incorrigible and was kept in a detention home where he continually made disturbances, evidently to attract attention.

Eventually he was discharged from this home because he was too much of a problem, and was placed on probation. Then he ran away and during his journeys he stole a quantity of golf balls and golf bags. He was finally sent to an industrial school. At this institution also, he was a disturbing influence and was given special study and attention. Chief among his offenses was a continual bidding for attention by making "bright remarks." One official reported that he was a "real entertainer in the dining room; creates disturbances at the table; tries to be a monkey; picks at other boys and tries to raise a fuss." After several unsuccessful attempts to escape, he finally made an unobstructed getaway from this school.

During his freedom he wandered all over the country, hitchhiking and riding freight trains. Arrested as a tramp in a large city, he was sentenced to serve thirty days in jail. Next he hitchhiked to another city, and according to his own claims he worked there for six months. This employment, however, could not be verified. He was later arrested in another part of the country but was soon released, and after two months was again arrested and released.

The charges leading to his first penitentiary sentence included the following: entering two rooms in a hotel; stealing a large amount of clothing which he sold to various secondhand dealers; and after his arrest, setting fire to the city jail. In a confession he said, "I wanted to get something cleaner—it was not my intention to burn down the building—I have never been charged with a criminal offense." While in jail the prisoner, with two others, tried to cut his way out and in numerous ways created disturbances among the other inmates. Both he and other members of his family said that he had been on his way to the West Coast to join the navy at the time the present offenses were committed.

The person interviewing him upon admission to the penitentiary stated: "The subject showed considerable resistance and was uncooperative in all three interviews with him. He was untruthful about all information given, stating, in part, that his mother had died, that he had never been arrested or in a prison or reform school before; that he was a high school graduate, etc. It was not until the third interview that his true name was obtained. He is sullen, defiant, stubborn, and has a fatalistic attitude. He says he is willing to work but has never been able to get a job. He claims he never has had a chance. When asked why others could get along in prison and he could not, he stated 'some fellows haven't much pride.' Asked how he got money to travel, he smiled and finally said 'I played the races.' When asked about the future he said, 'no time to think of that; wondering whether I will get through the next day.' He has no vocational interests—'I am not interested in any work I have ever done, I like to travel.' He still likes to be the center of attention and is a non-conformist. Is of superior intelligence but even during the tests, he gave the opinion that he was bored with the whole procedure."

After his admission to the prison the prisoner was a continuous conduct problem. He was placed in solitary confinement thirteen times, a total of nearly 1500 hours; he was whipped six times (ninety lashes); he attempted to escape; and he twice inflicted injuries on himself. He misrepresented his history, continuously maintained an uncooperative, rebellious, agitating attitude, and apparently made no attempt to adjust.

A psychiatric examination indicated that he had been emotionally defective in personality and a behavior problem all his life, with poor chances for future adjustment. Regarding his reason for mutilation, the prisoner said, "The boss called me a bastard." He further commented that the boss made remarks about his relatives and "rode" him all the time. "I couldn't take that riding all the time," he said. His desire for rest was his other reason for cutting off his finger.

During his imprisonment the man was stubborn, sullen, and resentful of authority. Despite his better than average ability, he had never used it legitimately and no vocational interests could be elicited. Particular efforts were made to gain his confidence but without success. He had a deep-seated fatalistic attitude; he was convinced he had "never had a break" and "never will have." In the past punishment had not helped him to conform, and it was thought unlikely to have any different effect in the future. If he was placed under a patient but firm guard, it was possible he would settle down, but the prospects for his adjustment, both in prison and in the community, were regarded as poor. It was agreed that if his present attitude continued he would be a dangerous community risk.

R. C. K.

P. Mixed	M:30:S:10	+1	'64–1 (47)	2:2:12
Paranoid		+10	'9468237–1 (61)	4:3:8

When this patient was first seen as an outpatient he complained of "nervousness." This was manifested by recurrent tenseness, weakness, insomnia, and mild epigastric distress during periods of emotional tension. The symptoms had been gradually increasing in severity since childhood. Apparently he had also had vague paranoid ideas and increasing depression. He was admitted to the psychiatric unit as a prophylactic measure, since the possibility of a developing psychosis was considered an important factor.

The patient went through the seventh grade in school but then stopped, feeling that he could educate himself. When he was 11 his only sister, who was 6, died; his symptoms dated from that time. He had always been considered shy and retiring and spent much time reading books and magazines, but he had a good many friends and attended church regularly. Sometimes he went on dates in the nearby community but his mother always waited up for him and he did not feel he could stay out late. He operated several farms with his father, working without a salary of any kind beyond the produce of the land. He was eager to introduce new farming techniques but could not convince his father that this was necessary. He objected to farming because it was a "lonely" occupation.

On admission he showed an unusual degree of self-confidence in his ability to do anything he tried. While in the hospital he was sociable toward other patients and cooperative with the nurses, but he usually preferred male companionship. He dressed neatly, smiled and talked freely. He was preoccupied with various methods of obtaining a release from his home environment, saying that his somatic complaints were caused by his problems at home. Although he had that much insight he failed to understand his limitations for the other occupations he was considering. He improved promptly upon his admission to the hospital. The symptoms disappeared completely. He was reassured about his physical condition and soon became eager to leave to go on a vacation and then possibly to enter the interior decorating business with a cousin. It was apparent that he was completely dominated by his parents and to a certain extent was making a conscious effort to break the domination.

B. Pri., Child. M:14:S:74 +5 '64–9213(43) 3:4:12

About two months before admission this boy had enticed two 8-year-old girls to go under a bridge in a lonely locale, where he made attempts at sexual intercourse. The girls were persuaded to accompany him under the threat of a gun which he pretended to have in his pocket. A medical examination indicated that the girls had not actually been raped, but one had suffered minor injuries and emotional shock. Put on probation, a month later he and two other boys on bicycles rode around two little girls, threatening them with sexual assault and using profane language. There had been no other abnormal behavior in his history except that he had become increasingly "nervous" in the past six months, his mother reported, following the return of an illegitimately pregnant sister to his home. There was no evidence of previous sexual misbehavior.

He had finished the eighth grade with a scholastic average of C and had shown considerable interest in school sports. He had got along well with fellow students and teachers, and he had had a few dates with girls. An older boy companion had recently been apprehended on a sexual assault charge. The patient was a "star scout" and had been regarded as a "model boy," particularly in contrast with other members of his family. The fifth of nine children, he was said to have always been independent in his thoughts, feelings, and actions. He handled his own money, which he earned from a paper route, and built model airplanes. He was kind, thoughtful, and usually cheerful. His home life was described as "confused" by the social worker. His mother appeared to be stable, but she was overly solicitous and talked endlessly in a rambling, supercilious fashion. Aside from the unmarried sister who was pregnant, the rest of the children had not shown any outstanding behavior deviations.

On admission the boy was alert, and there were no peculiarities of behavior except fingernail-biting, but he was obviously apprehensive about what might happen to him. He answered questions freely up to a certain point, when he became mute. He was depressed and fearful but eager to cooperate, and his behavior was that of any normal boy. The study seemed to indicate that his misbehavior was sporadic and possibly very largely influenced by the high delinquency rate of the neighborhood and by the actions of his older companion. Arrangements were made through a social agency for his placement in a foster home where there would be an opportunity for him to make new and more desirable friends.

B. Psth., Path. Emot. F:48:M:16 +12 6423'8719–(55) 5:4:16
Paranoid

The symptoms of this patient on admission were crying spells, which had occurred often since the marriage of her oldest son, marked nervousness, inability to concentrate, and many somatic complaints, the onset of which had been insidious. During her entire adult life the patient had had alternating periods of depression and excitement and had shown hypochondriacal tendencies. Her marriage had been a failure. Her husband had deserted her for twelve years, and his return four years before admission had upset her considerably. After two of her sons were drafted into the army the patient had lived with her oldest son. When he married, the patient had been unable to adjust to his wife, and she had finally been forced to leave her son's home. The patient believed that her daughter-in-law had turned her family against her. When the allotment from her two sons in the service stopped, she had to find work, but because of her nervousness and crying spells she was unable to hold any job.

The patient said that her health had always been poor. Twenty-three years before admission her husband had infected her with gonorrhea, for which she had apparently been successfully treated. She was a ninth-grade graduate at age 14 and married when she was 21. After her husband deserted her and she was left with three small children, she had been supported by relief most of the time. A pleasant person of average intelligence, she was friendly toward others but easily offended. She frequently repeated that she was well liked and friendly, but people outside the family regarded her as a queer, "mentally unbalanced" person.

On admission her main thoughts were concerned with paranoid ideas about her son and her husband, who she felt were against her. When she was moved to another room she became disturbed and resentful. She was well oriented and appeared intact in intellect, but she broke down and became emotionally upset to the point of crying during most of her interviews. Cooperative in general, she was pleasant and cheerful most of the time and talked very freely. It was only when an attempt at psychotherapy was made that the symptoms became markedly obvious. Her improvement was slight, and the patient gained very little insight into her problems. When she was discharged to her son there was little prospect of any permanent change in her condition, but with some tolerance and aid from her sons it was felt she might make a marginal adjustment.

Alcoholism M:30:S:14 +3 64287'93–(57) 2:11:7
Deteriorated
B. Psth., Path. Emot.

The patient had gone on a "drinking spree" about eleven days before admission. The incitement for it, according to the patient, had been the refusal of a welfare office to give him relief funds. In the days following, he drank a great amount of alcohol; on the morning of admission he began to get "the shakes" and went voluntarily to a general hospital. From there he was brought to the psychopathic unit. He complained of a buzzing in his ears and said that he had had these spells twice before. He also said that he had experienced hallucinations in one of the previous spells. He had begun to drink heavily seven or eight years before.

He was described as a good-natured, friendly, and easygoing person. He had a leg defect which caused him to limp. Much of his trouble he attributed to sensitiveness over the limp. He had a ninth-grade education and was an itinerant worker. Not many facts were known about his past history because no one was available who had known him. Apparently he was a shy person who nevertheless got along with people fairly well. Independent and stubborn, he was always restless and on the move so that he did not keep any job for very long.

In the hospital he showed evidences of a neuritis but it was not severe. The findings also indicated some deterioration. He apparently had begun to recover from the present bout, and although he had been disoriented earlier he was not so at the time of admission. He was, however, depressed and evidently felt considerable distress about what he had been doing. On the other hand, he certainly had inadequate insight and his manner was evasive. He was restless, agitated, and appeared to be under tension. He was cooperative around the ward and gradually became better physically. He showed some interest in joining Alcoholics Anonymous, but as he recovered from this bout he also recovered his self-confidence and became more inaccessible, less interested in help.

P. Hys. F:18:S:30 +9 6432'7891- 5:8:13

Two days before admission, while returning from a wiener roast, the patient noticed severe pains in her eyes followed by a few minutes of total blindness. Later she developed a headache, dizziness, nausea, and vomiting. A local physician treated her with ice bags, and she was taken to a general hospital. She said that when anyone touched here eyeballs it made her sick all over. By the time she was transferred to the psychiatric division her sight had returned to the point where she could see although her vision was blurred.

She had had no previous attacks and there was no contributory evidence in the past medical or psychological history. She was an eighth-grade graduate at age 15, and after going to high school for two months she had refused to continue. She had an I.Q. of 93. She said that after leaving high school she had wanted to live without having any responsibility, staying out as late as she wanted to and doing nothing for herself. Her attitude led to difficulties with her parents, and she left home to work as a domestic, but she did not enjoy the work and never remained long in any one position. She had always been headstrong, demanding her own way and reacting to any form of authority with temper outbursts. She was a slovenly worker and neglected her room and her personal appearance. Often she would go to bed without removing her clothes. She had a tendency to steal and to lie, and other members of her family considered her "boy-crazy." In her spare time she read confession magazines and indulged in autistic thinking. Just before the present admission she had been staying with a girl friend. She was no longer welcome there, however, and since her parents lived on a distant farm she really had no place to go.

In the hospital she quickly regained her sight. The staff was impressed with her great suggestibility—she would quickly adopt any explanation offered her but at a superficial level only. Because of this she was difficult to help. She was discharged to her sister but did not seem basically improved in her ability to meet life's situations.

P. Anxiety State F:29:M:5 +2 6'43879-(41) 2:10:11
Alcoholism

Six days before admission the patient, her husband, and several friends went on a drinking party that lasted for four days. While the patient was sobering up she became nervous and upset, pacing the floor in an agitated manner, wringing her hands, saying that she was afraid, and asking, "What am I to do?" Her husband encouraged her in the belief that she was "losing her mind" and wanted to send her to a hospital. According to a sister who brought the young woman to the hospital, the present episode was an anticlimax, for in the past she had suffered from more severe attacks. During one of these she had spent several weeks in a hospital. Her husband continually told her that she was losing her mind, and the sister believed this was the main cause of all the trouble. While recovering from a period of alcoholism the patient would regularly neglect her home, her children, and her personal appearance. Between bouts of drinking she was entirely normal and was a good housewife and mother.

At age 14 the patient had been attacked by a married man and since that time had been afraid of being molested. She had, for example, worn sanitary pads continually and carried a penknife whenever she went out on dates. When she told about this she cried, and apparently this fear was somehow related to her present trouble. At the end of the eighth grade her father had compelled her to leave school because he did not believe in "learning." Her husband was a truck driver and, when he was not drinking, was a steady worker. The patient appeared satisfied with her economic level. Before marriage she had had many dates, but afterward she had not gone out of her way to make friends. She and the husband were known as "smootchers," and anyone who would furnish liquor for a night was a friend of theirs. She was easily swayed by her husband, although she did not get along well with him and was afraid of him. She tended to be somewhat dramatic.

On admission mild evidences of alcoholic neuritis were noted in the neurological examination. Mentally, the patient showed no evidence of delusions or hallucinations. All she wanted, she said, was to "get a good rest," so that she would not have any more "nervous breakdowns." Her thinking capacity was fair and she was, if anything, euphoric. Nothing was wrong with her mind, she thought, she was "simply nervous and exhausted." She was neat and clean, alert and attentive. The drinking she repeatedly denied, in spite of the unmistakable history. In the hospital she got along well and was entirely satisfied with her stay. When she left it was against advice, but she gave the reason that the hospitalization was too expensive.

Ps. Paranoid F:34:M:15 +7 648273'19- 4:6:9

For two years the patient had been troubled with weak eyes, insomnia, and restlessness. She had always been an irritable, cranky person and had scolded her husband frequently. For a year and a half she had had ideas that some people, especially her neighbors, her husband, her stepson, and her stepdaughter, were saying that she was a poor mother and an unfaithful wife. She believed that the county attorney was after her, and she had talked about jumping into the river. These general symptoms became so marked that relatives advised her to come to the hospital.

Born in Norway, she had attended school through the eighth grade there, coming to the United States at the age of 18. She did housework until her marriage at 25. A sensitive, self-conscious, hard-working person, she had never shown any particular ambition. She had always thought that men "talked about" her.

In the hospital she showed a pronounced disorder in her mental content, with fixed paranoid delusions. She said, "My neighbors are trying to break up my home. They tell my husband to put poison in my coffee." There were also auditory hallucinations. She appeared slightly depressed and occasionally cried. She knew she had a nervous trouble and that was the extent of her insight, but she was logical, attentive, and cooperative, mixing well with other patients in spite of her ideas. About a week after her hospitalization she experienced delusions about the nurses and demanded that they stop talking about her. She was discharged to a state hospital with an uncertain prognosis.

Twin F:15:S 64'8297–1X (55) 5:22:4

The school counselor who referred this adolescent girl to us did not mention any personality problems but said that the student was attending a girls' vocational school and did not like it. She reportedly had a "high I.Q." and an interest in academic training, especially in art and English.

In the first interview she was very reticent but later talked readily about her dislike of cooking, which she was studying in school. Her twin, who attended the same school, liked it very much. They came from a deprived home background and were living in a church institution. She proved to have superior intellectual ability and an aptitude in English equal to the upper fifth of college freshmen. Her interest in writing was discussed, and she brought in several poems and one story she had written.

A transfer to an academic high school was recommended, despite her guardian's opinion that she should attend vocational school because she would have to earn her own living as soon as possible. A follow-up report indicated that she had attended the academic high school for two years, and then the twins had moved to another city where they had relatives. Before moving she had been in trouble once with the juvenile court because of shoplifting but had not been removed from school. Although in these two years following the MMPI measurement she was not sent to a correctional institution, her total adjustment and her social relations in school and in the community could be called precarious.

D. F. C.

Ps. Sz., Paranoid F:38:M:8 +1 '6483–92(51) 5:5:25

This patient's paranoid ideas became obvious for the first time about thirteen months before admission. When she arrived to visit her husband at the town where he worked she told him that people "planted" by relatives and close friends had followed her on the bus. Her visit had been preceded by two agitated telephone conversations with her husband, and when she arrived she told him that five years previously she had had sexual relations with another man while she was recovering from an operation. The next day when her husband waved goodby to her she mistook the wave to mean that she should leave home, and she boarded a train to a distant city. When she telephoned him he persuaded her to return and for a while she was normal. Later she again began to get peculiar ideas, chiefly that people were talking about her. No reassurance helped her. At about this time she became pregnant and although she was much happier, her basic ideas continued. After six electroshock treatments over a period of six weeks she was vastly improved, but three or four months later the symptoms again appeared.

The patient was a college graduate. Both she and her husband had been working. Shortly before the onset of the symptoms she had obtained a new and better position in which she had replaced a man but because she felt that other employees resented her taking the job, she resigned. A week later the present illness had its onset. She had always been a stable, extroverted, successful person. Her husband and she had been compatible, active in church activities, and successful in social and occupational fields.

On admission the patient's attitude was one of suspicion and apprehension, making it difficult to establish rapport with her. When questioned about any personal subject she would reply, "I have no problems physically or mentally. I am entirely normal, and consider this whole thing ridiculous. I did not ask to come to this hospital. I was forced to come. My personal life is my own affair, and I would rather not discuss it." She would then smile and change the subject. On other subjects her replies were normal, her attitude sweet and pleasing, and in all other ways she was cooperative and relatively well adjusted. She was finally discharged to go to a state hospital.

Ps. Sz., Paranoid M:49:M:1460 +9 6'48319–(63) 4:8:18

At the age of 48 this patient developed ideas of grandeur, saying that he had won the war by himself and that he was receiving messages from Churchill, Stalin, and others. He entered the hospital as a certified patient.

He had an elementary education. He served all through World War I and rose from the ranks to lieutenant. At one time he had been a heavy drinker. He worked in a factory for a time after demobilization, then as a temporary civil servant. He did not settle down to a permanent job for any length of time and always avoided work if he possibly could. He was married and had two children.

Diagnosed as having paraphrenia, the patient underwent a course of electric convulsion therapy. He improved for a short time but then relapsed. He is still in the hospital, still grandiose and unwilling to work. M. V.

Schizoid F:32:S 648′7<u>923</u>–(47) 2:8:8

A discharged WAC, this woman came to the counseling center for advice on how she could best use her training privileges under the GI bill. After her period of service she had returned to her home town, where she had resumed work as a bookkeeper and store clerk, a job she did not find interesting. She had hoped her service experience would get her out of a rut and into more satisfying work.

She did not complain about any obvious difficulties at home or in the community but said she found it difficult to meet people and felt inadequate and insecure in her relations with others, particularly those her own age. She asked in the first interview about some kind of personal development or speech training "to get me out of myself." She also considered business training in a nearby city or, as a final choice, in her own community. In a later interview she discussed a plan suggested by her pastor to take training for religious secretarial work, a course which included study of the Bible, office procedures, and public speaking.

Four months later she still was considering the religious training course but was having trouble getting approval from the Veterans Administration for it. Meanwhile some attempt had been made to get her into group activities with the Y.W.C.A., but getting transportation was difficult for her and she did not follow through. At the time of our follow-up interview she inquired about a dermatologist, believing that improvement of her skin might help her "personality."

This young woman remained self-supporting and did not to our knowledge become a community problem, but she continued to be unhappy and a problem to herself. She did not prove very accessible in counseling interviews, and the prognosis for a really satisfactory adjustment was poor. D. F. C.

Ps. Path. F:28:S:31 +3 64′97–1(45) 7:5:15
Paranoid +24 46<u>391</u> <u>28</u>′7–(39) 9:8:18

In the past seven years, after her graduation from college, the patient had held at least ten different jobs, for the most part as a teacher. Between these short-time employments she spent some time in a state hospital. All her life she had had difficulty getting along with people. The particular episode leading to this hospitalization began while she was still in the state institution; there, on several occasions, she went to a priest, claiming that he was the only one she felt like turning to. After her discharge she still visited him occasionally. A year before the present admission he called the police because the patient became unruly while trying to borrow money from him. Again, three days before the present admission she went to him to borrow a dollar. At that time she was agitated and excited and he called the sheriff, who found her so disturbed that she was taken to a general hospital immediately and kept under heavy sedation until the present admission.

Her past physical health was excellent. She had been a WAVE but had been discharged from the service within three months. In general she had made excellent grades in her schoolwork. She finally lost her teacher's license because of the highly irregular behavior she exhibited. She claimed that she had left her teaching jobs because of jealousy on the part of some one or other of the faculty or the school board. In one place she was accused of stealing money from the student's lunch fund. This was the particular occasion for her loss of her license to teach. She was described as having always been "quick on the trigger" and unable to take criticism. She had never had any friends and had not gone out on dates; she had been regarded as "peculiar" while in college and had walked about the campus ostentatiously reading poetry to herself.

In the hospital, as the initial sedation wore off, she became exceedingly agitated, pounded on the door of her room, and demanded to be released. She believed she was in the hospital because her parents wanted to keep her from going to a state institution. She was well oriented and her sensorium was intact but she had no insight whatsoever into her problem. She remained uncooperative and agitated for ten days and had to be kept in the disturbed section. She gradually improved, however, and was able to go to the regular ward. However, she still showed rigidity, a paranoid attitude, and general immaturity. She again and again became disturbed and had to be sent back into the disturbed section. She was finally transferred to a state hospital.

P. Mixed M:29:S:17 +5 6′729-4 3:1:8

The illness of this patient began six months before admission. At the time the patient was making an unsuccessful attempt at farming. He owed money, and he knew that if he did not have a good crop he would lose the farm. About this time he fell, striking his head on a stone. There was a short period of unconsciousness, followed by a headache that lasted for 24 hours. Nearly a month later he began having pressure feelings over the top of his head and headaches which went back through his head. He complained of seeing double and had his glasses changed several times. When he looked at things about him he noted a blurring of his vision. His memory began to fail, and he became unable to concentrate or to make decisions. When he came to realize that he would not be able to meet his financial obligations, his worrying and brooding induced acute insomnia, general fatigue, and anorexia. Fearing that he was losing his mind, he came to the hospital on a voluntary basis.

There was no previous mental upset, and except for a possible injury from the fall his physical history was not contributory. The patient had been brought to this country from Norway when he was 4 years of age. He had finished the eighth grade at age 16, and although he was a very good student, he had been forced to discontinue his education for financial reasons. He had worked as a chef in a short-order restaurant and had then taken up farming on his own. Although he had got along fairly well the first year, he had then begun to run into debt. A meticulous, ambitious person, he apparently had always been somewhat effeminate and introverted, and he had few outstanding personality traits. At the time of admission he was engaged to a schoolteacher and planned to marry her when he became financially secure.

An extensive study on his admission to the hospital failed to show any evidence of a neurological disorder. Greatly concerned about his physical state, he also worried about the possibility that he was losing his mind. He was able to accept reassurance about the aftereffects from his fall. He also needed reassurance that he did not have a brain tumor. He was given new glasses, a psychological evaluation, and vocational advisement, and he responded exceedingly well to these procedures. He was discharged with the advice to go into some line of work other than farming, preferably in an occupation not requiring the qualities of an extrovert.

Ps. M-D., Manic F:32:S:21 +1 6819′473–(53) 3:8:11

One week before admission the patient became hyperactive and restless. This was the most recent of many similar attacks dating from age 13. The attacks, characterized by excessive laughing or crying, hyperactivity, and insomnia, were usually associated with the menstrual period and had at first occurred several times a year. When she was seen in a clinic at age 14 her parents had been advised that she would "outgrow the attacks," and the intervals between them had increased until the spells occurred only once in every year or two. The severe stage of the attack usually lasted six to twelve days, and the patient was not kept from her work for more than a month. On several occasions she had required hospitalization, but at other times the family had cared for her at home.

She was a graduate of high school and a beauty school. She had average intelligence. She worked as a beauty operator in a shop owned by two older sisters, and she had a part interest in the shop. A cheerful, happy individual, she enjoyed people and had many friends.

The neurological examinations and history were negative. The patient was well oriented but exhibited a marked volubility. She realized that hospital care was needed during her hyperactive attacks, and she was resigned to them. She quickly adjusted to the ward routine, talked with everyone, and discussed everybody's problems, including her own. She wrote many letters to the staff and frequently requested permission to leave the hospital. She improved markedly, and by the time she was discharged she had probably recovered completely from the present illness. It seemed that a constitutional predisposition might have been a factor in her illness since a brother and a sister were emotionally unstable and overactive, and two uncles had committed suicide.

Ps. Sz., Simple F:20:M:65 +21 68213 794′–X (47) 5:20:6
+48 823 61′749–(47) 4:15:11

This young woman's symptoms, severe weight loss, anorexia, and a marked lethargy, had begun nine months before admission, two months after she was married. Suddenly she began to lose weight, her appetite diminished, and she lost interest in housework and in her surroundings. The patient and her husband were living in the home of the husband's parents and all the members of the family cooperated in trying to get her to eat and to feel better, but without success. Occasionally she complained of headaches; these seemed to be related to "overeating," and often she refused to eat in order to avoid this pain. She lost interest in sexual relations, and menstruation stopped. The patient's local physician decided that she was regressing, in spite of every effort to build her up, and he referred her to the hospital.

The young woman's previous health had apparently been satisfactory, and there was nothing to indicate the reason for the onset of the present illness. After she completed the eighth grade at age 17, she kept house for her brother and occasionally worked as a waitress or a dishwasher. Friends described her as quiet, pleasant, serious, friendly, sensitive, kind, and thoughtful. She did not mix well in groups, usually preferring to sit by herself, and she had relatively few friends. She was also known as secretive and somewhat stubborn, and she was never a good housekeeper even at her best. She liked dancing and movies.

On admission the young woman was severely emaciated and looked ill. There was no definite evidence supporting Simmonds' disease or any other organic disorder. The patient was chiefly concerned about her illness, not only the present complaints but her long-standing unhappiness and her attachment to her mother. She was depressed and there was a hint of a paranoid trend. There were no gross disturbances of mentation. Her intelligence was low normal. She had had previous attacks "something like the present one," but "I got well when I wanted to," she reported. She appeared cheerful. She stoutly resisted all attempts at psychotherapy on the basis that she had an organic difficulty. She hid her food and made every effort to avoid eating. She showed a number of obviously hysterical symptoms. Because of her resistance and her apparent lack of assets, little was accomplished with her and she was finally discharged to go home in almost the same condition that she was admitted, except that forced feeding had increased her physical well-being.

Ps. Paranoid F:46:D:60 +5 6'8243-9(43) 5:8:18

This woman was referred to the clinic by the welfare board because she had been making such a nuisance of herself. She had lost her job as secretary in one of the state offices and had found it impossible to obtain other employment. According to her, a definite attempt was being made to keep her from getting a job. During the first interview she complained that it was impossible for her to find an employer who did not make sexual overtures, and at times she had been sure that some of her employers were attempting to hypnotize her in order to gain sexual relations. She was also troubled with severe insomnia and persistent crying spells and was finding it nearly impossible to go into public places because "you just can't be treated like a southern lady."

Her family background was marked by poverty. As a child she had been undernourished and had had severe feelings of inferiority because of having to wear hand-me-downs. She gave little information about her adolescence, but it was apparently marked by feelings of loneliness. Following her schooling she married, was divorced, remarried the same man when she found herself pregnant, then divorced him again. She never gave a reason other than incompatibility for the divorces, although there was a definite indication of an unsatisfactory sexual adjustment. At this time she took a business course and then worked as a secretary, making every sacrifice for the welfare of her daughter. Rather curiously she was very happy when her daughter married, even to the point of refusing to stay at the girl's home, feeling that she would be a burden to her daughter and son-in-law. Her problem came to a head during the war when she was employed by the civil service in a psychiatric unit of the army. She evidently became very warmly attached to her psychiatrist-employer but refused to recognize her emotions. A period of confusion followed, which resolved itself into a feeling that the psychiatrist was trying to seduce her. From that point on her symptoms developed.

Because of the nature of her case it was thought inadvisable for the clinic to take her for therapy. Despite this she came in for a number of sessions in which she would chat about her problem; generally she broke into tears, and this was followed by a distinct feeling of relief. After half a dozen such sessions, she was employed outside of town at a summer resort and got along exceedingly well for a three-month period. Then another blowup came. She returned to town and was seen half a dozen times; then she left town again. We later heard from her that she had finally found a job where "the people know how to treat me like a lady." It was our feeling that her paranoid pattern remained essentially unchanged but that she felt accepted in the social situation. Much of the problem would probably diminish as she resigned herself to the full significance of the menopause.

A. S.

Ps. Paranoid M:35:M:63 +18 6827 413'9– 4:15:7

About six months before admission the patient developed misgivings about his wife's behavior. His ideas centered around the feeling that she was unfaithful to him and that she was attempting to poison him. To substantiate his suspicions, he misinterpreted casual occurrences, but at the same time he felt enough doubt in his mind so that he did not greatly elaborate on his apprehensions. Later when he began to feel pain after meals, he wondered if it might be due to poison placed in his food by his wife. As his anxiety increased he suffered from insomnia. Physical studies revealed no organic symptoms, and he was referred for psychiatric study.

There were no previous personality disturbances and his general health had always been good. He had left home at age 16, and after terminating his education in the second year of high school, he had worked at odd jobs, earning a precarious living. A commonplace, pleasant person whose judgment and intelligence were considered adequate, he got along well with people. His wife was a somewhat inadequate person, whom he had married after she became pregnant. There were three children at the time of admission, and the family was reasonably well adjusted.

The patient's chief concern in the hospital was with his forebodings about his wife. Because of bizarre experiences he claimed to have had with her, he believed that she might be sexually perverted. The patient revealed some feelings of guilt and an increased interest in religion. Even though he admitted that his ideas might not be correct, and he hoped that they were not, they stayed with him. No gross defects of sensorium or intellect were apparent. Although he was unhappy, anxious, and worried, his general manner was pleasant and friendly, and he discussed his problems willingly with an apparent desire for help. He ate and slept well, entered into the ward activities, and mixed with other patients. Although reassurance helped him considerably, the improvement was only temporary. At the time of discharge he was possibly somewhat better, but there was no reason to feel that any real change had been effected.

P. Psychas. F:23:S:280 +10 6842′3791–(45) 3:0:29
Schizoid

This student was very disturbed and presented a variety of complaints, the chief being compulsions about her clothing. She felt compelled to change her clothing several times before going out and even then was dissatisfied. She would hunt for weeks to get a blouse that had exactly the right line across the shoulders, and when she found it, she would wear it until it fell apart, fearing that she could not find another like it. The clothing compulsion was not her only complaint. She had marked anxiety reactions in almost every social situation. She daydreamed much of the time. Rather surprisingly, she was fairly well adjusted sexually. She summed up her situation in the first interview: "I live from day to day and pray that I won't get ill. I am afraid that I antagonize people. I don't want to show off, but I do. I want to have friends. I am an extremist—very happy or very sad. I need people, but I don't know how to approach them."

There was no way of verifying the family history; the girl's report was the only source. She was an only child and brilliant (I.Q. 150). She described her father as rejecting her, frequently to the point of borderline brutality. Her mother seemed to have played little part in the girl's life; she was apparently unable to understand her daughter. Both parents wanted her to grow up, get married, and spend her life in comparative mediocrity. This was in extreme conflict with the girl's ambitions. She was highly idealistic and "soaked up" such things as philosophy. For example, as a second-quarter freshman in college she talked her way into a senior philosophy course and stood head and shoulders above the rest of the class. Her adolescence apparently was a period of confusion. She never felt accepted by any group. After finishing high school, she worked intermittently, saving up to go to college. Between jobs she wandered from place to place—sometimes traveling around the country by bus, sometimes staying with friends. Once she was in a hospital for attempted suicide, and she spent approximately a year in a private hospital devoted to the treatment of gifted neurotics. There she felt accepted for the first time in her life. Eventually, however, her behavior proved intolerable and she was "expelled."

At first the client was disturbed to find that the therapist was a man; however, she recovered quickly and blurted out a long series of negative feelings, frustrations, hopes, and despairs. Underlying all these was a persistent feeling of defeat. Because of her disturbed condition, she was taken for several interviews in quick succession. She rapidly developed a dependency relationship with the therapist but this was not consistent. At times she was definitely antagonistic but once having vented her spleen became friendly again.

During this period she was classified by her housemother and dormitory mates as a "holy terror." "Terror" was probably the more adequate part of the sobriquet; the entire dormitory was afraid of her because of the way she lashed out at anyone for an imagined intrusion into her private affairs. She took benzedrine to overcome the depression which kept intruding itself, and this resulted in further social ostracism when it became known around the dormitory. It was felt, however, that suspension from school with the consequence of having to return to her home entailed too much danger of suicide.

Therapy continued for several months in which the client might be seen several times during a given week; she also indulged in innumerable phone calls to the therapist at the most improbable hours. At times she was very demanding of the therapist and in one instance cursed him roundly for a full five minutes because she believed he had deliberately broken an appointment. The therapist remained calm and when she paused, asked, "Do you feel better?" She smiled and said, "Yes," and the first of a sequence of fruitful and insightful sessions followed. Her adjustment scholastically and socially became much better and there was every evidence that the problem was going to come to a successful resolution. Unfortunately the client then began to develop "a terrific crush" on the therapist. This put her into some conflict, and she could not continue contacts because of her embarrassment. On the other hand, her emotional problem kept driving her toward him. She compromised with telephone calls, frequently as many as four or five in a given day. These gradually tapered off as she found herself more and more. She was not seen during the last three months she was in school, but favorable reports were received about her.

Her money finally exhausted, she returned home. The family situation again brought out considerable tension. She continued to write the therapist at monthly intervals, her letters giving evidence of a gradual decrease in tension. She resumed college much against her father's wishes, and when last heard from was attempting to gain admission to a college away from home. It was felt that this girl would not be able to resolve her problem completely without the benefit of further therapy. A. S.

Ps. Paranoid **F:49:S:42** **+3** **6′8432–79** **6:8:15**
Ps. Sz., Paranoid

The patient was admitted to the hospital because of marked suspiciousness, possessiveness, and delusions of persecution. A severe attack of scarlet fever at age 12 had left her with such impaired eyesight that she had had to leave school at the eighth-grade level. Although it was felt that this illness had been in part responsible for her development into a very selfish individual whose life was centered in the family home, she had shown no abnormal behavior until at the age of 30 she had replaced a slightly defective diamond from a ring of her own with another more perfect stone of her mother's. Upon her mother's death a few years later she was profoundly depressed for many months, and later she began to have temper tantrums that were set off by minor domestic disturbances. Developing into an overly meticulous housekeeper, she left the house infrequently, and then for only brief intervals. Although she rarely used them, she bought jewelry and clothes in excess. Always a snobbish person, she restricted her friendships to her old schoolmates. At 43 she became hard of hearing. Her general suspiciousness gradually focused on her father, a man well known and liked in his community. She accused him of threatening her life, spending her money, and leading an immoral life. She also suspected her brother of petty thievery. As her general line of thought became obvious and apparently dangerous the family brought her to the hospital for study.

The patient had above average intelligence, and her family was in the upper middle-class level. Her only discoverable ambition had been to take care of the family home. Selfish, egotistical, and emotionally immature, she was accustomed to having her own way. The woman had hoarded certain articles, but she had spent money freely since she had no concept of its value. There had been no love affairs or sexual relations in her life, and she had never expressed any interest in marriage.

In the hospital she appeared as a neat, somewhat obese woman. Her answers to questions were adequate and to the point, but she would have nothing to do with other patients. Her emotions were labile, and she was easily aroused to anger. Her thinking capacity was poor, and she could do only the simplest arithmetical problems. Her delusional system was very fixed, and her suspicious attitude was so marked that she would not leave her ring with hospital authorities for safekeeping. She had no hallucinations. A court order, which a brother obtained three days after the patient was hospitalized, changed her behavior from antagonistic to overly sweet, and all her expressions became exaggerated. Although she continued to refuse to associate with other patients, she said that the hospital had changed her entire outlook and refused to listen when her previous delusional statements were quoted to her. Her extreme gratitude for the smallest favors and her repeated mention of how well she had been behaving were interpreted as being part of a deliberately assumed pattern directed toward obtaining an earlier release from the hospital. She remained unapproachable, and there were no further changes up to the time of discharge. It was felt that she should be admitted to a state hospital, but because her behavior was so apparently normal it seemed unlikely that such a commitment could be made. She was discharged to the care of her father.

Ps. Paranoid M:30:M:38 +4 6'847-1 6:7:14

The present episode began about a month before admission when the patient had told his wife that other employees of the factory where he worked were doing trivial things that led him to suspect they were all against him. At first he felt that they were trying to bring about his discharge, but later he got the idea that an outside gang was trying to bring legal action against him as a "germ-spreader." He discussed the matter with the assistant superintendent of the factory, who recommended a rest. During the time he was on vacation he watched the factory, and the normal activities of others came to have a significant meaning for him.

The past medical history was not particularly contributory. The only family difficulties were concerned with the patient's inability to keep a steady job; after satisfactorily completing high school he had sporadically held jobs at a low economic level. Described as "effeminate," he had been considered somewhat different from other members of his family—while his brothers had worked in the fields he had helped his mother with the housework, and because of this he had been rejected by the male members of the community. He was unusually sensitive and was more ambitious than the other members of his family. His married life was fairly satisfactory. He had two daughters and an infant son. His sexual adjustment was adequate.

A poorly systematized, shifting set of delusions of persecution characterized him in the hospital, with the persecutors changing from time to time as well as the reasons for the persecution. Most consistently he thought that the persecutors were after him because he was a "germ carrier or an international spy." In some way he associated the other patients with these persecutions, maintaining that they had all had plastic surgery, and that they were in the hospital under assumed names. At times the idea that his food and cigarettes were doped made him a feeding problem. When discussing his problems he was tense and showed a mild panic reaction. He never took an active part in ward activities. He was discharged for transfer to a state hospital.

Ps. Sz., Paranoid F:19:S:99 +8 68472'31- 5:14:10

Two years before admission, when this girl was in high school, it was noted that she was listless, talked to herself, and did poor work. She became involved with a homosexual group of girls where she took a passive part. At home she had violent temper outbursts and was irritable and cross. On the recommendation of a physician she was sent to a state hospital, but in a few months when her parents found her unhappily placed among very disturbed patients they took her home and tried to keep her there. For short periods she made a fair adjustment, but then she would become irritable, critical of others, and subject to outbursts of temper in which she would throw things. More than once she threatened to kill her mother, and she accused both parents of being cruel, filthy in habits, and immoral. The delusions were constantly shifting and involved various people. She claimed that her body was not built right—the bones were too small and she was built "more like a boy than a girl."

In high school the patient took an interest in dramatics and poetry but always seemed a misfit and made few friends. She developed a crush on a woman teacher and believed the teacher was directing her ideas and activities. Of average intelligence, she nevertheless showed poor judgment and always lacked energy. She liked to put on boys' clothes and to slouch around, and she was careless of her appearance although she was decidedly feminine in figure and posture. Her attitudes regarding sex were peculiar; for example, she believed men had designs upon her and assumed that all girls who were popular with boys were "bad." Her homosexual activities apparently had been brief in duration and purely incidental to her associations.

The patient stated that she came to the hospital for insulin therapy, that she had "schizophrenia with feelings of unreality, inability to concentrate, and hallucinations." Declaring that she knew she was homosexual because she "looked more like a boy" than a girl, she said, "I'm cold with boys and attracted to women." She further volunteered the information that she often felt pleasure at watching women undress and had fallen in love with several women teachers. "I could knock her down in order to have her," she said of one. Many of these ideas were obviously picked up from her extensive reading of books and magazines on psychology. It was difficult to determine which ideas really belonged to her basic personality. In temper outbursts she would yell, stamp her feet, and say, "Don't come near me. Everybody makes fun of me." She misidentified other patients, and she was not friendly with them. At first pleased that she was to receive metrazol treatments, she said after having four that there was nothing wrong with her and she would "have no more of them." She would have the authorities investigate her home, she said, and give her protection against her parents. She was discharged to go to a state hospital. The long history of her poor adjustment before this illness indicated a poor prognosis.

B. Psth., Path. Emot. F:17:S:75 +1 6847'239–(43) 1:11:7
P. React. Depr.

During the year and a half preceding admission the patient had been living away from home because of a disagreement with her stepfather. During this period she had been in repeated trouble with authorities, twice as the result of inebriation and later because of a common-law relationship with a 24-year-old man. She was finally sent to a reform school; she was transferred from the reform school for psychiatric study on a court order.

The patient had had a continuous headache for the past few years. Her father, an irresponsible drunkard, had been cruel to his wife and children, but after her mother divorced him she married another man who was not much better. The patient had always been self-conscious about her teeth, her facial features, her height, her clothes, her father's behavior, and about almost everything else that could be mentioned. She thought that wearing braces to straighten her teeth had spoiled some of the best years of her life. She had always dreamed of having a pretty face and of wearing pretty clothes. She claimed that "everybody" teased her about her appearance. The girl considered sex a "dirty subject" and resented any discussion of it. Her quick temper had frequently got her into trouble. Of average intelligence, she had been a fairly well-behaved girl until the onset of the present pattern of misbehavior. Since her difficulties with the police she had had many nightmares, all referring either to being pursued by police or to seeing a field of snakes.

On admission she showed some paranoid tendencies, mostly about her appearance. She believed she had two entirely opposing personalities, one for good, one for bad. During the interviews she was obviously very much on guard, and she stressed the fact that she was a depressed, undesirable person who was becoming insane. She did not feel she had done anything wrong "compared to what some girls do," but she showed deep concern about being sent back to the reform school, even to the point of threatening suicide. After a course of insulin shock therapy her moods became more normal, and her behavior in the hospital improved until she accepted ward routine fairly well, but her defensiveness did not decrease, and no therapeutic rapport was ever established. She was finally returned to the reform school. Her condition seemed the result of a long-standing maladjustment in an unfavorable familial and social environment, and of deep inferiority feelings since childhood.

B. Psth., Path. Sexuality	M:27:M:20	0	6847291'3-(69)	1:14:8
		+13	427816'3-(67)	2:8:7

The patient was admitted on a court order following his attempt to rape one of his sisters. During the attack he had beaten her severely. The present illness was the culmination of a long-standing personality disorder; the earliest evidences had appeared at age 8 when the patient had begun to masturbate. He also claimed to have had sexual intercourse with one of his sisters. While in the navy he was diagnosed as psychoneurotic. After his discharge from the service he continued to be so irritable and hard to get along with that he could not hold a job for any length of time. He went on frequent drinking sprees during which he squandered all his money, and he claimed to have assaulted five girls in the last five years.

After completing high school he enrolled at a university, but a year later he switched to a technical course at a vocational school. Two months before the end of the course he dropped out of school, and after working as a machinist for a time, he joined first the army, then the navy. A sociable and out-of-doors type of person, he was dependent on others. He was generally considered kind and thoughtful. Before the first of the drinking sprees he had seemed to be stable, cheerful, and generally easy to get along with, but the irregularity of his employment and schooling indicated a persistent personality defect. He had also served several workhouse sentences, and there was a long history of hypochondriasis. At the time of admission his wife was considering a divorce. There were two children.

When admitted to the hospital the patient was deeply concerned about his sexual difficulties, pleading for help in overcoming them and blaming his troubles largely on his navy experiences. He felt that he should be helped not punished, and he was eager to amplify on this idea. Pleasant and cooperative, he was eager to participate in group activities. In view of his history it was recommended that the court consider him a psychopathic personality under the provisions of the state sexual psychopathic law.

Ps. Sz., Cat. F:30:M:176 +26 6'87–319 (53) 3:12:9

Shortly after the patient was married, two years before admission, her husband was alerted for overseas service, and five weeks later he was forced to leave without having an opportunity to say goodby. The patient returned to her parents' home and almost immediately began to display erratic behavior, with intermittent periods of depression and irritability during which she wrote lengthy, illogical letters to her husband. When her husband three months later wrote suggesting a divorce, her behavior became more deviant, and throughout the next year she had frequent spells of loquaciousness with irrelevant and suspicious mental content. At these times she was inclined to be extravagant with gifts and purchases, and she neglected to eat or sleep. Hospitalized for four months at a private psychiatric hospital, she was released when her husband returned; shortly thereafter she was notified of divorce proceedings. Once more she became talkative, delusional, slanderous, erotic, and assaultive, striking and scratching her parents and talking about being raped by doctors in various hospitals.

There had been several previous psychotic upsets, one ten years before admission when she was unable to write her final examinations at college because of severe abdominal pain. She also had experienced severe depressions after the deaths of two friends several years before the present difficulty. Her first actual psychotic upset had occurred five years before the present admission when she had experienced hallucinatory threats to kill her. She had been in a private hospital for three months during that attack. When well, she enjoyed an active social life, traveled widely, and was a very acute, able business woman. She had been known as a stable, cheerful, highly intellectual person with qualities of leadership and self-reliance.

In the hospital she was well oriented, her sensorium and intellect were clear, and her replies to questions were correct and logical, but her stream of thought was often interrupted by the interjection of irrelevant and delusional statements about doctors, sororities, male anatomy, religion, rape, and communism. She showed a marked flight of ideas. On occasion she screamed and became assaultive.

Her appearance was disheveled and careless, her manner superior and hostile. Her condition varied considerably from day to day, and on some days she was almost normal in behavior. After electroshock therapy, and later a course of subcoma insulin, there was a slow improvement with frequent remissions, but she finally improved enough to be discharged to her mother for a trial at home. It seemed likely that she would recover from the present episode, but it was equally likely that there would be future ones.

P. React. Depr. F:37:M:35 +5 6′87214 39–(61) 3:3:13
Ps. M-D., Depr.
Ps. Postpartum

During the last months of a recent pregnancy the patient had begun to have headaches, dizziness, and fears about the coming delivery. After a normal delivery three weeks before admission, she suffered from severe headaches and insomnia which, she said, made housework impossible. She lost interest in her child, her family, her friends, and her home; she became withdrawn, seclusive, and silent. At the time of admission she complained that she had been seeing shooting lights and black spots, her tongue felt paralyzed, her memory was poor, her legs and arms felt useless, and she was tired and weak and did not care what happened.

The patient had always been nervous. She had had two previous "nervous breakdowns." During one in late adolescence she was "jumpy and always on the go"; the other, when she was 21, followed a thyroidectomy and occurred during the course of a pregnancy and miscarriage.

She had completed the ninth grade. She had not experienced difficulties in school and had left "because it was difficult to get from my home to school." She got along well with the teachers and her schoolmates. Her intelligence appeared to be in the dull normal range. After six years of helping at home on the farm, she married. She was known as energetic and ambitious. Although she liked to visit with people, she always kept her troubles to herself. She had had thirteen pregnancies with seven miscarriages. At the end of each pregnancy she had felt depressed and useless, but until the present admission she had been able to recover fairly well from these feelings.

On admission the patient was found to be somewhat obese but in good physical condition. She was concerned about her symptoms and felt she was losing her mind. Her orientation and general mentation appeared to be adequate. She was somewhat retarded and seemed depressed, indifferent, and apathetic. During hospitalization the retardation gradually disappeared. Recognizing the importance of the pregnancies as a precipitating factor in her illness, she decided to limit them in the future. At discharge she was actively planning to resume the management of her home and was looking forward to caring for the baby and for her other children.

P. Anxiety State F:32:M:22 +2 687234'19–(66) 3:13:10
P. Psychas. +20 '718342–(61) 3:3:19

Shortly after the birth of her second child the patient began to experience a series of symptoms. Among these were weakness, fear of imminent death due to heart trouble, palpitation, and insomnia. She felt that her physician had not properly attended her before and during the delivery of her child and that she had suffered cardiac damage. The attacks of fearfulness were accompanied by an inability to sleep and frequent crying spells. She became especially concerned with feelings of guilt about her "past sins." This pattern had been present for one month at the time of admission.

At 18 she had had what she described as a severe attack of rheumatic fever and had been hospitalized for five weeks. She had returned to an active life, however, and had had no symptoms of heart trouble in spite of the fact that she had been employed in an occupation demanding physical labor. She did have mild attacks of asthma.

The patient's home life had been chaotic. Her parents were separated when she was 12. Her mother's moral standards were very low; her father finally died in a mental hospital. One brother spent periods in a reform school. The patient had left school after completing one year of high school and after that time had been employed as a waitress and barmaid until her husband's return from overseas duty. She was described as friendly, socially active, and a good mixer. Except for brief outbursts of temper she was cheerful, frank, and friendly with people; she had accepted responsibility and had been a good manager in her home. Her husband was rigid in religious convictions and in this he differed from his wife. The patient had had extramarital relations while her husband was overseas and had submitted to an abortion. Her husband did not know of this.

In the hospital the physical examination, including heart studies, was negative. The patient was depressed and showed mild anxiety at the time of admission. She was well oriented and her sensorium was clear. She spoke freely and was frank and open at all times. She gave the general impression of mild depression and apathy. She was chiefly concerned with her chest pain and she worried about her heart. She believed her heart to be so bad that it prevented her from all but a minimum of activity. With complete examinations and careful reassurance, she came gradually to recognize that stress and nervous tension had contributed to her problems. She tried to mix with other people and became very friendly. At the time of discharge she had fairly well regained control of herself and was actively planning how she would manage her home affairs. Apparently one factor in her difficulty had been a fear that her husband would learn about her behavior during his absence.

Ps. M-D., Depr. F:53:M:29 +3 68'724–(47) 1:10:8
Paranoid

Two weeks before admission the patient's husband noticed that she was extremely nervous and was easily upset by petty matters. She talked excessively about her inadequacies and cried for no reason. Reassurance from various people brought only temporary relief. A physician told her she was only experiencing menopausal symptoms, and following hormonal injections she showed marked improvement for a few days. Two days before admission, however, she woke up screaming, accused her husband of trying to kill her, and ran out of the house. From that time on she believed that he was poisoning her food and trying to get rid of her. She also thought the neighbors built fences to keep her away and turned their backs on her. On the morning of admission she tried to jump off the sun porch, and when prevented from doing so, she screamed for help because she felt that her husband was about to kill her. She called the police to arrest her husband but when they arrived she made no accusations against him.

There had been one similar episode twenty years before. In the interim she had been somewhat nervous, restless, and high-strung, worrying unnecessarily, and becoming readily agitated. Her general health had been good. A graduate nurse, she had been a night supervisor until her marriage at age 33. She had always been ambitious and energetic and had exercised sound judgment.

In the hospital she was well oriented, and her sensorium and intellect were intact. She was agitated but cheerful. Her mental content was predominantly self-accusatory and self-depreciatory. She showed marked paranoid trends, and she expressed many fears concerning the cause and outcome of her illness. Apparently she had no hallucinatory experiences. At first she was moody, cried often, and was talkative about her troubles, and during this period she did not mix well with the other patients. Gradually she improved and became more stable, finally making an excellent adjustment and recovery from the present episode.

P. Anxiety State F:29:S:60 +19 687′249–1X(66) 1:24:8

This woman became depressed, developed numerous bodily complaints, and suffered from insomnia and a fear of illness following an operation on her mother for cancer. She entered the hospital as a voluntary patient.

The patient was the second of five children. Several members of the family were "nervy." She attended a business training course on leaving school and then worked as a clerk in an accountant's office. At the age of 19 she had an affair with a man; then she was engaged to a student of theology for six years. She developed ideas of guilt about her earlier indiscretion following an interview with a psychiatrist at an outpatient clinic.

She was diagnosed as being in an anxiety state and underwent a course of electric convulsion therapy and an intensive course of psychotherapy. There was temporary improvement, but she again became depressed and unhappy a few months after her discharge. However, she managed to keep her employment.

M. V

P. Hys. F:45:M:37 +16 6874′23 91–X 7:19:11
Mental Deficiency

About seven years before admission the patient struck her back against a door knob and thereafter experienced pain in the lower spine. She was pregnant at the time and the pain was at first associated with weakness and palpitation. Since she continued to have some difficulty in walking, she finally came to the hospital for neurological study. There were minimal neurological findings and the patient very markedly improved with suggestive therapy. As soon as she went home the pain returned. She was readmitted at least once more and was given faradic stimulation of the abdominal wall. With this suggestive therapy she again improved. However, at home again, she was able to do little if any work and became depressed, especially after the death of a child. She was then readmitted in the present admission.

After completing the sixth grade, she left school at age 13. Her I.Q. was between 50 and 60. She worked on a farm and did housework until her marriage at age 28. Divorced from her first husband, she remarried thirteen years before admission. She had been interested in gardening and flowers and had always liked to work on the farm. Never a very social person, she did attend church regularly. Her second husband was undependable, especially in the early years of their marriage, and occasionally he struck her when she inquired about the late hours he was keeping. In more recent years, the couple became better adjusted. The patient's parents and her husband failed to understand her illness and were very unkind in their attitude toward her.

In the hospital there were a number of neurological findings but nothing that would account for the patient's complaint that she could not walk. Abdominal pain and rigidity appeared whenever she tried to get up out of bed or a chair. She expressed a strong desire to get well so that she could walk and do some of the work on the farm with her husband, but she did not seem really worried about her symptoms and was entirely relaxed in her confidence that the staff would help her. There was some depression and apathy but certainly these were within ordinary limits. She responded inadequately to questions, probably consistent with her low intelligence. The interviews were frequently interrupted by her complaints about her abdomen and extremities. In spite of every effort to get her up, she remained in bed and even with faradic stimulation improvement was transitory. It seemed that her child's long illness and death, added to difficulties deriving from her deficient mentality, were the chief factors in the illness. She was discharged unimproved to stay for a while in a rest home while social service workers attempted to find an environmental adjustment that would permit her rehabilitation. It was possible that in addition to other problems, she had a spinal cord disease and a central nervous system disorder.

Ps. Sz., Paranoid M:22:S:13 +1 6879′43–2 1:10:6

The onset of this young man's illness was insidious. He had first been under psychiatric observation at age 15 when his teachers had noted that he appeared dull and showed marked inferiority feelings. Their attempts to encourage him resulted in overbearing and impulsive behavior on his part. A psychiatrist who saw him when he was 16 said, "The patient's personality difficulties are attributable to the home situation. The mother is domineering and selfish, the father indifferent, while a bright older brother puts him to shame." The patient's I.Q. was 85. It was recommended that he drop out of school, but his parents did not agree. Later at a C.C.C. camp the boy made a borderline adjustment but gradually began to show seclusive and peculiar behavior. At times he walked in the snow or on frozen ground in his bare feet and otherwise improperly clothed. He became suspicious of others and made threats against officials. Later, at an army camp, he made homosexual advances to another young man and a fist fight followed. His family resisted the idea that he was mentally ill until he made sexual advances to his mother. On the following day he was admitted to the hospital for observation.

Although the patient's schooling was exceedingly irregular and included failures in a number of grades, he finished two years of high school. Slow in sexual development, he shaved at age 22 only once a week. He had never been at ease with girls and had worried about masturbation. Apparently he had always recognized that he was somewhat defective intellectually and had referred to himself as a "dumbell."

Shy and seclusive, he was exceedingly self-conscious. He had a strong religious tendency. On the ward he was neat, quiet, and courteous, seemingly preoccupied and little interested in his surroundings. He asked for many interviews and was never satisfied, continually returning to ask additional questions. Although he had no obvious hallucinations, he did have bizarre notions. One of his beliefs was that he had high intelligence and was the possessor of ideas that people were trying to take from him and use to gain fame and wealth. He was certain that in a few days he would be superintendent of the hospital. He was concerned about someone who as an experiment was trying to murder him by putting dope in his food. There was something wrong with him and "maybe I am mentally ill," he said, yet this statement was not substantiated by other evidences of insight. Although he never actually struck anyone, he threatened to do so on several occasions. Eventually he was transferred to a state hospital.

Ps. Sz., Paranoid M:39:M:50 +30 '689-(51) 4:8:15

Four months before admission the patient heard voices advising him to quit his job and leave town. Because of his withdrawal, nervousness, and inattention at work, he was actually unable to continue in his job and he went to a general hospital for a week. His condition was recognized and an institution recommended, but his family would not act on the suggestion. At times nearly normal, he gradually became increasingly preoccupied, although he remained tractable and harmonious with his family. He remained at home until the present admission was precipitated by increasing "strangeness" and silence.

The past history was noncontributory. An eighth-grade graduate, he had had some trouble in learning, had always been overconscientious, but had been considered reasonably well adjusted. His chief interest was in his home, and he had no hobbies. The patient and his wife appeared to be well mated. They had six children.

In the present admission he was mildly confused and withdrawn. Most of the time he assumed an attentive listening attitude, showing impatience when disturbed. He was oriented as to persons but not as to time and place. When he could be induced to pay attention, he answered questions lucidly and briefly. He showed suspiciousness and was reluctant to discuss the voices he obviously heard. Six electroshock treatments changed his reactions markedly. His sensorium became clouded but he showed more gregarious behavior, especially toward the nurses and the women patients. Gradually these actions were replaced by more normal behavior. In the last week he admitted to no hallucinations. Because he did not appear to be fully recovered, however, he was sent to a state hospital for additional observation.

Ps. Sz., Mixed F:35:S:98 +19 6'89–3127 4:12:12

About five years before admission the patient developed menstrual irregularities, and the condition was associated with a loss of interest in her surroundings. Claiming physical illness, she would retire to her room for several days where she either went to bed or sat staring into space. Each attack lasted about a month and was followed by a period of relative activity, but her conduct did not return to normal. She continued to be withdrawn and seclusive, was unable to hold a job, and refused to do any work about her home. Her habits became increasingly slovenly; she bathed infrequently, wore dirty clothes, and insisted on wearing silk dresses which she would not allow to be washed with the family laundry. No one was allowed to enter her room, which was extremely dirty and untidy. A year before admission she became upset and angry about the marriage of a man ten years her junior; she said he had been kept from marrying her because other people had separated them. There was no basis in fact for this attitude.

The patient was of low normal intelligence, but she completed the second year of high school, with a very poor record. After leaving school she worked as a domestic and until her present illness she had a satisfactory work record and was thought of as a conscientious worker who took her responsibilities seriously. In the small town where she lived she apparently was regarded as a completely normal person. The family existed at a low socio-economic level but her background was otherwise average.

In the hospital the patient was inaccessible, and it was extremely difficult to penetrate her inner thoughts. Although the hypothesis could not be confirmed, her conduct suggested that she was experiencing hallucinations. There were vague delusions of persecution, as indicated by the fact that she said she had left one church to join another because people were talking about her in her own church, but she never enlarged upon this point. There was a blunting of affect and inappropriate moods during her discourse. Though she was not a nursing problem, she took no active part in ward activities and for the most part sat by herself staring into space. There was little improvement during her hospital stay, and at times she showed excitement characterized by misidentification of people about her and by active responses to visual hallucinations. She was discharged to a state hospital.

Ps. M-D., Manic	M:26:S:41	+1	68′9147–(63)	2:15:8
Ps. Sz., Paranoid		+25	′92–3716(55)	5:11:5
Deteriorated				

The patient was admitted to the hospital because of nervousness and excitability. He also complained of a speech difficulty. The illness dated from about five months before when it had become increasingly difficult for him to get along with other people. He had been in several fights at parties and dances and had fought with a married man after dancing with the man's wife. This episode seemed to precipitate more intense symptoms of nervousness and excitability with increased psychomotor activity and mild delusions of grandeur. He had a suspicion he was hypnotized by neighbors so that they controlled his speech.

He had been in good health before the present illness. There were no past nervous episodes, although he had been nervous and excitable as an adolescent. This tendency was not severe but it resulted in his rejection from military service. Graduating from high school at the age of 18, he had spent all his life on a farm. Schoolwork had been difficult for him. He said, "My father has always been hard on me." He had attended school parties, however, and had taken part in numerous activities. His conduct had been good though he said he had secretly felt some suspicion and resentment. He worked hard on whatever task he was faced with and became angry when frustrated.

In the hospital his intellect seemed slightly disturbed though his sensorium was clear. He had a poor supply of information. There was a slurring of his speech and a questionable Romberg. The general psychometric studies also indicated the possibility of some sort of brain damage. In spite of these findings the staff could not state positively that there was organic brain deterioration. He had poorly systematized delusions of grandeur and mild paranoid trends. Typical of these was the following: "People bigger than I and with more money are beating me out of opportunities." His main trend of thought centered around becoming important and making money. He was given both electric and insulin shock treatments. His speech became worse and there was a marked mental retardation. In other ways he showed some improvement, however, took part in ward activities such as card playing and dancing, and was at times alert, overactive, and boisterous. He improved gradually and at the time of discharge was considered well enough to make an adjustment outside the hospital, though he was obviously not completely recovered.

Ps. M-D., Manic F:15:S:74 +14 689'47–X 1:26:5

This girl was admitted on a voluntary basis because of an acute excitement that had been present for several days. The symptoms dated from a month before when the patient told her mother that the hired man had forced her to have sexual relations with him. This had also occurred previously, the girl said. At times the patient had appeared bewildered and confused and had talked incoherently. She expressed feelings of impending disaster and identified the hired man with the devil.

A junior in high school, the girl had always been competent socially and had formed many close friendships. Despite her slowness in learning she had earned good grades. She had not begun to have formal dates with boys. In general she had appeared to be a completely adequate girl.

In the hospital she was overactive and overproductive of ideas. "Call Dr. Kildare. I see God in heaven. I see light. Biology. Find Satan. Find Gabriel. Put light together and get plant life. Biology." Apparently she was experiencing auditory hallucinations. Disoriented, she could not identify the people about her. She was euphoric, and her appearance was disheveled and untidy. In the first 24 hours in the hospital she experienced urinary incontinence. Gradually she became better and her discourse was somewhat more rational. In a little more than a week she was spending part of her time on the open ward. As soon as it was established that she was definitely pregnant a therapeutic abortion was advised. This was performed and was followed by a short period of overactivity and elation. By the time of discharge the patient had gained good insight and was apparently recovered from the present illness.

B. Simple Adult Maladj. F:31:M:33 +4 '689713– 6:1:12
Suicidal
Paranoid

The patient was admitted to the hospital on a court order filed by her husband. Although they had been jealous of each other for many years, the actual difficulty between the patient and her husband began about twelve months before admission when the patient became resentful because another couple who were visiting them suggested a change of partners. The patient complained that the other man had attempted to force sexual relations upon her, and she became angry because her husband and the man's wife were incredulous. She suddenly went to her mother's home, where she remained for three weeks. During that interval she wrote a letter to her husband, threatening suicide. On her return home she was overly critical, slept poorly, and was very suspicious about her husband's everyday life. In one suicidal effort, she attempted to cut her wrists but was restrained by her husband, and shortly before admission when she threatened to drink lysol he locked her in her room overnight. The next night he awakened to find his wife striking him on the head with a shoe and screaming.

There were no previous periods of illness or psychological upset. A high school graduate, the woman had married shortly after her graduation. Although she was self-reliant, conscientious, and hard working, she also was stubborn, frequently talked about others, and was known in the community for her bad temper. Never satisfied with her station in life, she always seemed to enjoy taking part in an argument, and although in general she was cheerful in the company of others, she cried easily when upset. Her husband said she had always been jealous of him, and in the last few years they had had numerous quarrels. At the end of these the patient would run from the house and go down the road until her husband caught up with her and brought her home. The husband had relatively few friends, was overly serious, and also was noted for his bad temper. There were six children.

On admission the patient's chief concern was that she might have permanently lost the good will of her family. Although she blamed herself for her troubles she said that she had been "forced to do" what she had done, and that she felt her husband had discriminated against her and no longer cared for her. There was a moderate retardation in her thinking, and she became tearful whenever she spoke of her family difficulties. She showed little spontaneity in thought. She cooperated well on the ward, but occasionally she was sarcastic toward other patients and displayed some irritability. Although toward the end of her stay she seemed willing to accept some help in planning for the future, she was not very receptive to psychotherapy. In a joint interview with the patient and her husband they both agreed to consider each other's personality in an attempt to avert major difficulties in the future.

Ps. M-D., Manic F:47:M:22 +1 6<u>89</u>7′2<u>34</u>1–X(61) 11:18:4

The patient's symptoms on admission were excitement, extreme talkativeness, irrationality, and general hypomanic behavior alternating with brief periods of marked depression. The onset was sudden. Two months before admission the patient experienced an attack of severe abdominal pain. No organic disorder was found in the medical examination and the pain soon disappeared. During the next weeks she was nervous and excitable and had increasing periods of depression. She complained of headache and her appetite was poor. Six days before admission the abdominal pain returned, but a medical examination again proved negative. The physician recommended psychiatric hospitalization in view of the hypomania.

The past history showed no previous episodes of this sort. A cheerful, energetic person, the patient was a leader in her community. She had good intelligence. In her family a considerable number of persons had had mental difficulties of one sort or another. The patient's 13-year-old son, apparently subnormal mentally, had made things difficult for the patient, and she had complained to her husband, demanding that he do something. She had insisted particularly that her mother-in-law, who had lived with them for 25 years, be moved to a rest home. When this was finally done, the patient felt considerable guilt about the whole affair. The menopause began about the same time, and she developed an aversion to sexual relations.

When first seen the patient was excited, and her thoughts were racing in a disordered fashion. She showed circumstantiality and a flight of ideas, with loosely arranged delusions about "taking over" and "reforming the world"; she also had mild paranoid trends. Her elated moods would suddenly be broken by brief weeping spells. The present pattern appeared to be merely an exaggeration of her usual psychological state. She had some insight and wanted to see a "psychiatrist doctor." Her improvement was rapid; she quieted down, talked more rationally, and developed better insight. She was discharged greatly improved. The present episode, it was thought, had run its course.

Ps. Paranoid F:23:M:36 +16 6897′421– 1:12:9
Ps. Postpartum

One month before admission the patient had become irritable and restless, with psychomotor retardation, depression, and apathy. She began to be afraid that her husband would leave her, and she suspected him of infidelity. She also had the fear that he was going to kill her in order to collect her insurance. About two weeks before admission she told her husband that a big industrial company was planning to do harm to her. She thought that people looked at her peculiarly. The day before admission she had become so acutely agitated that she had torn off her clothing and had thrown the silverware off the table.

Seven years before admission, while employed by the industrial company, the patient had been hospitalized with a knee injury. Acutely ill for two weeks, she had been delirious and had run a high temperature. She had received considerable compensation for this injury, part of it after a court action. The patient's mother some time earlier had also been engaged in a lawsuit against a public utility company because of the accidental death of the patient's father.

An eighth-grade graduate at age 15, she had left school to go to work in a factory; she had also been a waitress for a brief period. Before her marriage she had been more than a moderate beer drinker. Although she had always been suspicious, jealous, easily angered, and irritable, she was a good housekeeper, and she got along well enough with her husband, although her family had never liked the man and they accused him of drunkenness and of mistreating the patient.

In the hospital her mental content was dominated by a fixed systematized delusional system. She believed that the industrial company was planning to get even with her because of the compensation suit, and she thought that possibly her husband was a member of a clan. She was afraid that he intended to kill her for her insurance. She said that a Filipino had left some banjo strings on the front porch as a warning of a plot to do physical harm to her. Unhappy, depressed, and frequently on the verge of tears, she recognized that she was mentally disturbed, but she did not doubt the veracity of her delusions. Although she was never unpleasant, she was moderately asocial. Her suspiciousness and anxiety made it difficult to help her, but she did get somewhat better. She was finally discharged to the care of her husband against the recommendation of the staff, after he had signed a release relieving the hospital of further responsibility.

B. Simple Adult Maladj. Suicidal | F:21:M:8 | +1 | '69372–(53) | 3:2:6

About fourteen months before admission the patient became nervous and irritable and began to have difficulties with her husband. She was depressed, sulky, and insecure. About a year before admission she took twenty aspirin tablets, more to gain sympathy than as a suicidal attempt. For a while she was in constant conflict with her relatives by marriage and with her own parents. Feeling that her husband had never shown her enough affection and attention, she finally took nine grains of phenobarbital and was admitted to a general hospital, from which she was transferred to the psychiatric unit.

Her previous physical health had been good. She had been nervous from an early age but this nervousness apparently had never been very noticeable. An intelligent girl, she went to a business college for a couple of years and then did stenographic work until she married. After her marriage she continued working as a clerk. She was friendly and thoughtful toward others although she was described as shy. She was avocationally active in art.

In the hospital the physical and neurological findings were negative. She was free of delusions and hallucinations and appeared entirely normal. She explained the suicide attempt as a "lapse of my mind." During the examination she was open, friendly, cooperative, and appeared eager to get well. She said that she had been "tricked" into coming to the psychiatric unit and considered that most of her troubles had a very rational basis. While in the hospital she seemed to make fair progress in more realistically evaluating her home situation. She was discharged to attempt to re-establish her home and she was to continue outpatient contacts. The prognosis was not felt to be particularly good, however.

Ps. Sz., Hebe. | F:36:S:18 | +1 | 69'48 123–(47) | 4:8:15

Eight years before admission the patient had become incoherent, had thought of killing her parents, and had expressed fears of being kidnapped. She had been exceedingly confused, expressing the idea that she had a dual personality. At times she had refused to eat, apparently because she had believed her food was poisoned. She had been committed to a state hospital where she remained until the present admission for the surgical treatment of an abdominal growth.

No information about her past history or personality was available. At the time of admission she had many delusions of grandeur, among them that she was married to a prominent physician, that she was the head of a large chain of beauty shops, and that she was a graduate "doctor-nurse." She was euphoric and without insight, but she was well oriented as to time, place, and person. Her vocabulary indicated that her intelligence was above average. There was no evidence of a depressive or agitated state. In fields other than those relating to her delusional ideas, her stream of thought was adequate. Although she was interested and cooperative in the interview on admission, her manner was condescending. Her progress in the hospital was uneventful. She adjusted adequately to the hospital activities. After an uneventful recovery from the surgery she was again transferred to the state hospital.

Ps. Invol. Melan.	F:59:W:48	+1	69′487–X (53)	3:17:14
		+30	′2349– (34)	2:3:14
		+47	′317248– (51)	1:1:18

This patient had been nervous most of her life, but in recent years this nervousness had increased. When her youngest daughter married and left her alone, she began to feel useless and developed urinary and fecal incontinence, after an initial period of "colitis and hypertension." In the ensuing years she underwent intensive psychotherapy but continued to worry and lose interest in her work. Her depression was accentuated when she was asked to resign from the job she had held for 25 years, and when she heard that one of her major investments had failed, leaving her with little financial reserve. She began to develop guilt feelings and although she had previously been very active, she lost interest in all her activities and in life generally.

She had been healthy until four years before admission at the time of her youngest daughter's marriage. She did well in school and graduated from normal college. When she was 16 her mother died and a year later her father died also. Her mother had been an invalid before her death and the patient had had to assume responsibility for most of the household while she was still in school. She had high intelligence and was, as a rule, very active, liking to keep busy. She had been compelled to teach school to support her family of two children after her husband had left her. He later died.

In the hospital she was worried about her financial and occupational difficulties and thought about them a great part of the time. She said that things looked bad and she blamed her present predicament on "terrible things" she had done years before. Her sensorium and intellect were intact. She was fidgety and cried easily but was cooperative and logical in her stream of thought. Electroshock treatment helped her. She forgot about the "sins" that had previously bothered her so much and was discharged to live with her mother-in-law, with whom she got along very well. It was felt that the probability of a recurrence was moderately high.

P. Anxiety State M:20:S 6'971234–(62) 5:4:19

This college student came in with complaints of eye tics, jerking of his shoulders, and feelings of tension in new situations.

He had had a tense and dominating mother and a passive father. The youngest in his family by ten years, he had led an overprotected and generally sheltered life. His brother had had chorea and had received considerable attention from the family because of this illness. One of his brother's symptoms was a jerking of the limbs and it seemed likely that the patient had mimicked this behavior as a means of maintaining his dependence on his mother. The boy seemed to have been characterized by considerable sexual immaturity.

During the interviews there was very little evidence of the presenting complaint, but the patient seemed to develop a great dependence upon the therapy. He was overly conscientious. In the course of his therapeutic development there was a gradual release of his hostility toward his mother. This was accompanied by an improvement in his ability to deal with his problem. He was seen in a series of group sessions over approximately a six-month period. C. K. A.

B. Psth., Mixed M:31:M:28 +2 '6973–(57) 9:2:21
P. Psychas.

The patient had begun masturbating when he was 5 years old and had continued ever since. Until fourteen months before admission, he claimed to have had intercourse with his wife three or four times daily and to have masturbated sixty times per week; he also went out window peeping several times a month. During the past fourteen months he had refrained from intercourse, but he said he had increased his rate of masturbation to 80–120 times a week. Further, he had been window peeping at every opportunity. Readily excited sexually, he was irritable and destructive until he could have an orgasm. He demanded that his wife be dressed in a manner that excited him and angrily left his house without his supper if she was not so dressed. He forgot prudence and morality when sexually excited, and he made clever plans for sexual gratification. He thought of knocking girls unconscious and masturbating on them but presumably never executed his plans. He devised schemes such as having his wife advertise for domestic help so that he could have women in his home and watch them through specially prepared peepholes. He had an obsessive desire to eat certain foods, notably candy, pop, and ice cream.

He had had great difficulty in school, repeating at least three grades, and had left at age 18 after failing the ninth grade. He had been the captain of teams in several sports, however, and had repeatedly been elected president of his class. For a while he worked as a common laborer and then got a somewhat better job; he was promoted a number of times and apparently did fairly well. He had always been a sociable, well-liked person, although in school he had felt "dumb" and ignored when in a group. He was shy with girls and was childishly egocentric. He had some feminine traits but these were not extremely marked.

He showed compulsive behavior, manifested by having to check and recheck things to make certain that they were in order. His early home life had been relatively good, though the other men in the family apparently had also tended to be overdriven by sex. He had three boys of his own and loved his wife and children; there was no evidence of infidelity. His financial judgment was very defective.

In the hospital the physical examination was relatively negative except for a moderate degree of immaturity in the development of secondary sexual attributes. His mind was occupied with the sinfulness of spilling seed, and he worried about whether or not he would get well. There were no obvious defects of sensorium or intellect. He seemed reasonably well informed and intelligent. He claimed he had no craving for sexual excitement while he was in the hospital. He constantly asked to see his wife and children and repeatedly wanted to be reassured that he could leave by a certain date. Ten shock treatments did not seem to change him appreciably. He left the hospital with the strong determination to continue the good behavior that characterized his stay there. The staff could not clearly classify the case, though the dominant factors seemed to be more in the nature of obsessive compulsive characteristics than anything else. It seemed significant that the present hospitalization did not represent a particular exacerbation of his usual behavior and the fact that he had got into so little difficulty over the years was evidence that he had controlled fairly well, in a social sense at any rate, whatever abnormalities were present.

M:21:M	'698–2 (55)	1:4:14
	9'43–67 (57)	5:1:15

Referred first by a veterans' organization as an applicant for training in engineering, this man appeared to be pleasant but earnest and he took the test results very seriously. His interest tests showed a low engineering interest and a generally indefinite profile except for a positive interest in purchasing and in sales. After counseling and a discussion of the test results he changed from engineering to business administration.

More than two years later he returned, saying he wished to talk about a change in his college course. He appeared anxious, excited, and full of ideas, most of which were related to the teachings of an economics professor. He said that after taking this professor's course, he could not think of going into business to work for a capitalistic enterprise. In two subsequent interviews he discussed his anxieties and also his relationship to his wife and her family; the latter had means, whereas his own family had a history of financial dependency. An MMPI retest showed a high Ma score, and another interest test indicated a shift away from business and purchasing toward personnel and public administration.

He changed his major to personnel and social science, believing when he did so that he would later work for the government, since he could not subscribe to the philosophy of private enterprise as it is practiced today. By the end of his college course he considered this period a "very adolescent stage," when he was unduly influenced by one person. He said he now realized that "one can work in business without agreeing with everything that is done," and he was willing to take any beginning job which would provide experience for future work in personnel or industrial relations.

At one time the patient had seemed almost paranoid in his reactions, but the MMPI did not indicate that pattern, and his subsequent attitudes suggested that he would achieve a satisfactory adjustment if given a reasonably favorable job opportunity. D. F. C.

Ps. Sz., Paranoid	F:34:M:24	+5	6′98341–7	9:6:14
Ps. M-D., Manic Ps. Sz., Paranoid	F:40:D:5	+3	4′82–(49)	8:2:22

The patient, whose conduct had always been unpredictable, left home a week before admission, saying that she was going to a class reunion. A few days later her husband received a letter postmarked from a distant town, in which she said she was traveling about with a girl friend. Then the husband was called by the sheriff of that town to come after his wife. She had been diagnosed as psychotic by a local physician. On his arrival the husband learned that the patient had engaged a lawyer to prosecute a man who was, according to the patient, responsible for her pregnancy. She was not, however, pregnant. She had come into contact with the sheriff when a hotel clerk had asked her to pay her bill and she had made a scene.

The patient had had meningitis as a child. There were no residual findings for this. In the ninth grade she had left school without any apparent reason. She then took a business course and worked as a stenographer. After a few years of successful office work she lost interest and took up scout work. Becoming overly active at that time, she made unusual demands on her family. While she was attending a summer school, she became pregnant and later bore an illegitimate child. After that she worked as a housemaid. Until her marriage, which occurred two and a half years before admission, she had always been unpredictable and had not discussed her thoughts with anyone. There were outbursts of temper whenever she was crossed. She had few friends and spent most of her time reading or just sitting about the house. During the period of overactivity preceding the illegitimate pregnancy she "ran around with a fast crowd of young people," bought things she could not afford, and began many projects which she never finished. After this period there was a depression. She stayed in bed and refused to see anyone. This depressed period ended with the birth of the child. After that time she had mild ups and downs until the present admission.

In the hospital the patient expressed the belief that she was pregnant and gave a bizarre story of an "affair" with a strange man. She had paranoid ideas about her family and her husband, and she misidentified many of the patients.

She thought the lights were movie cameras, and she had a vision in which she saw the Holy Father and the Son. She frequently quarreled with other patients and had to be isolated. Discharged to go to a state hospital, she received electroshock therapy there and was out of the hospital for a short time. However, she soon returned with a manic spell. She was later discharged.

Seven years later she was readmitted to the psychiatric unit after having had two more hospitalizations, with shock therapy, at state hospitals. In the second admission she was also paranoid, having many ideas of reference, though she was not as severely disturbed as she had been during the first admission. She completely lacked insight and was incoherent and voluble. She appeared euphoric. Among her expansive delusions was the belief that she was engaged to a Russian pianist and would inherit a large estate. Again she was transferred to a state hospital.

Ps. Sz., Cat.	F:49:D:52	+45	'69874-2 (72)	4:13:7
Paranoid		+59	9'64-31 (59)	4:5:11

About eighteen months before admission the patient's father died. She had been unusually closely tied to him. Some time later a spiritualist told her "how to contact the dead." After that time she experienced hallucinations, hearing her father's voice and writing down material he dictated to her. At first this "post-mortem contact" occurred only at night, but she became worse and began to hear accusatory and warning voices as well as her father's voice. She worked day and night transcribing her father's words and became physically run-down. At times she would stand rigid for long periods in unusual postures. Occasionally she would run through her apartment, apparently running away from something. During the week before admission she spent a period of two or three nights without sleep, attempting to escape hallucinatory threats by running about and hiding. On the morning of admission she appeared to be in a catatonic state.

The patient had graduated from high school and had worked until her marriage at age 30. Her marriage ended in divorce five years later and after that she lived with her mother and supported her mother and one daughter. She had good intelligence and a high level of energy output. Probably she had been somewhat overactive; she had many interests and was gregarious and friendly. It was always important to her to be well thought of. She was actively interested in religion and in mysticism.

In the hospital she was hallucinatory, disheveled, and distraught. The threatening voices she heard made her so concerned about the welfare of her family and friends that she sought a means of communication with them and attempted to telephone them. In many of her conversations she interjected denials of any dishonest or promiscuous behavior in apparent response to hallucinatory voices. She was unstable emotionally, predominantly depressed and agitated. Her condition did not change until she was given shock therapy two weeks after admission. After five treatments she was much better; no longer hallucinatory, she continually insisted upon going home. After fifteen treatments she was somewhat agitated but self-possessed, cooperative, happy, and cheerful. At the time of discharge she was almost completely recovered from the acute episode and was probably her usual mildly hypomanic self.

Ps. Invol. Melan.	F:45:M:57	+2	'7–<u>63</u>(61)	6:6:15
Suicidal		+55	'42–9(61)	7:1:22

This woman's illness began two months before admission during a cross-country drive with her husband. They were on a vacation following the sale of their business. She did not enjoy the trip and when they reached their destination she became restless, agitated, and unhappy. Her conversation centered around the wrongs she had committed in the past and she wanted to see a minister about them. When she began to develop physical ills she consulted a physician who declared her to be in good health. Her husband decided it would be wise to return to their home city. On the way the patient jumped out of the car when it was moving at a high speed. She gave this as her reason: "I'm not worthy of my husband and he's been too good to me all my life." Hospitalized briefly for bruises and lacerations, she recovered and the couple resumed the drive home. It was noted that she was quiet and withdrawn and the feelings of unworthiness continued.

The past history indicated little of significance. For about a year there had been a series of episodes in which she awoke at night, felt afraid and short of breath. These attacks were relieved by hurrying outside into fresh air; eventually they ceased and no basis for them was discovered. Heretofore, she had been an alert, sensible, efficient, hard-working person. Not usually difficult to get along with, she could be curt toward people with whom she differed. She was painstaking in her activities. She was moderately religious and emotionally stable as far as could be determined.

In the hospital there were marked self-depreciatory feelings. She felt she had "done no good" throughout her life and had been a burden to her husband, and she wondered if "anyone will punish me for being so unworthy." Her sensorium and intellect were clear. She was deeply depressed, was retarded in her replies, and cried a great deal. Sometimes she became agitated and restless. The problem was complicated by the discovery that she was a diabetic. After a series of electroshock treatments she showed a general improvement in her mood and activity. In fact, after seven or eight treatments she became overactive and euphoric. Still later she seemed to return to her usual personality and was discharged with a good prognosis.

P. Mixed F:57:M:11 —1 '7128–4 1:2:6

P. Mixed F:58:M:106 0 7'21638–94 (59) 2:3:9

The illness of this patient began a little more than a year before admission when she became dizzy one night while working and feared she might have a stroke. From that time she became progressively more worried about her condition until she was finally hospitalized for two weeks of physical studies. She was also depressed. Later she underwent another hospitalization for eleven days and was given electroshock treatments. The depressive symptoms increased following this treatment, and after another period of attempting to live with various relatives and to relax, she voluntarily entered in the present admission. She feared that she might "go insane and do something to myself or to others."

The past history contained a long list of medical procedures. Included were an operation for the removal of a tumor from her breast, a hysterectomy, and a unilateral ovariectomy. For one period she had what was called a nervous heart.

The patient's childhood had been chaotic. When she was 9 days old her mother died and she was "farmed out" to first one relative and then another. In the second year of high school at age 16, she quit to go to work. School had never interested her. Her marriage took place when she was 17. Her five children were a heavy burden on her. Three sons were in the army and she worried about them excessively. Considered a capable person, she had got along well with people, had engaged in social activities, and apparently had led a fairly normal life.

In the hospital she appeared to be cooperative and was willing to talk readily. On further observation this proved to be more apparent than real. At times she behaved in a clearly haughty manner and showed annoyance with staff members and other patients. She was unable to see any possible relationship between her symptoms and emotional factors. Initially she made a fairly good adjustment, but she soon began to express dissatisfaction and annoyance with minor details of the hospital routine. She asked for special privileges and when these were not granted she became unhappy. A close relationship could not be established for therapeutic treatment, but she did improve considerably in the hospital. The home conditions were modified somewhat, and it seemed that she might make a satisfactory adjustment in the future.

P. Anxiety State M:26:D 713'26849–(59) 3:9:11

This staff sergeant was referred from the psychosomatic ward where he had been under observation for multiple complaints including a cough, stomach "churning," and "heart skipping beats." He was aware of constant tension, both physical and emotional.

The sergeant's early life had been dominated by a rigid, arbitrary, unaccepting parent. His father, a German-born physician, was still active in his profession at 78 years of age. His parents got along poorly, his mother being passive and solitary. The patient obviously was strongly identified with his mother. In spite of the almost constant tensions, he insisted that his childhood had been happy. His high school and occupational careers were not unusual except for his failure in both instances to live up to his parents' high expectations and his own considerable abilities. A marriage he had entered into at 23 had been annulled after a few months because his wife "had cooled off and was two-timing" him. An ingratiating person, he professed an intellectual breadth which he did not possess, and he seemed actually to be narcissistic and shallow.

Under brief and superficial therapy, the sergeant was able to accept and discuss freely his hostility against his father and, in a secondary degree, against the army. He gave up his original plan of continuing in the army and was ultimately discharged from the service in a relatively stable emotional state.

A. T. K.

Ps. M-D., Depr.   M:48:M:27   +22   '7183–9X(41)   14:1:25

The patient was admitted to the hospital with complaints of nervousness, tiredness, periods of vertigo and tinnitus, and peculiar sensations in his chest and extremities. The symptoms had been present for about six months and had become so acute that he could not perform his work but remained at home and did nothing. He did not want to meet his former business associates because he felt so ill at ease. He believed that his condition was the culmination of a long period of nervousness over the years.

The patient's past physical and psychological histories were not helpful. He had come from Russia as a boy and had gone through the eighth grade in school. He had always worked hard and had been very active. He had no close friends, his only acquaintances were business contacts. A withdrawn person, he was not particularly cheerful. He had been married about twelve years before admission and got along fairly well with his wife.

In the hospital he was agitated and anxious about his trouble, and he had various suggestions of his own about what was wrong. He was distinctly hypochondriacal and somewhat irritable. There was marked volubility and rambling. His dress was neat and during his first few days in the hospital he cooperated fairly well. Eight shock treatments brought no marked change. A manic tendency appeared and he left the hospital against advice because he felt he had recovered sufficiently to return to work. He had many ideas of the vast amount of work he could perform in a few days. His wife tried to persuade him to remain but felt that if he insisted on going home she would be able to handle him. The case was not at all clear diagnostically but the prognosis was thought to be reasonably good.

P. Mixed   M:25:S:38   +6   718'3942–(49)   1:4:16

The complaints with which this young man came to the hospital had been present for eight or nine years; he summarized them under the term "feeling of tension." Among the symptoms was a tightness in his head and in the muscles extending from his neck down into the trunk. He also had a feeling of pressure in his eyes. These were not accompanied by pain. He believed the people around him could see that his eyes were glassy and staring; he also saw other people's eyes "as glassy." This bothered him considerably. The tension feelings increased when he was among strangers or under emotional stress. Four years earlier he had had what was called a "minor nervous breakdown." This had come on suddenly, "like a cloud going over my mind." Things had seemed unreal, he had been depressed, and his thought processes had appeared to slow down. Nevertheless, he had continued to work, and after three or four months the condition had cleared spontaneously. He had visited several clinics during this period and had sought the aid of numerous physicians and chiropractors.

A high school graduate, he had earned good grades in school and had taken an active part in sports. He had wanted to attend a university but had been afraid to enroll because of his symptoms. The patient's mother said that he had been a "model boy." After high school graduation he held various odd jobs, shifting quickly from one to another. The reasons for these changes were not clear. Apparently he had no vocational ambition. Beginning in high school, he had many heterosexual experiences and he felt considerable guilt about these. He went out with a number of girls, never becoming actually engaged but having sexual intercourse with each one. He said that he had also been intimate with "plenty" of pickups and that after such experiences his feelings of tension, along with the depression, heightened. One homosexual experience had occurred when he was 16, and he said that he had felt guilty afterward but that the experience had not left a lasting impression.

In the hospital the thoughts uppermost in the young man's mind were concern about his condition and desire to get well. He constantly talked of his "nervous tension" and all its various aspects. What his friends would think troubled him greatly. On the ward he appeared normal and was apparently completely at ease, although he himself said that this appearance was "just a front." His troubles had begun as a functional disturbance, he believed, but had continued so long that there was now some organic involvement. Partly because he had his own ideas about what he needed, he was difficult to work with. He constantly asked for hypnosis, sedatives, and other similar treatments. He felt that the rest in the hospital had helped but that his basic condition was unchanged. With this point of view the staff concurred.

B. Psth., Asocial   M:18:S:14   +1   71′863 29–(67)   2:9:5
P. Psychas.

About twelve days before admission the patient had been accused of stealing a considerable sum of money from a church. Part of his regular duties in the church service had been to take the money from one section of the church to another. On this particular day the patient walked out of the church with the money and went home. When confronted by detectives, he readily confessed his guilt but could not explain his actions. He had apparently not planned the crime beforehand and did not need the money. His room was examined and a large number of library books, a stethoscope, a number of hypodermic syringes, and other stolen articles were found.

Up until the third grade he was apparently a normal child but then he began to behave peculiarly and was placed in a special class where he was characterized as willful and stubborn. Later when he was returned to regular classes, he did well enough but was never accepted by his classmates and demanded attention to the point of exhibitionism. He had never had any close friends and had worked at only a few odd jobs. Having an active imagination, he talked continuously. Easily hurt and angered, he was markedly effeminate in character and probably this had led to additional rejection by his group. An illegitimate child, he had lived with foster parents most of his life.

In the hospital he was quiet and withdrawn but not obviously abnormal in behavior; he was not worried, anxious, or tense. His sensorium and intellect were clear. There was no evidence of an emotional disturbance. He conducted himself well though he did seem to assume a braggart attitude. His effeminacy impressed the personnel as his most outstanding characteristic. During his time in the hospital he attempted to learn to dance and play the piano. No real understanding could be reached of the basic mechanisms that were operating. It seemed possible that the feminine factor was important but he would form no close rapport with anyone and his volunteered information was not at all helpful.

P. Psychas. M:30:M:41 +9 7'2–148 3:2:6

The patient had always had a fear of high places and of water. He dated the present illness from about a year and a half before admission. At that time he had purchased a second-hand car and because it had a poor ignition system he was worried that it might catch fire. As the illness progressed this fear extended to other objects, and at the time of admission he was afraid that he might start fires by touching objects with his expectoration or by papers dropping out of his pockets. The compulsive features of his illness were first noticed shortly after he was married, about a year before admission. In time it became necessary for him to check and recheck barn doors to make sure they were locked. He felt he had to return to a room he had just left to make certain that a fire had not broken out. He became afraid that he might be assaultive toward others, and he began to worry about possible accidents to his wife. His own health was of great concern to him, and he feared that he might contract a cold which would end in pneumonia. Although he recognized his fears and compulsions as "silly," nevertheless he was unable to free himself from them.

He had stopped school after the eighth grade and had remained thereafter on the farm. From age 15 to age 24 he had worked for his father, receiving a spending allowance but no regular salary. He had then worked as a hired hand until he and his brother had rented their father's farm. He said that he was mechanically minded, but he had not made a special hobby of this interest. Sensitive, friendly, good-natured, and generous, he apparently had been able to adjust in groups. His judgment was good. He described himself as easily hurt and said he lacked self-assurance. The patient had known his wife all his life and had courted her for three years before their marriage; except for religious differences, which were very important to them, they would have been married much sooner. They had had frequent sexual relations before marriage, and they were sexually compatible. Largely because of his fear that the religious differences might cause problems, the patient did not want children.

On admission the thoughts uppermost in the patient's mind had to do with his illness: "I worry about everything. I am afraid for my wife, afraid she will get lost, afraid to have her gone. I make a lot out of nothing." He was oriented and apparently intact in mentation. He described himself as depressed, and at times he cried. While he enjoyed farm work, he felt he had never been truly happy and rationalized by saying, "I guess it looks greener across the road." Without the courage to make a definite plan, he thought of suicide. Sober, reserved, and generally cooperative, he made a satisfactory ward adjustment, and he was always able to admit the absurdity of his obsessions and compulsions even though he could do nothing about them. There was a basic rigidity in his personality that prevented much progress in helping him. He was discharged somewhat improved, with the recommendation that he have shock therapy if his improvement was not sustained.

Alcoholism	M:43:M:20	+3	72168′934–(78)	3:7:10
		+19	6749′2813–(57)	1:3:15
		–41	27′4618 39–(69)	2:4:7
		+55	′6279–(57)	2:2:13

This man was admitted to the hospital because of nervousness, insomnia, and chronic alcoholism. Although he had been drinking since age 14 he had not indulged to excess until he was 25 years old, after he had been married two years. Shortly after the birth of a second child he lost a job he had held for five years; then he began to drink almost continuously. His wife took the two small children and returned to her parents, leaving the patient alone. He continued to drink for at least two more years and was unable to work steadily. Later, however, he was reunited with his family and moderated his drinking enough to hold a job, although he continued to drink occasionally and was constantly in debt. After joining Alcoholics Anonymous some time later he remained sober steadily until a few months before admission, when he was working under great stress, was worried about his business, and was anxious about his obligations. This he was sure had caused him to "fall from grace." In the last two months he had been almost continuously inebriated.

An eighth-grade graduate, he became a skilled workman and eventually a contractor. Above average in intelligence, he was extroverted, made friends very easily, and showed considerable drive and enthusiasm. On the other hand he was always quick to assert his independence and he showed ill-concealed resentment toward people he felt inferior to him. He was sensitive to criticism, direct or implied, and unusually sensitive to minor disappointments.

In the neurological examination at the hospital he was essentially normal. Physically there were some evidences of hyperthyroidism, although this was not clinically significant. The patient was chiefly concerned with his desire to overcome the drinking habit and get back to work. As indicated psychometrically, there was borderline evidence of intellectual deterioration. There was no gross evidence of a disturbance in intellect, however. He was cheerful, complacent and confident, cooperative, and appreciative of the opportunity for treatment. That alcohol was an escape from facing failures he recognized and while in the hospital he renewed his association with Alcoholics Anonymous. He became very confident that he would stay "dry." The prognosis was considered fairly good in view of the fact that he had had such a long spell of relative abstinence in the past.

P. Psychas. F:27:W:29 +5 72 318'46– 9:7:15
Mental Deficiency

Although the patient had always been meticulous and orderly, disabling compulsive behavior and obsessive thoughts had appeared about four years before admission. Among other things she became afraid to stay at home by herself, she feared that dishes had been washed in poison, and she repeated things over and over again. She also had obsessive ideas, of which the impulse to jump from a neighbor's windmill was characteristic; this urge was so strong that the patient avoided the vicinity of the windmill. Her appetite became poor, she grew irritable, her children upset her, and she repeatedly washed her hands. As the symptoms became more acute she spent most of her time in bed reading the Bible. Completely bewildered by her symptoms, she became depressed and worried about losing her mind.

From the time she began school at age 6 until she dropped out of school in the seventh grade, the patient had never actually passed a grade, although she had been moved along from one grade to the next and had always been interested in her schoolwork. Her I.Q. was 63. Her first child was born before her marriage, and subsequently she had two other children. Shortly after the third child was born her husband died, and the early symptoms of her illness appeared soon after his death. Although she was very shy with strangers, she was socially not badly adjusted. She had no hobbies and no interest in such pastimes as sports; her only activity outside of her home was attendance at a church. Before the development of the symptomatic pattern she had been a relatively good housekeeper and not too inadequate as a mother.

In the hospital she was very troubled about her symptoms. She had insight into the irrationality of such compulsive behavior as scrubbing the floor three or four times a day, or in doing the dishes over and over, but she was unable to do anything about it, and she could not explain her reaction to the windmill or her impulse to throw herself off it. She disclaimed depression and suicidal wishes. During interviews she cried frequently, especially when she described her fears, and although she felt that hospitalization would be beneficial, she still feared losing her mind. Her answers were relevant. She was a cooperative, pleasant person, but her reactions in general were passive. Her behavior on the ward was normal. Although her restricted mental level was apparent in ward activities, she engaged in games and made acquaintances. The woman was of German extraction and a marked language handicap in addition to her low mental level put her at a disadvantage. Some of her apprehensiveness disappeared during hospitalization and after social service study of the home situation, she was discharged. It was thought likely that she would be able to continue at her borderline level of adjustment.

P. Anxiety State M:29:M:7 +1 7′23418 69–(43) 8:1:23
Schizoid

About ten months before admission the patient began to experience anxiety. A few months earlier he had been discharged from the navy, where he apparently had been very tense and nervous, although he said that his discharge had been prompted in part by high blood pressure. After his discharge he worked as a filling station operator, but he found the work a strain. After the sudden onset of the anxiety he became unable to sit still and experienced palpitation and difficult respiration. A physical examination indicated that his heart was all right and his blood pressure normal, but this did not reassure him. After three electroshock treatments he improved considerably, although the cloudiness that immediately follows shock treatment became a constant symptom. This feeling of mental cloudiness was the reason for the present admission.

Before his service in the navy the patient had never had any health or psychological difficulties. A high school graduate, he had been especially interested in mechanics. He felt that he worked better on his own than with people, and he had never been a very sociable person. He showed a marked dependency on his mother. Married, he was the father of two children. At the time of admission the patient was the center of a family conflict in which his sisters, his wife, and his parents were pulling the patient toward several mutually inconsistent activities they wanted him to undertake.

In the hospital he was concerned about his difficulty but did not appear deeply depressed. On several occasions he showed some anxiety, but most of the time he was apparently free from it. He needed continual reassurance from clinicians and nurses that he would be all right and that things would be worked out satisfactorily. There was a poverty of ideation and a marked lack of spontaneity in his speech, suggestive of a schizoid process. It was recommended that he and his wife get away from the family circle, possibly on a farm where environmental stresses would be at a minimum, but in view of his schizoid trends the prognosis remained poor.

P. Mixed Paranoid	F:36:M:13	+1	'7243–(55)	5:2:18
P. React. Depr. Suicidal	F:38:M:37	+2	'436 218–(49)	9:5:18
Ps. M-D., Depr.	F:38:M:32	+2	'67–3(47)	3:5:11

The patient was brought to the hospital by her husband because she kept asking for an overdose of barbiturates or an operation on her brain to relieve her of worry and confusion. For several years she had become increasingly more withdrawn, had shunned her family responsibilities, had lost interest in her personal appearance, and had worried excessively about the behavior of her 12-year-old son. Under psychiatric care, she had received two electroshock treatments, but the course of her illness had not been much affected.

Her previous health had been good. There were no past psychotic episodes. After she completed high school and a commercial course, she worked as a secretary until she married her husband at the age of 20. Her early social life had been limited. Her marriage represented her only real love affair. Neither in personality nor in behavior had she especially deviated from others.

Although she talked freely and was perfectly clear and oriented, she had a tendency to fix her attention on too simple and too obvious explanations of the underlying cause of her illness. At the time of admission, while still under the influence of barbiturates taken at home, she said that she must have paranoia, and that she was in need of a brain operation. At times she refused to recognize that any problem existed. She adapted well to the ward routine, although she tended to be dramatic and demanded the doctor's attention in childlike ways. Her behavior seemed entirely normal; the illness was apparently a mild depression with suicidal ideas and veiled hostility, probably broadly paranoid. After a trial visit with her husband she refused to come back to the hospital and was discharged against advice.

Two months later she was readmitted, having again become depressed and apathetic. Again she talked freely and was chiefly concerned with getting well. She could not understand how she "got into such a fix," and she still blamed everything on insignificant causes. With electroshock therapy there was a gradual improvement, and she was discharged to be followed in the outpatient department. About a year later she was again admitted with the idea that she was losing her memory because of the shock treatment. She now had a definite dislike for crowds. Her third child had been born about three months before admission, and she had developed feelings of inadequacy about her ability to care for it. Her physician had advised her readmission for further shock therapy. In the course of psychotherapeutic interviews she expressed some feelings of guilt regarding her choice of her present husband instead of a rival, who had later died, and she also discussed the fact that she had worried some about her son's tendencies to be homoerotic.

B. Psth., Path. Sexuality M:24:M:9 —19 7'<u>26</u>8<u>14</u> <u>39</u>-(57) 1:10:7
P. Psychas.
Alcoholism

Shortly before admission the patient was apprehended by the police for entering and rifling an automobile. When searched he was found to have with him women's undergarments and United States mail not belonging to him. He admitted having stolen the clothing and the mail from an apartment house. Later he said he had been stealing undergarments for several years and had practiced exhibitionism for the last twelve months. Previously an alcoholic, he had been court-martialed on several occasions while in the armed forces for episodes related to drunkenness, but, he said, he had overcome the alcohol problem. He was a passive, dependent person when sober but under the influence of alcohol he was belligerent and aggressive. He had never adjusted well socially and was known by his associates as an "odd" but friendly person. There was a close attachment between the patient and his mother. He and his wife were not compatible, largely because of the alcoholism and because of the patient's poor handling of money.

He had left school at the end of his junior year, after doing very poorly in his studies and failing to socialize adequately. Before entering the armed services he had had two jobs, holding each for only a short time.

In the hospital the patient was worried that his marriage might end in divorce. He recognized that he had a severe problem and was eager for treatment. He was well oriented and there was no evidence of psychosis. He was neat and tidy and had average intelligence. Projective and other tests indicated a neurotic make-up. Under the circumstances, since the patient had been sent to the hospital by the court, no attempt at psychotherapy was undertaken. He was discharged back to the court with the recommendation that he be supervised and that a long-time psychotherapeutic program be planned for him.

Ps. Sz., Cat. M:28:M:37 +32 7'<u>26</u>89-4 (55) 7:7:12
Ps. Toxic

Six weeks before admission this young man had experienced an attack of influenza; he had seemed to recover uneventfully although he had complained of being unusually tired. Four weeks later he learned that the farm he had been renting was to be sold and this worried him. He consulted a lawyer about his contract; and when leaving the attorney's office, he noticed his landlord sitting in an adjoining room where he could have overheard the conversation. Immediately the patient began to have trouble sleeping and felt that everyone was against him except his immediate family. Sedation given by his physician brought little relief. One night he woke the household to announce that he was going to be a minister and at least help himself and seek forgiveness for his sins. He became absent-minded and confused; for example, he told his mother that he had been out with a couple of neighbors who actually had been dead for some time. He felt sure he had done something wrong but could not tell what it was.

Except for a nervous breakdown at the age of 15, there were no previous psychotic episodes. At that time he "saw Christ." Apparently recovery occurred in about two months. He had difficulty learning in school and left before the end of the eighth grade. He then farmed, first with his father and later on his own place. Although he had few outside interests, he was characterized as being friendly, at ease, and consistent in his work and obligations. There was no evidence of sexual deviations, and he and his wife appeared compatible. Intellectually he was dull normal.

In the hospital the patient had religious delusions. His hallucinations included several sensory fields—he smelled malodorous vapors, saw a shaft of light, and told of voices that spoke to him. He constantly repeated, "I know what's right and I know what's wrong. I know. That's the way it works." Another frequent remark was, "If it weren't for electricity, everything would fall over. I hold your hand. Electricity goes from my body to yours. That's the way it works." His replies to questions were inadequate and occasionally he was mute. Apparently he tried to be cooperative and affable, but his attention span was short. He frequently gesticulated dramatically. The MMPI was given at a time when he had improved and was apparently normal. Therapy consisted of eleven shock treatments and resulted in his almost complete recovery from the symptoms. It was agreed that he might have similar attacks in the future.

Ps. M-D., Depr. F:50:M:5 +2 72813'46– 4:4:18
P. React. Depr.
P. Psychas.

Six years before admission, following a pelvic operation, the patient became depressed, sullen, worrisome, underactive, and apathetic. She experienced difficulty in thinking and in doing things, and she was bothered by weakness, fatigue, a sore throat, dysphagia, and other somatic ills. She wondered if these might indicate a morbid disease and also feared she might "go insane." A number of physicians treated her without apparent success and finally she became so ill that she was admitted to the hospital.

At 20 the patient had contracted syphilis; she was given antiluetic treatments for five years and occasionally thereafter. The only other obvious contributory factor in the past medical history was a hysterectomy for a fibroma, which was the point of onset for the present symptomatic picture.

Her early development was apparently normal. School did not interest her, but she finished the eighth grade at 15 and then went to work. She began a nurses' training course but gave this up. Before her marriage she had several sexual experiences and three pregnancies terminating in abortions. Known as an honest, hard-working person, she had a tendency to moodiness, hypochondriasis, and minor phobias. She had never told her husband about the syphilis. She and her husband were compatible. She had had one child and a number of spontaneous abortions.

On admission the patient was somewhat obese. There were no findings of consequence in the physical or neurological examinations, which included spinal fluid and blood Wassermann tests. Psychologically she was concerned that she might have a serious organic disorder and thought that perhaps the syphilis accounted for a part of her trouble. She was well oriented and appeared intellectually intact. In general depressed, she talked freely and without evidence of retardation. She was neat, pleasant, and cooperative. A few days after admission she began to ask to return home. She left the hospital against the advice of the staff.

Ps. Sz., Cat.	M:19:S:270	+14	728134'96–	2:10:15
		+52	721843'69–	4:11:18
		+113	2431'78–9	1:7:17
Ps. Sz., Cat.	M:19:S:4	+3	7'4231–9	2:1:20

About two months before admission this young man began to show progressive concern about his bodily organs. Upset whenever he thought they were not functioning correctly, he became more and more disabled. He gave up his job and began to attend a university, but he worried excessively about whether he had selected the right vocation and he felt he was a failure. These feelings culminated in an attack of panic that led to a general hospitalization. For a period he was mute and showed posturization and an apparent break with reality. After he was returned to his home, the abnormal conduct continued, he made several attempts at suicide, and he was finally admitted to the psychiatric unit.

At age 15 he had suffered a "nervous breakdown" of six months' duration, not as severe as the present one but otherwise similar. Always a sensitive, retiring, introverted, shut-in boy, he leaned heavily upon his family. He had completed two years at a university, doing satisfactory work. He felt inferior to his older siblings, particularly because they were able to work their way through school while he was not. He had a strong desire to "keep fit" and he overevaluated the benefits of athletic prowess. His habit of masturbation worried him and he feared it would lead to insanity. He had no special friends and had never had a girl friend.

In the hospital he was observed to be a thin though not unattractive boy.

At first he was mute and would not answer questions, turning his face away from the examiner. He took no interest in his personal appearance. He was apathetic, tense, and inactive. A few days after admission he began to answer questions and gradually was induced to take some interest in the ward activities. However, the retardation was still obvious. Later he said that he had given up a lot of "fool ideas." Typical of these were the belief that he had a bad odor and the conviction that he had "lived a very wicked life" and was the "cause of all the other patients becoming sick." Some of his ideas he retained, however. For example, he feared that his intestinal tract might become stuffed with food, and he would refuse to eat unless he had an adequate bowel movement. Sometimes he refused food so long that he had to be fed by tube. One day he announced he would die on the next Saturday. When Saturday came he was lethargic and mildly stuporous. After 36 hours he was up and around again.

At the time of discharge he appeared considerably better. He was, however, not deeply changed. He said that he now felt his talents in art, music, and poetry might be of real value and that he no longer thought of these as effeminate. The discharge was temporary, and he was to be readmitted in three weeks. During these weeks at home he behaved well enough but had difficulty downing solid foods and complained of weakness. His second stay in the hospital lasted only four days, and he was eager to be discharged. Careful instructions were given to his family, and he was advised to undertake a limited amount of schoolwork.

P. Psychas. M:29:S +5 728′3–96 (65) 3:5:11
P. React. Depr.

The patient's chief complaint was the feeling that he was attractive to men. In addition he was depressed over his tendency to "fall for" attractive men. He struggled against this urge and was anxious and disturbed about it. "As soon as I feel that way toward someone, I clamp on it." He reasoned that he must be somewhat attractive to girls, since he had many girl friends and dates, but he believed he did not have the "proper reaction to girls."

As a child the patient had had no marked contributory experiences. He had always been fairly well adjusted and socially accepted. His I.Q. was 100, and he completed high school at 18. Then for two years he worked on a farm. For some time he had felt that he was attractive to men and had assumed strongly masculine behavior as a defense against being noticed as unusual. For example, he became a truck driver and learned to swear and "act tough." Once when intoxicated he had a heterosexual experience; otherwise he had been impotent heterosexually. He disclaimed having any homosexual experiences. For a while he drank heavily but one night a friend snapped a picture of him. "I saw the picture," he said, "and I was so disgusted, I have not since been drunk." He deliberately lowered his voice to avoid possible feminine tones. He participated in church activities and sang in the choir. Active sports had never interested him.

On admission the patient's complaints centered almost wholly around his desire to be freed of his ideas about men. Approximately a year before the present two interviews, he had suffered an even worse depression; he had been suicidal and seriously disabled. He read some "philosophy" and decided to seek aid for his problem. It took many weeks to carry out this decision because he was afraid "they would point their finger at me." In the interviews considerable effort was spent in reassuring him that his feelings would not lead, necessarily, to insanity or to criminal activities. He benefited from the reassurance, and it was agreed he might continue to make a reasonably adequate adjustment.

P. Psychas. M:43:M:52 +4 72831'69–(51) 3:7:7

The patient had always been a quiet and pensive person. He had felt a great deal of jealousy, especially toward his wife, but had kept these feelings to himself. For about a year and a half whenever he picked up his carpenter's hammer he experienced tendencies toward assault. This had not really troubled him until the last three weeks. During those weeks he had periodically "felt" the word *kill* in his mind. This caused insomnia and an impairment of normal processes. He told his wife to hide all the knives in the house and not to remain alone with him because he might kill her or someone else. He became irritated by passing cars and said, "Whenever there is a car there has to be a person."

At age 18 he had received a head injury that resulted in strabismus and progressive blindness of his left eye; this eye had been completely blind for the past six years. He had had occasional abdominal pain for the last five years and epigastric distress along with still other somatic complaints.

The patient was a high school graduate and had done well in school. For about a year he had done all the housework for his mother while she was bedridden; this occurred when he was about 9 years old. After high school graduation he worked on the farm and at various jobs, chiefly as a carpenter and a mason. He was engrossed in his work and never cared for recreation; he was often restless and easily irritated. He had always felt that he had been mistreated while he was acting as "maid" for the rest of the family.

In the hospital the neurological and physical examinations were noncontributory. He was mainly concerned with his jealous feeling toward his wife; this was mixed up with his resentment and the "feeling" of the word *kill* in his mind. His sensorium was clear and his intellect unimpaired. He appeared restless but there was nothing unusual about his stream of thought, his attitude, or his manner. He adjusted to the hospital with little difficulty, though he had insomnia for a couple of weeks. He seemed to be relieved considerably by just talking over his troubles with attendants. He was examined with narcosynthesis, but little of note was discovered. Gradually his problems, while still present, became less irritating to him and he was fairly comfortable. He was discharged after an arrangement had been made for him to continue in the outpatient psychiatry department.

P. Hys. M:45:M:25 +3 72831'96–(67) 8:4:13

This man had a twenty-year history of depression and pains in his head whenever he got depressed and worried about anything. He entered the hospital as a voluntary patient.

He was the third child of a strict and rigid father and a "nervy" mother. He had an elementary education. Subsequently he became a hall boy, valet, and coach painter. He had a nervous breakdown at the age of 18, which he attributed to witnessing a fatal accident. He married at 23 and had one child.

He was diagnosed as having anxiety hysteria and his condition improved after a course of electric convulsion therapy and suggestion treatment under cyclonal sodium. M. V.

Ps. M-D., Depr. F:46:M:25 +1 72'836–49(47) 6:8:5
P. Psychas.

Three years previously the patient had noticed marked nervousness just before her oldest son came home on furlough. At the end of his visit she became still more nervous and upset, and she had frequent choking spells. She experienced severe difficulty in breathing, particularly when she had guests for supper. At such times she retired to her room "for fear my head would go to pieces." The fear developed, for example, that if she took a drink of water she would choke to death. She stopped reading newspapers, she said, because she might read of a murder and that would give her ideas of harming someone, especially her children. These symptoms continued until admission.

There were no other previous psychotic episodes except a minor emotional upset when she was 21. She was an adopted child. Always quiet, shy, sensitive, "too" good and obedient, she had had few playmates and had lived in a make-believe world. Until her marriage she did not know that her parents were not her "real ones." She worried then because she did not "belong to anyone." Shy in school, she stammered and reddened when called upon to recite. At her marriage she was total ignorant about sexual matters, was frigid sexually, and did not desire intercourse as often as her husband did. Otherwise they were compatible.

The patient was sad and depressed when admitted to the hospital, wept frequently, and was shy and quiet. She was well oriented. Her insight into her problems appeared to be fair; she felt her trouble came from an inability to express her emotional feelings. She showed some improvement but was agitated and asocial on the ward. Apprehensive about electroshock therapy, she refused further treatment after four shocks. Her husband took her home against advice. She had improved slightly before the discharge.

P. React. Depr. F:36:M:24 +2 72'8361–9(41) 3:2:12

This woman was admitted because of nervousness, depression, insomnia, anorexia, nausea, and vomiting, all of which had been present since the beginning of her sixth pregnancy. Following the delivery there was a brief improvement, but she soon became increasingly irritable, lost her appetite, and was unable to sleep. Always a worrier, she was now more than ever easily disturbed, and she cried when excited or when awakened by noise. Her local physician administered sixteen shock treatments on an outpatient basis, but when she showed no improvement and experienced memory impairment and inability to think clearly she was brought to the hospital.

The past history included no evidence of a previous mental illness. She had had a gonococcal infection at the age of 17 and had been treated for this infection before her marriage. Shy and secretive even as a child, she had preferred to read or daydream rather than to play with other children. Since her marriage her husband had become her close confidant and she showed a great deal of emotional dependence on him. According to him, she worried too much. Apparently she had been promiscuous sexually at the time she acquired the gonorrhea. Before the end of her senior year she had left high school and had lived at home on her parents' farm until her marriage.

In the hospital there was no certain sign of organic involvement although there was an area of analgesia on the left side. She was cooperative but markedly nervous and easily fatigued. She exhibited deep concern about the possible harm done by the shock treatments, and remorse about her past sexual indiscretions. She disclosed that she had an 11-year-old daughter who was feeble-minded, and this was apparently connected with her guilt feelings. Her sensorium was clear but her intellect did appear somewhat affected with respect to memory. In the course of the hospitalization her memory for recent events returned, and she began to show an interest in her surroundings and to anticipate returning home to resume her household duties. At the time of discharge she seemed to be recovered from the attack. In view of the long history of minor maladjustment, it was felt that the future held some difficulties for her. In general, however, the prognosis was considered to be good.

P. Psychas. F:38:M 7283′614–(51) 5:12:7

This housewife wrote down as her reason for coming to the counseling center, "Don't like and feel unfitted for present occupation." She was extremely upset and unhappy and felt that if she could work outside of her home for a while, she might get along better with her family. The home included her husband, who was a business executive, and her young son.

She proved to have average ability, highly cultural interests (sometimes related to escape motives), and a low interest in other people and their welfare. She complained of compulsive reading which prevented her from doing her housework or carrying out any schedule. The reading had no meaning for her and she did not care what she read, but she could not pass a book or a magazine without picking it up. She showed considerable bitterness toward the demands that marriage makes on a woman, objecting to changing her name, not having money of her own, and the like. Later she exhibited real antagonism toward her husband for his failure to make either her or himself happy. Her physical complaints centered around "rheumatic" pains and "stiffness," but her physician considered her physically well.

She used several counseling interviews very well and developed some insight. It was a painful process for her, however, and she occasionally missed appointments after discussions which verged on her own responsibilities. She did not discuss job possibilities after the first interview. She took her son to a child study center and later she went to a health center for massage and exercise. She asked if she could return later for more interviews but did not return after discontinuing them in the midst of these other activities. The child study center reported that the son was a very disturbed child, and plans were being made to take him out of the home as much as possible. The mother did not follow through the contacts there either, however, and very little work could be done with the parents.

D. F. C.

Ps. M-D., Depr. F:61:M:47 +9 728'<u>36</u>14–9 8:5:13
Suicidal

This woman's first symptoms had appeared thirteen months before admission, following her son's departure to live in another state. This son, to meet a payment for a large debt, had given a mortgage on his parents' house. A week after he left home the patient developed depression, irritability, daily crying spells, and hypersensitivity to noises. She withdrew from outside activities and found it difficult to do household tasks. She also had epigastric discomforts, dizziness, and headaches; she ate and slept poorly; and there were suicidal thoughts.

A previous psychotic upset at age 35 had followed the birth of her second child. Similar to the present pattern, this attack had been less severe. A hard worker all her life, she was devoted to her home and fond of her children. She was conservative, planned well, enjoyed parties and dances, and was kind and considerate. Her schooling had been intermittent and brief. She and her husband, a carpenter, were compatible and, in general, their family life was satisfactory.

On admission the patient's chief complaints were restlessness, epigastric discomfort, depression, unnecessary worrying, and inability to do her housework. During examinations, she frequently cried; she recognized the presence of depression and attributed it to her son's absence. She was pleasant and cooperative, only moderately agitated. Although quiet and retiring, she adapted herself readily to the hospital routine. Toward the end of her hospital stay she became much more comfortable and optimistic. However, she retained a fear of "losing her mind" and wondered if her ambition and zest for work would ever return. She was discharged improved and with the expectation that she would become steadily better.

Ps. Sz., Cat.   M:31:S:107   +12   72′84–1 (61)   5:3:14

This man showed signs of a disturbance at the age of 23 while he was in the navy. He was very retarded and slow in performing routine actions of everyday life. There were some catatonic features and a tendency to repetitive action. He spent three months in a hospital where he was treated by electric convulsion therapy. He improved and returned to work but six years later re-entered the hospital in the present admission. By now he was unable to keep his appointments and complained of an inability to concentrate. He was solitary, appeared hallucinatory, used stilted language, and showed signs of compulsive thought. He was retarded in matters of daily routine, spending hours in dressing, eating, and the like.

He was the oldest of seven children and received an elementary education. A good conversationalist, he was keenly interested in classical music and intelligent subjects. He had been nervous as a child, overanxious about trivialities. On leaving school he was employed by the general post office as a wireman. He joined the Royal Navy at the age of 23 and was discharged with psychoneurosis without having seen active service.

He was diagnosed as having schizophrenia and was treated by courses of modified insulin therapy, triazole, and electric convulsion therapy. His condition improved. M. V.

P. Psychas.   F:38:M:59   +10   7284136′–9   7:7:15

P. Psychas.   F:41:M:92   +9   23417′86–9X   10:3:21

There had been a previous admission for this patient (first MMPI) with a complicated illness that included many obsessive and compulsive symptoms. Although the patient had had a fear of dirt since adolescence, it had not become obvious or caused her discomfort until about the time of the first admission when she began to withdraw from social events because she was afraid of "germs." Her husband had noted that she washed her hands frequently, but when he remonstrated with her she had had a temper tantrum. In addition to numerous somatic complaints such as headaches and dizziness, the patient had become despondent and irritable. After the previous hospitalization she had been temporarily relieved, but the symptoms had returned. She insisted that her husband move away from their home town in order to avoid relatives and others in the community, who she thought had venereal diseases. The symptoms had nevertheless increased to the point where she would not leave her house or allow anyone else to come into it. When her husband came home from work she ran away from him because she was afraid of germs on his clothes, and she exhausted herself scrubbing the house, her body, and her clothing. She felt so constantly tortured and depressed that she was willing to submit to almost any procedure for relief.

She recalled that at age 13 she had the impulse to wash her hands after touching such objects as door knobs. A venereal disease pamphlet, which she read at age 19, made her apprehensive about "catching a dreadful disease," a subject in which she was abnormally interested. In other respects her judgment and intelligence were good. She had always been clean and meticulous in her personal habits. A capable person, she had worked as a part-time schoolteacher to augment the family income. Emotionally she had never been happy. Her childhood had been miserable, with many events which gave rise to feelings of insecurity. Even as a child she had thought, "What's the use of living?" On the other hand, until the present illness, she had enjoyed popular fiction and such community affairs as dancing. Sexual matters gave the woman a feeling of shame, and she said, "I liked babies until I found out where they came from." Although no basis for her apprehension was established, she had recently become concerned about her husband's relations with other women, fearing that they had a venereal disease. She denied any concern about masturbation, or homosexual, extramarital, or premarital relations. She was not overly religious.

In the hospital the thoughts uppermost in the patient's mind were concerned with her phobias and compulsions. Although she was apprehensive and anxious, she was well oriented and in most ways appeared entirely normal. No amount of investigation elicited any background for an adequate understanding of the disorder. Because of the severity of the symptoms and the fact that they did not respond to ordinary approaches, a frontal lobectomy was performed. While she retained some of her delusional ideas, she was sufficiently relieved to live a fairly normal life. She was now more restless, however, and showing some irresponsibility, she left her husband and moved about the country.

Ps. Invol. Melan. M:48:S:7 +3 72841 36'9– 2:5:14
P. Psychas.

The patient was depressed and worried, had "numb" feelings in his head, and was bothered by hearing and speech difficulties and insomnia. He had been a chronic worrier all his life, but this had not interfered with his work until about a year before admission. At that time religious matters began to bother him and he feared that his acts, however trivial, might be sinful. He became indecisive, each decision requiring inner debate. Distraught and desperate, he went to a physician who prescribed "shots," which helped for a while, but soon the excessive worry reappeared and in addition he developed a "numb" feeling behind his eyes, which he noted was aggravated by worry and was alleviated whenever his attention was distracted. He had other physical symptoms also. He began to avoid people and to neglect meals, his ideas became obsessional, and, unable to work, he spent many hours in bed. Until the present illness his life had been relatively uneventful, without any particular factors that had apparently contributed to the present illness.

The patient was known as a hard worker who "minded his own business" and always kept his worries to himself. He was religious and had little social life. After leaving school in the seventh grade, he became an itinerant workman.

Eventually he bought a small bit of land but at the time of admission he was in debt for more than $1000, and he was very worried about this. Never able to form close relationships with women, he showed evidences of sexual conflict.

In the hospital most of the patient's thoughts concerned doubts about the suitability of his actions from a religious standpoint. For example, once when repairing a fence he inadvertently nailed two boards across each other. This aroused in him fear that his act might be construed as a desecration of the symbol of the cross, and he tore the fence down. He was harassed by obsessional sexual thoughts and saw sexual significance even in inanimate objects. A door latch clicking into its opening, for example, reminded him of the sexual act, and he believed that when he closed a door he aided and abetted this "dirty business." Frequently he was compelled to change the position or appearance of things to destroy fancied resemblances to "sinful" objects. He considered suicide but abstained because "it would be sinful to carry it through." He said he recognized that his worries were the source of his trouble. In the hospital he remained quiet and cooperative but was depressed and worried so about conditions on his farm that he was finally permitted to return home. It was recommended that he live a broader life. He left the hospital little improved and the prognosis was guarded.

Ps. M-D., Depr.	M:42:M:17	+1	728436'19–(71)	5:7:18
		+14	'24783–(57)	4:2:24
Ps. M-D., Depr. Suicidal	M:42:M:9			
P. Mixed	M:42:M:52	+6	427'3819–(59)	4:5:22
		+19	'4873–(51)	5:5:21

This man was troubled by inability to concentrate or to sleep and a feeling that he could not continue to work. He dated this illness from ten years before when he had a number of somatic difficulties. Since then the symptoms had been irregularly present. Two months before admission it became unusually difficult for him to continue at his job. He said, "I feel like a machine on which I can't find the right button to push in order to make it get into action." Several mornings he returned home from his office and went to bed. At times he broke down and cried. He consulted a psychiatrist but discontinued treatment after a few interviews "because I felt much better and thought I could lick this problem by myself."

When the patient was a junior in college he began to feel depressed and quit school for one year. During that time he was seclusive and avoided his friends. He took a job, however, and later returned to college with no further difficulty. During his boyhood he had always felt different from others, although the actual points of difference were unclear to him. Successful in his work, he was not affected when one of the men under him was advanced to a position superior to his, but later when he himself was promoted he exhibited tension and nervousness. Of a pleasant disposition, he was a fairly social person, yet he never formed deep or lasting friendships. He had five children and the family appeared to be a relatively happy one.

In the hospital the patient was oriented and apparently normal in sensorium and intellect. His discourse indicated self-condemnatory thoughts. He had insight about the emotional aspects of his illness, yet he did not understand how he could have developed the problems he felt he had. His adaption to the hospital routine was good and superficially he seemed normal. Somewhat casual psychotherapeutic efforts led to improvement. There was considerable evidence of dependency and some conflict in sexual matters. At the time of discharge he was nearly recovered from the episode. He went home, got a good job, did fairly well for three months, and then suddenly regressed. He came back to the hospital after being found under his car in what appeared to be a suicidal attempt. After a short stay he again was apparently well and left, only to return in another three months with the same problem.

Ps. M-D., Depr.   M:25:M:139   +2   7284'3916–(59)   2:4:20
Schizoid   +113   6247'8319–(61)   4:2:20
Paranoid

About the time he was discharged from the navy the patient became tense, restless, and unable to relax. He felt compelled to begin work immediately. A lawyer, he began to help out in his brother's office, but he was indecisive, unsure of himself professionally, and felt the need of more training. He obtained a fellowship, but when he began to work he obviously had considerable doubt about his ability to make a good showing. As the doubt became progressively worse, he expended more and more effort, to the point where he was spending most of his waking hours reading or working. His anxiety mounted until he was unable to work efficiently. A vacation gave him temporary relief, but with the approach of his return to work he became tense and anxious. Depression and mounting agitation completely incapacitated him, and he was finally admitted to the psychiatric unit.

There had been no previous breakdown. The patient had been a very good student and adequate socially, but he had always been obsessed with the desire to make a good showing. He had had to make the best grades, know the most people, and be the most popular student. On several occasions, however, when he had been the principal speaker at a school function he had been so overcome with anxiety he could not speak at all. He had never used tobacco or alcohol, and was known as a moderate person. His family background was poor. A number of members of his family had been psychotic or very obviously neurotic. His mother was an ineffectual person who had tried to control her children by weeping and by demanding sympathy rather than by firmer, more positive methods.

72 846'319–

In the hospital the patient was moderately depressed, somewhat agitated, perplexed, extremely defensive, and markedly concerned about being hospitalized. There was such retardation that it was difficult to get a satisfactory idea of his thought content. Over and over he referred to the "mess I've gotten myself into." He did not refer to his condition as illness, but rather as a punishment for purported misdeeds which he never named directly. There were indications that suicidal ideas were present. After admission he rapidly became worse. Heavy sedation was necessary to give him a few hours of sleep. He developed a hand-washing compulsion and his hands became raw. There was no improvement with insulin subshock, and the treatment was changed to electroshock therapy with grand mal seizures under which he rapidly lost his depression. Within several weeks he became somewhat euphoric, and he developed an obsessive desire to find the cause of his illness and to make up for all his supposed wrongs to his wife and his family. His delusional system remained, taking on a more paranoid character in which he suspected the staff of being against him. He was finally discharged for transfer to a veterans' psychiatric hospital.

P. Mixed	F:36:M:120	+2	72 846'319–(41)	3:12:12
Epilepsy		+95	478'296–(37)	1:8:13
Alcoholism				

The patient was admitted to the hospital for diagnostic evaluation of epileptiform attacks and for help with her chronic alcoholism and her spells of acute panic crystallizing about a fear of epileptic attacks. The first disturbances of consciousness had been noted when she was 15 and had consisted of feelings of confusion and one "blanking out" spell. At the age of 17, after the deaths of both parents within a period of weeks, she had the first of a series of fainting spells which continued during the next two years. Usually she fell, bruising herself; her eyes rolled; she bit her tongue and urinated. Feelings of unreality and shyness followed. Between these more definite spells she had "queer feelings" which sent her into a panic because she feared she might faint. By age 21 she was afraid to venture out-of-doors by herself and she stayed at home, cared for by a devoted elder sister. She began to drink because it calmed her. At the time of the hospitalization she had had only one or two "real seizures" in the past two years, but because of her fears and alcoholism she was incapacitated as a wife and mother.

The patient's father, a kind and indulgent man, was popular and active in the community. Her mother was a lenient, quiet, and retiring person. They were both old when the patient was born and she was never disciplined. As a child she had severe temper tantrums. At one time she refused to go to school because she said the other girls picked on her, and she forced her parents to hire a tutor for her for six months. Sex was never discussed in the home and she always felt embarrassed with boys, considering herself too tall and skinny. She married at

20, but her husband, who was in the navy, was gone frequently and for long periods of time. They had two children. Shortly after her marriage her sister, who was slavishly devoted to the patient, came to live with her and acted as housekeeper and obedient servant to all the patient's demands.

On admission to the hospital the patient was neatly dressed, pleasant, and cooperative, except for several episodes of panic. During these she became extremely childish in manner, cried, shook violently, and demanded much reassurance. During the hospitalization she had no seizures. The physical findings were compatible with a convulsive disorder but the evidence was not conclusive. Twice weekly over a period of three months she was seen for psychotherapy. She was able to accept the interpretation that the panics were not necessarily related to epilepsy but were a long-standing reaction pattern carried over from childhood and applied to similar frustrations in adult life. She was encouraged to broaden her activities and make short trips away from the hospital alone. The patient was told that the doctors were not convinced that her seizures were epileptic but that she would be given medication to help prevent their recurrence. Her relatives were interviewed and an attempt was made to help them see how they played into the hands of her dependent, infantile demands. The patient improved steadily. Several months after discharge a letter to her therapist said that she was still relatively free of fears and was optimistic about her future adjustment at home, where she was living with her husband and without her sister E. B.

Schizoid F:18:S 728'4963-(39) 7:6:8
'9736-(37) 8:3:13

This college freshman was referred by her dormitory counselor because she was seclusive, seemed unhappy, and expressed unusual ideas about herself. She also had talked to the dormitory counselor of her difficulty in making up her mind about an occupational choice.

In the dormitory she had kept herself apart from the other students; she had been the butt of some of their jokes and had been unable to take these jokes in her stride. She was given to going off on long walks by herself and to daydreaming and general abstracted behavior.

In an extensive series of interviews over a six-month period, she went through several stages; first she gained in the ability to face herself more realistically, then she carried through into some fairly deep exploration of her negative attitude toward her mother and her younger sister, and this seemed to lead to a release from her tension and her need for an escape mechanism. At the end of the series she had made several friends and was participating more in college life. In addition she reported a considerable reduction in her daydreaming and an increase in actual planning. The second MMPI was taken near the end of the counseling interviews. E. S. B.

Ps. Sz., Paranoid	**M:23:S:61**	**+3**	**728 61'34-(59)**	**1:8:13**
Suicidal		**+9**	**'3146-(55)**	**4:3:19**
Ps. Sz., Paranoid	**M:23:S:41**	**+2**	**'7684 23-9(59)**	**2:5:19**
Suicidal				

This young man's father asked that he be admitted because of peculiar behavior. The patient had become seclusive, and six months earlier he had been especially perturbed when the girl he had planned to marry suddenly married one of her other friends. He said that he almost committed suicide at that time. His family noted that his work in dental school fell off markedly, and he began to develop ideas of reference. One day when an instructor questioned his judgment in treating a dental patient he became angry. Following this incident he had hallucinatory experiences and paranoid attitudes. The instructor who had questioned him and the "town" were especially against him, he thought. Later on a train he decided that passengers were singing dirty songs about him. At another time he asked a policeman for a gun "to kill myself." For this he was jailed and when the youth's father went to see him he called himself "a failure in life and a disgrace to the family." He was brought from the jail to the hospital.

The patient was bright and interested in sports and outdoor activities; there was no evidence of peculiar behavior before the present illness except that for eight or nine years he had found it difficult to urinate in an open men's room. He had resorted to masturbation as a relief from abdominal pains but seemed not to be worried about this habit. Sexual intercourse with two women had apparently left no regrets or guilt. Described as somewhat shy, secretive, and easily offended, he nevertheless had many friends.

When he arrived at the hospital, he appeared to be exhausted, did not speak spontaneously, and answered questions only after a long delay. He had auditory hallucinations and suicidal wishes. After insulin shock treatment he lost some of the more obvious signs of his illness. He then had doubts about his previous paranoid ideas, yet he did not clearly give them up. Eventually he expressed a desire to leave the hospital and to return to school. Before his first discharge, he became deeply engrossed in bridge and played late into the night. He was sociable, talkative, and friendly in the last days of this admission. Discharged, he spent several weeks at home and appeared relatively normal. He took a job and worked at it satisfactorily, but still the family felt he was not back to his usual self. Gradually he became nervous again. When he began to collect knives and guns in his room, his family had him readmitted. Shock treatment was used. He recovered somewhat, then regressed, and was finally transferred to a veterans' hospital.

B. Simple Adult Maladj.	F:22:S:36	—30	72'8631-(51)	3:5:15
P. Psychas.		+60	'2713486-(50)	7:4:21

This girl came in initially for vocational advice. Since her sister had previously been treated for an acute panic of psychotic dimensions, the girl was given the MMPI as part of the test battery. During a discussion of the test results, she admitted that she was suffering from intermittent periods of depression, which she attributed to her inability to find a profession. She also felt that she could not contribute with any spontaneity to normal social situations.

She described her family life as being fairly satisfactory, and she said the parental treatment was that of the average home. This was in direct contradiction to the report given by her older sister. During her life she had been in close contact with the older sister, who had led the way in childhood activities without giving the patient a sense of being dominated. She had accepted this role of the minor actor so successfully that it came as a distinct shock to her when she found out her actual potentialities—she had an I.Q. of 146. She had gone through college unaware of her capacity, which was so well concealed that she was given the sobriquet of "Plain Girl."

During the interviews treatment was largely superficial; an attempt was made to direct her toward a vocational goal more in keeping with her ability. The therapy was terminated when she left town, with both the therapist and the client feeling that not much had been accomplished. Despite this, the MMPI scores show a change of approximately one standard deviation in the direction of improvement in the aberrant scores. It is believed that when she finds a satisfactory life situation, her adjustment will improve. A. S.

P. React. Depr. M:29:M:10 +1 728'63419– 5:5:12

Since the age of 19 the patient had had a tendency toward depression during the summer. In these spells, which usually lasted four or five months, he worried excessively about his farm work and had great difficulty getting his chores done. As the load of work lessened the spells gradually subsided, and during the winter he was well, active, and full of energy, plans, and optimism. During the summer of his admission the spell had been unusually severe, with marked weeping spells, and his local physician had referred him to the psychiatric unit.

Except for gonorrhea, which he had contracted several years before, the past medical history was negative. He had left school in the middle of his second year at high school, having decided to go out and earn some money, but after two months he had returned home. Shortly afterward, his depressive episodes began. A good worker and a successful farmer, he had always wanted to run a big dairy farm. At age 23 the patient had married a schoolteacher and the two got along fairly well, except that he was too much attached to his own family. She described the situation by saying, "He is married to his family." Although they had always wanted children, he had been distressed when he learned of his wife's pregnancy shortly before his admission. His wife was much upset by his depressive episodes and had threatened to leave him unless he improved.

In the hospital he spoke freely about his unhappiness and his strong desire to end it all. He said that he had lost interest in everything, and he was inclined to talk extensively about that fact. He blamed his father for his difficulties, saying, "I would like to get away from him. I'm too dependent on him. I want to use my own ability, but my father won't let me." He said he felt better when he was away from his parents, but he doubted his ability to get along away from them. There was no peculiar behavior except for his tendency to weep frequently. He entered into ward activities after a few days and improved very rapidly. In planning for the patient's discharge a social worker interviewed his wife, his father, and the others concerned, and it was decided that he and his wife would move to another community where he would attempt to run a dairy farm. The patient accepted these plans as his own and looked forward to their execution.

B. Psth., Asocial   M:34:M:14   +5   7286'43–(49)   4:8:10
Schizoid
P. Psychas.

During most of his adult life the patient had exhibited peculiar behavior characteristics including seclusiveness and inability to conform. To evade being drafted he attempted to assume the role of a conscientious objector. Unsuccessful in this pretense, he was later discharged from the army as a psychoneurotic. The army record mentioned "battle fatigue." A few months later he was taken into custody for attempting to borrow $100 at a bank, while offering a $100 bill as security. His wife said that he had collected paper money with certain serial numbers because of their sentimental value. Both of them had made a practice of eating at various restaurants and not paying the checks. They had also charged items at department stores under assumed names. He had many get-rich-quick schemes and constantly sent away for articles which he might sell. The patient and his wife had finally been arrested for forging a $15 check in order to pay for opera tickets. The patient complained of fatigability and occasional insomnia.

After high school the patient had gone through one year of business college. A very irregular worker, he had held numerous jobs. Sensitive and belligerent, he was also seclusive and a poor mixer. Within the limits of their peculiar behavior, the husband and wife appeared well suited to one another.

On admission the patient readily rationalized and was not especially disturbed over the fact that he was in the custody of the court, but he was excessively concerned about the disposition of his property and about the whereabouts of his wife. He was certain that his mother-in-law was controlling his wife's activities, and he attempted in every possible way to get in direct touch with his wife. He recognized the deviant nature of some of his activities, but he had well-systematized rationalizations for them. In the face of any frustration he was impulsive and irritable, but he was in good contact with reality in other ways. After being served with the notice of his wife's petition for divorce he became agitated, did not sleep, and wrote dozens of letters asking for help. He continually asked the staff, his minister, and his attorney for advice. He requested that he be allowed to enter a period of praying and fasting, but continued to eat when told to do so. By the time he was to be discharged from the hospital he had mapped out a plan of action that depended on his being placed on probation by the court. In that case he intended to go to another state and contest the suit for divorce. He was returned to legal custody to await his disposition by the court.

Schizoid	M:23:S:35	+9	728643'19–(67)	2:15:11
P. Psychas.				

This man became depressed, lost sleep, and developed ideas of unworthiness and guilt. He entered the hospital as a voluntary patient.

He was the second of three brothers. As a youth he had been solitary, studious, and introverted. He was a bright boy. He joined the Royal Air Force as a wireless mechanic on leaving school at the age of 18. He then became an educational instructor until his demobilization.

He was diagnosed as having schizophrenia with a depressive onset, and he underwent a course of modified insulin therapy and electric convulsion therapy. His condition improved. M. V.

P. React. Depr.	M:43:M:32	0	72864'319–(67)	4:14:13
P. Psychas.		—22	278'964 31–(63)	4:7:11
Alcoholism		—42	27864'13–(61)	6:12:11
Suicidal		?	2'76–91 (47)	5:4:12

The illness of this patient dated back approximately ten years. At that time the patient noted a marked increase in feelings of inferiority and anxiety, insomnia, and general depression. He felt that twenty years of work as a service station attendant had contributed to his illness. The demands of the public annoyed him at times, and he felt that his work was monotonous and unpleasant. Because of this he resorted to excessive drinking, at times drinking himself into unconsciousness. This behavior created a strained family situation which gave him a sense of guilt. While he said that his wife was "grand and understanding," it became hard for him to look at her directly. In his job and in other associations he became uneasy and insecure. An attempt at suicide was thwarted when a meter reader found him unconscious in the basement of his home with the gas jets open. Although he went back to work, the seriousness of this suicidal attempt seemed formidable to him. He continued drinking and evaded people. Three years before admission he was given a series of electroshock therapy but derived little benefit from it. A vacation did nothing to help him. One attempt to stop drinking ended in a debauch. Once more he went to a private hospital for additional shock treatments. At the time of the present admission the chief symptoms were still a lack of confidence, anxiety, nervousness, and depression.

7286'4931–

A high school graduate, he began work as a service station operator immediately after finishing school. Although he remained at this job for more than two decades he had few aggressive qualities that would help him in his work. He himself said that self-assertion was very difficult for him. Known as a vacillating, indecisive individual who always left things undone even though this caused him great distress and anxiety, he was also immature, inadequate, and extremely dependent. While he appeared to be above average in intelligence, his wife, apparently the aggressor in family affairs, ruled the family.

In the hospital the patient was depressed, although his orientation and intellect appeared to be intact. Showing no evidence of delusions or hallucinations, he discussed his problems eagerly, attributing them to "tenseness and anxiety." The patient responded so favorably to additional electroshock treatments and to some psychotherapy that he felt ready to go back to work. However, it seemed unlikely that under the strain of everyday, routine work, he would be able to overcome completely the personality defects of such long standing.

Ps. Paranoid	F:29:S:5	+2	7286'4931–	2:4:10
Ps. Paranoid	F:29:S:16	+994	728'4136–9 (43)	0:5:14

Over a period of thirteen years this young woman had shown mild personality upsets of a paranoid nature. The first indication of a disorder in her thinking occurred in high school, when she expressed the belief that people were not telling her the truth and were purposely deceiving her. Concurrently she had difficulty sleeping. She was referred to the school psychiatrist and was able to continue school without interruption. During four years in the university, there were evidences of relatively minor disorders, which brought her in contact with a university psychiatrist. At one time, after a tornado in a neighboring town, she expressed feelings of guilt and depression because she thought she was responsible for the disaster. At the onset of the present illness she was in charge of a school library, and apparently the responsibility was too much. Decisions were difficult for her to make, insomnia developed, and she became depressed, expressing ideas of personal responsibility for the war. She was unduly concerned about the birth of a child to a close relative and expressed ideas of jealousy. Preceding her admission to the psychiatric unit she had spent two months in a private hospital.

In school she had studied hard and had had no particular learning difficulties. Following the conclusion of her training in library science she had worked at a number of places, sometimes changing jobs because she had been discharged for psychological reasons. Apparently she had never been well adjusted. Self-conscious and introverted, she had never been out with a boy, and although she had many acquaintances she had known relatively few girls very well. She had never enjoyed social gatherings, although she had attended church meetings regularly. She was described as distrustful, sensitive, suspicious, and self-conscious.

In the hospital paranoid ideas dominated her mental content, and she felt that the world centered around her. Accordingly, she believed that the psychiatric unit existed for her sole benefit, with the other patients hired to stay there to make it appear real to her. She was oriented and apparently psychologically intact except for her delusional ideas that she was being watched constantly and that people were deceiving her. For the most part placid and pleasant, she occasionally showed some irritability and impatience, but she showed little emotion when discussing "touchy" subjects. Her stream of thought was coherent but at times vague. She was cooperative and friendly. At the end of five days she was discharged to her mother against the advice of the staff. Two months later she was readmitted of her own volition, but when she failed to respond to six subconvulsive shock treatments her family became convinced that state hospital care, which had previously been recommended, was indicated and she was transferred to a state hospital.

P. Psychas. F:28:S:127 +5 7'2893- 1:7:4
Mutilative

This young woman was admitted for plastic surgery on her abdomen because of ulcers that were the result of self-inflicted wounds. In a previous admission to the surgical service for treatment of the ulcers, she had shown peculiar behavior, irritating her wounds, tearing off dressings, and stubbornly nullifying all attempts to permit the skin to heal. She was so clever and sly that it was some time before staff members discovered she was frustrating their efforts. Among other things she introduced a needle into the anterior abdominal wall.

Eight years before admission the patient had a radical mastoidectomy which healed slowly because of constant irritation. Next she had an abscessed tooth removed and she caused osteitis by probing with an applicator.

She was described by her sister as a sociable, likable person with many friends. However, she had always had a habit of picking at herself; she seemed "to have to be doing something." Strongly dutiful toward her parents, she had never made any close men friends, although she seemed to enjoy masculine company. Her father, a drunkard, had frequently been abusive to the patient. He accused her of being responsible for the death of her mother, to whom the patient had been deeply attached and loyal. Never an interested student, the patient had left high school at age 17. She then went to work and earned a fair amount of money, which was spent mostly for hospital bills.

When she was admitted to the psychiatric ward the most obvious finding in the physical examination was the mass of scars and fibrous tissue around the abdomen and the mastoid. She was concerned about her family and could not forget the accusations her father had made. The situation at home following her mother's death had been intolerable for her, and she felt she could not return to it. With reference to the self-mutilation, she said she tried at first to restrain herself but then went ahead. When asked what she thought about while doing this, she said, "I sometimes—oh nothing much. I just do it." Later she admitted, "I sometimes get pleasure from the pain. I feel relieved afterward." Her I.Q. was about 85. She was passively resistant to therapy and skillfully effective in preventing any approach to her problem. She was finally discharged with little improvement, although physically she was healed and improved. A recurrence of difficulty in some form was predicted for the future.

Ps. M-D., Mixed	M:19:S:116	?	7289′6–(55)	4:4:16
Schizoid		+114	′46398–(47)	3:0:22

About a year before admission the patient attempted to join the army air corps. It was not known whether he was rejected because of a small hernia or because he was working in an essential war industry, but the experience precipitated a marked personality change. When he came home for a few days shortly after his rejection his family noticed that he was extremely quiet, but they assumed it was because he was tired. In addition, he had lost interest in social and sports activities. At the time there was nothing bizarre in his actions, and he returned to his war job. After working three days he quit without explanation, and when his mother learned indirectly about it three weeks later, she went after him and had him admitted to the hospital. When she found him he was unkempt, depressed, and worried, and he made many remarks about his being "no good." While being brought back for admission to the hospital, he suddenly developed severe abdominal cramps, which lasted about 45 minutes, and on admission there was still mild abdominal tenderness and pain.

A "model boy," he had graduated from high school as salutatorian in a class of more than a hundred students. In every way he had been a normal, responsible, conscientious, sensitive, and thoughtful boy. At the time of the onset of his illness he had been saving money for college. He had always taken disappointments hard and had remained unhappy about them for more than the usual length of time. For example, about two years before the present illness he had injured his back while playing basketball, and his disappointment over being kept out of a later game had been so great that he had cried a good deal about it; his whole reaction had been greater than was normal. There were no obvious contributory factors in the family relationships.

On admission, ideas of guilt were uppermost in his mind, and he believed that certain acts of other people and some newspaper articles referred to him because he was no good. His thinking capacity was fair but retarded. Although he smiled at times, he claimed not to feel happy. He recognized that there was something wrong with his mental outlook, but he felt that nothing could be done about it, and his only suggestion was that he should die. During the first two weeks of hospitalization he was almost inaccessible, but after convulsive shock treatments and encouragement to talk under partial narcosis, his depression disappeared, he took part in various ward activities, and he became slightly hypomanic. At the time of discharge, it was felt that he was, if anything, a little too elated.

P. React. Depr. F:32:M:51 +2 72'91384–(47) 4:3:16
Twin (see 2731 48'6–)

Four weeks before admission the patient gave birth to a second child. In the latter part of the pregnancy she was irritable and restless. Seven days after delivery she was told to remain in bed and rest because she was showing some hypertension. She became depressed and anxious about her heart and her general condition and developed anorexia and insomnia. Her first pregnancy had been uneventful. The patient was an identical twin and her sister had been seen a year before in the same clinic with a similar symptomatology also following the birth of a second child.

The patient's past health had been good and there had been no previous problems like the present one. The patient was a registered nurse. Her intellectual level was better than average. Her husband and she led an active social life. Before the present depressive episode she had seemingly been well adjusted in her social and domestic life. In fact, the general background material on her was almost entirely bare of any factors that might have contributed to the present illness.

In the hospital she was depressed and worried about the depression as well as about her heart. She was well oriented and her sensorium and intellect were normal. Although she claimed to be jittery she appeared composed. Her thoughts were orderly. She was well mannered and it was easy to talk with her. From the first she was eager to "get well and go home." She had a kind of superficial insight, expressed in her statement that her problem was simple after all. The feelings of inadequacy and depression continued for five or six weeks and then she began to lose at least the edge of the affect. She developed a much more active interest in getting out of the hospital and in making specific plans for her home life. Her twin sister, who had been in the psychiatric unit twice in the last year, was admitted for a third time just before the patient was discharged.

P. Anxiety State F:20:S:35 +1 7291'836–(45) 3:3:15
+40 '237 619 84–(43) 3:4:14

This girl's complaints were numerous. She felt that she could not concentrate, she tired easily, and she was irritable. It was difficult for her to maintain social relationships; she said, "I was grouchy and some of my actions were considered queer by my friends, but I could not help doing them." For a while she felt that the irritability was associated with her menstrual periods, but as the problem intensified, she realized that it must result from other factors.

As a child she had always felt lonely and unwanted. This feeling was intensified by such incidents as this: at the family dinner table one evening when she had come home bubbling over with events to tell about her day in school, she was cursorily informed that unless she had something to contribute to the family group, she should remain quiet. She began to withdraw socially. In high school she derived satisfaction from scholastic excellence but was continually oppressed by the feeling of not belonging. This problem was partially resolved when she entered an occupation which forced her into some social contacts, but when she went to college the feeling of being "left outside" returned.

The therapeutic process was somewhat lacrimal, but she took the sessions seriously and participated to the best of her ability. Insights came readily once she broke down her reluctance to talk about a given area. Following the termination of therapy, she was seen for two interviews a month apart. In these she resolved two fairly simple problems; one concerned religion and the other, her relationship to her boy friend. A month later she sent back a report of progress which indicated marked improvement, but the therapist's feeling that residual tensions were still present was substantiated by the client's showing on the second MMPI. A. S.

Ps. M-D., Depr. M:47:M:71 +1 7′29618–(39) 4:10:9
Suicidal

For a few months before admission this man was nervous, tired, slept poorly, perspired excessively, and felt tense. This pattern was followed later by crying, hypochondriacal complaints, and feelings of hopelessness. Fear of death and suicidal thoughts developed also. No apparent basis for the illness was elicited. His physician advised him to continue working, which he did, but he could not concentrate efficiently.

The patient was a congenial person of above average intelligence. There was a history of four similar mental upsets in the past fifteen years, each requiring two to three months' hospitalization. In his normal intervals he was cheerful and friendly, well liked and respected by everyone. He was open, truthful, and responsible toward his family and society. He was happily married and had one daughter. A first marriage had ended after four and a half years of unhappiness and discord.

On admission the patient made a good appearance, was cooperative, and talked spontaneously about his illness. He looked depressed and said that he felt hopeless and thought he was going to die because his stomach had stopped functioning. Full of regret at being a financial burden to his family, he had suicidal thoughts. He was well oriented, his stream of thought was orderly, and his memory was somewhat defective. Fluctuating between cheerfulness and depression, he was, however, depressed most of the time. At first there were numerous hypochondriacal complaints. Eight electroshock treatments had almost no effect. Because of his tenseness and depression he was given a prolonged narcosis treatment, which was discontinued after five days. He was somewhat more relaxed and showed steady improvement thereafter. At the time of discharge he was so much better that it seemed likely he would continue to recover from this attack.

P. Psychas. F:19:S:60 +5 $73\underline{28}4\underline{16}'$–(39) 3:2:23

This student was referred for therapy by her mother because of the girl's anxiety about persistent thoughts and fears. She was afraid that she might pick up a pair of scissors and kill somebody. She was worried about the meaning of love and complained of a feeling of insecurity and a lack of self-confidence. In addition she noticed a persistent ache in the back of her neck. This latter had its origin one day while she was making a speech, when it seemed to her that her neck was jerking and at the same time she realized she was "nervous." From this point on she began to dread meeting social situations because of the fear that her neck might begin twitching. The problem became acute when she was invited to a wedding out of town. At the time she had been "cramming" for final examinations, and she found the wedding a strain, suffered severe headaches, and broke down completely the following day.

At first the patient reported her childhood as a fairly happy one, but as the therapy progressed she described feelings of loneliness and of being unwanted by her social group, particularly following adolescence. This was accentuated by the fact that her family moved about a good deal at this time, further defeating her efforts to make social attachments. She compensated for this by throwing herself into public speaking, in which she showed considerable proficiency. In college this mechanism stood her in good stead for a while, but the emptiness of her life caught up with her in the consequent breakdown. She summarized her problem in this way: "As a child I think I acted much too old for my age. I think I had the attitude that I had to grow up. I was always too serious about things. Now I have to be grown up, but it seems that I have missed one phase of my life, therefore I couldn't meet the situation."

The patient entered readily into the therapeutic situation and developed good insight into her problem. She quickly perceived the relationship between her problems and the unsatisfactory social situation. As therapy progressed she went out of her way to put herself into awkward situations in order to learn how to handle them. Moreover she insisted on following through in all these situations to prove to herself that she was not running away from anything. Toward the end of the therapy she resumed college and registered for a course heavier than either the therapist or her parents desired. Some anxiety still persisted in her fear of what might happen, even though there was no situation that she had been unable to face.

A. S.

P. Psychas. F:32:M:6 +2 $'7\underline{38}\,\underline{69}$–(68) 4:1:23

About fourteen months before admission the patient discovered the body of one of her relatives after he had hung himself in his home. In spite of the great shock of this discovery, she told no one but let others find the body. A week later she had a miscarriage. About four or five months later she began to experience such severe nervousness that she would have to drive to her mother's home to stay all night. Gradually she withdrew from social contacts and was afraid that she was becoming insane and that she would harm her children. She hid all the knives so that she could not use them on anyone. Just before admission she had spells of violent crying, vomiting, nausea, palpitation, and trembling whenever her husband even suggested leaving her alone. A week before admission she jumped from a moving automobile in a panic, suffering abrasions from the fall.

She was a high school graduate at age 17 and after that was busy keeping a house, raising a family, and in general enjoying life. She was an active, extroverted person, friendly and social. She managed her home and children well and showed no defects of judgment. The marriage seemed to be a happy one and the two children were healthy and well adjusted.

In the hospital the patient kept up a constant stream of conversation and appeared generally overactive. She felt that she could have done something about her fears long before if she had just made up her mind and if her husband had not been so easygoing. In spite of her smiles and effervescent manner she had a feeling of inner tension, and rapport with her was difficult to establish. She kept on the move, constantly cheering up the other patients, laughing, and talking. She continued on a superficial level throughout her hospitalization. She and her husband decided that there was no need for her to stay longer and she was discharged against the advice of the staff. She was improved superficially but was basically unchanged.

P. React. Depr. M:23:S 7'41238–96 (57) 5:9:12

Extreme apathy in all fields of interest was the dominating complaint of this youth, a university student. Fear of his parents, particularly his mother, was another difficulty for which he sought help from the university therapist.

The youth's father, a country doctor, was an austere, remote person toward whom the boy, from his earliest years, had felt fear. The mother, although overprotective, inspired fears in him also.

At the beginning of the treatment sessions the student expressed a great deal of conflict over his desire to marry and his fear of displeasing his parents. He was lackadaisical in manner and attitude, disinterested in the life about him, and dependent. Treated over a five-month period in six interviews, with the therapist assuming chiefly a supportive role, he began to show definite improvement. His interest in school and other activities heightened noticeably, and his fears lessened measurably. At the end of this period the student felt equal to facing his parents with the announcement of his plans to marry soon. C. K. A.

Ps. Sz., Paranoid F:42:M:46 +4 '746–139 (68) 1:4:6
+43 '879–463 (63) 0:6:11

The patient had begun to believe that her husband was not faithful to her and that people were talking about her. This pattern had appeared four years before admission and in the interim she had shown a progressive decline in social activities and had become increasingly irritable. Their home life became so unsatisfactory that the husband asked for psychiatric evaluation and treatment of his wife.

The past medical history showed a long list of vague somatic complaints with several episodes of medical treatment. An eighth-grade graduate, the patient left school at age 14 and worked at odd jobs until her marriage at 18. Before her present illness she had enjoyed sports and other social activities, though she was somewhat shy and sensitive.

In the hospital she was chiefly concerned with her present status and with the future of her marriage. Her sensorium and intellect were intact. She was depressed and had very poor insight. She needed constant prompting to continue talking and she exhibited considerable blocking in her speech. She was cooperative but nervously defensive and apprehensive. Even after twelve electroshock treatments she continued to believe her husband was unfaithful to her and never became willing to discuss her problems at all completely. She did admit that she had always been of a suspicious nature and that she and her older sister had never trusted each other, having scarcely spoken for the last seven or eight years. Since she had always had borderline paranoid tendencies and had never made a really good adjustment, the prognosis was poor. She was discharged for a trial period at home.

P. React. Depr.	M:28:W:26	+13	74812 36'9–(55)	8:9:19
		?	12 738'469–X (59)	11:7:19

The patient entered the hospital with a depression, insomnia, and somatic complaints that had become progressively worse over a period of two and a half years. The origin of the depression went back to his wife's death in childbirth after six months of marriage. The child had also died. Because of premarital relations with his wife, the patient had felt considerable guilt about her death. In time this feeling had lessened in intensity; but the oppressive guilt returned a year later following sexual relations with another woman. Just before admission he had taken five sleeping tablets in one night, attempting to control his insomnia. He complained of a failing appetite, persistent diarrhea, and regurgitation of food. He had also begun to drink fairly heavily.

He had had one previous period of depression eight or nine years before, from which he had recovered spontaneously. His mother described him as having been a "good boy." He had few friends and always "came right home after school." He had difficulty with his schoolwork and repeated a grade or two. Always shy and reserved, he had been dependent on his parents and had never become really mature. Conscientious in his work, he tended to drive himself, because, he said, "I was afraid that the foreman would get after me if I did not work hard."

On admission he presented the picture of an agitated depression. He sat on the edge of the bed, did not speak spontaneously, and stared at the floor. His thoughts were centered on the death of his wife and on his somatic complaints. There were no gross disturbances of sensorium or intellect. He had little insight and believed that if he could once again sleep properly he would recover. He did not participate in the activities of the ward and kept saying he wanted to go home with his folks. No improvement occurred until after six electroshock treatments; then the depression seemed to leave him and he slept better. He was discharged considerably improved, but the probability of future attacks was recognized.

Ps. Sz., Mixed	F:28:M:18	+1	76'284–(43)	5:7:15
Suicidal		+15	'742–1(49)	3:3:15
Ps. Sz., Hebe.	F:28:M:22	+6	'467–(57)	2:4:19

Three months before admission when this young woman gave birth to her first child, she was happy and pleased but extremely anxious about her duties as a mother. Overzealous about the baby's needs she neglected all her other household duties. She became depressed and believed that she was covered with lice and was contaminating everything and everyone she touched. To prevent her infant from getting lice she tried to suffocate him; then she attempted suicide in remorse. These severe behavior changes appeared about three weeks after the delivery. The patient thought that the lice were a punishment because she had permitted intercourse while still bleeding following the delivery.

In the young woman's past history there was one questionably psychotic episode that had occurred immediately after her marriage when she and her husband had both seen lice. The young bride was cured in two or three days. The difficulty with her husband's corroboration of the story was that he was subsequently discharged from the navy for psychiatric reasons. The patient was of low normal intelligence. Primarily interested in her home and in reading, she described herself as shy and self-conscious. She would not, for example, attend church on Sunday because she felt she "stood out." Her self-consciousness was directed at her clothes, her teeth, and her hair. A generally cheerful person, however, she had not appeared to be unhappy.

In the hospital she was apprehensive and completely concerned with the lice. When asked to indicate what she saw she pointed to pieces of dandruff, lint, and the like. "Getting the lice," she believed, constituted a grave wrong to her husband. She was depressed and showed a schizoid affect. She was completely unable to recognize the delusional nature of her fears. After shock therapy she improved markedly and was willing to accept the idea that she was not infected with lice if the doctors and nurses told her so. Nevertheless, she was obviously still attentive to the lint and compromised by referring to "that darn lint." When discharged to the care of her husband, she had a poor prognosis.

Only a week later the young woman was readmitted. Her husband said that when they drove away from the hospital, she appeared happy and cheerful, but as soon as they arrived home she began to clean the house vigorously and insisted that all the rooms be fumigated. Immediately, also, she began to "see" the lice, and within a day or so became upset, began to cry, and returned to her former state. During this hospitalization she received seven electroshock treatments and seemed to improve again. When she was crossed, however, she became assaultive, screamed loudly, and once struck a nurse. After this episode she was extremely apologetic and tried to behave acceptably. Again she was discharged with a poor prognosis.

P. Anxiety State M:25:S 781236'4–9 (69) 4:13:6

This private came to the psychiatrist of his own volition and requested a transfer to a "base nearer home." His tensions and irritability, he complained, had mounted so that he annoyed all the men with whom he worked. They, in turn, misconstrued things he did and said. He had no army friends and found soldiers "vulgar." Because of two previous hospitalizations for psychoneurosis, he had already been disqualified for overseas duty.

The patient, a slender young man, manifested pressure in his speech and was a chain smoker. He was restless and his hands were noticeably wet with perspiration. Born to high-strung, excitable, hypochondriacal parents, he was one of six children. Well provided for and "very happy," they were a clannish group who seldom made social contacts with the outside world. The patient was a lifelong nail biter, and in earlier years he had been much disturbed by somnambulism and bad dreams about the deaths of family members. He had felt inferior when he was with other children and he had refused to eat or visit with children other than his siblings. Paradoxically, the patient's school record was good. He engaged in no athletics, but his marks were above average and he participated in the debating society and in student council activities. In addition, his preinduction social, sexual, and occupational adjustments were apparently good.

The problem was that the patient had no motivation for making a successful military adjustment. His superior capacity as indicated by his work record and his score of 139 on the Army General Classification Test contrasted markedly with his poor performance. After he talked out his hostility and aggression against the army during several sessions he was returned to duty and was not heard from again. A. T. K.

P. Hypo. M:47:M:22 +6 7812364'9–(51) 6:8:12
P. Psychas.

The patient's condition at admission was apparently the outgrowth of a lifelong personality deficiency. The symptoms were chiefly "nervousness," a marked fear of committing suicide or harming others, and apprehension that he might be attacked if left unprotected. In addition, he had gastrointestinal complaints. The present illness had begun with anxiety experienced preceding the birth of his last child, when he feared that bad roads might make it impossible to drive his wife to the hospital. Shortly before he had suffered the loss of four cows. He began to lose interest in his farm work and became sloppy and careless in his activities and personal habits. A quarrel in which he was threatened by an aged, senile neighbor brought on a severe emotional state, characterized chiefly by fear and hallucinatory experiences in which he saw faces.

His past history was marked by many somatic complaints, for which he had received various treatments. In the fifth grade he left school "because it was too hard." After that he did farm work and farmed for himself. His intelligence was in the dull normal range. Hypersensitive even as a child, he had had to be excused from the classroom before a teacher could physically punish another pupil. He was self-conscious and had always been regarded as extremely immature. His wife and he appeared compatible. They had eleven children, the somewhat unwelcome outcome of their religious attitude toward birth control.

On admission the patient appeared in good physical condition. Well oriented, he was apparently about as capable mentally as he had ever been. His emotional immaturity was very evident. He exhibited a peculiar physical activity in which he threw back his head and made sweeping arm movements without vocalization. The therapy consisted chiefly of careful reassurance along with good physical treatment. Finally he brought out in discussion his fear about the outcome of masturbation. The patient appeared to improve significantly and it was felt that after continued psychotherapy he would be able to adjust again at his previous level.

P. Mixed	F:23:S:68	–5	78132'496–(55)	4:4:15
		+62	78213'64–(53)	4:6:15

Since infancy this young woman had suffered from spastic paraplegia of her lower extremities, and because of the paralysis she felt inadequate, self-conscious, and unable to make a normal adjustment to her life situation. Further troubles, present most of her life, included severe headaches brought on by an emotional upset or by eyestrain, eye soreness and burning whenever she did close work, constipation, and insomnia. Ever since reading two years earlier a book on the subject of insanity, she had felt she was mentally ill. Many of the symptoms described in the book fitted her case, she believed.

After graduating from high school, the patient spent a year in business college; she was an average student but was absent frequently because of headaches and the paralysis. Her chief ambition was to marry and have children. Regarded as cheerful and friendly, she appeared to enjoy life and to get along well with people. She disliked receiving sympathy or any partiality because of the paralysis. Crowds made her feel conspicuous.

On admission the young woman's dominant thoughts centered around her desire to be accepted as normal. She maintained a calm and composed appearance but confessed to inward nervousness. She was certain that she was mentally ill, and she felt this was due to social inadequacy. There were no bizarre features in her behavior. Her I.Q. was 116. The initial apprehension and depression continued throughout her hospital stay, but on the ward she entered into all activities with zest and was cheerful and cooperative. She was especially interested in the other patients and their problems and she made many friends. During her hospitalization she tenaciously clung to the notion that some day she would walk normally and even dance, in spite of the fact that the paraplegia, from a medical standpoint, was not subject to treatment or to improvement. Because of this insistence that she was basically normal or would become so, she was not very accessible for psychotherapeutic work. Crutches and braces were provided for her and the social worker worked on the problem of outside adjustment so that when she left the hospital she would have a job she could handle. At discharge there was little change in the basic picture, but the patient was hopeful and expectant of a reasonable adjustment in her new job as librarian in an institution.

P. Hys. M:16:S:6 +4 7813′62–9 5:6:11

About a week before admission the patient left home when his father ordered him to return some baseball equipment he had stolen, and he was not seen again by his parents until his discharge after the present admission to the hospital. Three days before admission, when he was found by a sheriff of another county supposedly suffering from amnesia, he claimed not to know who he was or to remember anything about himself. He was transferred to the hospital from the jail.

A hard-working, industrious, and active boy, he had always been successful in finding and holding odd jobs, but he had been a disciplinary problem both in school and at home. Resentful of any form of discipline, he talked back to his parents and disregarded school regulations. Socially he was somewhat withdrawn and uncommunicative. His mother had tended to "baby" him, and he resented her oversolicitude. He had not been a severe behavior problem, however, and until the present series of events he had done nothing that had brought him into contact with the law.

In the hospital he was obviously in good health, and there were no contributory neurological findings. Although he was completely oriented and intact for the period after he was picked up by the sheriff, he denied knowing his own age or identity, disclaimed any knowledge of current events, and was undisturbed about his apparent amnesia. He did not speak spontaneously and his answers to questions were short. If left alone he was completely quiet and comfortable. Though he was not actively resistant, he clearly gave the impression that he did not want to lose his amnesia, if in fact he was amnesic. By the use of a free association technique his name was ferreted out, and his parents were notified. He was obviously disappointed to see them, and immediately after his identification by them he professed the complete return of his memory. He said that it was like coming out of a dream. There was no way of determining whether he was a true amnesic or whether the situation was faked. Considering his basic psychological type, however, and the problems that he had, he was more likely truly amnesic in the hysterical sense. He did not remain in the hospital long enough for a real assessment of his problem.

P. Hypo.	M:21:S:18	+14	7814632′9–(47)	7:9:18
Mental Deficiency				

This patient was admitted to the medical service with numerous vague somatic complaints referring to most parts of the body, including abdominal pain, blood in his stools, inability to sleep, heart leakage, inability to pass urine, and nocturnal emissions. Depressed over these symptoms, he had been unable to work efficiently for a two-year period. There had been no previous psychotic episodes, but since his father's death six years earlier he had shown increasing anxiety, and a fear of death had been present whenever he became ill.

He had left school in the seventh grade at age 16; he had repeated the first grade. His I.Q. was 58, but it was felt that this score may have been lower than his best ability because of a loss in efficiency due to his anxiety. He was exceedingly dependent on his mother, had few outside activities, and was secretive, very suggestible, and superstitious. He daydreamed a great deal about his somatic complaints and needed much sympathy and general reassurance. Two years before admission he had had sexual intercourse with two different girls, and since that time he had become greatly concerned about "frequent" nocturnal emissions and masturbation.

In the hospital the physical and neurological examinations showed some abnormalities but nothing consistent with the extent of the patient's complaints. He was chiefly concerned with himself, and it was difficult to get him to talk about anything other than his pains and somatic troubles. He expressed a fear of impending death, and occasionally he cried briefly. His sensorium and intellect were intact, but he answered questions with a very limited vocabularly. He was ill kempt in appearance. Seclusive with other people at first, he poured out his problems once rapport was established, going out of his way to tell about his troubles. Since nothing could be done with him psychotherapeutically and since the family situation did not permit much modification, he was sent home to his mother with no particular recommendations.

Ps. Sz., Simple	M:23:S:69	+1	782134′6–9	7:13:20
		+68	′4182–7	4:1:19

Weakness, fatigue, malaise, ideas of reference, weight loss, delusions of having cancer, frontal headaches, and insomnia were first noted by the patient about nine months before admission. He felt that the symptoms came from cancer of the head, back, and thorax, which had impaired his memory. Because of his belief that a lack of memory made it impossible for him to converse intelligently, he began to avoid his friends. When a car came to his farm he was always afraid it might bring friends with whom he would be compelled to talk. When he went to bed he was unable to sleep because he began to hear noises resembling automobile and airplane motors. In explanation of a 25-pound weight loss he said, "I just didn't feel like eating." He did not believe he was capable of doing as good work as other people, and he thought that neighbors were talking about his peculiar behavior and were commenting on the fact that he was "so dumb."

The eleventh child in a family of thirteen, he completed the eighth grade with average marks. Until age 21 he had lived on his parents' farm. Since then he had been farming with his brother, although the patient had not been enthusiastic about leaving home and did not particularly like farm work. At 21 he had become infatuated with a girl and had paid her considerable attention for six weeks but the affair had broken up. According to the patient, he was "not good enough for her." Since that time the patient had gone out on occasional dates, but his interest in girls had not been as intense as it had been formerly. A steady, reliable person who had always displayed good judgment, he was also shy, reserved, and slow to anger.

On admission the patient showed definite psychomotor retardation. The delusion that he had cancer which could be cured by electricity was evident, but the hallucinations about automobile and airplane motors could not be elicited. While he was in the hospital he was well oriented, and he had no obvious ideas of reference. His general mood was one of depression. He was apathetic and listless, with a marked dissociation between his thought and his mood, and his ideas about cancer were told without any evidence of a change in affect. He made a fairly good adjustment, and by the time of his release there had apparently been a complete remission of the symptoms. At discharge he had made tentative plans for the future.

Ps. Sz., Paranoid M:26:S:5 +2 78213'46–9 4:5:21
P. Psychas.

This young man's complaints included a peculiar sensation in the back of his neck and a general personality change. The former difficulty had been present for years, but his concern about it had recently sharpened. He said the sensation was more prominent following masturbation, a compulsive habit and one of his major problems. The masturbation gave him little pleasure, but he could not free himself from it. People "stared" at him, he claimed, and knew "what kind of person" he was by his eyes. He was afraid of "going insane" and sought advice from physician after physician.

His previous history contributed little of significance, physically or psychologically. Always shy and retiring, he had made no friends outside of his immediate family. He had spent some time in a C.C.C. camp. He had never had a girl friend, although he once had sexual relations with an older woman who apparently made the approach, an unsatisfactory experience. In school he was slow but managed to graduate from high school in the normal time. His work history included only a clerking job in his father's store.

On admission the patient was deeply concerned about what other people thought of him and so tended to avoid them. Vague and rambling in his stream of thought, he answered questions indefinitely and inadequately. No gross disturbances other than those indicated in his complaints were detected. Outwardly he adjusted well to the ward, but whenever examined more closely he presented a typical picture of inward discomfort. He was discharged to the care of his father without having changed appreciably.

P. Anxiety State M:32:M 7821346′9–(59) 2:5:18
P. Psychas.

This airplane pilot was referred by his flight surgeon because he was suffering from anxiety attacks associated with an inability to concentrate and a general loss of interest in his duties. The attacks were panic-like in nature and were precipitated by situations involving crowds or closed places. His difficulty had its onset in a German prison camp during the war. On his nineteenth mission his plane had been shot down and he had been under close surveillance for about six months. At that time his fear of crowded places and confinement had crystallized. After one year he had escaped from prison but the anxiety, insecurity, and tension never completely left him.

The man's childhood history showed sporadic bed-wetting to the age of 10 and an early tendency to run away. When he was 16 he left home for good. His parents, farmers, were very religious, but the main source of dissension in his home had been the patient's refusal to have anything to do with farm work. An aggressive individual, he had had a successful career in aviation because of his own initiative and drive.

The officer was immaculately neat. Although he was superficially poised and confident, this was clearly a façade. He soon showed evidence of psychomotor retardation and emotional depression. He tended to have repetitious combat dreams and was completely unable to come to grips with his work. The patient was sent to a general hospital and he was later retired from service. A. T. K.

P. React. Depr. M:33:M:22 +1 78213649′–(65) 2:9:12
+21 ′2748–(55) 5:0:18

Although considered a nervous person most of his life, the patient's first overt symptoms appeared several months before the present hospitalization when he experienced nausea and vomiting. At the same time he began to have crying spells which he could not explain. He became gradually more depressed, listless, and lethargic. For a while he worked harder than he had previously, but he felt that his brothers were better salesmen than he, and became withdrawn and antisocial. Realizing that something was wrong, he asked to be admitted to the hospital as a voluntary patient.

The past history was not helpful except that he had always been a "nervous" eater and had been intermittently nauseated for five years. In school he did poor work and stopped from a lack of interest at the age of 16. He held many odd jobs but always avoided those with responsibility. His usual social response was complete agreement: "Anything you say, let's not argue." In the hospital he was cheerful and pleasant but jumpy and somewhat inaccessible. He realized he was sick and wanted to get well but said that he "was very happy at the hospital." He showed only passive interest in the life around him, though he became oriented to the daily routine and appeared to enjoy the ward activities. He was well liked. When he finally left he was feeling much better, yet he still had an underlying anxiety and tenseness. The present episode seemed to be merely an exacerbation of a constant maladjustment, not previously incapacitating possibly because he worked with his two brothers and was protected by them. The prognosis was judged uncertain.

P. Anxiety State M:22:M 782149'36–(69) 7:11:?
Drug Add.

The patient, a first lieutenant, was referred for psychiatric clearance before demotion procedures were instituted against him because of his fear of flying and his refusal to fly. He had served a tour of combat duty overseas, during which he flew 85 fighter missions in 150 combat hours. The first symptoms had appeared while he was overseas and they had gradually become more serious until he was completely unable to tolerate flying duty.

A slender youth, he was limp in posture and indifferent in attitude. Besides various vague somatic complaints, he said, "I don't give a damn for nothing any more." He found himself unable to sleep and unable to wake up. The discussions of flying experiences among his fellow instructors aroused acute anxiety feelings. Constantly trying to get out of teaching assignments involving flying, he either appeared late for duty or complained of illness.

His family history indicated alcoholic tendencies in his father. The patient was an only child. His school performance was average and he finished high school, but his occupational history showed a lack of incentive and poor judgment. Most of his earnings had been made by playing in bands and in connection with this work he used alcohol, marijuana, and benzedrine to excess. His married life was unsatisfactory, and he had resorted to physical aggression against his wife on several occasions.

The patient was sent to the air force regional hospital where he was discharged from the service. No follow-up material was available. A. T. K.

P. Psychas. M:23:S:110 ? 78234′169–(73) 5:8:17
Suicidal ? 728436′1–9(76) 6:7:18

The onset of this young man's illness was insidious. It had first appeared about seven years before admission when he was in the second year of high school. At that time he began gradually to withdraw from the normal activities of a high school boy into a moderate seclusiveness. This was evidenced by an increase in studying and a decrease in recreational participation. He began to seek treatment for a "weak heart" and he had compulsive feelings about suicide and homicide. He described these as "wanting to run people down with the truck," or "wanting to stab someone with a knife." He sought various types of medical treatment, including a short series of interviews with a psychiatrist. Believing he had schizophrenia, he read many books and articles on that subject. When he was admitted to the psychiatric ward, the outstanding symptoms were homicidal and suicidal impulses, feelings of unreality, and depression.

Except for his "never having been strong," the past medical history was not contributory. He graduated fourth among 32 students in his high school class. His particular interests at school had been scientific and medical books. After high school he worked sporadically, usually helping around the farm. Always a shy, quiet, well-mannered boy, he was eager to behave properly, showed no aggressiveness, and, in fact, was considered a passive person. There was no evidence of any heterosexual interest.

The patient was short, physically somewhat unattractive and forlorn, but organically in good condition. His conversation indicated dejection. He showed no gross disturbance of mentation or sensorium. During the weeks of his hospitalization he began to talk more freely, relating a mass of material about what he considered to be early sex perversion. "Enjoyed watching other people's bowel movements," "loved young boys," were examples. He associated his perverse interest in bowel movements with the job assigned to him of getting rid of his mother's excreta when she was bedridden. He had obviously ambivalent feelings toward his father, a long-standing feeling of inferiority and sibling rivalry, and frustrations of various types. He gained a kind of verbal insight but did not markedly improve. He returned to his home but it was expected that he would later need to be committed to a state hospital.

P. React. Depr. F:21:S:54 +6 ′782 46–9 7:6:15

The present illness dated from a few months before admission when this young woman was in an automobile accident. Although neither injured nor unconscious, she felt jittery and shaky. Later she confided to her family that she thought the accident had changed her; she felt different. During the summer she worked as a nursemaid at a lake resort. Her sisters noted that her letters became progressively less lively and when she returned home she showed moodiness and depression. Unable to look for another job, she sat in a corner and cried, developed marked insomnia, had severe nightmares, and appeared agitated. When these symptoms continued her family brought her to the hospital.

Following an attack of infantile paralysis when she was 5, the patient lost the partial use of one leg. In spite of a number of surgical procedures to repair the leg she continued to limp. She was very self-conscious of this physical impediment. A high school graduate, she spent a year and a half at college but left because she lost interest in schoolwork. Then she worked at various jobs until her present illness. After her illness when she was 5 she had been overprotected, the family never allowing her to make decision or judgments on her own. In fact the family had so limited her activities that she lost her initiative and confidence in herself. Her sisters, however, called her a "show-off." She never confided in any family member. Subject to fairly marked mood swings, she had never been interested in boys and had had very few dates.

On admission the neurological examination yielded nothing except for findings attributable to the paralysis of the right leg. She showed no severe content disturbance, and the main difficulty seemed to be in affect. She was withdrawn, depressed, and moody, exhibited a great deal of indecisiveness and self-accusation, and was convinced that she herself was the cause of all her difficulties. However, she made no attempt to adjust or help herself. Her thinking was definitely retarded, she was apathetic and listless. Her resistance to psychotherapy made that approach difficult but she steadily and slowly improved so that at discharge it was felt possible she would recover sufficiently to make an adequate adjustment.

P. Psychas. F:31:M:26 +157 782'<u>46</u>3–9 (57) 8:4:22

Nervousness and marked fears relating to clothes and uncleanliness brought the patient to the hospital. These symptoms first appeared about ten years before admission at the time the patient was married. Feeling guilt about a premarital sexual experience, she thought it was wrong to wear white at her wedding. After marriage she continued to worry a great deal about this sexual experience and about the use of contraceptives. She became afraid of broken glass and needles, feeling that such objects would stick to her clothing and then harm other people. She developed the idea that she had poison on her clothing which would harm others, and she also had a fear of blood and unclean clothing. After her first pregnancy she began to look compulsively five or six times to make certain that she had locked the doors at night. She was depressed and cried frequently. Her physician advised medication for hyperthyroidism, which made the symptoms worse. About a year before the present admission her children had contracted scabies. This was very upsetting, and added to the normal requirements of the five children she had by that time, the rigorous program she undertook to cure them made a heavy burden for her. Her phobias increased and she began to "grow weaker and weaker." A thyroidectomy improved some of her physical symptoms, but her mental symptoms were more acute. She became suspicious and jealous of her husband and their maid, with whom she thought he was flirting. She was afraid to hang her clothes out of doors because they might not be her own when she brought them back inside. Her husband finally brought her to the hospital because of the disorganization of the family resulting from all these symptoms.

The patient had always been shy and quiet. She graduated from high school, doing average work. She never worked for her living and was married at age 21. Her husband, a high school sweetheart, was the only romantic interest in her life. Her interests were limited to housework and reading. Fond of her husband and children, she got along well with others except for her husband's family, whom she considered shiftless and worthless. She was a Catholic and believed in Catholic teachings firmly and literally. She seemed to have been faithful to her husband both physically and intellectually. Her husband, who did not understand her illness, had tried to talk her out of her fears with "common sense."

While in the hospital the patient did not express many of her fears, but she was upset about having to wear a used gown over her slip when she went for X-rays. She washed her slip several times and did not wear it again for several days. Of average intelligence, she was usually quiet, shy, and a little depressed. Pleasant to talk to, she derided her phobias, saying that they were silly but that she could not overcome them. She was neat and tidy, perhaps to an unusual extent. Her general background and marital problems were discussed extensively with her. She was apparently relatively comfortable under the hospital routine and at the time of discharge appeared considerably better.

P. React. Depr. M:33:S:16 +1 '782496–(57) 4:5:15
Ps. M-D., Depr.

This patient's illness began approximately a year before admission but became particularly severe half a year later. Just before the onset the patient had been turned down by a girl he wanted to marry. He immediately developed some physical complaints of a gastrointestinal nature which was diagnosed as an "irritable colon." A month later, without any obvious reason, he sold his entire herd of cows, which was known to be a very fine one and which he had spent years building up. He gave various reasons for this act, but they were not deemed appropriate by people who knew him. Two weeks later he regretted the sale and developed fixed ideas that he had done "something terrible." He expressed the idea that his friends would think he had made the sale because the cattle had become diseased. He lost all interest in his business and showed psychomotor retardation.

The patient's early life was uneventful. He had lived on a farm and was a high school graduate, earning excellent grades. After high school he enrolled in a number of special courses in agriculture. Known as a hard-working man, he had considerable drive and ambition, his intelligence and judgment were well above average, and he had been a successful farmer and dairy man. He took an average interest in social activities and was moderately interested in the opposite sex.

When admitted to the hospital he was at first defensive about accepting treatment and hospitalization and insisted he could go home and would be all right in a few days. However, he soon adapted to the routine and by the time of discharge appeared to have made a fairly complete recovery. Whether he was changed deeply was uncertain, however, because he was not receptive to psychotherapeutic investigation.

Ps. Postpartum P. Psychas. Schizoid	F:28:M:67	+19	78 26′4319–(49)	2:14:8

This patient became depressed during the second week of her confinement after the birth of her second child. She was admitted to the psychiatric hospital because of occasional outbursts of violence when she wanted to kill her baby.

She had a university education and was a teacher before her marriage. After the birth of her second child she discovered that her husband had tuberculosis of long standing.

She was diagnosed as being in a puerperal state and underwent a course of electric convulsion therapy and modified insulin therapy. Her obsessional preoccupation with doing injury to her family persisted for some time. She had hallucinations, hearing voices telling her to kill herself or someone else. She improved, and according to a recent report by the psychiatric social worker she finally made a complete recovery. M. V.

Ps. Sz., Simple	M:31:M:63	+1	78′2693–4(61)	5:9:13
		+19	7′8–4(59)	4:8:10

The present group of complaints appeared one year before admission when the patient's family and associates noted marked behavior changes. Whereas previously he had been frank and open, he now became secretive, self-centered, and depressed. Sensitive to criticism, he at times showed anger but never violence. As he became more and more nervous, he worried and developed anorexia. Startling dreams marred his sleep. The contents of the dreams he never revealed. Fearful of being talked about or criticized, he refused to go into crowds. He realized that there was something wrong with his thinking but "couldn't figure it out." Finally he decided he was losing his mind and came to the neuropsychiatric department for help.

There was no history of a previous physical or psychological illness. Until the end of the seventh grade, he did well in school. However, in the eighth grade he failed and could give no explanation for this change in achievement. Although he wished to continue school, he stopped to go to work on his parents' farm. Later he rented a large farm for himself and managed it well. Described as a shy person, he was slow to take the initiative in making friendships, but once the first contact was made he was friendly and warm. He seemed to learn new things slowly, but on the farm he worked industriously and took pride in having a good field. Open and truthful, he was apparently not subject to mood swings. The patient and his wife appeared well adjusted and there seemed to be nothing in the home situation that contributed to the patient's illness.

On admission he had delusions and hallucinations. He appeared to be entirely composed, but one felt that he was wondering whether he should reveal what he was really thinking. Something was wrong with his recent memory and his thinking ability, he felt, but there was no proof of this. In spite of a willingness to discuss his illness he remained reserved and somewhat abstracted. There was a fairly definite depression, although it was not marked. During one period of sudden restlessness and nervousness he had to be placed in a disturbed ward. After that he suddenly changed, however; he mingled with other patients and seemed to feel at ease. When he was finally discharged to the custody of his father and his wife he was markedly improved. Nevertheless, there was no evidence of any profound changes.

P. React. Depr.	F:29:M:42	+1	78 2694'31–(59)	2:11:9
Schizoid		+118	7'8426–3 (49)	1:7:12

Less than a year before admission this young woman began to experience feelings of unhappiness, which she described as "desperate spells." Without apparent cause or explanation, the spells increased in number and severity until she lost interest and pride in her home and in her role as a farmer's wife. She said that along with the fading interest in her home she noticed in herself altered feelings toward her husband and her 3-year-old daughter. No longer did she feel love for them, and she grew indifferent toward sexual intercourse with her husband. She also developed somatic complaints. Seeking advice from a number of physicians, she was treated in various ways but without alleviation of the symptoms. Gradually she became worse, was greatly upset, and cried almost constantly. The physician then treating her suggested that she seek admission to the psychiatric unit.

As a child the patient had been sickly but had never been under a physician's care until the appearance of the present problems. There were no previous upsets of a psychological nature. Her early life was unhappy. The father, a drunkard, was finally committed to a state hospital and the mother and eight children were left to fend for themselves. After graduation from the eighth grade, she left school and took a job as a waitress because of the unhappiness in her home. Later she worked as a housekeeper and at similar posts. For a year she went with a man who did not return her affection. After breaking with him she met and married her present husband. The marriage appeared harmonious. She described herself as a serious person and a hard worker, but one who enjoyed "having a good time." She did feel some inferiority to her husband. This bothered her since she did not wish to be rated as inferior by him or by his family. She tended to be aloof and somewhat introverted, not at all aggressive.

On admission she was severely depressed, believing there was no hope for her. She had some tendencies toward delusional and hallucinatory experiences, but these were never really clear. Although she described the hallucinations as definitely visible to her, she always seemed to appreciate their unreality. These images were snakes, which she not only saw but smelled. She was cooperative but had little insight and believed that her illness was probably inherited from her father. She showed a definite desire to get well and to cooperate but was rigid. At discharge she was improved although far from recovered.

Ps. Paranoid M:59:M:15 +1 '78312469-(63) 1:2:18

Three months before admission this man had begun to accuse his wife of flirting and to quarrel with her. The wife claimed her husband had struck her on the head, causing lacerations of the scalp. Immediately, she said, the patient had been remorseful and they had agreed to call the injuries accidental. The wife did have partly healed head wounds, but the patient denied the story and claimed that his wife had injured herself in falling down the stairs. Some weeks after this event she had spent two weeks in a hospital for jaundice. During this period the patient began to brood over domestic affairs and visited a former neighbor whom he accused of having an affair with his wife. Then he became nervous, tense, and overexcited; he told long, detailed stories about his past marital difficulties and his present suspicions. He expressed the fear that he might lose control of himself and commit either suicide or homicide. At this point his daughter applied for his admission to the psychiatric unit.

The past history, obtained from the patient, was so extensive that it was difficult to select a few details. The periods of jealousy dated back to his courtship days. A reserved person, and very dependent, he had always been overly conscientious, bashful, and ill at ease, he claimed. He was considered kind and fair, but rigidity was one of his outstanding traits. Outside of his home and business, he had no hobbies or interests. The patient's wife was a friendly, open, warm person. In contrast, he was considered cold, aloof, and shy. They first became acquainted when he was 16. He remembered her for fourteen years and then began a formal courtship. It was his opinion that she was "desperately" in need of a man. He accused her of trying to "seduce" him during their courtship, and of flirting with an old "flame" during their honeymoon. He was voluble about all these points, citing events too numerous to mention.

On admission this story was all that could be elicited from him. He talked continuously, refusing to abbreviate or curtail his account of his marital history. He repeated events again and again, apparently forgetting completely that he had narrated them before. He seemed to be impelled to bring up delicate matters even when they were irrelevant to the story. For example, he insisted upon telling about a man who "broke my wife's maidenhood when she was 15." He discussed these affairs indiscriminately with patients, students on the service, and doctors. If not permitted to talk, he became restless and annoyed. After a few weeks he began to behave better and after consultation with his attorney it was decided that he should be discharged and released from the court order. When he left the hospital he was considerably improved.

P. Hypo. M:25:S:27 +4 7842′1936– 1:3:19
P. Psychas.

About a year before admission the patient noticed weakness, insomnia, and difficulty and slowness in thinking. About the same time impotence during an attempt at sexual intercourse made him fear that there was a decline in his strength and sexual powers. When he later noted a sensation like a worm crawling on his penis he developed the fear that he had contracted a venereal disease.

There was no contributory event in the previous history. The man had always lived on a farm, and his chief interests had been hunting and trapping, which had also been a source of income for him. A high school graduate with a good scholastic record, he was a cheerful, even-tempered, intelligent, and sociable person. Although he met others of his own sex comfortably, his desire for female companionship was frustrated by his extreme bashfulness. As a result he lived in a state of tension, with this desire as the basis for a great deal of autistic thinking.

On admission his chief content, which kept him upset and agitated, was exemplified in this statement, "It feels as if a little worm were crawling on my penis, and that's how they tell me you feel when you get a venereal disease." His inability to give a clear-cut account of his daily routine was apparently the result of a retardation in thinking, but by psychometric determination he was of normal intelligence, and he could do routine tasks without defect. He had a peculiar gasping respiration which became more marked when he was interrogated by a number of examiners. He was given reassurance that he was in good physical condition and that his problems would clear up. With hydrotherapy his insomnia disappeared. Very contented in the hospital, he was disappointed at his discharge, but at that time he seemed to be well enough recovered to be able to adjust to society.

Ps. Sz., Paranoid M:32:S:19 +1 7842316′9–(69) 2:8:16

Six years earlier, the patient said, he met a woman who transmitted an "antagonistic Nazi force" into his mind. Ever since the moment he first "met her eyes," this "force" tried to propel him into "Nazism"—which he defined as the use of narcotics and the practice of homosexualism. As a result, he had been unable to do anything worthwhile, even though he had not given in to these "Nazis," he said. In the light of these delusions, he frequently made bizarre misrepresentations. He was convinced that he was continually fighting against this force and being terribly punished. As to why he alone was singled out for this punishment, he was vague. The symptoms gradually progressed in intensity until they completely dominated his mind and he could concentrate on nothing except this "force."

Except for the fact that he had contracted gonorrhea eleven years before admission, there was no obvious factor in his past history that appeared to be contributory. A high school graduate, he made a good school record and took a job in a small company. He was doing well enough until he was charged with petty larceny and put on probation. After that he held many jobs, "from dishwashing to welding and gambling," as he stated it. Most of his time he spent at bars and pool halls, in the company of the woman who, he thought, wanted to make him a Nazi. His intelligence was well above average. A likable person, he was, however, stubborn and quiet, and he made few friends. After he graduated from high school he began to drink, was sexually promiscuous, withdrew from his family, and spent most of his time loafing.

In the hospital the most striking symptoms were the bizarre delusions of reference and, to a lesser extent, the hallucinations which followed the same trend. Well oriented, he was mentally intact in other ways. Not only did he show no insight into his psychological illness, but he was completely unapproachable on the subject of the "force." While he was indifferent to the activities of the ward, he got along with everyone. It was decided that he was at present relatively harmless and there was nothing that could be done for him within the limits of the available therapy. He was discharged to stay at home, after his mother had been warned of the possibility that he might become dangerous in the future.

P. Hypo. M:24:S:21 +3 '7893–2(57) 7:4:18
Mental Deficiency
Deteriorated

On admission the patient complained of a weak and sore back which had been present for as long as he could remember; it had recently become so marked that he could not work at all. He had been admitted to a hospital for crippled children when he was 16, and a thorough study at that time indicated that the back pain was due to bad posture.

Although he said that his past health had been very poor, there was no evidence that he had been organically weak or frequently ill. He was born with a large meningocele, which was attached to the lower occipital region. This was surgically removed when he was 3 weeks old, and although his recovery was uneventful, the patient thereafter appeared mentally retarded. He attended school until he was 18, at which time he was only in the eighth grade. He explained his inability to get along by referring to his back pain. After leaving school he worked as a dishwasher and cook's helper in a restaurant. When he was asked to substitute for the cook, his back pain and other nervousness became more pronounced. Mostly he spent his spare time at home doing household duties one would expect of a girl of similar age. His mother told him that he was more like a girl than any of his brothers. He had few friends of either sex and few hobbies, crocheting, reading, and seeing movies being almost the only ones. Shy and retiring, he was apparently ignorant of subjects that would ordinarily concern a young man of his age. His back pain prevented his participation in anything active.

On admission there was no evidence from the neurological examination that indicated a definite remnant of the meningocele. The patient's chief concern was nervousness and the back pain. If one did not particularly refer to these, he seemed to forget them too, and he did not appear overly concerned about his illness when the subject was not brought up. He was cheerful and pleasant, with certain feminine characteristics in his manner. His I.Q. was 74 and psychological tests gave some positive evidence of organic brain damage. During his stay in the hospital he showed little improvement. Faradic stimulation of his spine resulted in some decrease in his complaints about the pain. At the time of discharge he had changed very little. It was felt that there was a fair possibility of some sort of cerebral defect. The patient was inadequate and immature and these factors had to be considered also in what was a bad prognosis, although he was not mentally ill in any usual sense of the term.

Ps. Paranoid   F:37:D:10   +5   '789 32–(72)   7:3:18

The patient was admitted to the hospital with the obsessive feeling that she was pregnant and had been for nearly three years. She also had hallucinations and delusions of influence and reference. The apparent beginning of the present illness was a hallucination three years before admission of seeing a former boy friend. She "saw" him many times after that. Then came the idea that she was pregnant, and this persisted in spite of the normal continuation of her menstrual periods. Seven years before this idea appeared she had married for the second time, having divorced her first husband earlier. A shiftless fellow who did not support her, the second husband had an 11-month-old child by his first wife who had died. After the patient, who had no children, was told by a physician that she could not have a child of her own, she wanted the custody of this child, but her husband would not agree. It was after this that she developed the idea that she was pregnant. She came to feel that she could do only a small portion of her housework at a time and then had to rest. Her stomach was upset much of the time. Her husband, disgusted with her "laziness," finally divorced her.

The patient had no previous psychotic or obvious nervous upsets. In school she had failed in the second and fourth grades and finally withdrew in the seventh grade. She became a waitress and continued at that until her second marriage, which had been a fairly compatible one until the development of the present symptomatic picture.

On admission the patient expressed much concern about her condition. She told a vague story of long-standing ideas of reference and influence. "A man" had been near her constantly (in spirit), she said. She was convinced that he had made her pregnant, and no amount of reasoning or explanation could change her mind. Her sensorium and intellect appeared unimpaired. Her stream of thought was normal, and her answers to questions were logical and straightforward. She joined in ward activities, associated freely with other patients, and in general got along well in the hospital. Extensive gynecological consultations and reassurance did not affect her delusion. She requested discharge and left the hospital with the recommendation that she have shock therapy later if she did not improve.

P. Hypo.	F:26:S:49	+4	8123 764′–	8:13:9
		+40	231 4876′–9	6:8:12

This young woman's difficulties began a year before admission when she contracted a severe case of what she considered to be "flu." The symptoms were severe headaches, fever, chills, nausea, vomiting, dizziness, and aching bones and muscles. She developed bilateral parotid swelling. This condition confined her to bed for a month; during this period she was miserable, constipated, and unable to swallow anything but water. She lost twenty pounds. Following this illness the symptoms of nervousness, constipation, mucous stools, headaches, and multiple somatic complaints persisted and finally she voluntarily entered the hospital.

In her past history there was no evidence of any pertinent medical condition earlier. The patient finished the eighth grade when she was 13, having been an average student. Although she wanted to be a nurse, for economic reasons she hired out to do housework. A man much older than she, a widower with five children, persuaded her to live with him and help care for his children. After three years she began to have sexual intercourse with this man, with a normal amount of satisfaction. At first she was ashamed, but his promise to marry her salved her conscience. When she became pregnant the man's attitude changed and he began to drink heavily. He became abusive and beat her severely after the child was born, calling her obscene names and cheapening her in front of his children. Finally she was forced to leave his home and she moved in with her sister. Repeatedly she returned to the man in order to see her child, and each time he abused her. He was now eager to marry her but she refused. She did not take the child from him because he threatened to kill himself if she did. A neutral person, she seldom smiled and had never been able to get people to like her. She said that she had always helped her neighbors but "they would never help me."

On admission she was well oriented and apparently intact in mentation, although she complained that her memory had deteriorated. She had peculiar visual hallucinations in which a form, vague, indistinct, and white, would flash into her field of vision. What this was she could not decide but felt it was significant. She was mainly concerned with herself and her troubles. She gained little insight into her problem. The treatment centered mainly around social service aid in improving the home situation and in encouraging her to make plans after she left the hospital. She became somewhat better and was finally discharged to live with a relative until she could obtain work.

B. Psth., Asocial   M:43:M:37   +14   '81<u>24</u> <u>63</u>–(51)   8:3:25
Alcoholism
Paranoid

The patient was referred to the hospital for a pre-sentence investigation; he was charged with violence toward his wife. Five months before admission he was in a car accident and suffered a lumbar vertebral fracture and multiple contusions and abrasions. His car was demolished and his driver's license was taken away from him. He was put into a heavy body cast and sent home from the hospital after a few days. From that time until the present admission he had been unable or had refused to work. He also had not interested himself in reading or any other activity. According to his wife he was unhappy, irritable, and depressed. The precipitating incident resulting in court intervention occurred when his wife had spent a few hours talking to her daughter downstairs and had then come up to go to bed. The patient would not allow her to come in the room and insisted upon her leaving the house.

The patient had been a farmer all his life with the exception of the last two years, when he had moved to town and had done common labor. He had been barely able to support his family. He had never taken any responsibility in raising the children or running the house. He also used alcohol excessively whenever he had an opportunity. His two brothers were notorious drunkards. His I.Q. was 84. He was an agreeable, passive person but had never occupied anything more than a borderline position in the society about him.

In the hospital he was mainly concerned with what he was going to do when he left the hospital and with the injustice done him by doctors, his wife, the judge, and several of the townspeople. He was mildly depressed and hypochondriacal. There were some psychometric evidences for psychological deterioration; however, the neurological examination did not indicate extensive damage. He changed very little and because of the long history of inadequacy and the rigidity of his character the prognosis appeared poor for anything better than the borderline adjustment characterizing him before the present illness. It was even doubtful that he would again be able to reach that adjustment.

Ps. Sz., Paranoid F:33:D:46 +2 '8147369–X(57) 11:1:26
P. Psychas.

This woman was troubled with an obsessive fear that someone was planning to harm her. The first symptoms appeared a month before admission when a friend telephoned her and in the course of the conversation told the patient, "Take good care of yourself." A few days later, at a bowling alley, a man told the patient's little daughter to be careful and not get hurt. This disturbed the patient a great deal. She began to feel uneasy around people and thought they were plotting against her. As the fear developed that she might be harmed while at work she twice left in the middle of the day. One night she thought children were screaming nearby, and sometimes she heard rappings on the windows. Two days before admission she became so frightened that she asked a friend to come over to protect her.

During the second year of high school the patient had a psychotic upset and could not continue school because she felt as if she were in a daze. Others said she appeared sleepy, and she lost interest in her work and in people. This episode lasted for three months. She did housework and other varied jobs thereafter. Competent at managing her affairs, she took good care of herself and her daughter after she was divorced. Although she made friends easily and was considerate of them, she was described as sensitive and seclusive, and it was easy for her not to take advice from others. There were times when she would stare into space and become entirely unresponsive. Never much interested in men, she married because her friends thought "it was the thing to do." Because of her husband's affairs with other women she divorced him after five years. At the time of the patient's admission he was involved in a divorce from his second wife, by whom he had three children; the patient said that she would remarry him and take care of his children if he asked her to do so.

In the hospital her thoughts were centered around her fears, and she wanted to go home to care for her daughter. She was very defensive and said, "If I have done something to anyone I am sorry." Her memory was good; her intelligence appeared to be low average. Her insight was poor, and she could not reasonably account for her fears. She spoke well, usually rapidly. Often staring into space with a blank look on her face, she was apprehensive and fearful of everyone. In a few weeks the fears lessened in severity and she adjusted well to the ward routine. At the time of discharge she seemed entirely well. There were minimal findings suggesting the possibility that she had had an obscure toxic condition.

B. Psth., Path. Emot. F:22:M:57 +31 817296'34–X(63) 0:17:14
Suicidal
Deteriorated

The patient was referred to the psychiatric hospital from a general hospital, where she had been taken after an attempt to commit suicide by carbon monoxide poisoning. Three months before admission, after her husband had entered the armed services, she had become increasingly depressed. This depression was accentuated by the fact that her husband had been a great disappointment to her and there had been marital discord. The monoxide poisoning was severe. She had been in a coma for three days and at the time of admission there were extensive neurological findings indicating damage to the nervous tissue.

Her past health had been good. Since early childhood she had been considered "high-strung." She completed two years of high school and then ran away from home, working at various jobs for six months. Upon her return home she was disinterested in schoolwork and in most other things. She ran off with a boy for a while and exhibited an almost utter lack of responsibility. When she returned home after the escapade, it was found that she was pregnant and the couple were married. During the first year of her marriage she had attempted suicide by taking iodine but prompt treatment saved her from hurting herself. It was said that she had always been friendly, thoughtful, and kindly toward others but moody, irresponsible, and immature as well.

In the hospital she was markedly depressed and concerned with the futility of the future for herself and her children. She considered her husband worthless but said she still loved him. She had no definite delusions or other bizarre mental aberrations. Her sensorium was relatively unclouded. Her intellect was presumably impaired though there were no obvious signs of this. She was logical and adequate in thought and response. During the two months of her stay she gradually showed improvement and she lost some of her neurological disorders. She was given intense psychotherapeutic interviews and when she left the hospital she appeared completely relieved of her depression. She was actively planning for the future. While the immediate prospect for adjustment appeared good, the long-time prognosis was considered questionable in view of the history.

Ps. Sz., Hebe. F:24:S:40 +4 81934'726– 5:9:15
Suicidal +77 mos. '439–(43) 1:0:20

Four months before admission, following a short period of depression and decreased activity, the patient took sixty grains of phenobarbital. After treatment for this poisoning at a general hospital she was transferred to a psychopathic hospital where the case was diagnosed as schizophrenia. Although she was uncommunicative, she was depressed and complained of unhappiness, frustration, and dissatisfaction with her family situation. She was released after a forty-day hospitalization, but continued restlessness and irritability and the expression of bizarre ideas in a jumbled manner made it necessary to admit her to the psychiatric unit for study before her transfer to a state hospital.

Four years before the present episode she had a brief period in which similar symptoms occurred, and during that time she attempted suicide by taking fifteen grains of phenobarbital. After a few months' rest she recovered spontaneously from that attack.

A graduate of a business college course with a very good curricular and extracurricular record, she had gradually moved up in her work until she was earning a good salary. An intelligent, energetic, cheerful, sociable, outgoing person, she was, however, stubborn and insistent on having her own way. Although she had always appeared to be happy and optimistic, she had never been able to give complete expression to her inward feelings. The patient had reacted strongly to an unsatisfactory home life in which there was a great deal of quarreling and dissension. Her father was an uncommunicative, unstable person who spent most of his salary on himself rather than on his family. A half brother was sought by the law on a charge of petty larceny.

In the hospital she showed a vague, shifting, unsystematized delusional state with mild ideas of reference. For example, when she noted that a magazine cover was reinforced with brown paper, she inferred that the magazine had been altered to make it refer directly to herself. Although she seemed happy and elated, it was felt that there was an underlying depression. She was silly and facetious, with a tendency to be circumstantial, rambling, and incoherent in her conversation, but there were no definite evidences of hallucinatory or systematized delusional states. At times she was noisy and tended to disrobe. As she gradually grew worse she developed a marked erotic trend, and she was finally transferred to a state hospital.

Ps. Sz., Paranoid	F:32:S:46	+5	819′6327–	6:13:9
		+94	2813′467–9	4:5:10
Ps. Sz., Paranoid	F:33:S:25	+9	2381′476–9	6:9:8

The patient had been mentally ill with many ups and downs over a period of fourteen years. Her complaint on admission was, “I’m nervous and mental. No one tries to help me, and no one gives a damn.” In describing her first hospitalization seven years before the present admission, in which she was diagnosed as having a manic-depressive psychosis, the woman said, “I felt wretched and sorrowful, different every minute with different kinds of pain. I paced the floor and ate nothing. At times I was so noisy that they had to tie me down.” At that time there was a history of attempts at suicide by drowning. For the past two years she had been on parole from a state hospital, but the summer before admission she had become irritable and had developed many body complaints, particularly referring to the rectal region. Anal surgery for the removal of polypi and fissures had increased her irascibility and paranoid trends to the point where she had become a problem at home, throwing things, crying easily, and blaming others for her trouble.

She was an eighth-grade graduate at age 15 and had worked satisfactorily on her parents’ farm until her first breakdown, getting along well with her family and having the reputation of being a good worker. She had had few men friends and had never been engaged to be married. During her earlier years she was said to have been socially interested and active, enjoying parties, dancing, and other activities of teen-age children.

821347'69–

In the hospital she was sullen and depressed with many temper outbursts in which she accused her family and the medical staff of treating her "like a dirty shirt. You ignore me and you blame me for things I cannot help." At various times she gave belching, bad heritage, and lack of proper treatment as the cause of her illness. Her dominating desire was to get well, marry, and have a family. She admitted to marked sexual desires and said, "This mess I'm in is what I get for leading a decent life." As a patient she was demanding and difficult; she wanted to go home, but when she was told that she could go, she insisted that the staff was trying to throw her out. When the faradic stimulation treatments she asked for were not given immediately she became vituperative, but after a few shock treatments she refused more. Because of the long history of illness and the difficulty in handling this patient, a prefrontal lobectomy was performed. After the completion of the second stage of the operation she was more sociable, laughed more readily, was definitely more responsive, and was appreciative of the attention given to her. At times she still showed seclusiveness and dejection, and had rages. Although she continued to insist that the future was hopeless, she was somewhat encouraged by reassurance. Her manner of speaking improved, and she was less biting and sarcastic, but her posture remained poor, and she looked down at the floor when talking to anyone. She said, "I want to earn my own living, and I don't think I can this winter. More than anything else I'd like to get married and have a home of my own." When she was discharged to live with her sister, it was recommended that she return to the hospital later for study.

Four months later, she was readmitted, and according to her sister she had not got along too well in the interim. She had been inclined to worry a great deal, had been depressed, especially in the morning, had made contradictory statements, often elaborating on one subject for hours at a time, had been difficult to satisfy, and had found inactivity distressing. Inconveniences had been hard for her to take gracefully, but she had cried on only one or two occasions. In the opinion of the staff, her behavior was distinctly improved. Although there was a measurable decline in her intellectual functioning on this admission, the gain in general behavior balanced her loss in adaptability.

Ps. Invol. Melan.	M:61:M:39	+8	821347'69–(43)	3:15:18
Deteriorated		+11	2471836'–(57)	3:6:16
		+33	21376'48–9(45)	4:4:16

Ps. Invol. Melan.	M:61:M:35	+1	824761'3–9(53)	2:19:14

A few months before admission this man began to complain of failing eyesight. He said he no longer could see clearly, he had difficulty reading, and light hurt his eyes. Four different physicians after examining him found nothing wrong with his eyes, but he continued to complain. Concurrently, the patient's wife and his associates began to notice personality changes. In the past he had always been active, interested, and successful in his work. Now he lost interest in his business and in the four farms he owned and managed; he no longer cared to mingle with his friends; and even visitors to his home made him feel ill at ease. His memory, which had already been failing, became markedly worse. Previously careful and even close with his money, he now seemed to want to spend large sums on doctors and medicine. He became careless of his dress, insisting upon wearing one suit all the time; he sat around his home inactively, mumbling to himself and scratching his head so constantly that scalp sores appeared. It was difficult to induce him to leave his bed, and he told the nurse he had hired, "I want to lie here and worry." Agitated at times, he would pace the floor for hours. In conversation he rambled from one subject to another, without finishing a thought. He told his wife, "Box me up and send me to the asylum," and he threatened suicide, asserting that his family would be "better off that way." There were no previous psychological upsets.

An intelligent person, he attended college, where he took a two-year business course; he liked it and did well. He became a salesman and then an office manager, rising steadily until he was well off financially and on a fairly high social level. He had a reputation as a man of sound judgment, with a facility for getting along well with people. A hard worker, he had a burning ambition to make as much money as possible. He led a "fast life" as a traveling salesman until his marriage. He "chased with the gang," drank heavily, and "had a good time." He was interested in sports. An admitted trait of his was stubbornness, and he said also that he had always liked to have his own way. In the past he had not been given to depression nor had he been hypochondriacal. He had put off marriage until late in life, possibly because of his absorption in his work and in the accumulation of money. His wife was much younger than he and, in his words, "extravagant" and full of "millionaire ideas." She was, in fact, a forceful and domineering woman.

In the hospital the patient was found to have elevated blood pressure, and there were evidences of arteriosclerotic changes. He was concerned about his health and sanity, and when asked what he did all day, he said, "I just sit and think about how I'm going blind and losing my mind." Given careful rest treatment and later four electroshocks, he showed so much improvement that his wife took him on a vacation. Two months later he was back on the ward. In the interval he had become foolish, was very depressed, talked solely of death and of "losing my mind." This time, following several electroshock treatments, he again showed some improvement but, finally, was sent to the state hospital.

P. React. Depr. M:21:S:41 +2 82'1637–4 7:10:7
Suicidal

The main symptom that brought this patient to the hospital was a tremor, most marked in his upper extremities. In addition he was depressed and dissatisfied with his present existence. The physical symptom dated from about nine years before; at that time a few neurological findings led to a provisional diagnosis of functional neurosis, disseminated sclerosis, or a postencephalitic syndrome. In recent weeks the patient had become deeply depressed and had thought of suicide, chiefly because of the poor compensation he received from his farm work and because of the persistence of the tremor.

In the past history there were vague stories about a severe illness in his early infancy, but the exact nature of that illness could not be determined. The patient had left school in the seventh grade, presumably because the family moved about so much that he could not keep up with his studies. For the ensuing eight years he had worked without compensation on a farm where the hours were long and his employer extremely demanding. The patient had always had difficulty getting along with boys and girls his own age, and he tended to seek the company of older people. He had never gone with girls, and he felt uncomfortable in their presence.

His general appearance was best described as eunuchoid. He was beardless, there was a definite gynecomastia, his testes were small, and his pubic hair was female in distribution. There was a persistent low basal metabolic rate; X-rays of his skull led to some doubt about whether the pituitary was normal. There were a few scattered neurological findings of a general nature. Although the patient was eager to find the cause of his tremor, and if possible to get help, he preferred not to discuss his many worries, and he was not readily accessible to psychotherapy. He was unhappy on the farm, chiefly because the social opportunities were so restricted. His intelligence was low normal. His interests were feminine, but there was no clear-cut sexual inversion pattern. He never entered wholeheartedly into ward activities, but although he was occasionally sullen, his care presented no particular problem. Efforts were made to place him in some new line of work and to get him into a larger community. No final decision could be made about possible organic pathology.

Ps. Invol. Melan. F:57:M:8 —6 8231'4679–(41) 8:7:13
Paranoid

The admission complaints for this woman were depression and marked feelings of jealousy directed toward her husband. For two years, the patient said, she had the feeling that she and her husband were drifting apart. When they were together she believed he stared at younger women "more than was proper," and she misinterpreted minor incidents and relationships with other women. As a result of one of these misinterpretations she felt as if "a sharp knife had pierced my abdomen and I had a feeling of fear which I could not explain." She was unable to eat because of "strange feelings in my stomach," and her weight dropped from 137 to 90 pounds. Placed in a private hospital, she was given six electroshock treatments. These helped her and she was discharged, but the symptoms recurred before long. When her husband left for his office in the morning, she was frequently obsessed by questions such as these: "Where is my husband going? What is he saying to that girl?" At night she picked quarrels with him accusing him of infidelities. When the patient learned that her husband had signed the permit for electroshock therapy, she became really upset.

Ten years earlier the patient had experienced an artificial menopause, apparently with the deliberate intent of avoiding the difficulties of the natural menopause period. Following this she had lost all sexual desire.

After two years of college she worked as a teacher and as a telephone operator until her marriage. She was active in club work and was considered an authority on antiques. Before her marriage she had been highly independent, had worked her way through school, and in other ways had expressed forcefulness and self-sufficiency. A rigid person, she tended to be domineering except toward her husband, who usually made the family decisions. She seemed to be frustrated by this and unable to handle the hostility she felt toward him.

In the hospital the patient appeared to be composed and almost cheerful part of the time, but occasionally she cried and beat the bed with her fist. Aware of the unreality of her husband's "unfaithfulness," yet she was unable to rid herself of her jealousy and suspicion. There was a marked hostility toward him, and she repeated frequently, "Oh, how I've suffered. He should be suffering instead of me. He is the cause of all my troubles." Others of her emotional difficulties, she believed, were due to an endocrine imbalance. The first two nights in the hospital she caused a considerable disturbance because of crying and loud claims that "nothing is being done for me." As days went by she showed some improvement but no appreciable insight. She rejected psychotherapy as fruitless and requested to be discharged so that she might attend a "clinic" in another state. The marked rigidity of her personality and her rejection of the various plans to help her made treatment difficult, and against advice she was discharged.

B. Psth., Mixed M:24:S:43 +4 824 173′96–(63) 2:11:18
Suicidal

This young man was admitted because of depression, personality changes, and attempts at suicide. These symptoms appeared two months earlier when the patient became nervous and unable to sleep at night but was exhausted in the daytime. Dropping out of college, he began to date a different girl each night and to drink heavily. He offered to marry a girl who was pregnant. During the last week before admission he made several feeble attempts at suicide, for example, drinking "nervine" and slashing his wrists. It was his own decision to come to the hospital, for he felt he needed psychiatric care.

The past medical history indicated that he was a forceps delivery, which had resulted in a deformed head and cyanosis immediately after his birth. Two years before admission he spent fourteen months in the hospital with poliomyelitis that left an almost total paralysis of his left leg and weakness in his right leg.

Until the age of 18 he planned to study medicine, then he decided to become a minister. In the draft he registered as a conscientious objector. He was in his senior year when the present illness developed. Known as a secretive, self-reliant, introspective, hypochondriacal person, he first showed an obvious interest in girls about a year before admission. He never seemed to feel a need for sympathy. He had held jobs but had always resented turning money over to his parents. His circle of friends was large.

On admission he was physically normal. In addition to the paralysis, there were cuts on his left arm, superficial in nature. In mental content he showed an excessive interest in women. He worried about masturbation and wanted to commit suicide to escape reality. His deformed leg caused him worry also. He had lost all interest in religion. Tests revealed an I.Q. above 130. Although apathetic, he appeared relatively normal except for his symptoms, was attentive and interested, and showed appropriate affect. Most of the time he seemed exhausted. His cooperation with the routine was poor, he was rebellious, and he flirted with the nurses. Much of his behavior was infantile and seemed to fit with the diagnostic concept of a psychopathic personality. After he lost some of the more obvious symptoms he was discharged with the note that his threats of suicide appeared more rebellious than genuine. It was recommended that he return to college under psychiatric guidance. About one year later he committed suicide.

Ps. Sz., Mixed Paranoid   M:23:S:16   +1   82467'3–X (49)   5:17:8

The family of this patient noted the onset of his illness about a year and a half before admission when he began to be introspective and to daydream with such intensity that he could hardly be drawn out of it. He neglected his personal appearance and in general changed markedly from his usual personality. He was hospitalized and diagnosed as having schizophrenia, probably paranoid. Given both insulin and electroshock therapy, he "improved, developed insight, socialized well with other patients, and was discharged." Two months before the present admission he showed signs of a relapse, again developing the same general pattern.

He had been born with a harelip and a cleft palate, which were repaired by the time he was 27 months old. There was, however, a residual slurring of speech. He was average in intelligence, and his school progress was satisfactory. He was social and interested in sports and did not have any noticeable personality defects. There was a suspicion that he had engaged in minor thievery. His parents said that some children had made fun of him because of his facial scars; he had never had dates with girls. The family was a happy one, and his older brothers had usually taken him with them, probably to protect him from other children.

In the hospital he was primarily concerned with getting out and going home. There were no obvious delusional tendencies and no evidences of hallucinations.

His sensorium and intellect were intact. The main symptom was a flattening of affect and an unwillingness to carry on conversation. He had an uneventful hospital stay, gradually working into ward activities. Before long there were no signs of withdrawal or other evidences of abnormality. He repeatedly said that he was eager to be discharged and to return home. The only complaint that persisted was an occipital headache. Although at the time of discharge he appeared recovered it was felt that the recovery was more apparent than real, probably a result of the simple hospital routine to which he could adjust. It was recommended that his family attempt to shield him by getting him into simple work activities and protecting him from unusual pressures.

Ps. M-D., Depr.	F:36:M:76	+2	8′26137–9 (39)	8:3:19
		+19	78′6239– (61)	4:4:9

According to her husband, the patient's first abnormal behavior occurred about three months before admission, when, as she was seated with her family, she suddenly cried out, "I am going to die! I'm going to die!" Then she began to cry. The local physician advised medicine for tachycardia and anemia, but these medications did not help. On several occasions she said, "I can't have any more children." She had been concerned with this idea from the time of the birth of her third child, although there was no basis for it; she already had nine children ranging in age from 10 months to 16 years. Tense and worried, she apparently feared some impending disaster. "Maybe God is going to punish me," she said. Much of her attention was centered around her heart, even though extensive studies failed to reveal any pathology. She began to suspect her neighbors of interfering with her children and she interpreted trivial incidents as having portent for her future.

The past medical history showed little of consequence. The patient finished a business college training course without difficulty and worked as a stenographer for a year before her marriage. Of average intelligence, she was considered to have good judgment and to be efficient in working and planning. She was interested in her social life, home, and friends, but she had no intimate personal contacts. Very seldom did she complain and she appeared to keep her worries to herself. She was devoutly religious, increasingly so just before admission. The couple had tried a number of methods of birth control but had abandoned each one because of the husband's objection to the nuisance. She felt bitter toward him for not helping to limit the family, especially since his salary was hardly sufficient to meet their needs.

On admission the patient appeared wholly normal, but as she became less on guard in the new surroundings, she expressed many grossly abnormal ideas. She believed that she was in the hospital to be punished for not having been a good mother and that the staff was to decide whether or not she should die. She felt she was discriminated against because of her religion. On the other hand she was well oriented after the first few days and her general intellectual abilities and sensorium seemed unaffected. At all times she appeared dejected and unhappy and she cried frequently. She could never accept the idea that she was emotionally ill. There was a definite psychomotor retardation, and at all times she reacted with distrust and suspicion. Treated with electroshock therapy, she at first made a fairly rapid recovery, but after the third week this initial gain was lost and there was little change in her behavior. At the time of the final discharge she was to try living at home for a while.

Ps. Invol. Melan. F:51:S:57 +32 8261′7349– 7:12:14

Apparently the patient was fairly well adjusted until two years before admission when her mother died of cancer. After that event she became extremely irritable, grew emotionally labile, and was usually depressed. Her interest in church and social activities disappeared. When she discovered an area of irritation under her lower dentures, which she believed to be cancer, she became progressively more agitated, pacing the floor by day and lying awake at night. Before the present illness she had been in excellent health.

After receiving an eighth-grade education she had helped her parents with farm work until she was 23, and since then, with the exception of a brief interval as a hotel cook, she had worked as cook and housekeeper for five bachelor brothers. An independent person, she had never confided in anyone and had never had many friends, preferring to remain by herself. Her ethical code was exceedingly high. Men had never found her very attractive and she gave as her reason for being single the fact that no man had ever asked her to marry him. For two years before her mother's death the patient had been unable to leave the house because of her responsibilities to the invalid.

On admission she appeared much older than her 51 years. Her blood pressure was somewhat elevated, and she had a bromide rash; in addition, moderate arteriosclerosis was present. Except for these findings, there was nothing helpful in the general physical and neurological examination. Although otherwise she was entirely intact mentally, she had a fixed, unsystematized delusion that cancer permeated her entire system, and she attributed her weakness, peculiar pain, and other complaints to "poisoning in my system." No amount of persuasion or reassurance could convince her that she did not have cancer, and she was resigned to the fact that she was dying. At times she became agitated and restless, picking at her clothes and face, and appearing generally uncomfortable. With further observation and study it became apparent that the depression and agitation were basically more significant than the cancer phobia. She was given endocrine therapy and a general physical build-up program, but since therapy could not be very effective because of the fixity of the delusional ideas, she was discharged with the advice that she go to a state hospital.

Ps. Invol. Melan.	F:55:M:22	+1	826′3714–(47)	7:8:12
Ps. Sz., Paranoid				
Deteriorated				

About four months before admission the patient began having headaches and nightmares and became apprehensive. She received medical attention but did not improve and developed paranoid ideas toward the physician. She had spells in which she reverted to her native language and visualized friends she had not seen for years, at the same time not recognizing her close present friends. Paranoid delusions about her common-law husband also appeared. Occasionally she was incontinent of urine and was obviously disoriented.

At one time she had had syphilis, which she had contracted from her first husband. This had apparently been cured. Otherwise she had been physically healthy. The patient was in the fifth grade when she left school. Since then her only occupation was domestic work. She was of low normal intelligence and in many ways backward. Her husband "always took care of everything." Socially she got along well and was moderately active. A sensitive person, she was often hurt by the actions of her husband. Any tendency to aggression apparently was inhibited by feelings of inferiority and general passivity. She was known as being "quick to forgive," fond of sympathy, and moody. Her first husband was burned to death, an accident which she witnessed and which upset her deeply. Following this loss she stayed with her mother for two years, then began to live with a domineering and inconsiderate man who became her common-law husband. By her first husband she had fourteen pregnancies; four of these ended in miscarriages or resulted in children that died in infancy. One child died at age 17, possibly of congenital syphilis.

Except for a positive reaction to a Kline test there was no admission evidence to indicate an active syphilitic process. She appeared to have numerous scattered ideas, suggesting a flight of ideas. She had incoherent hallucinatory and delusory experiences of a general paranoid nature. She was perplexed and fearful, laughed and cried without provocation. She had little insight into her condition. Electroshock therapy brought little change and she was discharged to a state hospital.

Ps. M-D., Depr.	F:35:M:32	+1	$8\underline{267}43'1$–9X (47)	3:22:8
Schizoid		+31	′67–91 (47)	4:3:16
Suicidal				

This patient had been well until the birth of her first child about five months before admission, when she became apprehensive about her ability to care for the child adequately. Her attitude toward it then changed from meticulous care to carelessness. She developed the delusion that she had unalterably injured the child and that it was doomed to be a hopeless misfit as a result of her negligence. She had ideas of infanticide and suicide. She indulged in self-depreciation, feeling that she was stupid and incapable. Ideas of reference led her to think that everyone knew of her sin and that she had brought shame and scorn on everyone associated with her.

At school she had been a good student and had graduated from high school at age 15. She then took some business training and advanced her position until she held a supervisory job with a good salary. A shy, introverted child, she had always felt inferior because of her family background and, to a certain extent, because of her personal appearance. She had married a man she was temperamentally unsuited to, and she had not looked forward at all happily to the possibility of motherhood.

In the hospital she was concerned chiefly with the delusion that she had injured her child, and she was voluble with self-abuse. She believed she ought to be jailed and was doomed to eternal damnation. Well oriented, she was clear in sensorium and intellect. At first she was seclusive, crying frequently and staying by herself. With shock therapy she showed rapid improvement. At the time of discharge she was much better but there were still schizophrenic characteristics in her behavior that made the prognosis guarded.

Ps. Sz., Cat. F:41:S:85 +20 8269′71<u>43</u>– 1:14:5

For two months this patient had been ill with depression, agitation, crying spells, fever, insomnia, and bizarre delusions. The first evidence of difficulties had appeared when there was a sudden decrease in the amount of food she ate. Several days later she had an unprovoked crying spell and refused to talk, but she finally went to work. That evening at home she suddenly became agitated, paced the floor, screamed, and cried; then she ceased talking altogether and became rigid. The family physician prescribed sedatives, but when she again became agitated she was placed in a private hospital for three weeks. When she went home again, the pattern was repeated and she returned to the same hospital, this time for two weeks. There she was overactive and developed some fever. Given medication, she did not improve and, finally, was referred to the psychopathic hospital.

Eleven years earlier the patient had suffered a "nervous breakdown," characterized by a refusal to talk, rejection of food, rigidity, visual hallucinations, crying spells, and fears. This episode apparently had been precipitated by her attempt to leave home. That illness had lasted six months. In school the patient had done fairly well and had finished the eighth grade. Next she had done housework and later she had been employed in a factory. This factory work, which was on the skilled level, was satisfying to her. She lived with her father in a rented house, sharing expenses. Her mother was dead. If the patient had ever expressed ambition to change her mode of life, it was not known. Always "self-conscious" and feeling that her friends were not interested in her, she stayed at home a great deal. She was meticulous about her housework. Not only had she never had men friends but she had expressed no interest in them.

On admission the patient was full of delusions of sin and guilt. For example, she saw stains on her bedding and wondered if she might have contracted a venereal disease. Later she worried that she had injured herself seriously in the past and thereby upset her mind. She protested frequently and spontaneously that she was clean in mind and body. She questioned the sincerity of her friends. Many of her statements were accompanied by peculiar facial grimaces and motions. Often she refused to answer questions and struck odd postures. She was always well oriented, and her memory was good. Never assaultive or destructive, she was cooperative. With five electroshock treatments she improved somewhat and the treatments were stopped. She then became more depressed and more agitated. Five more treatments were given and again she improved. She remained irritable, however, was profane and obscene in language, and refused to leave the disturbed ward. A very direct and outspoken interview with her was followed by improvement; apparently this talk had also shown to her satisfaction why her hospitalization had been necessary. At the time of discharge she was still emotionally unstable and appeared tense and self-conscious. It was recommended that state hospitalization be considered because of the serious possibility of a relapse or recurrence.

B. Psth., Mixed M:22:S:126 +6 82713'694– 3:11:7
P. Mixed
Deteriorated

Four years before admission the patient had suddenly had a series of convulsions, losing consciousness during each. He had been studied in a general hospital, where a diagnosis of subarachnoid hemorrhage had been made. Apparently he had been delirious for a time and aphasic. After recovery a visual field defect persisted. He was first seen in the outpatient neurology service three years before admission and the only remaining symptom at that time was the visual defect. He was again seen in the outpatient clinic four months before admission, when he complained of pain in his eyes, impaired visual acuity, and a number of other somatic disturbances.

The patient had never been in good health, although there was no history of any clearly identifiable illness. "Leakage of the heart" was typical of the disorders he was alleged to have experienced. A high school graduate and a good student, he did stenographic work and was employed at various clerical jobs. He was stubborn and irritable, and he avoided crowds because he was ill at ease among others. He was not robust or athletic and did not have many friends his own age.

In the hospital the patient's attention centered principally around his physical complaints, which he described in great detail. He also hinted that some special problem was on his mind but at first he would not discuss it. After a while he confessed that he was worried because he had been masturbating almost daily and considered this an evil habit. He had also had a long-standing urge to have sexual contact with young boys or girls. He wondered if others might not have become aware of these ideas. He showed an inclination to misinterpret casual occurrences, although it could not be said that he had frankly paranoid ideas of reference. There was no gross disturbance of his personality.

He was querulous and frequently disagreeable, becoming angry over trifling matters. He was extremely fussy. He did not mix freely with other patients, and his chief amusement was in playing the piano. Reassurance about his somatic complaints did not lessen them. His obsessions about sex also did not respond to reassurance. He confessed that he had had the urge to swallow his semen or particles of feces. There was a possibility that he had a tumor on the brain and finally the left parietal and occipital regions were explored surgically. No evidence of a tumor or a clear-cut abnormality was disclosed by this procedure although the cortex was not uncovered. In general he became better adjusted to the hospital routine and apparently would have stayed longer if the staff had permitted it. No real understanding of his condition was gained by the staff, and though he was more comfortable at discharge he was really little changed.

P. Mixed F:25:M:224 +10 82714369′–X(41) 4:21:9

This young woman's presenting complaints were "nervous spells," chronic anxiety associated with almost daily episodes of choking, palpitation, and the like for three to five years, and a feeling of repulsion for sexual relationships with her husband. Her first "spell" occurred a year before admission. At that time her husband found her lying on the floor crying. When he spoke to her she did not recognize him and was apparently disoriented. She mistook him for her previous husband and thought he had come to take their son away from her. In subsequent spells the patient also misinterpreted the environment and re-enacted memories, usually unpleasant childhood scenes. She had no recollection of these spells afterward.

The patient's father died before her birth, and because her mother could not afford to keep the child, she was placed in an orphanage at the age of 4. After her mother's death, when the patient was 5, she was taken from the orphanage by her legal guardian and placed in a series of foster homes. The longest placement up to the age of 10 was for two years with a strict couple, whom the patient disliked. From age 10 to age 15 she lived with her guardian and worked for her. At the death of the guardian she roamed about for a year and then married. This early marriage soon ended because she could not stand living with her husband's family. Following the divorce she was promiscuous for a short period but did not enjoy it, felt disgusted with herself, and suddenly stopped. Later she felt exceedingly guilty. The patient later married a second time, not because she loved the man but because she "did not want to disappoint him." The patient regarded herself as a person who always gave in to others, lacked self-confidence, felt inferior, could not do anything properly, never "looked good," and was often eyed critically by others.

When admitted to the hospital the patient was an attractive, bewildered-looking girl. Although fully cooperative, she was depressed and showed little spontaneity. Her conversation consisted mostly of responses to questions and she showed no evidence of having any insight. The patient was seen twice weekly in psychotherapeutic interviews and encouraged to join in all the ward activities. She expressed a fear of sharp things but otherwise she fit into the ward routine well. During one of her "spells," in which she misinterpreted the situation as a threatening one and misidentified all the people around her, her therapist was called and brought her out of it by the use of strong suggestion. Fully oriented again, she denied any memory of the incident. Her behavior in interviews was characterized by passivity, and she conveyed a feeling of helplessness. The therapist felt obliged to make active attempts to help her, only to be constantly frustrated by gaps in the patient's memory of experiences and feelings.

There was a gradual improvement during her stay in the hospital, and just before going home she seemed more interested in making the best of her marriage. However, she still had little or no insight. The staff felt the patient was an immature, poorly integrated person who at times probably "dipped into and out of psychosis." After leaving the hospital she was seen a few times over a four-month period for supportive therapy. There was no further change in her condition but she continued to feel somewhat better than before hospitalization and was no longer troubled by "spells" of dissociated behavior. E. B.

Ps. M-D., Mixed F:41:S:101 +28 8273641′– 4:13:13

Many years before admission, the patient had suffered a "nervous breakdown" of short duration as a result of learning that her favorite brother had tuberculosis. During the following year she had spent all her money and time in taking care of the brother. After his death the patient's mother had had an emotional upset, and for the next nine years the woman had devoted herself to her mother, a demanding person who required the patient to be at home most of the time. Eventually both the patient and her mother had been committed to a state hospital, where the mother had died a year after commitment. Released on parole, the patient had continued to be depressed, nervous, agitated, and worried, and because of the persistence of these symptoms she was admitted to this hospital for psychiatric study. At one time she was found to have tuberculosis, but after considerable study it was decided that the lesions were inactive.

She had never been strong and had had numerous colds in addition to nearly all the usual childhood illnesses. A high school graduate, she had been the class valedictorian. For several years she had taught school but had had to stop teaching to take care of her family. She had always worked hard, but before the onset of the present episode she had had outside interests and had made an adequate social adjustment. There was very little money in the home, and the patient had resented the fact that she and her brothers had been given inadequate opportunities after her father bought a farm on which they had had to live. Very early she had been described as being "a bundle of nerves, eccentric, and overscrupulous."

In the hospital she talked mostly about her worries and the unpleasantness of her past—for example, the hardship of walking long distances. Her constant complaint was that because of her past hardships she was suffering unbearable mental torture that she did not deserve. She had no delusions or hallucinations. Although she appeared depressed, she was well oriented and intact intellectually. At times she was agitated and paced the floor, wringing her hands. Her answers to questions were logical and to the point, but she always brought every conversation back to her early life. She cooperated only under great pressure and changed very little in the hospital, finally being discharged to a rest home.

Ps. Sz., Simple M:17:S:66 +10 827'4– 5:9:15

The onset of this boy's illness dated back five years to an appendectomy. Given several enemas before and after the surgery, he developed a fear of these. Once he lied to a nurse, claiming that a bowel movement had taken place although this was not so. Since that time he had been constipated, bowel movements occurring only every second or third day. He sometimes felt as if he were "filling up inside," he said. A year before admission the boy's teachers noticed that he was studying a great deal more than usual, yet appeared to be learning less. When invited to play games or to attend movies he said, "I have to study." Several times he expressed the idea that he "might go insane." Twice he ran away, returning in a few days; finally he refused to attend classes because, he said, "I'm not learning anything."

All this time the boy was living in a state school because his mother was in a state hospital and his father had been adjudged incompetent. His grades were slightly below average, even before the present illness. The head of the school described him as quiet, mild-mannered, diligent, and meticulous about his work and his appearance. Well liked, he mixed with other students but never made close or intimate friends. When angered he would become sullen and withdrawn. He was never a disciplinary problem and was well behaved. Boxing was his main sports interest.

On admission the boy said that he saw "inhuman, ugly creatures at the end of the hall." He made it clear that these did not bother him, nor did they talk, "they just walk up and down." Otherwise his sensorium and orientation appeared clear. His tested I.Q. was 85, but there was a considerable scatter in the intelligence test data. He was apathetic. Although he had some insight into the possibility that he was mentally ill, he believed that the illness was largely due to constipation. He spoke very little and then only when prodded, was slovenly in appearance, and had a fixed, evasive manner. At first he was dissatisfied with the hospital routine, but as time went on he made a few acquaintances and showed more friendliness. Most of the time, however, he kept to himself. During the last few days of the hospitalization the patient suddenly lost most of the gains made and again became apathetic and asocial, withdrawing from ward life, sitting in his room, and appearing to brood about his condition. When questioned he would reply, "Why don't they let me out of here? They don't know what's wrong with me and they don't give me any treatment." He thought heavy labor outdoors would cure him. He was finally transferred to a state hospital, having improved little.

P. Mixed	F:26:M:45	+2	8274631′-(47)	3:11:12
Schizoid		—108	8247163′-(47)	2:11:9

Six years before admission, at the time the patient had her first child, she was attracted to the attending physician and on two occasions after the child's birth she had sexual relations with him. As a result of the experience she gradually developed guilt feelings, and although she suppressed them, she suffered from insomnia and became increasingly nervous and tense. About a year and a half later she decided that something her husband was discussing at a family gathering had to do with her condition, and as the conviction that she was actually losing her mind swept over her, she suddenly felt pressure and tingling sensations in her head, palpitation, and tachycardia. Shortly after that she told her husband about her affair with the physician, and although he apparently forgave her, her symptoms became progressively more acute. Her obsession with the idea that she was insane grew to the point where she thought people were comparing her with her mother, who had been in a mental hospital. She had constant fights with her husband, and she grew so negligent of her domestic duties that he finally sent their son to live with his mother and the patient to live with her foster parents. Since that time he had made no effort to see her.

Since she had always done well in school, the patient would have attended college except for financial difficulties. During her school days she had always been well liked, but she had few social contacts after her graduation. From early childhood she had tended to withdraw from people, and she had always been sensitive and shy, as a child hiding in closets when visitors came to the house. She had always had a feeling of stigma because of her mother's illness. Her childhood had been spent among several sets of foster parents. Although it was her mother-in-law who had helped promote the patient's marriage, she also appeared to have been instrumental in arranging the separation of the patient and her husband and child.

On admission she made constant reference to her vague symptomatology and to her feelings of guilt, insecurity, and depression. She frequently expressed the fear that she would go insane as her mother had, and she said people still compared her to her mother. Although her I.Q. was 128 and she was mentally clear, her insight was poor. She clung to the idea that she had had a serious nervous "breakdown" and that, without special treatments to cure it, she would go insane. Although she enjoyed occupational therapy she was shy and withdrawn in activities with other patients. During the hospitalization her somatic symptoms improved but they were always with her. Four electroshock treatments produced no appreciable change, although she finally did show an interest in making plans for her future, and simple reassurance was enough to convince her that she would be able to work again and possibly become independent. She was improved on discharge and was to be followed in the outpatient department.

Ps. Sz., Cat.	M:23:S:33	+6	$8\underline{27}4\underline{6'3}\ \underline{19}-$	4:11:9
Suicidal				

Four months before admission the patient had developed symptoms of withdrawal, dissatisfaction with his work, and marked anxiety, after being unjustly accused of spreading a rumor that friends of his had stolen some beer. In consequence, he was more or less shunned by many members of the community, and his reaction had been to lose interest in his work, to become dissatisfied with farm life, and to grow markedly preoccupied. Two days before admission he had suddenly expressed fears of death due to heart trouble and had been taken to a general hospital; from there he was transferred to the psychiatric unit.

The early history was noncontributory. He had discontinued school at the eighth-grade level, and with the exception of a two-week period when he was employed by the highway department, he had worked on his father's farm, where he did his work well. He enjoyed being with people, showed a moderate interest in sports, and often went to community dances. He made friends impulsively but was somewhat sensitive in his relationships with others. He was easily discouraged. His immediate family showed a poor tolerance for excitement of any kind, and as a result of the patient's illness, his mother found it necessary to remain in bed most of the day.

On admission he believed that he was in danger of dying and that excessive worry about his life on the farm and his unattained ambitions was responsible for his heart trouble. His only hallucinatory experience was on an occasion when he "heard a strange voice." His orientation was intact, his general knowledge was good, and he was mentally unimpaired. Although he was unhappy, apprehensive, and pessimistic, he believed that help was available and that his case was not hopeless. Accessive and cooperative, he frequently demanded reassurance that his heart condition would not be fatal. There was a vagueness and a lack of logic in the picture that he presented of himself. At one time there was an increase in his preoccupation, lack of interest, and feelings of inferiority and self-pity. Once he developed a mild panic state, during which he insisted that his parents be called. He complained of severe weakness, insisted that his brain was getting foggy, and said, "I don't want my parents to think they failed me."

When his anxiety, unrestrained behavior, and regressive playfulness became uncontrollable, it was necessary to put him in a disturbed ward. There, under faradic treatments he improved somewhat. Later, however, he attempted suicide by choking himself with a towel. His trends became more bizarre, and he insisted that he was the devil and not human. There were other less severe suicidal attempts. Since he was not improving it was recommended that he be transferred to a state hospital, but his father insisted on taking him home for at least a few days.

Ps. Sz., Paranoid	M:32:M:103	+1	$827\underline{631}'4-(67)$	3:13:13
Suicidal		+99	$2'\underline{1783}4-9\,(63)$	4:6:22

The patient came into the hospital with the complaint of hearing voices for the last year and a half. In spite of the voices he had managed to continue working for some time but recently had found it more difficult and had been asked to resign. The voices carried on endless conversations among themselves, as well as addressing remarks directly to the patient. Typical of the remarks made by them were these: "You're not as bad off as you think you are" and "You're a poor kid." They adjusted comments to the circumstances, giving a running commentary on all that the patient did and saw. He felt that the voices could read his mind and that they had been "put there as part of some treatment a psychiatrist arranged." Also disturbing to him was a chronic "faraway feeling."

The patient's father, a professional man, was described as "kind but preoccupied" and highly successful. The father had developed an ulcer and had blamed it on the worry caused by his son's difficulties. His mother was also described as kind but very strict, old-fashioned, and nervous. She dominated and overprotected the patient. Both parents were ambitious for him and a high premium was placed on education and position. The patient showed fears in early childhood and signs of a further disturbance were evident at the age of 13. Taken abroad by his parents he was overly anxious and perfectionistic in adopting the language of the country where he attended school for a year. Later he returned to the United States to finish high school and college. Never a good mixer, he continually longed to go abroad again. The "faraway feeling" first occurred at the age of 15, the morning after his first experience with masturbation. His schoolmates told him he acted as if he were in a daze. He returned to Europe for postgraduate work and there met his future wife. When he came back to the United States he worked hard, seven days a week, and studied on the side. One of the several physicians he consulted for the "faraway feeling" told him that he had schizophrenia. Until the present illness he and his wife had had a happy marriage and he had held jobs compatible with his superior intellectual level.

In the hospital the patient was found to be a large, soft-spoken man, with a blank, staring expression. His voice had a flat, unresonant quality, which added to the impression he gave of passivity, resignation, and distance. He was cooperative and deferential toward the examiner and seemed concerned about his symptoms and about whether he might be thought to be a homosexual. However, he had no insight, believed his voices were real, and invented vague and illogical explanations for their existence. He was seen in frequent psychotherapeutic interviews but these were felt to be unsuccessful in helping the patient to deal with his disturbing thought content. Preoccupied on the ward, he was seclusive and given to outbursts of self-accusations and anxiety. He made frequent suicide threats and attempted to slash his throat. After insulin treatment his paranoid trends became more marked and his contact with reality more tenuous. Concomitant electroshock therapy was tried. Following two of these combined treatments he stated that he no longer heard the voices. This type of treatment was discontinued when he expressed the fear that a homosexual assault had been made upon him while he was unconscious under shock.

A course of fifty insulin comas was finished. The second MMPI was administered five days after the last coma. The patient said that he felt better and wished to leave the hospital and resume work; his wife was eager to have him home again. The staff felt that there had been no fundamental improvement but that he might be able to adjust to the outside world on a highly schizoid level. Seen for a follow-up study a year later, he appeared dull and a little suspicious and reported that he was still not able to work or to study in any profitable way. E. B.

B. Psth., Mixed M:34:M:39 +4 8279'641– 7:13:7
P. Hypo. +29 2178'639– 3:5:11
P. Hys.

Four years before admission the patient had complained of paresthesia involving the lower extremities. After an attack of syncope that followed these symptoms he underwent a thorough study at a clinic. Because he was a house painter by profession, an extensive investigation was made for evidence of lead poisoning, but there were no positive findings. After the patient left the clinic the symptoms continued and, to complicate the picture, depression and irritability developed, with gradually mounting insomnia. He had not worked for the four years.

At the end of the second year in high school, the patient went to work in order to help his mother support the family. He had been a painter for thirteen years before the present illness. Of low ambition and energy always, he had feelings of inadequacy and was shy and easily discouraged. Lacking any interest in sports, he preferred to read. As a child he was closely attached to his mother, feared and disliked his father. His wife, who was four years older than he, was intelligent and aggressive and assumed full charge of the family affairs. The couple appeared compatible. There were no children.

In the hospital, as at the clinic, no evidence for lead poisoning was discovered. The patient, however, believed that a diagnosis of lead poisoning had been made in the previous clinic study. His wife had been shown an X-ray, he said, and "there was a puddle or clot of lead right in the base of the brain." According to his story, his wife had been told that the doctors were trying to "dissolve that lead." He said that he had been unable to work and had constantly reproached himself for "sponging" on his wife. Convinced of his worthlessness, he said, "I am the biggest loafer in my town." His speech was slow and deliberate, and he showed considerable circumstantiality in his sequence of thought. There were no gross defects of sensorium or intellect, however, and he was eager to please and cooperate around the ward. Much urging, however, was necessary before he would make contacts with other patients, and he was subject to spells of crying, especially in front of visitors from his home town. During hospitalization he became much better and was encouraged to return home and try to resume work. Plans were made to help the patient change jobs.

P. Hys. M:56:S:45 +1 '831247–(63) 3:7:21

The patient was in good health until six months before admission when he began to experience sudden feelings of pressure in the lower cervical region, followed by generalized muscle weakness and "pressure." The attacks lasted for just a few seconds, but they became progressively worse and the weakness was eventually so severe that he would fall to the ground during an attack. He never lost consciousness and was aware of what went on around him during the spells, although he had trouble speaking. He was sometimes able to "shake off" the weakness by sitting down to rest but more often he sank to the ground, lying there for one or two minutes until the weakness left. The attacks never occurred while he was in a reclining position and there was no pain connected with them.

Except for these attacks, his general health and physical condition had been unusually good. There had been no previous psychotic or obviously neurotic upsets. He made normal progress in school through the eighth grade and then left both school and home because he could not get along with his mother, who was more stubborn and headstrong than he was. He became an itinerant farm hand and traveled around the country for 23 years, making only enough money to care for himself. Several times he returned to his mother's farm and stayed for a few months but he never offered any financial help or assisted her in any way. He was of average intelligence but lazy, and he said he lived only for the present. He had few outside interests and was secretive, stubborn, and irritable about anything that required his attention. Because of these traits he had few friends.

In the hospital he was chiefly concerned about his illness, saying that he was eager to get well and go back to work. There was no gross disturbance in his mental content. He was well oriented and appeared intact in intellect. He was mildly depressed, though this was apparently superficial. He had no insight and tended to be reticent about his past and about what he was thinking. He was somewhat dull and restless and spent most of his time lying in bed or reading. He showed little change in the hospital, remaining stubborn and irritable. It was felt that the present illness might be related to his insecurity about the future. No neurological findings appeared and there were no attacks during his stay in the hospital.

P. Psychas. M:31:S 837164'2–X (73) 4:16:18
P. Anxiety State

This soldier asked for help, complaining of irritability, extreme agitation, and general nervousness. He was constantly fatigued. Doctors had labeled vague pains in his legs "arthritis." At the time contact was first made with him, his unit was being combed for men qualified for overseas duty.

Both his parents were foreign-born and had seemingly made a good adjustment. The patient was the youngest of a closely knit sibship of five. The only significant neurotic traits in his childhood were severe temper tantrums and somnambulism, which lasted until he was 12 years of age. Above average in intelligence, the patient had made a fair record in school and had finished one year of college. A competent clerical worker, he was rated as steady and diligent by his employers. Socially he was considered to be a good mixer.

8'372164–X

A swarthy man with numerous blinking and shrugging tics, he was restless and overtalkative during interviews and at times his emotional reactions were quite inappropriate to his thought content. It was felt that he was a neurotic person who had made a fairly good adjustment throughout his life, but who presented in his prominent muscular tics signs of impending "emotional decompensation." He was disqualified for overseas duty. With sporadic psychotherapeutic interviews, he was able to make an adjustment until his discharge to civilian status. A. T. K.

Ps. Sz., Cat.	F:30:M:49	+37	8'372164–X(57)	10:15:17
Twin				
Ps. Sz., Cat.	F:30:M:22			

This woman was admitted because of mutism, posturizing, gross hallucinatory and delusional ideas, and echopraxia. The patient, an identical twin, had been hospitalized four years before the present difficulty at the same time that her twin sister was emotionally ill. Both received shock therapy and made good recoveries. The patient remained well until she received a telegram informing her that her sister had again become disturbed and had been hospitalized. At this news the patient became apprehensive of her own condition and began to complain of anorexia and insomnia. The condition grew worse. One week before admission she remarked to her husband, "Take me some place before I lose my mind," and she developed fears of hurting someone. Then the admission complaints appeared.

With the exception of their illnesses four years earlier, which were similar to the present ones, the twins had experienced no particular difficulties. They attended the same schools and graduated from the same university. Both earned excellent grades. They secured jobs and lived together until they became ill. After that the patient married a man who was a Catholic, adopted his religion, and became active in church work. Her twin was also married. At the time of the patient's admission her sister was recovering from her second illness.

In the hospital the physical and neurological examinations were essentially negative. The patient was accessible for only brief periods; usually she was mute and sat in the same position for hours. She was actively hallucinatory and her utterances were bizarre. For example, she said, "There's an earthquake out there. Just a minute and I'll go out and let the log in." Her speech was incoherent and irrelevant. After electroshock treatments, she improved rapidly and began to show interest in ward activities and to gain some insight into her illness. At the time of discharge she was well along the way toward recovery but the prognosis was felt to be poor. She was readmitted nine days later, having almost completely regressed. She was given more shock therapy and further psychotherapy. When discharged for the second time, she had a good contact with reality and had developed fairly adequate insight into her difficulties.

P. Hys. M:33:M:60 +17 '83 91–X(47) 13:3:23

This man fell from a tree while at work. He was away from work for six weeks but received no hospital treatment. Since then he had suffered from severe headaches, each lasting several days. He complained of "pressure" on the left side of his head, the side on which he fell. About a year later he had hallucinations, seeing "children playing" and the like. He neglected his appearance and behaved in a strange manner. He was certified and entered the hospital in the present admission. Improved, he left two months later. Two years later he was readmitted as a voluntary patient.

He was the second of three children and left school at 15 to become a quarryman. Later he worked for the general post office and was promoted to a linesman.

He was diagnosed as having hysteria, conversion, and in addition to the usual routine physical examination, he was subjected to a thorough neurological examination. The report of this said, "The evidence is conclusive, there is no organic intracranial condition and one must assume that his symptoms are of psychological origin." M. V.

B. Psth., Path. Emot. F:15:S:15 +1 '84–2(61) 3:1:24

For the past two years this girl had had severe and uncontrollable temper tantrums. The tantrums were precipitated by situations in which she was not allowed to have her own way. Her attendance at school became irregular and she did not get along with her teachers. The tantrums, however, were confined to her home and directed at her mother, whom on several occasions she threatened to kill. The patient was taken out of school and a job was obtained for her, but she stayed on it for only a short time, and it was finally necessary to take her to juvenile court, from which she was remanded to the psychiatric unit for study.

There were no previous episodes of psychological or physical disturbance that seemed contributory. The girl had apparently led a normal social life until the onset of the symptoms, although she had had few friends. She had completed the tenth grade and until the last two years had done well in school. Known as a daydreamer, selfish, and not altogether truthful, she was also "spoiled," according to her older sister. Her parents were separated. Her father was an undesirable person, and her mother, while more responsible, was nervous.

On admission the patient was grossly normal, although she said she had a dominant thought which she would not express. No one was able to find out what she meant by this. Except for the tantrums she was emotionally controlled. She completely lacked insight into her problems. Neat in appearance, she was fairly pleasant most of the time, and she adjusted well although she responded slowly to orders. The staff always had a feeling that she either was not telling the truth or was evading certain issues. She did not get along well with the nurses and resented their corrections of her behavior. She expressed a profound hatred for her mother while under sodium amytal, but this set of attitudes could not be discussed with her. Finally she was discharged to live with a sister. The staff felt that if the next five or ten years could be bridged, she would probably get along fairly well. No real progress was made in understanding this patient.

Ps. Sz., Paranoid   M:19:S:87   +20   8′4172–   4:5:22

The illness of this young man appeared suddenly two months before admission when one day he accused his parents of being "out to get him." Later he had periods when he was in a trancelike state. "He sat motionless with eyes rolled inward or outward," according to his father. Partially recovered for a week or so, he then abruptly expressed the idea that a gang had a "bad influence" on him, controlling his speech and thought. One night he left home, announcing his intention to live with neighbors.

There was no known precipitating factor. The boy grew up on a farm and attended a country school. After one year of high school he left at age 15 to work on his parents' farm. Never considered shy or reticent, he had many friends, enjoyed sports, movies, and dancing, and played several musical instruments by ear. His friends and family had thought of him as stable emotionally, although he had always been somewhat overconcerned with body development, proper diet, and general physiological functions.

On the ward the patient was shy and at times withdrawn. For the most part he was conventional in appearance and behavior. He did not speak spontaneously. He had systematized vague delusions, such as, "I get kind of mixed up in my mind on account of dope. I guess they were jealous of me. I used to catch on faster than the other guys and now I'm slower. I haven't felt good for a couple of months. I look older than my years. I'm 19 as far as I know. Someone is trying to stagger my mind." During interviews he sat in an attitude of listening and, when questioned, insisted that the examiner must also have heard some messages in the Morse code about "something going on in another city." His thought was difficult to follow because of the lack of connecting phrases and also because of his extreme vagueness. His delusional systems changed but always contained the concept of forces acting upon him in a mysterious way. On one occasion he became panicky and was transferred to a disturbed section, where he became inaccessible, laughed inappropriately, and posturized. After that he gradually improved. Just before discharge he wanted the police called because, he said, "electric needles are being shot through my heart and my intestines are being squeezed." Such delusions and his other ideas were impervious to all approaches. He was discharged with the recommendation that he go to a state hospital.

P. Hys.   M:18:S:182   +18 $8\underline{42}76\underline{39}'1$–(53)   1:8:17
P. Mixed
Schizoid

This youthful patient's complaints, at the time he applied for outpatient psychotherapy, consisted of many fears and an inability to concentrate. He feared the dark, dogs, and heights; he was afraid that someone would break into the house at night and that he might become a homosexual. Enrolled in a business course at high school under the GI bill, he had been missing many days because of extreme restlessness and inability to concentrate. To relieve his worried feeling he took to drinking but feared that it was becoming a habit. During the war he had been overseas and had not adjusted well to army life. Depressed and homesick at one time, he requested to be locked up in a hospital because he felt he needed security. After his discharge he returned home to a disturbing family situation, and his fears and worries became even more acute.

Since early childhood the youth had always had various unreasonable fears and temper tantrums. He had a lifelong career of minor delinquencies, petty thievery, sex play, and traffic violations. After the seventh grade he did poor work in school. At that time the family moved from the country, where he was in a one-room school, to a city, where he attended a large junior high school. The gang activities among groups with different foreign backgrounds caused the patient much fear and he suffered a certain amount of bullying. This did not prevent him from making friends of both sexes, however, and he frequently went to shows and dances.

The patient was Catholic and observed all the rituals of the church carefully. He prayed compulsively. He was considered the black sheep of his family on his return from overseas, but the whole family was apparently disturbed and there was little family coherence. The patient described the family situation, when he was younger, as being dominated by his father, who "ruled his wife and children with an iron hand." However, at the time of the patient's application here, his parents' roles had been reversed, and his mother was said to browbeat his father. At this time his father was seen as a small, passive, ineffectual man, who felt his son to be a burden. It seemed fairly clear that the father was identified with the boy in his rebellion against the mother, and the father felt his wife's nagging was responsible for the boy's illness.

Weekly interviews were arranged for the patient, but half of the appointments scheduled were broken. When he did come he spent the hours giving dramatic accounts of his sins and symptoms, with voluble expressions of repentance. After breaking an appointment he would plead to be given another chance, saying he needed help desperately. At one point the case was closed after he failed to keep an appointment. Later he appeared and begged to be given one more chance. He gave fear of heights as his reason for not keeping his appointment, since it would have been necessary to drive across a high bridge and he lost his courage at the last minute. During the interval when he lost contact with the clinic he was arrested for drunken driving. After this arrest his probation officer urged him to renew contacts with the clinic.

A conference of several social agencies involved with this boy made it clear that the patient did considerable manipulating, using his needs and fears to persuade people to make special allowances for him, to pull strings, and to give him an endless number of last chances. A short time later the boy again failed to come for an appointment without notifying his therapist and the case was then closed in spite of the patient's further protestations. It was felt that although his problems were serious his motivation for help was insufficient for the clinic to justify continued work with him. E. B.

B. Psth., Path. Emot. M:32:D 8427'936–X(69) 2:21:8
Alcoholism

The patient had been a solitary drinker for periods over the sixteen years before the present interviews.

He came from a home where he was the favorite son of a nagging mother. A very large man, he had had good physical health. He was particularly resentful of the favoritism his father showed to the patient's older brother. There was a long history of jobs he had lost because of his aggressive behavior. In the air force his record was marred by numerous episodes when he was AWOL. He had had a very unsatisfactory marriage, apparently broken up because of his drinking.

Therapeutic work with this man was not satisfactory since he was extremely dependent, self-pitying, and unable to come to grips with his problems. He showed a great deal of childish resistance and an extraordinary degree of immaturity. Nearly everything he said was in the general category of rationalization. He stopped treatment after only seven interviews, spread over about four months. C. K. A.

P. Psychas. F:30:D:22 +2 8437'219–(53) 6:6:16
+28 78'42693–(49) 5:2:13

This woman came to the clinic because she had been having difficulty in a language class. She found that she was unable to join the group which sat at the front of the classroom and carried on a discussion in French, although she had had four years of the language in college and had come from an early environment in which French was spoken frequently. She got a feeling of panic every time the idea of her joining the group was suggested, and this caused her to lose sleep. Although she stated definitely that this was the only thing bothering her, it quickly became manifest that she was having trouble in making social contacts; she had the feeling that her friends were imposing on her from time to time and she was not able to identify herself with either the regular college students or the group of so-called "mature students." Although she would not admit it, she had definite feelings of loneliness and a desire for male companionship which frightened her. This caused her to feel some conflict because she had "avowed celibacy" for the rest of her life.

Since the woman was most secretive about much of her childhood, no adequate anamnesis could be obtained. It became apparent that the family situation was one of little friendliness and warmth, and that the present family relationships were uncomfortable due to differences of interest. She was intelligent (I.Q. 135) and had finished college with comparative ease. Then she taught at the grammar school level and, after several years of teaching, married an older man who had children by a previous marriage. The marriage was not successful. She felt that her husband had been very unfair in the demands he had made on her to assist him in his business. He treated the children in the same manner, and they had to work without remuneration. She felt that the children were too sensitive and that their father was stifling their growth by forcing them to participate in the business. She became pregnant but was encouraged by her husband to have an abortion. She had guilt feelings about this, and she began to believe that her husband had plotted this for his own ends—if she were to have a baby she could not assist him in his business. As this idea developed in her mind, the marital friction increased. She obtained a divorce and returned to school in order to work on an advanced degree.

During counseling the client was most defensive. She wanted an immediate solution for her problem, feeling there was little point in going into her background for causative factors. She could see no relationship between her early life, including her marriage, and her immediate problem. As therapy progressed this defensiveness increased rather than decreased, and, therefore, therapy was terminated by mutual consent because of a lack of progress. During the last session she said that the best solution to her problem would be retiring to intellectual and social isolation. Her plans were to dress in a drab fashion and to cultivate only such social liaisons as were necessary to carry on her professional activities. The therapist expressed doubt that she would find this a solution to her problem, and suggested quite an opposite approach. She rejected this idea, and the end of the hour was marked by near acrimony on her part. Thereafter, she averted her eyes whenever she saw the therapist. She did, however, take the final MMPI, returning it about a week later when the therapist was out of the office. Despite the feeling of the therapist that nothing had been accomplished, there was an improvement in the scores of the MMPI, and more marked improvement on another personality test she took. The Pt and Sc scores, however, remained almost unchanged.

She was not seen for about six months, and nothing was known of her activities during that time. Later the therapist met her accidentally and the change in her appearance was manifest. She was an attractive woman, dressed in such a way as to set off her charms to the best possible advantage. She greeted the therapist cordially but made no attempt to strike up a conversation. A comment made by a friend of hers indicated that she was obtaining some sexual outlet. It was felt that the rigid personality still existed and would be present until she had further therapy. A. S.

B. Pri., Child. M:13:S:30 +4 84639′712–(53) 3:13:11
B. Psth., Asocial

This boy was hospitalized when a probate judge recommended thorough study after he had made a violent scene in school. The incident began when he refused to do an assignment and was sent to the principal. Enraged and excited, he tried to fight his way out of the principal's office. In the ensuing melee the patient hit the principal, threw the furniture about, and threatened to jump out of the window. The incident occurred shortly after the patient's mother had gone to visit another son. At the same time his father, who lived alone, visited the home and bestowed gifts and attention on an older sister but had nothing for the patient.

A few months earlier the lad had had a bitter experience when a neighbor killed most of his pigeons, which he appeared really to love. Following the fight in school he was taken to the court by the police and later his mother threatened him with reform school. He replied that he would kill himself if that happened. At this time the judge recommended study in the psychiatric unit.

At various times in his life the boy had had temper tantrums in which he locked himself in his room for hours, raged, and cried. Moody and willful, he had never made friends and insisted on his own way always. His contention was that he "didn't care to have any friends." He did few chores and took no interest in sports or cooperative games. His school achievement was marginal and he was in the seventh grade when the present pattern of behavior appeared. The pigeons were all "that ever loved me," he said tearfully. Suspicious of adults, he was defensive in general. The lad was the ninth of ten children. Much conflict between the parents had ensued because of the mother's reluctance to bear so many children. When the patient was born his father, who preferred girls, had been disgusted. A year later, when the mother gave birth to another unwanted child, also a boy, the father left the home and from that time he supported them with only enough money to avoid being jailed. The patient disliked all his siblings. One older brother had committed suicide while in the army. In general, the other children appeared normal.

The boy was small but well developed. A likable lad, he often gave the impression that his aggressiveness was a false front and that he would really like to be friendly and warm. He was alert and his responses were rapid, but he became irritated at frustration. Of high average intelligence, he was logical and adequate in his thinking. In the hospital he was often moody, but for the most part he got along well with other patients and the nurses. On two occasions he refused to eat but abandoned that conduct when it brought him no attention. Once he precipitated a fight with his roommate, threw things, and when attendants intervened, bit one of them. It was difficult to work with him and no real contact could be made. After considerable study of the boy and his social environment, it was decided to discharge him to a foster home.

B. Psth., Asocial   M:16:S:13   +10   '84 67–13   3:5:10
Schizoid
Paranoid

About six weeks before admission the patient had twice struck a friend in the head with a hammer because the latter had "stolen" another friend from him. The patient said that he had been seeking revenge on this boy for about two months, and when he found his opportunity he had attacked from behind. The other boy had staggered but had succeeded in getting away, and although the patient was not angry at the time, he did not know what would have happened if his friend had not been able to escape. He believed that the boy was afraid of him. In relating the story of the attack he showed no concern, either for himself or for his victim.

There was no definite history of any previous difficulty. A junior in high school, he got along well with his teachers and other students, but he did not make friends easily and tended to be secretive and self-reliant. Most of the time he was cheerful, although he had a bad temper and occasional fits of severe anger in which he cried and shook, but he had never previously hit anyone or broken anything.

On the ward his mind was chiefly occupied with the desire to get home by Christmas. He said that the friend he had attacked had stolen his favorite companion, and that jealousy and hatred had occupied his mind most of the time after that. He was complacent about the fact that he might have seriously injured someone. Although he felt self-conscious and expressed the idea that people were talking about him, there was nothing clearly delusional about his behavior. In general he showed no defects of mentation. Work on the ward appealed to him more than going to a trade school. He said, "I never had that terrible feeling against anyone before, and don't think I will again." His answers were brief and to the point, although frequently he was evasive. He was quiet and cooperative as a rule, talked little, and tended to stay by himself. He said in one interview, without any sign of emotion, that he had used a hammer in his attack because he had not wanted to get "scratched up." On another occasion he remarked about the friend he had attacked, "He spread stuff about me," but the patient did not support this statement or elaborate on it. When he was discharged to the care of his mother it was with the advice that he not return to his home town. Relatives were warned of the seriousness of his behavior and they were advised to seek aid if he showed any suspicious actions.

B. Psth., Path. Emot. F:17:S:19 +3 '84672–(74) 5:8:11
Suicidal

The patient, admitted to the neurological service in a coma, had taken seventeen tablets of pentobarbital because she felt that life was not worth living. She had been considering suicide for two months. For three years she had been in love with a 31-year-old man. The original relationship had begun with a mutual interest in horses. The patient had planned to run away with him, but when her parents discovered the affair they insisted that she never see him again. She had agreed, saying, "You'll be sorry." On the day she attempted suicide her pet mare, a gift from the man she was in love with, had been sold. She had then stolen the sleeping tablets. After taking them she had called the man to tell him what she had done and had gone to his home, where she had collapsed.

The girl had grown up in a small town and had lived with her parents in an adequate home until she had begun working at age 14. There had been no necessity for her to leave home or to go to work, but she had been a poor scholar, had hated school, and had finished only the seventh grade. She had always been a retiring child and had never liked to play with other children. She liked animals and did not care whether people liked her or not. A moody, quiet, and stubborn person, she had always had her own way in everything.

After her recovery from the coma she was composed, oriented, and cooperative. Her greatest concern was the necessity of giving up the man she was in love with. Tears came to her eyes when she talked of him, but she had no further thoughts of suicide. Her I.Q. was 83. She improved markedly and was happy and enthusiastic about her future plans. She was less stubborn than she had been, and she washed her own clothes for the first time in her life, although it was a task she had previously refused to do. With close supervision by the social service there was a fair possibility that she would make a good adjustment in spite of her immature personality.

P. Psychas. M:16:S:23 +15 '8467 23–(61) 5:2:19
Schizoid

The patient, who had engaged in masturbation from age 11 to the time of admission, thought that people could tell he had the habit and that it altered his appearance. Masturbation caused him such great mental anguish that he became withdrawn, did not go out much with his friends, and worried excessively about his "sins." Each time after he confessed to a priest, he worried about the sins he had forgotten to mention. Two years before admission the boy developed compulsions to check faucets, lights, and doors, and after he left the house he often came back to ask his mother if he had broken anything on his way out. His previous interest in hunting and fishing was greatly diminished.

The only particularly contributory factor in his past history was an extended fast during Lent when he was 12 years old, but when he became thin and sallow he gave up the fasting at his parents' request. He completed three years of high school with considerable difficulty, and his compulsions finally forced him to leave school altogether. He was meticulous and slow, and he gave up a number of odd jobs on the grounds that he was not doing the work properly. He had to do everything perfectly. As a child he had been a "model boy," never getting into any of the scrapes his brothers had. He had always been more attached to his mother and sisters than to his father and brothers. People liked him, although they made him the butt of jokes. He had always been a dreamer. He had never manifested any interest in girls.

In the hospital he was greatly concerned about his worries and compulsions but did not seem overly preoccupied with them. He was interested in sports. A good conversationalist, he was cooperative and friendly but thought he could get along better at home than in the hospital. He realized that his actions and worries were foolish and felt they were the result of his "bad past." It took him eight hours to do the MMPI. He changed little while in the hospital.

Schizoid M:16:S 846792'31–X(57) 0:27:6
87964'321–X(61) 0:17:5

The school counselor referred this case to the counseling center, saying that the boy had ability and liked to work with his hands but had no idea of what he wished to do. His school grades were high in craft courses but low in academic ones. No personality or home problem was mentioned, but the boy himself wrote as his reason for coming to us, "I would like to know what I am best suited for and why I cannot get along well at home."

Both the psychologist and the physician learned that he was very unhappy at home because of his stepfather. When he reached 17 he hoped to get away from home by enlisting in the army. In the first interview his conversation was coherent and fairly fluent, and he was able to use the situation to discuss the possible solutions to his difficulties. He considered these alternatives: immediate enlistment on his birthday, finishing the semester at school and then enlisting, or finishing his high school course. After tests and vocational reading he decided he would consider occupations such as engraving, jewelry repair, and stone setting as well as the repair of small instruments. He wanted to find out what training opportunities the army could offer along these lines. When he left, we said we would be glad to talk with his mother if she wanted to come in for a conference.

We had subsequent interviews with the client six, eight, and fifteen months after the first contact, and one interview with his mother, at her request. The army rejected him, presumably because of poor vision, although this was corrected to 20/20 by glasses. He acquired a new interest in high school and came in one day to show the marked improvement on his report card. An MMPI retest reflected some improvement, but the psychotic scores remained high.

The client completed high school and looked for a job. He did not attempt to take any additional training immediately nor did he leave home. At one time after he had been out of work for several weeks, he came back to ask about his college aptitude and especially his aptitude for engineering. His college aptitude scores were average and better than would have been predicted, but he later dismissed the college idea, saying he did not like mathematics well enough to take engineering. Again he considered short courses at a school of aviation or a school of engraving and design. He continued to be unrealistic in his discussion of training, its financing, and the mechanics of making the arrangement. He responded moderately well to counseling interviews on a temporary basis but his total life adjustment remained precarious. D. F. C.

Ps. Sz., Paranoid F:28:S:62 +2 84 72 13'69– 4:11:17

The patient dated her illness from seven years before admission when she first experienced the sensation that people were staring at her with eyes "like balls of fire," and at the end of six months she had the same reaction to everyone in her family. The idea developed that people were watching her and talking about her in her absence, and she began to avoid all social contacts. A brief hospitalization was of no benefit to her, and later she was studied in several medical clinics, one of them treating her for retroversion of the uterus. After that time she experienced dysmenorrhea, with abdominal discomfort between periods. She said that because her family thought there was a moral cause for these disturbances she had begun to have "sensual thoughts." A psychiatrist had her admitted to a state hospital, but she complained of noise and requested dismissal after three weeks. At the present admission she had numerous physical complaints as well as what she called "sensual sensations and visionary trouble," memory difficulty, and inability to concentrate.

There was nothing of note in the past medical history. During her childhood she was in general a well-behaved, affectionate, and likable child, and in high school she had apparently been a normal person with many friends of both sexes. A very good student, she had graduated from high school at age 18 and after that she and a girl friend had traveled about, working in another state as domestics. The patient, who had been raised in an extremely moral home atmosphere, suddenly began to engage in many previously forbidden social activities. She had two sexual experiences and believed that she had been doped with an aphrodisiac. After nine months of this life she returned home.

The patient was a tall, neat, fairly attractive girl. She was obsessed with her complaints and refused to meet anyone's gaze, stating that at times other people's intent looks seemed to paralyze her and that if she attempted to meet their eyes her own pupils dilated in wild stares. When she first experienced a "sensuous touch" while sleeping with her married sister, it felt like a shock over her abdomen and made her jump. Her sister felt a similar shock. Because of this experience she would not touch the hand of a streetcar conductor in giving him a token. She believed that people made insinuating remarks concerning her "visionary trouble," such as "Good for you, my eye." There were no gross defects of intellect or orientation. She complained of depression as a result of her present condition. On the whole, her moods were appropriate, her thoughts logical, sequential, and coherent. She wanted treatment, asking for insulin treatment in particular, but shock therapy failed to make much change in her behavior, and she was finally discharged to the care of her family.

B. Psth., Asocial F:16:S:78 +1 847'2639–(53) 4:10:8
Suicidal

The patient had been involved in numerous petty larcenies. These had come to the attention of her mother chiefly during the past two years, but the patient said that the thievery had been going on as long as she could remember. She always knew she was stealing, but she had no feeling of guilt about it. There had also been numerous escapades in which she had left home for several days at a time, claiming to have stayed with a girl friend. She had also skipped school to visit her father (her father and mother had been divorced when the child was one month old). In spite of her truancy she had managed to get through the freshman year of high school but had then left school. She was excessively interested in boys and wrote "mushy" letters to many boys she scarcely knew. About seven months before admission she had attempted suicide by taking some pills a doctor had given her mother. Sick for a few days, she had recovered without ill effects. Apparently the only person who had much influence over her or in whom she confided (with the possible exception of her real father) was a boy she had been dating for more than a year.

Her past physical and mental health had been good. She was above average in intelligence, but she did not have good judgment about money and other matters. Although she wrote many letters, she mailed only a few of them. It was difficult for her to keep her attention on any one thing for long. She had never confided in her mother and appeared uneasy when her mother was around. Meeting strangers upset her and she was obviously insecure with them. Until two years before admission, when he got in touch with her, she had not known who her real father was, but she had decided after meeting him, "I'm just like he is." She had always felt she was not wanted by her stepfather and her mother. Her mother was very strict, making her wear "Victorian" clothes and forcing her to attend church.

In the hospital she was chiefly concerned with her belief that she was not wanted at home and that her mother and stepfather would be happier without her. She felt she was of no use to anyone. Her emotional tone was that of a person who seemed "always on edge," and she jumped when anything unexpected happened. She said that her "thinking is all mixed up—don't click with myself," but in psychiatric terms, she appeared normal, and there was no disturbance, no bizarre behavior. She preferred to be alone, but in general she was not a problem in hospitalization. While no real progress was made in psychotherapy, social service efforts in her behalf provided a foster home and some rearrangement of the plans for her future so that at the time of discharge, it seemed possible that she would make an adequate adjustment.

P. React. Depr. F:22:S:14 +14 8473 216′9–(26) 7:12:19
B. Psth., Path. Emot.
Suicidal

Three days before admission the patient had consulted the college counseling bureau about the results of certain psychological tests. These results upset her severely, and she was immediately referred to a psychiatrist, who after a brief interview asked that she be admitted to the hospital. She was depressed and while awaiting admission made two suicidal attempts.

The past history contained nothing in the way of physical or mental illness that seemed pertinent. The patient had lived with foster parents after her mother had been committed to a state hospital when she was very young. Her father died when she was 9. Her early years were marked by a longing to be returned to her family and she eventually developed a feeling that she had been the cause of her mother's illness. Later on she was emotionally disturbed when an uncle attempted physical sexual contact with her. At age 15 she had relations with a brother, who forced her to promise loyalty to him. She was a superior student in high school but was not popular and had few close friends. At college she continued an intimate correspondence with her brother and was involved in numerous emotional episodes. Several men had sexual relations with her, and others, after showing great affection for her, denounced and insulted her. She developed a complicated guilt feeling, believed that she was "basically evil," and felt anxious because she feared she would commit "evil acts." Her foster parents said that although they had loved her and had tried to do everything for her, she had rejected them.

In the hospital she professed no confidence in her moral or intellectual ability; she was deeply depressed and blamed herself for her troubles, saying that she had never done anything creative or constructive. She was sullen and quiet and after being presented at a staff conference, became markedly disturbed and hysterical. After a while she adjusted and quickly became normal in behavior. Apparently she had undergone an acute depressive episode and had recovered. The staff felt, however, that no real change had been effected and that basic maladjustment was very likely to characterize her future behavior.

Ps. Sz., Simple M:19:S:13 +6 84'<u>76</u>9–13X(47) 2:19:10
Mental Deficiency

The patient had never made an adequate economic or social adjustment, but his problem had become particularly acute in the last seven months, following his discharge from the army after two and a half months of service. In the army the slowness and difficulty with which he learned had been exasperating to his superiors, and he had been the brunt of other men's pranks and jokes. Although he felt resentful and aggressive toward his tormentors, he made no attempt to retaliate. On his return home he found that his family no longer tolerated him around the house. Forced to support himself, he worked at odd jobs, usually manual labor, and wandered about the state, but his slowness and his inability to keep up with other employees made it impossible for him to keep a job. On several occasions he was jailed for vagrancy, and he was finally sent to the hospital by the court for evaluation.

His physical health had been good, but he had always been maladjusted. He had completed the tenth grade at age 16, but he had been passed from the eighth grade chiefly because he outgrew the seats. His I.Q. was 80. Although he gave as his reason for leaving school the fact that "the boys were pawing him around," the principal said he was too lazy and sleepy to attend. He had never had close friends and was particularly shy with girls.

In the hospital he was unkempt and was obviously more dull witted than his measured intelligence indicated. His crude, boisterous, and ill-mannered behavior made him obnoxious, but he was usually happy, giggling and talking loudly without apparent reason. If corrected, he became angry and sulked for long periods. He was cooperative, and in examinations he worked as well as he could. He had difficulty adjusting to the group and was shunned when he attempted to enter into activities and conversations. His clumsiness and lack of social grace was always a disadvantage. Occasionally he showed resentment and jealousy toward more popular patients. Commitment to a state hospital was recommended although his behavior was never frankly psychotic, and there were no severe breaks with reality.

B. Pri., Child.   M:15:S:39   +6   '8479–2(39)   2:13:18

This boy's misbehavior was almost lifelong. At school he was a problem child; he had disrupted classroom routine as far back as kindergarten and he had no friends and made no effort to win any. The lad's father, his brother, and his school acquaintances rejected him as being "dumb." In one boarding home after another he failed to adjust in spite of many efforts to help him. A mental hygiene clinic closed its file on him, declaring he was beyond their help. When his father was deprived of his custody the boy, as a ward of the state, was admitted to the hospital for psychiatric evaluation.

The boy's I.Q. was 90. He experienced considerable difficulty in learning to read, showed no interest in sports, had no hobbies, and in general disliked school. Apparently he tried to attract attention through his misbehavior. He was described as secretive, stubborn, and untruthful. The physiological and neurological examinations were negative. The boy's home background was poor. When he was 3 his mother died, leaving him to the care of his father, who was described as "dull and nervous." The father had always rejected the child and, in any case, was a most inadequate person.

In the hospital the boy showed no apparent aberrations of mental content. Although boisterous and disrespectful, he was cooperative during interviews. He was well oriented. Fully aware of his misbehavior, he nevertheless seemed unconcerned. He had little regard for the feelings of others and was insulting and insubordinate. During his stay in the hospital there was no change; he continued to be disturbing, broke the rules, and annoyed other patients. There was no really normal behavior at any time. After general arrangements were completed for social work follow-up and supervision, the lad was discharged to be tried in still another home placement.

B. Psth., Path. Sexuality   M:27:S:14   +2   '84793–2   6:0:24

At the age of 20 this patient had had his first homosexual experience with a 50-year-old man, and since that time he had had repeated experiences with other men. The incident leading to his apprehension was a homosexual episode with a minor, a ward of the state, who had also had previous homosexual experiences. The patient had lived in many communities and had developed a group of homosexual friends in each locality, but his experiences had apparently been the result of mutual desire rather than of seduction.

After high school graduation the patient had attended a Seventh Day Adventist college until he was expelled for smoking, possessing obscene literature, and forging a small check. Always immature and dependent on his home, he had never been wholly self-supporting in spite of many unsuccessful promotional schemes to make money, such as an advertising bureau. Although he had held numerous positions he lacked the ability to stick with any one project. He had had some heterosexual experiences at age 18.

In the hospital he discussed his homosexual experiences freely and expressed the belief that because his sexual drive was not strong it was something that he could control. He was not entirely honest, but when he was caught in contradictory statements, it seemed in no way to disturb him. His I.Q. was about 150. Although he was entirely cooperative and normal in his behavior on the ward, his immaturity and lack of stable assets were very apparent. Because the staff felt that he did not present any real danger to society he was not recommended for commitment under the psychopathic personality law, and when he was returned to the court for disposition, it was with the general recommendation that he be considered sane and not dangerous to society.

Ps. Sz., Paranoid M:36:S '849–273 (55) 4:11:14

This patient asked to be admitted to the hospital to escape "enemies" who were trying to kill him and to steal his inventions. He had tried to evade them by fleeing to the next state, but after seeing so many cars on the road with license plates from his home state, he assumed they were trying to drive him off the road, and he headed in another direction. His car broke down, and when he tried to set it on fire, he was apprehended by a sheriff. It was suggested to him then that he seek admission to the hospital.

This veteran was a skilled worker and before his service in the armed forces he had worked steadily and without difficulty. He served in the navy and the army and received honorable discharges from both. He then held several jobs, claiming he left each one because of other employees' jealousy of his ability and the antagonism shown him. Shy and timid, he rarely went out on dates. His mother was said to have been "queer" and his father had left home years before, leaving no address.

During several interviews, the patient expressed ideas of grandeur and delusions about people trying to kill him, to control him by electricity, or to steal his inventions. When discussing these, he showed little or no affect. Insight was completely lacking and he was unable to give any clues about the precipitating circumstances of his panic state before admission. He regarded the hospital as a haven but participated only passively in ward activities. Shock therapy was recommended. W. M. H.

Ps. Sz., Simple F:32:M:20 +2 ′86–3 (63) 5:12:9

For three years before admission this woman had been showing gradually increasing seclusiveness and withdrawal. She neglected her household responsibilities, refused to care for her child and her husband, often skipped meals if no one else did the cooking, and lost a great deal of weight. Spells of nearly normal behavior, lasting one or two weeks, were invariably followed by longer periods when she remained in bed. Occasionally she complained of sickness and abdominal pain. At times she did not respond to questioning, did just the opposite of what she was asked to do, burst into inappropriate laughter, and threw clothes at her husband. A year earlier she had been hospitalized briefly but without effect.

The past medical history was not significant. A sensitive child who demanded her own way, she had retired to bed whenever displeased or frustrated. Members of the family accepted this behavior and babied her a great deal. During the second year in high school she stopped because, she said, she "liked to stay home." Her school progress was otherwise normal. At one time she thought she would like to be a nun, but after she left school she decided in favor of marriage and a family. Prone to violent temper tantrums, the habitually became, even before this illness, sullen, morose, and ill if things did not go well. Her husband was a farmer and the marriage was said to have been a perfect one until the present illness. There were two children.

In the hospital the patient was withdrawn and unresponsive for several days. She was apathetic and disinterested in life around her; she answered questions only after much prodding and then in monosyllables. She had periods of inappropriate grimacing. After much questioning she admitted hallucinatory experiences. The details of these could not be elicited. Her general appearance was that of a deeply retarded patient. After a short while she became somewhat better but never entered into ward activities and spent much time staring into space. She had to be urged to eat or to leave her room. She was unkempt and sometimes showed catatonic behavior. Electroshock therapy brought about definite improvement, which increased until the time of discharge. She was transferred to a state hospital definitely improved but still manifestly ill.

Ps. Sz., Paranoid F:22:D:67 +3 86 1′23479–X (53) 2:18:4
+31 48′9263– (45) 5:11:6

The patient dated her illness from about six months before admission when she had met an army sergeant who exerted great power over her mind. She had sexual intercourse with him on several occasions and then he told her that such a love affair would not last and such actions should cease. She believed that he had people in all walks of life watching her to see if her love was worthy. Because of her worry about the people she presumed were watching her, she became irritable and restless, sleeping but a few hours each night. A physician prescribed a sedative and referred her for psychiatric study.

At the time of her divorce two years before admission she had a nervous breakdown and was for several months under the care of a psychiatrist. Details of that illness were not known. As a child her interests had been largely athletic in nature. She was especially good at speed skating and swimming. A good student, she nevertheless did not complete high school. After her divorce she worked at various clerical jobs; she always gave the appearance of being well adjusted and had a friendly, warm manner. Haphazard in her handling of money she frequently borrowed after spending all her own money. She did not make friends readily because she was suspicious of the people she met, a trend far more marked in recent months. She felt that people who attended church were hypocrites. Married to a soldier at age 18, she claimed that she had married merely to get away from home. The marriage was not satisfactory in any respect and was terminated by divorce. The patient had one abortion during the time she was married. Subsequent to the divorce she had intercourse with a married man but moved away from the neighborhood because of gossip.

In the hospital she was somewhat apprehensive but on the whole composed. There was some fluctuation of mood and her expression was subtly indicative of suspicion. She realized that no one believed her delusions about someone following her, but she repeatedly stated that it was true. She had no insight, and she was chiefly concerned with the people following her and with the conviction that the sergeant wished to check on the validity of her love. She improved somewhat during her stay, was given insulin and electroshock therapy, but on the whole changed very little. She was discharged to her home but the prognosis was not considered to be very good, though it was possible that she would be able to remain out of an institution.

B. Pri., Child. M:15:S:21 +1 8'612 394-7 (71) 2:13:12
Mental Deficiency

Apparently the first sign of trouble with this boy appeared about a year before admission when he was living with a married sister. The presence of the boy irritated his brother-in-law, and relations were strained to the point where the boy was sent to live with an aunt. She found it "impossible to handle him," and his behavior caused him to be expelled from school. He was then placed in a farm home, where he was rejected because of his deceitfulness, his failure to do assigned chores, and his unkempt appearance. Other placements lasted a relatively short time. In one instance he was said to be cruel to farm animals and to indulge openly in masturbation. Another couple had no real complaints against him, but they "couldn't like him." He was finally sent to the hospital by the child welfare agency handling the case for a general appraisal.

His mother had died when the boy was very young. Until his father's death, the two of them had lived at a county infirmary. The boy was usually cheerful, although there were periods when he sulked. He wanted to work on a farm, but there was a repeated history of cruelty to farm animals. He did not like school, and he had always been a poor student. Baseball was his main interest, but he enjoyed "talking" and "movies." In personal appearance he was usually dirty, with eruptions on his face, numerous warts on his hands, and an offensive body odor.

On the ward he was alert and interested in the activities, taking part in games without undue shyness. His I.Q. was 79. He said he was in the hospital "because I don't get along with people and they don't get along with me," but he mixed fairly well with others around the ward. He did his routine duties with cheerfulness and with little urging. At times he was reprimanded for teasing the nurses or for quarreling, but on the whole he was well behaved. Dental hygiene and treatment for his skin and eyes improved his physical appearance. After study and social work investigation, he was sent to another farm home placement with the recommendation that he not be returned to school.

B. Psth., Path. Emot. F:31:M:30 +17 8612473′9–(61) 8:14:13
Ps. Sz., Paranoid
Mental Deficiency

The patient was admitted to the hospital because of fits of anger, headaches, crying spells, a fear of cancer, and a number of somatic complaints. The onset of this pattern dated back about four years to the birth of her second son. At that time she noticed that she had a purulent vaginal discharge and she complained of pelvic pain. Five months before admission she complained of paresis of both legs. These complaints continued to the time of admission in spite of a series of electroshock treatments at another psychopathic hospital. She had previously enjoyed good physical health. However, she had always suffered from attacks of palpitation, had been chronically constipated, and had been generally a nervous person.

She completed the eighth grade without great difficulty though her intelligence was dull normal. She worked only at housekeeping and before the present illness, appeared to have been moderately well adjusted and happily married, although quiet and passive. There was a peculiar history of sexual promiscuity involving several men during the same evening about eighteen months before the present admission. A criminal assault charge was filed following this event but no convictions were obtained and all participants were exonerated. The patient was amnesic for the event at the time of admission.

In the hospital she was dull and apathetic. She had many somatic complaints. Her sensorium and intellect were clear. There were no hallucinatory experiences and the delusions seemed to be chiefly somatic. She cried frequently and claimed to be constantly worried, but she did not appear so as one watched her. Her stream of thought was slow and her responses were vague. She had a disheveled and sad appearance. She spent most of her time watching other patients, rarely entering into conversation or activities. During her stay she developed no insight into her illness and continued to be unresponsive and withdrawn. She feared that she would be sent back to a state hospital. She was discharged for a trial at home with a poor prognosis.

Ps. Sz., Hebe. F:26:S:81 +9 8613′472– 3:11:10

The patient's illness apparently began about five years before admission during convalescence from a uteritis, when she had vague fears, uncertain visual hallucinations, and a feeling that she was different from others. These gradually subsided, but thereafter the patient noticed that she was easily fatigued and experienced difficulties in thinking. After a recurrence of the symptoms three years before admission she began to withdraw from reality, slept poorly, had shaking spells, and felt she was generally cracking up. The various medications she tried apparently helped her. A year before admission she renewed an old friendship, became engaged to the man, and had sexual relations with him. Her mental state became more bizarre, with gruesome delusional experiences, auditory hallucinations, and ideas of reference, in which she felt that people were reading her mind. At times she believed her parents were going to poison her and other times she was afraid that she might kill someone.

After she had graduated from high school with an excellent record, she had attended a Bible school for two years. Her two ambitions were to become a traveling evangelist and to play the piano, but for five years before admission she had lived at home and her only employment had been giving piano lessons from time to time. She had never been interested in domestic work, preferring outdoor sports. A friendly, imaginative person, she was sensitive about the attitude of others toward her, and although her elderly father was a minister and she occasionally occupied his pulpit, she had apparently not been overly religious. The patient said that she had always been the favored one in her family because of her "weak health."

Her mental content in the hospital was incongruous. In addition to bizarre ideas about people reading her mind and about "things coming down upon me from the skies," she said that she "had to fight to keep my head straight—something was in my head." There were no demonstrable hallucinations, and no obvious paranoid trends. Well oriented, she showed some difficulty in concentration and thinking, and she appeared indifferent toward her illness. She had only shallow insight, if any. Although she said that her main difficulty was "fear," she was unable to amplify on this. She had ideas of reference and auditory hallucinations, most of which were derogatory, but she was inclined to keep them to herself. In general she was a rigid, indecisive, and unapproachable person, and at the time of discharge, although she was probably somewhat better, no real change had been effected.

Ps. Sz., Cat. M:21:S ′86143–7(51) 6:9:16

This patient was first seen for a psychological evaluation before a prefrontal lobotomy. At that time he was catatonic, manneristic, and inaccessible in interviews and in testing. One month after the operation he was seen again and, at that time, was oriented, in relatively good contact, friendly, and cooperative, and he responded well to testing. He appeared very dull and passive, however, was emotionally reduced, and sometimes smiled inappropriately. The MMPI was given at this time.

The young man apparently had always been backward, shy, and retiring. He had a twelfth-grade education and was considered an average student. In school he took little part in group activities and was solitary in his habits. He entered the service directly from school. In the army he made a passive adjustment until the onset of his illness, when he stared into space, was asocial and seclusive, and admitted to ideas of reference and hallucinations. After failing to respond to continued hospitalization and varied treatments, including both electroshock and insulin shock therapy, he was approved for the prefrontal lobotomy.

Although he was in much better condition after the operation, more responsive and cooperative, and seemed definitely improved, he still showed residual effects of his illness and the prognosis was guarded. W. M. H.

Ps. Sz., Mixed F:20:S:42 +7 861792'34– 7:13:7
Paranoid
Mental Deficiency

About two years before admission the patient began to complain of headaches and insomnia, and she became firmly convinced that her brother-in-law was saying unkind things about her. Her emotional state alternated between depression and euphoria. The symptoms remained unchanged for about a year, and then she developed feelings of guilt after having had sexual relations with a young man she had been acquainted with for only a short while. Seven months before admission she began to be afraid of remaining in a dark room by herself, and in addition she was troubled by terrifying visual and auditory hallucinations. She insisted that the neighbors talked about her. It became impossible for her to go into crowds, and she began to experience periods of agitation and frequent bouts of crying. She believed she could read people's minds. A month before admission she expressed the fear of insanity.

The patient's I.Q. was about 80. She had been in a special class in grade school, finally completing the equivalent of the eighth grade at age 16, and had made an unsuccessful attempt to attend high school. In school she had behaved poorly and had resented the teachers, in part because of her shyness, sensitivity, and feelings of inferiority. She showed a certain amount of vanity and an apparent need of sympathy. She had tried working in a small factory and had taken care of children but her efforts were so unsatisfactory that she had never been steadily employed.

In the hospital she was self-depreciatory, stating that she had "made a mess of her life," and it disturbed her that she was unable to concentrate or to interest herself in anything. She said she could sense where people were by using mental telepathy. Voices frequently spoke to her, describing the happenings of the day and how her relatives felt about her sickness. Sometimes sexual topics were discussed vividly. The hallucinations were further described by the patient as "one side says one thing, another side says another." She had visual hallucinations in which she saw a man in dark clothes, and she was often terrified by the appearance of animals. She wondered how it would be possible to commit suicide, and she was concerned because her illness had made others miserable. She thought that people called her "dumbell" and "crazy." Her general information was very poor, and she was unable to perform simple arithmetic. Her ideas of reference and delusions of persecution were unshakable. She described her illness somewhat disconnectedly as being due in part to "a misplaced coccyx and a leg injury." In a 24-hour interval there would be periods of elation and depression that might alternate several times. There was one period in which she became so disturbed that she had to be put into a special room. During this time she was in a state of acute excitement, refusing to eat, sitting on the floor, disrobing, and carrying out other regressive behavior. She insisted that her food was poisoned and that she was being given drugs in order to kill her. She was finally transferred to a state hospital.

P. React. Depr. F:23:S:113 +4 86217′439– 5:10:14
Ps. M-D., Depr.

A year before admission this young woman, who had always been depressed about her physical deformities, showed a marked increase of this depression and began to weep and complain that "things seem to have changed" and no longer were real to her. It was as though she looked into a mirror, she said. Insomnia was a distressing symptom. Six weeks before admission she developed a fear of swallowing food "lest it go down the air passage." This became so marked that she began to lose weight. She also complained of pain in the left flank and lower abdomen. She had congenital deformations of both legs, for which she had undergone extensive surgery without satisfactory results.

The patient had always been self-conscious and insecure and had withdrawn from social contacts as much as possible, spending her time reading and drawing. From her earliest years she had tended to brood over difficulties and had tried unsuccessfully to find satisfaction in art work. Believing that people would dislike her because of her deformed legs, she had never attempted to make friends. The thought that she would never marry because of her legs disturbed her always.

In the hospital the examination revealed a hydronephrotic kidney with an apparent stricture at the urethral pelvic junction. Psychologically the patient was concerned about her physical deformities, feeling that life had little to offer her. She was preoccupied with sex and still disturbed by an unfortunate sexual experience when she was 10 years old. A fear of choking was a marked symptom, and she was depressed and hopeless. Although she cooperated with the examiners she had little faith in their ability to help her. She was fed by tube for a few days, then began to eat naturally. It was hard to keep her out of bed but eventually she showed considerable interest in occupational therapy and ward life. Frequent attacks of pain in her left flank and the left abdominal region were controlled by pilocarpine. Before she left the hospital, arrangements were made for her to teach art in a small school. Other plans were made to improve conditions in her home. She cooperated well and at discharge was much improved.

P. Hypo. F:34:M:27 +1 86 231'47–(61) 8:6:18
Mental Deficiency

Three years before admission the patient began to complain that she felt weak and tired, had pains in her neck, and had a choking feeling in her throat. She also took less interest in her housework and was content just to sit. A chiropractor gave her some electric treatments, which seemed to clear up her symptoms for two years, but about three months before admission she had a recurrence of the symptoms. In addition she was grouchy and irritable with her husband and children, punishing them for small and insignificant things. She lost interest in her friends and was careless about her personal appearance and her housework. Her symptoms became progressively worse, until just before admission, during an argument with her husband, she took up a knife and threatened to attack him.

She was an eighth-grade graduate and had lived all her life on a farm. Friendly, cheerful, and fun loving, she had no special hobbies, although she enjoyed dances and visiting with friends. Her relationship with her husband had been strained for the last two years. They did not have intercourse "very often," and her inability to do the housework properly angered him.

On admission to the hospital the patient's mental content chiefly concerned worry about her somatic complaints and a fear that she was losing her mind as her mother and sister had. She was neat and cooperative, but she gave the impression of being slow and dull. She was clear mentally but poorly informed, and she functioned at a low intellectual level. Her measured I.Q. was 67. Her emotional tone was stable, though she described herself as nervous. The recognition that she had nervous trouble was her only real insight. Her answers did not fit questions very well, but this seemed to be caused by a lack of understanding. No real change occurred during her hospitalization. The efforts of the staff were directed at improving the home situation and at preparing the way for her adjustment at a level more appropriate to her intellectual standing.

Ps. Sz., Mixed F:23:S:55 +46 86239 14'7–X 3:18:8

The patient had always been considered a little "queer," but this had been especially marked for the past two years. She first came to the attention of social agencies when she sent her father's diary and love letters to the superintendent of a state hospital where she had applied for nurses' training. In sending the private papers she had wanted to explain her poor record by showing that she had been mistreated. Her reason for wanting to take nurses' training was to learn modern contraceptive methods. She had been engaging in considerable sex fantasy and had disrobed in front of a window to attract the attention of passing men. Once she had enrolled in a correspondence club whose purpose was to assist members in obtaining marriage partners.

She was markedly antagonistic toward her parents. She had a congenital strabismus, but otherwise the physical and medical histories were noncontributory. A high school graduate, she had had great difficulty with her schoolwork, and when she had tried to continue with a postgraduate high school course her bizarre behavior forced the family to take her out of school. She had never shown "common sense," her thinking had always been vague and poorly formulated, and she resented criticism. She was jealous of her younger sister. Early in life she had been a masturbation problem.

In the hospital the general physical and neurological examinations were essentially negative except for a congenital heart disease that was not severe. There was evidence that she had not engaged in sexual intercourse. A marked dissociation between her mood and her apparent mental content was present; she talked about very private matters with no more emotion than if she were discussing the weather. On one occasion she nonchalantly requested tweezers to extract pubic hair with, stating that such hair was an abnormal finding in the female, and when the tweezers were refused she suggested that the doctor pull out the hair for her. She expressed great dislike for her parents, speaking of her mother as "that woman my father married." Her I.Q. was 82. She was voluble, rambling, disconnected, and careless of her personal appearance, and she frequently made queer facial grimaces. She tended to be dissatisfied with the hospital and was somewhat of a nursing problem. Gradually she became more suspicious and more seclusive, and she was finally discharged to go to a state hospital.

B. Psth., Mixed   F:16:S:15   +1   86471239′–(55)   5:8:13

Following a series of unsuccessful foster home placements, this young girl had been in the care of the civil correctional school for a year. Shifted from home to home in each foster home, she had been truculent, uncooperative, and defiant. Moreover, she had been subject to temper outbursts and had engaged in petty thievery. After placement in the correctional home she appeared extremely unhappy and depressed and had fainting spells that appeared to be hysterical in nature. It was difficult for anyone to establish rapport with her or to make any real evaluation of her psychological state.

The family background was so chaotic that the girl had been removed from the control of her parents at age 5. There was evidence that in a number of her earlier foster homes the patient had been poorly treated. It was impossible to decide how much of the difficulties in placement derived from the girl's misbehavior and how much from the kind of foster homes she had experienced. Her schooling was exceedingly irregular and the teachers complained that she had a low tolerance for any frustration. Her intelligence was in the low average range. She enjoyed sports and liked to read, cook, and go to the movies. Shy with people at first, she made a good impression because she "sized people up," figured out how to get along with them, and then began to use them for her own purposes. The social service report said, "She is confused and disturbed about sex and would like to know more about it. She was misguided by an aunt, teased and embarrassed by several foster siblings, and disgusted and horrified by her dreams and daydreams."

In the hospital the girl was reticent and offered almost no information spontaneously. Evasive, she suppressed information about herself and was only concerned about her present problems and her immediate future. Her belief that she was persecuted by an aunt seemed not to be necessarily delusional. Excitable and anxious, she was fairly cheerful much of the time, giggling often. She had a certain amount of insight; she admitted her difficulties in getting along, but her attitude was that no one would believe her no matter what she said. Plans were made for her to continue in school and also to work part time. The prognosis was judged uncertain.

B. Psth., Asocial	F:18:S:23	+3	86479'31–(53)	2:9:14
B. Psth., Path. Sexuality		+10	'748 96–1 (49)	1:8:9

The patient was sent to the hospital from a girls' reform school for observation and evaluation. At the age of 7 the girl had been placed in an orphanage, where she had been so unhappy that she had run away several times. At 14 she was sent to a foster home; there her foster father seduced her. She was then placed in another home, but at the age of 16 she was allowed to go to a large city to work. Her associates in the city were immoral and asocial, and she was committed to the reform school for sexual delinquency. In the school she was resentful, incorrigible, and antagonistic, and she spent much of her time in the "punishment cottage." On one occasion she escaped and was not apprehended for more than three months. She became friendly with a young Negro inmate, with whom she had frequent homosexual relations, and when discovery resulted in their separation the patient became so depressed and irritable that she put insecticide in a matron's coffee.

She had finished the ninth grade but had not liked school and had made poor grades. Then she had worked as a domestic and at other unskilled occupations. An energetic, quick-tempered person, she was unable to engage in any sustained activity, liked to dominate her associates, and had very poor judgment.

In the hospital she was primarily concerned with her future and was so eager to be helped that she told her story to anyone who would listen. Intact in sensorium and intellect, she was of low average intelligence and was mildly unstable emotionally. As to her homosexual activities, she said she was merely behaving as the other girls did: "All the other girls did it, and you would too if cooped up for so long." Although defensive, she was frank and logical in answering questions, apparently truthful and open, friendly, entirely cooperative, and responsive to constructive criticism. She adjusted well to hospital life and at least on the verbal level realized that much of her difficulty had been caused by her own misdoing. When she was returned to the school it was felt that if the patient was unable to make the necessary adjustment, her commitment to a state hospital as a sexual psychopath was not unlikely. However, the staff was somewhat optimistic about her adjustment.

Ps. Sz., Simple	F:32:S:90	+6	86497'1-(57)	2:11:12
		+59	6489'721-(43)	6:13:9

This patient had experienced repeated depressive episodes throughout her life. In school she was nicknamed "Cry-Baby" because she cried so easily. After the divorce of her mother and father she was depressed for months. A gradual increase of these general symptoms, with seclusiveness and inability to eat or sleep as additional complications, led to this admission.

At age 26 during a pregnancy out of wedlock she had become melancholic. The child was placed in an orphanage but the patient continued to be depressed and thought of herself as a "good" girl who had been tricked. Three years later she became pregnant again, was depressed, and said it would never happen again. This child she took to her mother's home but showed little further interest in it. At that time she also became seclusive and had frequent crying spells. At admission she was pregnant for the third time. Her mother had said she would not help the girl if she became pregnant again. This third pregnancy was by the same man as the second, but she refused to bring charges against him, although he admitted paternity and was willing to marry her.

A high school graduate, the patient had average intelligence. Employed at housework and other jobs, she was a fairly steady worker until the first pregnancy. After that she never held a job for more than a few months. Extremely dependent on her mother, she never showed much initiative. She was not friendly toward others and appeared ill at ease. She said that she had always felt inferior. A great deal of her time she spent in reading romantic fiction and in daydreaming. Her parents were divorced when she was 14 and both remarried. Two sisters showed more aggressiveness then she and both made successful adjustments to life, which apparently increased the patient's feelings of inferiority.

At the hospital her sensitiveness and feelings of inferiority obviously engendered ideas of reference. In other ways her sensorium and intellect were normal. There was an appearance of depression, but apathy was possibly the genuine state. She had no insight. Her replies to most questions were adequate and she showed little psychomotor retardation. In manner she was aloof and disinterested and she took little interest in her personal appearance. After a few weeks she became more open about her problems, but as the culmination of the pregnancy approached she was increasingly depressed and self-conscious. The baby was delivered while the patient was in the hospital. The birth was normal, but the patient became worse, more seclusive, self-depreciative, and impoverished in mentation. Remaining in her own room, she read and cried quietly most of the day and refused to engage in ward activities. At discharge she was transferred to another hospital.

Ps. Paranoid Schizoid	M:13:S:62	+21	'8671<u>42</u>3–(41)	5:3:28

The patient's illness began abruptly three days before admission with the appearance of delusions of a paranoid and somatic character. He believed that his neighbor was a Nazi spy who intended to poison the patient and his family, and that this neighbor had got control of the patient through hypnosis. "Heart attacks" and periods in which he said he was unable to breathe and had no pulse were ascribed by him to the poison. During this time he was extremely restless and was incontinent of urine on three occasions. There were no previous medical or psychological upsets with the exception of an episode six weeks before admission, when he developed a fever lasting four days and was more excited, talkative, and irritable than usual.

He had completed the seventh grade at the time of admission, but he had shown little interest in schoolwork, and his grades were poor. The family said that he had always been genial toward everybody, open, friendly, and well behaved. He did his farm chores conscientiously. He had relatively few friends and spent a great deal of time reading comic books and daydreaming. His family background was not good. There were twelve siblings, and the social worker reported the home filthy and poorly kept.

In the hospital the patient was preoccupied with his poorly systematized delusions, and talked at great length about them, but he was well oriented as to person, time, and place. When not speaking of his delusions he appeared entirely normal. During the first day he was restless and fearful, but these symptoms soon disappeared. He adjusted to the routine activities, although he was frequently insolent and disobedient toward the nursing staff. Sometimes he admitted that his delusions might be imagination, but he was never truly convinced. Occasionally he used profanity and talked of sexual matters. In many ways his indifference and compulsive behavior suggested an early schizophrenia. It was advised that his home environment be changed, and he was discharged to live with an older brother, with the recommendation that he be subjected to fairly firm discipline.

B. Pri., Child. Schizoid	M:14:S:30	+16	8'<u>67</u>2–3(47)	4:8:12

At the time the patient was admitted to an orphange six years before hospitalization, he was a problem child; he stole minor articles and was unreliable generally. At times he showed great enthusiasm for games or other activities but his interest receded as quickly as it began. On occasion he was sullen and withdrawn, resentful and uncooperative in the classroom, and slow in getting his work done. He daydreamed considerably. He ran away repeatedly and used unacceptable language, particularly in talking to a younger boy whom he keenly resented.

The patient had been placed in the orphanage after his parents had separated because of incompatibility. He progressed poorly in school, never showed any consistent interest in anything, and was usually on the fringe of group play. He had an I.Q. of 92. He had no evident qualities of leadership, but his classmates had elected him president of a boys' club in an attempt to make him more social. The opposite occurred; he became stubborn and inactive, vaguely blaming "politics."

On admission he was emotionally disturbed and withdrawn, and he never spontaneously expressed his thoughts or feelings. He appeared depressed and at times negativistic, but he had no obvious delusions or hallucinations. His sensorium and intellect were intact. When working in occupational therapy he finished every task to the point of perfection. His work was neat, and he was gifted with his hands, particularly in painting and drawing. His efforts to be friendly and interested in the work of others met with coldness because of his annoying habit of hanging over the chair of the person he was interested in. He had a basic need for affection and secure personal relationships, but the possibility of early schizophrenia was felt to be fairly important. He was discharged with the general recommendation of placement in a foster home.

Ps. Sz., Simple   M:28:S:29   +1   86721'93–X   2:18:7

The patient was brought to the hospital on a court order with symptoms of agitation, hallucinations, and general somatic concern. He had been well until two months before admission when he began to lose interest in his farm work, his dress became careless, and he sat around the house frequently crying to himself. Asked to do specific chores, he complied willingly. Two weeks before admission he experienced an hallucinatory episode involving a local man who the patient thought had taken on an unreal, ghostlike appearance. For the next two nights the patient heard noises in the walls of his bedroom. Ten days before admission he attended a picnic and thought he made unsuccessful advances toward a young woman—this could not be confirmed. His lack of success with the young woman bothered him, and he believed that something had been put in his whiskey to make him impotent. He decided that pain, which he thought was connected with a goiter, might explain his impotence, but two different physicians failed to discover genital abnormalities.

Eight years before admission he had had an attack similar to the present one. At that time he had lost weight, was nervous and tremulous, and complained of impotence. The condition was diagnosed as hyperthyroidism, and eventually he recovered. Otherwise he had been free of obvious nervous or mental illness. A hard-working, industrious man, with no specific hobbies, he was sociable with men but bashful and shy in the presence of women. He had always shown good judgment. An eighth-grade graduate, he had worked on his father's farm after leaving school, and he resented the fact that his father never allowed him to make decisions of any importance.

In the hospital his chief concern was with his assumed impotence and the abnormality he felt present in his genitalia. He also complained of a lump in his throat and a blurring of his vision. Otherwise, he was quiet and cooperative and showed no particular aberrancies. Occasionally he became restless and felt that he "just had to talk to someone about my sickness," but there was no disturbance of his sensorium or intellect. He quickly adjusted to hospitalization and made friends with male patients, but considerable reassurance was needed to relieve him of his worry about the possibility that he had a goiter or that his genitalia were abnormal. As his somatic concerns became less pronounced, he began to look forward to his return home. When he was discharged to the custody of his brother it seemed that the present mild episode had ended, but it was felt that the prognosis for a recurrence was not good.

Ps. M-D., Depr.   F:44:M:21   +3   86729'431-(30)   0:14:6

For twenty years the patient had suffered from depressive spells. She came to the hospital because of the ineffectiveness of any of the many types of therapy tried; she was frequently relieved temporarily, but nothing ever helped for long. Aside from this there was no more reason why she should have sought psychiatric aid at the time of admission than for any other period in the last ten years. The depressive attacks were not rhythmic or regular in appearance. On the average, four or five occurred each year, sometimes only one or two. Usually no precipitating events were identifiable, and sometimes events that might be expected to produce an attack failed to do so. A given attack was usually preceded by a gradual decrease in her working efficiency. She became despondent, cried easily, was indecisive, and spoke little. Sometimes she appeared dazed and failed to answer questions, and invariably she became neglectful of her personal appearance. "A blackness seemed to descend" upon her head, she said, followed by agitation and tenseness. If untreated, the attacks lasted from ten to fourteen days. In spite of the numerous kinds of therapy tried, "all that ever happened was I might get over the spells sooner." There were no suicidal tendencies and she always remained well oriented. She did complain of headaches.

A quick, alert person, she showed good judgment and an ability to plan and to handle money. She was self-reliant and well adjusted. Full of energy and interested in community affairs, she had held several offices such as superintendent of the Sunday school, and she was friendly and at ease with others. Friends considered her not overly sensitive. The patient and her husband got along well.

In the hospital the most pronounced impression given by the patient was dissatisfaction with her mode of life. She had not attained the level of living she had once hoped for. Financially and socially she was less well off since her marriage. She hated her house, was disappointed in her husband, and doubted his love for her. Everyone was against her and she was friendless, she felt. She admitted to the thought of taking her own life but felt that the Lord would not permit it. She cried frequently and without provocation. There was psychomotor retardation. Although she recognized that she was ill, she said that "something seemed to snap" in her head and she could not prevent herself from becoming depressed. There were occasions when she joined in songs and games with other patients. A short course of electroshock treatments was followed by immediate improvement. By the time of discharge the attack seemed to be over, and she was completely normal. The staff felt that no real progress had been made in understanding her difficulties or in developing a new approach for her treatment. General recommendations were made, however, for improving the family situation as a prophylactic measure.

B. Psth., Path. Emot. F:16:S:23 +1 86732'41–(49) 3:13:12
Schizoid

About two months before admission the patient experienced, while in church, strange, distant feelings in which she felt as though she were a year old. Voices sounded far away and her head was foggy. Subsequently, her symptoms centered on an inability to do her schoolwork. Her school grades for the sophomore year had not been up to her previous honor roll standard, and even before that time she had begun to have trouble. Unknown to her mother, she learned to smoke and to drink moderately.

She had always been shy and quiet. At the age of 4 months she had a severe attack of whooping cough. At age 11 she missed a half year of school because of crying spells, which ceased after the discovery and correction of a severe myopia. She had no hobby, work, or other interests except schoolwork. She was able to keep up a good front and was punctilious in dress and manner. She had had a few boy friends but denied having any sexual experiences.

On admission she was a nice-looking, somewhat apathetic girl. Constant in mood, quiet, and withdrawn, she was cooperative and relatively interested in ward activities. Her inability to maintain high grades in school, which she attributed to her inability to concentrate and to memorize, disturbed her. High grades were her only mode of self-expression. She desired to be extremely intelligent, but her average grades up to the time she had withdrawn from school were consistent with her I.Q. of 106. She was narcissistic and more interested in herself, her appearance, and her own feelings than in anything else. There were evidences indicating the possibility of an early schizophrenic pattern. An attempt was made to induce her to lessen her scholastic expectations and to develop more appropriate modes of self-expression.

Ps. Sz., Paranoid M:21:S:7 +1 867 423′19– 2:13:11

The patient, a university student, was apparently well adjusted until three months before admission when he began exhibiting bizarre behavior. His mother noted that he read intensively from books on philosophy and religion and neglected his schoolwork, spending most of his time thinking about religion. He believed that he was a new prophet and that it was his duty to convert others to his religious beliefs. Speaking at a student meeting on the subject of immortality, he wandered from the subject and the meeting took on the character of a revival meeting. His dreams were numerous and vivid. In one he was told that he must either become anti-Christ or a prophet of God. Hospitalized for eight days, he became somewhat better, and it was recommended that he visit an uncle's ranch in the West. There he filled out a draft board questionnaire in which he described his present job as that of a prophet who must lead the pacifists to invade Germany and, armed only with the Bible, must start a spiritual awakening in America.

An honor student, he had completed two years of premedical work at the time of the illness. He had, however, abandoned that educational line because he did not like "sick people" and had shifted to the college of law. Most of his energy had always been expended in study and in music. He also played golf and tennis. Never active socially, he did become a Y.M.C.A. leader. He felt inadequate in that role but continued because he considered it good for him "to train younger boys." A perfectionist in everything, he usually gave up in discouragement when he could not attain the high goals he set for himself. His friends had been few, and a year before admission he had acquired his first and only girl friend.

In the hospital the patient had many self-condemnatory and persecutory ideas of a religious nature. He believed that he had an evil eye and that unless he was completely destroyed he would become a dictator "through the immoral use of persecutory persuasion." Death was the only solution to his trouble, he reiterated, and unless he was killed the world would have a new dictator. His emotional tone showed blunting and dissociation. The assaultive behavior persisted; he threatened to kill several of the patients on the ward, and he frequently mentioned suicide also. Unchanged after some days, he was transferred to a state hospital.

B. Pri., Child. M:15:S:48 +13 867 49′321–(71) 1:14:5
Schizoid +19 89742′631–(63) 2:14:7

From the time he was 4 or 5 years old, the patient had suffered from recurrent attacks of abdominal cramps and diarrhea of several days' duration. These seemed to have been precipitated by episodes of "nervousness" induced by emotional factors in the environment. About two years before admission he became very irritable. He developed a suspicious attitude that people were talking about him and began to twist things that were said and done into a pattern of action directed against him. Toward members of his family he became so very aggressive that he would strike them or break furniture. He was always "telling off" somebody. Because he did not like school and because it interfered with his plans, he refused to continue the ninth grade and he isolated himself from everyone. His only desire was to be on his own where he could "live my own life as I want to."

A poor student, the patient had failed in the second grade and had consistently received poor marks. His main interest was in outdoor sports, and he read many books on physical culture. Music was his hobby and he spent much time writing cowboy songs and collecting records of western music. In general he made friends easily, was open and self-reliant, but was so extremely sensitive that he cried when other children were punished. His father had died when he was 10 years old, and since then the patient had been supported by his mother with the help of an uncle. His mother, who was overly concerned about the schooling of her three children, was extremely strict with the patient, and she had abused and beaten the boy.

When he was admitted he was so determined to escape from the hospital that he threatened to steal the keys or to choke himself. For a while he refused to eat or to cooperate in routine procedures. Emotionally unhappy and depressed, he claimed not to want sympathy, and when he was questioned he became extremely angry. His belligerence was so great that he had to be put into a disturbed ward for a few days. His recovery was slow, but he came to adjust fairly well. As he took an active part in ward activities, his stomach pains and diarrhea disappeared, and he appeared fairly normal, but when an attempt at giving him insight and positive therapy was substituted for passive hospitalization he again became extremely negativistic. His attitude that no one understood him and that he would be all right if left alone was so persistent that he was well adjusted only as long as he was merely allowed to remain as a member of the hospital patient group. Any attempt to change him, to talk to him, or to get him ready for discharge resulted in an exacerbation of his symptoms. With these emotional outbursts his stomach symptoms recurred. He showed marked improvement at the time of his discharge, although he did not want to leave the hospital and for the first time he listened to advice and suggestions. Discharged to the care of his mother, he agreed to find a full-time job, to engage in athletics and other outside activities, and to return once a month to the outpatient clinic.

Ps. Sz., Paranoid M:34:S:66 +6 8679241'3–X (67) 1:23:8

This client had not been able to work for a year, being handicapped in every activity by pains in his head, dizziness, and palpitations so severe that he was forced to spend most of the day resting. Told that nothing was physically wrong with him, he could not believe his symptoms had an emotional basis. He felt the illness might be caused by people who "fixed me up with the evil eye." He admitted that he worried too much about things. He seemed eager to have a listener, and so in spite of his apparent lack of understanding of psychotherapy, he was accepted for treatment on an outpatient basis.

The patient came from a disturbed family. A number of relatives had threatened or attempted suicide. The patient's mother told him early in life that he was an unwanted child and that she hated him. An authoritarian father threatened him frequently with the devil and hell. From his early years he was fearful, nervous, insecure, and was told by all his family that he was crazy. When fairly young, he had sex play with three of his five sisters and at least one homosexual experience. In school he did well except for a reading disability, which so disturbed him that he attempted suicide three times and once tried to burn down the schoolhouse. This was at the age of 14. At 18 he became emotionally withdrawn and developed strong compulsions and auditory hallucinations for a short time. At 30 he was worried by multiple physical complaints and many obsessive thoughts. In spite of his difficulties he had been able to work on various jobs at an unskilled or semiskilled level until the year before admission. He worked hard and tended to be anxious when jobs piled up that could not be done immediately.

In therapy the patient seemed at ease and talked readily with no blocking, but in a quiet, flat voice. As he talked at length about his symptoms, he dwelt first on hypochondriacal complaints which tended to be bizarre. He described an endless array of symptoms, from washing compulsions and suicidal preoccupations to fears of insanity, and he read to his therapist from long lists which he prepared on various aspects of his problems. He seemed to be a museum of psychopathology, and there was an absence of almost all factors in his general life picture that might be considered normal. After approximately one and a half months of therapy the doctor seeing him recommended that he be admitted to the hospital because of the possibility that he would act out some of his homicidal fantasies. He talked about getting even with all the people in the past who had done him wrong, and he told of plans to kill, mutilate, and dispose of the body of a prostitute who owed him money.

In the hospital the consensus of opinion, after further observation, was that it was unlikely any therapy would be of much value, and commitment to a state hospital was recommended. The patient and his relatives refused to agree to this and he was discharged against advice. A year later he reapplied for admission after having spent part of the interim in another hospital. He appeared to be much the same as before. Invited to join a group therapy class, he dropped out after one session. It had been too exciting for him, he explained.

This patient was much taken by the MMPI. He wanted to buy one for himself, saying, "The Minnesota test is the mother of all tests." He said he would like to be able to take it daily because of the new ideas it gave him, such as calling his attention to the fact that he stepped over cracks in the sidewalk.

E. B.

B. Psth., Asocial M:19:S 867942'13–X (51) 2:23:7
Drug Add.

This 19-year-old youth and another inmate have caused prison officials more trouble with petty disciplinary problems, it has been said, than any other inmates in the penitentiary. They hold the record for abusing themselves by making superficial lacerations on their bodies with pieces of razor blades, rocks, fingernails, and the like. This boy used a dirk knife to sever his right Achilles' tendon, and one month later he was treated for self-laceration of his arms, legs, and body.

The inmate was reared by his parents on a farm. Although he claims to have completed the seventh grade, he earned on tests a grade placement of only 4.9. He left school to "run around"; he traveled over the country as a truck driver and did a little plumbing work. First arrested at the age of 11, for forgery, the boy was next picked up at the age of 15 for burglary. For this offense he received a suspended sentence. At 16 he was sentenced to a state juvenile training school. Six months later he was given a furlough but was soon rearrested, this time for driving while intoxicated.

The prisoner's present sentence is five years for cattle theft. Twenty days after his arrival at the prison he was punished for creating a disturbance in the building. Twice in one year penalties were meted out for self-mutilation and once for agitating and using abusive language to the guards. The following year he attempted to escape and again mutilated himself. For further defiances he was later transferred to the isolation section and spent some time in the psychopathic ward for observation.

The prison psychiatrist reported: "The subject is emotional and unstable, and definitely a psychopathic personality; antisocial in thought and behavior; well oriented in all spheres; and no delusions or hallucinations could be elicited. He knows right from wrong and is legally sane and responsible for his acts."

The prison manager's summary differed slightly. He stated: "I do not believe that either this man or his companion are responsible for their acts, although the prison psychiatrist says they are legally sane. Both have been in and out of the psychopathic ward a number of times. Both men are now in isolation. These two men stabbed the inmate nurse in the psychopathic ward, after which they were transferred to solitary confinement. The subject was caught passing a letter to another inmate in isolation, threatening to kill the Negro porter working in isolation. Both of these boys are known users of benzedrine, and both will be institutional cases the rest of their lives." R. C. K.

B. Psth., Asocial M:25:S 86794'23–1X (65) 2:20:8
Mutilative
Mental Deficiency

The prisoner had a long record as a troublemaker. A list of his recent defiances included attempts to escape, repeated refusal to leave the building for work (each time he received thirty days in solitary confinement), severing the Achilles' tendon of his right heel with a dirk knife, and digging a hole under the wall.

The case record from a private agency indicated that the prisoner was an illegitimate child. Placed in an orphanage, he lived there until the age of 9. He had never seen his father. He was an unwanted child, and his mother had been listless and complaining through the pregnancy. As a child he was pale, thin, fretful, and irritable. He had temper tantrums and was said to be nervous and high-strung through his preschool years. At the age of 5 he would strike and kick during his temper outbursts. He feared being alone and liked the orphanage but was removed at the age of 9 because of his poor behavior. Frequently the temper outbursts were precipitated by his dislike of a piece of wearing apparel. Shortly after he was transferred to a boarding home, he changed from a shy, quiet child to a noisy, talkative one. After eight months in the boarding home he was returned to the orphanage for two years. From that time on he was shifted about from one residence to another until he joined the navy.

His school life was sketchy and unsuccessful. He was poor in all school subjects and particularly slow in reading. He disliked school, never applied himself, and paid no attention to the classroom work. When not permitted his own way in the schoolroom he screamed and yelled and if corrected became sullen and defiant. Three months before he was 16 he left school, not completing the seventh grade. One test showed an I.Q. of 81, another an I.Q. of 70. His work history was as erratic as his school history. For example, he worked as a common laborer for one month, then quit because he was "fed up on common labor." Taking a job as waiter, he stayed at that for two months; he left because he was "tired of the job and wanted to run around." After two months of work on a railroad in another section of the country, he left to go west to determine whether or not a patient in a distant hospital might be his father.

The young man's known criminal career began after an "undesirable discharge" from the navy for repeatedly being AWOL. His first arrest was for attempted burglary of a café; for this he received a ten-month jail sentence. His present offense was breaking into a barber shop, taking money and equipment, and, two hours later, entering an insurance office, taking cash. Officers arrested him the next day as he was walking down the highway. The prisoner felt that he was a victim of injustice and was convinced that money left him by his unknown father was being denied him. He resorted to burglary and crime in a desperate and confused attempt to right these wrongs. He lacked emotional attachments and had no loyalties. It was felt that in all probability he would not develop these while in prison. It was further judged, after an interview and observation, that this man was in need of therapy rather than punishment. R. C. K.

P. Hys. M:12:S:11 +6 '86947-13(39) 4:8:12

This boy had suffered from aphonia for two and a half years. The aphonia began following a tonsillectomy when the patient had said, "Good morning, Mother," and then had not spoken to her or to any other member of his family afterward. The rest of that school year he continued to talk in the schoolroom but he finally became completely mute and continued his schoolwork satisfactorily by writing. Severe punishments, threats, and bribes had been unsuccessful. For a year before the tonsillectomy, after running or playing hard, the patient had had attacks of diffused abdominal pain which were relieved by lying prone.

He started school at age 6 and was in the sixth grade at the time of admission. He had no difficulty with his studies and he was good at farm work, assisting on his uncle's farm at every opportunity. He was described as shy, quiet, and emotionally arrested, but he got along well with his playmates. His father was a chronic alcoholic who did not support his family; when home he was belligerent and obnoxious. At one time, when the child was 3, his father had kidnapped him in a drunken rage and had kept him for a week in his automobile. On the other hand, when his father was sober he was affectionate and generous. His mother was an emotionally immature, clinging person, depending entirely on her 15-year-old daughter to be the head of the household.

On admission to the hospital the patient showed an almost complete lack of emotional reaction. He was complacent and indifferent. No real notion of his mental content could be obtained since he did not write anything but very brief answers to questions. His I.Q. was 88 on the Chicago Nonverbal Test. He established an abnormally close and affectionate relationship with one of the older male patients on the ward and hated to leave when he had to be discharged to another department. He did not talk under sodium amytal. The patient appeared to have been unconsciously rejected by a very closely knit family group consisting of his mother and two sisters. Apparently this rejection occurred because the patient attempted to relate himself to his father. At the time of the onset of the mutism following the tonsillectomy, when he had said, "Good morning," his mother had said, "Your voice sounds like a girl." The secondary gain for him in the hospital seemed to have been tremendous. He was the center of attraction and received extra care and attention. Still mute, he was finally discharged to his mother.

P. React. Depr. F:27:M:71 +28 869′472–(70) 5:10:8

This patient became depressed after the birth of her third child. Her domestic life was not happy and she thought that her husband was not faithful to her. She entered the hospital as a voluntary patient.

One of five children, she received only an elementary education. She had always been delicate, having had rheumatic fever and a weak heart. She was somewhat deaf. At 19 she married a quarryman.

She was diagnosed as having a reactive depression and her condition improved after a course of modified insulin therapy. M. V.

P. Psychas. F:26:M:36 +3 8<u>69</u>47231′–X(59) 2:18:11
P. Mixed +18 8<u>372</u>6′4<u>19</u>–(49) 2:7:11
Suicidal

P. Psychas. F:26:M:83 +35 78'964231-(43) 3:5:18
P. Mixed
Suicidal

For at least two years before admission the patient had had repeated anxiety attacks, and after she was delivered of her third child by Caesarean section she had become progressively more irritable, nervous, and depressed, and also had begun to experience vague fears. When she developed thoughts of harming herself or others she forced her family to restrain her with ropes. She talked of attempts at suicide. As the episode progressed, she became preoccupied, lost interest in her family and in her personal appearance, refused to eat, and slept poorly. At no time did she have clear-cut delusions.

Her past health had been good. There were no previous emotional illnesses though she had had hysterical attacks following unpleasant situations. After high school graduation she had taken nurses' training, and before her marriage she had been a registered nurse. A friendly, cheerful, but somewhat frivolous person, she was described by her mother as having been a "tomboy," and by herself as having been a "spoiled brat," selfish and idealistic. Her general personality was characterized by immaturity. Her husband was a reasonably good partner but moody and not very sociable.

In the hospital the patient expressed strong compulsions to injure or kill herself and others. Outwardly she appeared composed, but she said that she felt she would burst and that her thoughts were mixed up. Well oriented and for the most part emotionally stable, she showed no retardation, no clouding of sensorium, and no defect of intellect. She said that she wanted to go insane, that she did not want to get well. Shortly after admission she tore off a window screen and made several attempts to assault nurses, which necessitated keeping her in restraints for a while. Under fairly intense psychotherapeutic interviews she became more realistic. It developed that she had ambivalent feelings toward her mother and her husband, a definite attraction toward her father, and a great deal of guilt about several unfortunate sexual experiences as a child. She was discharged but was readmitted the next day because of a suicide attempt, which she described as having been primarily a gesture. A course of insulin treatment was discontinued on her insistence, and she was again discharged after arrangements were made for her to continue in the outpatient clinic. It was felt that with adequate follow-up interviews the patient might make a reasonable adjustment in spite of the emotional instability and immaturity present from childhood.

Ps. Sz., Paranoid M:23:S:10 +4 86'97234- 3:10:8

The patient, a university student, was apparently normal until about six months before admission when he suddenly showed marked personality changes. He became excessively preoccupied with his own thoughts; he expressed the feeling that people were against him and that his fellow classmates were jealous of him; editors of the student newspaper were discriminating against him, he complained after he was denied a position on the staff. In addition, he showed hypersensitivity to noise of all kinds, and although he never admitted hearing voices, any noises irritated him. He wrote lengthy letters to newspapers and several to the president of the United States, expressing the belief that he would be able to lead the world out of the depression if given an opportunity. One month before admission he became assaultive toward his girl friend when she refused to go home with him because of his abusive behavior during the evening, and before a friend interceded, the girl was severely beaten.

Of superior intelligence, the patient had always been the center of attention. He had usually insisted on having his own way and his friends considered him conceited. Otherwise, there seemed to be nothing out of the ordinary in his history.

In the hospital he showed marked psychomotor activity. Unable to sit still for any length of time, he played games almost continuously and insisted on being allowed to go home. He had marked ideas of reference. Although he said that none of the staff members "had it in" for him, they "are not courteous to me." Typical of his expressed political views was this statement: "I solved the depression, but I was so young that people tried to undermine my idealism." When an attempt was made to discuss his problems with him, he replied, "I'm sitting tight. I've got plenty in my head which I'm not telling anyone about. There are times when I cannot concentrate because so many things run through my mind. I've been under a strain. The whole world seems to be against me. Right now the future looks black, but there is some hope left." He admitted that "things have not been exactly right for me the past six months"; nevertheless, he thought there was nothing seriously wrong with him and said, "I have had lots of funny ideas, but I guess I will just have to make up my mind to forget them all. I don't belong in any psychopathic ward." One day he expressed the idea that he was not on the psychopathic ward but that the other patients were placed in his room merely as part of his therapy. No appreciable change occurred during his stay on the ward except that he became more resigned to remaining there. He was discharged to go to a state hospital.

Ps. Sz., Paranoid	M:39:M:24	+1	869′724–3X (49)	5:20:9
		+24	–4281739 (49)	4:1:10

The patient's wife had noted a gradual onset, over several months, of overtalkativeness in her husband. Unusually energetic in applying himself to his work, he began to talk excessively about his business problems and to complain of being held back by jealousy on the part of the man over him. A week before admission he began to talk of "Catholics" following him because he had "meddled too much in other people's affairs." Then he became unable to work at all, sat for hours looking into space, and at times talked and acted strangely.

There were no previous psychotic episodes, and apparently the man had been unusually healthy. A high school graduate, he was well liked and active socially. Apparently, however, an important part of this socialization came about after he met the girl who later became his wife, for she took the initiative in socializing him. A conscientious and perfectionistic person, he was compulsive about finishing any task he once undertook. He was successful in sales work and friends described him as "always cheerful and friendly but secretive," and said that "he never talked openly about things."

On admission the patient appeared to be experiencing auditory hallucinations. He also expressed peculiar delusions. There was a disharmony between his affect and his mental content; he laughed heartily and inappropriately, and one of his statements was, "The most important thing is to make children happy. I've made so many people unhappy, what can I do for them now? I must get away where I can have rest and peace. The right for me is preaching the gospel." His most common affect was euphoria. Apparently unconcerned at being in the hospital, he had no insight into his illness. He was well oriented. It was difficult to determine his psychological state because of his circumstantiality and uncooperativeness. After a series of electroshock treatments he immediately began to change; he became subdued and was able to remember his recent bizarre behavior and the incident leading to the hospitalization. About these he said, "I can't understand how I happened to go off the deep end like that." The illness he attributed to the pressures of his work and to being away from home so much. In interviews he became reserved and guarded and gave the impression that he knew what his trouble was but refused to talk about it. In this stage he was inaccessible to psychological approaches, and this general condition remained unchanged until the time of discharge.

Ps. Paranoid	M:38:S:19	+1	8712346'9–(84)	1:12:15
Alcoholism		+9	7812346'9–(84)	0:9:18

This patient's illness began five years before admission, after four years of army duty. The patient became tense and anxious and developed paranoid ideas. One delusion was that others suspected him of being unfaithful to the United States. As a "sense of impending disaster" developed, with agitation, worry, fear, crying spells, and wringing of the hands, he resorted to alcohol. Hospitalized for four months, he returned home, but only for one month, and then was again hospitalized. This time he was discharged after only slight improvement. Eight weeks of "night-clubbing" followed, and then he began to suffer many hallucinatory and delusory experiences. For a year he attempted to write and also to resume study in a university. His inability to concentrate forced him to give up that experiment. Two weeks before admission he went on an alcoholic spree, threatened to jump from a high window, and ended up in the police ward of the city hospital.

The patient's childhood had been deprived and insecure. When he was 10 his father and mother were divorced after a long period of discord. Four years later his father and stepmother also separated. During these stressful years the patient was very unhappy. Following his graduation from high school he attended a university for two years, then did radio work before joining the army.

871'236 49–

A shy person, he was, nevertheless, extroverted and apparently well enough adjusted until the onset of the present symptom picture.

When first examined in the hospital the patient was well oriented and mentally clear. He was concerned with paranoid delusions which he recognized as false but which he could not shake. Able and willing to discuss his problems, he was from the outset cooperative and insightful. Apparently he had suffered considerably from feelings of guilt. The paranoid ideas were initiated in the army intelligence corps where he "was taught to be suspicious of others." There was a positive improvement during this hospitalization, and he was discharged finally after plans had been made for outpatient therapy. A few months later he was admitted to a veterans' psychiatric hospital.

B. Psth., Path. Sexuality	M:34:M:167	+8	871'236 49–(100)	0:16:3
		+140	6'91 834–	1:9:7

The patient was admitted for study under a criminal indictment because of homosexual activity. His sexual history began with accounts of mutual masturbation among a group of teen-age boys at a swimming hole. His first known homosexual experience occurred at age 20 when an older man initiated him. It was about this time that he realized males were more attractive to him than females. He had one or two other experiences before his marriage. He considered girls attractive but had little specific interest in them. He was married at age 25 but shortly after had a love affair with an 18-year-old boy. His wife discovered the alliance and divorced him after a bitter quarrel. The patient threatened suicide because the boy left him at the same time. He underwent a three-month psychiatric treatment but continued his occasional homosexual escapades, until at age 28 he was arrested for molesting two small children. Following the advice of some well-meaning professional people he remarried his wife but was eventually arrested again on a complaint of indecent assault. Under sentence for a prison term he was sent to the psychiatric unit before beginning to serve the term.

A high school graduate, he had done very well in school. After leaving school he was employed in white-collar jobs and was a fairly good worker considering the trouble he got into because of his sexual behavior. He was said to have been reliable, punctual, and efficient. He was average in intelligence and interested in a number of hobbies. Described as quiet and somewhat difficult to get acquainted with, he apparently lacked self-confidence and had a tendency to mild blue spells in which he was self-depreciatory. In speaking he was often blunt and tactless. His sexual relations with his wife, when they occurred, were normal and satisfactory to both. He emphasized that his most gratifying sexual experiences were heterosexual and that these occurred only with his wife. There were two children, and he claimed that it was during his wife's pregnancy that he resumed his homosexual activities.

The physical and neurological examinations on admission were negative.

There was no evidence of a hormonal imbalance. The patient conducted himself in a formally correct manner, showing only mild irritability on a few occasions. While in the hospital he seemed to become more open and comfortable and to develop some insight into his feeling of inferiority. There were no marked evidences of abnormal mentation or behavior. He was discharged on a medical reprieve for a probationary trial at home.

Ps. Sz., Simple   M:25:S:46   +5   87126'493–   1:10:5
Paranoid

The patient's problems appeared very gradually during the course of about a year. The environmental pressures acting on him had gradually increased, the latest event being the departure of his brother for the army. He and his brother had managed a farm together and had been very close friends. After his brother left, the patient became preoccupied, walking around in a disinterested manner and failing to respond to questions. He withdrew from social life, stopped going out with girls, constantly paced the floor, and complained of headaches. When company came to the house he retired to another room. He felt that people stared at him.

After the patient had finished the eighth grade, he had begun to do farm work. At one time he had worked for the W.P.A. but had been discharged after two days. He had always been somewhat sensitive, but he had been a friendly person who had liked to go to parties. He was known to be emotionally stable.

On admission to the hospital he admitted having ideas of reference, and in particular he thought people were talking about him and watching him. He showed psychomotor retardation. He would say, "I'm nervous. I've got a sour stomach." When asked why he had stopped going out to parties, he said, "Oh, no particular reason." Well oriented and mentally intact, he was neither happy nor sad. In appearance he was apathetic and indifferent, and the staff felt that he was on the defensive and that he was holding back a considerable amount of his mental content. At times he was slightly agitated and preoccupied. Once he informed the doctors that somebody was reading his mind. He said he was unable to work because he could not stand the cold, got too nervous, and tired too easily. He had no interest in hospital activities. He was finally transferred to a state hospital.

B. Psth., Asocial   M:14:S:30   0   8714263'9–X(57)   4:19:14
Suicidal
Deteriorated

This boy had been placed under state guardianship when he was 2 years old and had spent most of his life in various boarding homes and boys' schools. He had never adjusted well; his behavior had been poor, he had appeared sly and tricky, and he had bullied younger children. He had frequently run away, and he had stolen large sums of money from several foster homes. In spite of special tutoring, his inability to read was a big problem. In the reform school he was finally sent to he seemed to be suffering a depressive episode. He said, "Life is not worth living if I cannot learn to read," and he made two suicidal attempts. Given a special tutor for reading and a job in the print shop, he improved somewhat but not completely and was sent to the psychiatric unit for evaluation.

For years he had masturbated four or five times daily, apparently in a compulsive way. In the last few months he had experienced terrifying dreams. At age 11 the lad had had rheumatic fever. This recurred several times and greatly limited his physical activities. His parents had been judged intellectually dull, and his mother was known to be sexually promiscuous. Most of his five brothers and sisters were either maladjusted or in an institution for the feeble-minded. The boy himself was of low normal intelligence.

In the hospital he was found to have an enlarged heart, indicating a definite pathology. The neurological examination was grossly normal. Psychometric indications pointed to the strong possibility of an organic brain defect. He showed no gross disturbance in personality, emotions, or intellect, but he expressed much concern about his inability to read, a defect he insisted he wanted to correct. He worked hard at the MMPI and although his scores may not have been entirely valid, nevertheless there was an indication of better reading ability than he claimed to have. Disturbed and puzzled about his uncontrollable masturbation, he believed that it made him "dumber" than he really was. He frequently responded to intellectual problems with "I can't." He had a strong tendency to project all his troubles onto others, and he assumed little responsibility for his own behavior. During his stay in the hospital the boy changed little. He adapted fairly well to the ward and, with some pressure, lived within the rules. His behavior was immature, boisterous, and prankish. No good rapport could be established, and it was difficult to do anything psychotherapeutically to help him. It was felt that his reading defect probably had a generalized organic basis; the possibility of organic brain damage from rheumatic fever remained. The prognosis was considered poor. He was transferred back to the boys' training school.

B. Pri., Child.	M:14:S:87	+1	8716243'9–X (49)	4:21:20
P. Psychas.		+57	'47239– (47)	1:5:13

The patient was referred to the hospital by the court because of exhibitionistic sexual behavior. He had been involved in more than twenty episodes of exposure and exhibitionism. A complaint had been filed nine months before admission and another two months later. He was studied in the outpatient psychiatric service from the date of the second complaint until the time of admission to the inpatient service. Apparently he had made good progress under therapy and was being tutored for his marked reading difficulties when he was reported to the police for feeling an 80-year-old woman's leg and for masturbation. It was following this that he was referred to the inpatient psychiatric service.

Physically the patient had developed normally. His work in a parochial school was very poor. At the time of admission he was in the seventh grade. His I.Q. was 87. He had worked as a paper carrier and was very interested in sports. Superficially friendly and cooperative, he had always been a docile person but easily discouraged.

In the hospital his behavior was acceptable, although he talked very little and answered questions as briefly as possible. No abnormalities of behavior or mentation could be elicited. He was preoccupied with sexual fantasies and described his behavior in ways that made it sound compulsive in nature. He felt he had a problem but accepted no real responsibility in the situation. The early MMPI showed him to be very confused and disturbed and the F score indicated complete invalidity. His father read some of the items to him on the second MMPI and its validity was also questionable. He gained some degree of insight while in the hospital, partly through regular interviews and partly through interviews conducted under sodium amytal. It was felt that his association with an older boy who was also delinquent encouraged some of his tendencies. He was discharged after arrangements had been made to supervise him closely. The prognosis was poor.

Ps. M-D., Depr.	M:17:S:91	+1	87213469'-(53)	1:13:7
		+90	'2719843-(43)	3:1:15

The present illness of this patient began four months before admission, after the youth had worked six weeks for an airline. He had left high school in the junior year to take this job. In the course of the job he alternated every two weeks from one eight-hour shift to another. This irregularity of hours bothered the patient unduly. His sleep became irregular and poor and he began to miss many meals. His eyes bothered him and frontal headaches developed. Listless and disinterested in everything he was doing, he showed confusion at work and worried constantly about completing tasks that previously had been easy for him. Finally he could not make up his mind about whether he should continue work or go back to school. On the advice of a physician he returned to school. In spite of the complete cooperation of teachers and everyone concerned, he found it impossible to continue. His environment seemed unreal to him and eventually he was brought to the hospital on the advice of a local judge.

He had had no previous illness that seemed at all contributory. A serious and scholarly youth, he nevertheless had a keen sense of humor, was liked by his classmates, was neat, and assumed responsibility well. In fact, until the present illness, he seemed to have led an entirely normal life. His interests were athletics, radio work, and airplanes. The boy's father and mother were compatible and no serious problem seemed evident in his home life.

8721436′9–

On admission the youth suffered from self-accusatory ideas. Every small aspect of life loomed as an unsurmountable problem to him. He felt the future held nothing for him. Although he was apathetic and depressed, his mind appeared clear and logical except for this pattern of ideas. He showed psychomotor retardation, and he had to force himself to mingle with other patients. His illness, he thought, was entirely the result of his irregular hours. For the first three weeks he sat most of the time with both hands over his eyes. Toward the end of that period he had an acute depression in which he expressed suicidal ideas. On several occasions he was cheerful in the morning but lapsed into depression toward night. After electroshock therapy he lost much of this depression, began to take part in social activities, and at the time of discharge was fairly normal in behavior and appeared to have recovered.

Ps. Path.	F:28:M:67	+3	8721436′9–(43)	2:14:12
Suicidal		+18	8712463′9–(53)	1:13:10
		+58	72 84631′9–(53)	3:9:9

Nearly a year before admission this young woman had obtained a divorce from her husband. One month later she suddenly felt that "something was wrong" and she experienced an uncontrollable fear. "I couldn't explain the fear and thought I was losing my mind," she said. This feeling progressed so that she had an increasing sense of insecurity and became profoundly depressed. She noticed that she tended to withdraw, became irritable and restless, and was unable to concentrate on anything except the one thought that "I was going insane." A psychiatrist recommended a private hospital, where she received five electroshock treatments but only temporarily improved. Neither did a change of jobs help, and finally when the symptoms became severe, she was forced to stop working. She became sleepless, tremulous, and anorexic. There were no previous psychotic upsets, although she had always been a nervous person.

The patient's father was shiftless, and a family quarrel when the patient was 9 years old resulted in the separation of her parents. The social position of the family was poor and the patient was early conscious of discrimination against her by better class families. She was considered a "wild youngster." In her schoolwork she was one year ahead of her age group. At the age of 17 she became pregnant. She refused to marry the father, an 18-year-old boy. After the birth of her child she finished high school and lived with her father and mother, who were reunited. Later her father left the family again and the mother and daughter carried on a life of sexual promiscuity. At the same time the patient held jobs, one after another, working efficiently at each. She became, however, nervous and run-down. Finally she married a man who had been twice divorced. He was abusive toward her and she separated from him. Before her present illness she was just beginning to feel happy and contented, she said, and according to others' reports, she had indeed been fairly adequate in the support of her son. Superior and efficient in everything she undertook, she was suspicious of other people's intentions, had always felt inferior, and tended to parade her superior intelligence. Although variable in mood, she had generally been carefree and lighthearted and had taken nothing seriously.

When admitted to the hospital the patient was deeply depressed, anxious, and fearful. She was restless and suicidal. There were no obvious defects in sensorium or intellect. Possessed of some insight, she knew that she was mentally ill but was at a loss to explain her fears and anxiety. Neat, quiet, and cooperative in her conduct on the ward, she was fairly open and frank in discussions but tended to cover up her emotional unrest. After further electroshock therapy there was moderate improvement. Neither psychotherapy nor any other procedure shed much light on the exact nature of her illness. When she returned home she was to be followed in outpatient study.

P. Mixed F:16:S:6 +1 872'19346–(53) 3:5:11
P. Psychas.
P. Hys.

For several months this girl had suffered from a severe fear of dying and terrifying dreams, and in addition there had been nausea and vomiting. The symptoms were precipitated by the death of a neighbor girl, possibly due to an abortion. Immediately following this event the patient developed death fantasies in which she imagined herself dying of many and vague conditions; she also complained of "horrid dreams." During this time she ran over a dog. This was a severe shock to her and "snapped all those silly ideas out of my head. I feel normal again and things seem real." She did, however, continue to vomit a couple of times a day; and it was in this state that she was brought to the hospital.

As a child she had been delicate. An average student although not a hard worker, she was about to enter the senior year of high school. She led a normal life and apparently mixed well with both boys and girls. She reported that she had a "nervous breakdown" when she was 8 years old, which included a phobia about having sleeping sickness. Always easily depressed, she tended to daydream. She was described as egocentric, hypochondriacal, pessimistic, easily worried, and always demanding of sympathy.

On admission to the hospital she was well oriented, her answers to questions were normal, and in general she appeared intact. The chief thought content that seemed pertinent was her conviction that she might never get better and might die. What insight she had into her condition was largely verbal. She kept herself neat and clean and was cooperative. In spite of the many activities of the ward she often complained of being lonely and had many crying periods. There were obvious signs of immaturity but none of the gross fears she had previously expressed. At the time of discharge she was little different from what she had been at admission. In spite of the fact that no real understanding of her condition had been reached, her mother insisted upon her leaving against the advice of the staff.

P. Hys.	F:32:M:11	+1	87231′469–(49)	2:7:11
P. Psychas.				
P. Hys.	F:32:M:44	+15	231 6′4897–(53)	5:6:15
P. Psychas.				
P. Mixed	F:32:M:58	+3	8743261′–(49)	1:12:11

For the last two years the patient had become progressively more weak, nervous, and tense and had had persistent headaches, backaches, and occasional tremors. She had noticed feelings of unreality and an indefinite obsessive feeling that some sort of calamity was about to occur. There were occasional paresthetic sensations in her hands and feet, and she was anxious and apprehensive. For many years she had been constipated, she said, and had used laxatives and enemas extensively. During the last six months much of her hair had fallen out, she claimed. Recently her children had "got on her nerves."

The history showed one period of "aphasia." About ten years before admission she had also had an acute attack of "nervousness," but she had taken a vacation and had recovered in a few weeks. After two years of high school she had left to take a job doing housework. She had always enjoyed being with people until the onset of the present symptomatic pattern. She was married at 18 and had two children. The marriage appeared to be successful although the husband was a somewhat ineffectual person, and there was no exchange of confidences between the two.

On admission to the hospital the patient was deeply concerned about her complaints and her inability to control her emotions. She was well oriented, and there were no gross defects in sensorium or intellect. She was tense, alert, unhappy, and irritable. She adapted poorly to the hospital routine, was anxious and demanding, and had to be continually reassured about trivial matters. Several days after admission she had what appeared to be a mild hysterical paresthesia of the right arm. Against advice she left the hospital, remaining at home for sixteen days, and then was readmitted. At home she had developed more specific symptoms—fear of meeting people and apprehension at being left alone with her children because she might harm them. She said that the previous hospitalization had helped her and that she had returned to be "cured." She continued to be very immature, and a firm discipline was maintained in treating her. The therapist said at this time, "A childlike behavior pattern characterizes her method of adjustment." In two weeks she was discharged. Nine months later she was readmitted in an almost identical state. She still refused to discuss her more intimate thoughts. A new worry was that of death, and the old fear that she might kill her children persisted. She was difficult to treat and no significant progress was made before the third discharge.

P. Mixed	M:51:M:11	0	872361′49–	3:14:10
P. Psychas.		+17 mos.	728314′69–(67)	2:8:7

The patient had various somatic complaints and had been treated by a succession of physicians. Outstanding among the symptoms were dizziness, a peculiar congested feeling in his head, nervousness, and irritability. He lacked self-confidence and feared people so much that he tended to avoid them. These symptoms had led to a "nervous breakdown" six years previously. After that he never really recovered, remaining unstable and easily upset, and tending to neglect his business. At the same time the patient's wife had a series of pelvic operations, with a "self-prolonged" convalescence, and was plagued by a pattern of symptoms markedly similar to the patient's.

In all, the patient had only two years of formal education and stopped school at the age of 14 to work in his father's shop. After twenty years in this job he took up sales work and did fairly well until the onset of the symptoms. He had always been nervous, irritable, and impetuous. A zealous and expansive person, he had many friends and was known as goodhearted but selfish and somewhat thoughtless in his dealings with people. His lack of education contributed to his feelings of inferiority.

In the hospital the patient at first was preoccupied with himself and his many complaints nearly all the time. He had a host of peculiar somatic and nervous symptoms but showed neither extreme delusions nor hallucinations. He was excitable and generally expressive, but there were no outbursts of temper or other overactive behavior. A good conversationalist, he made an excellent first impression. However, when one tried to work with him he was stubborn and uncooperative in minor ways. Toward other patients he was selfish and overbearing. Although he improved somewhat in the hospital, the outstanding obsessions and the phobic reaction to crowds remained basically unchanged.

Ps. Sz., Mixed M:21:S 87246′139–(57) 2:14:12

Shortly before admission to the hospital this young veteran, while intoxicated, had broken windows in a garage and had set fire to a shack. There were earlier instances of his setting fire to buildings, and the patient reported dreams in which he had seen his father, mother, and older brother "burning in fire."

The son of oversolicitous, unusually strict parents, this man had shown a poor home adjustment for some time. An intelligent youth, he had finished half a year in college before this admission. Since early childhood he had manifested shyness, seclusiveness, and feelings of inferiority, and had daydreamed frequently. He had always been poorly motivated. Extremely passive, he nevertheless exhibited negativistic attitudes toward authority.

Information brought out in the psychotherapeutic sessions suggested that for this patient fire and burning represented punishment and ways of expressing hostility. The diagnosis was schizophrenic reaction, unclassified. After individual psychotherapy over a period of six weeks he showed no gain in insight and continued to be bothered by headaches, ringing in his ears, and inability to concentrate. He was then given a course of electroshock followed by insulin shock therapy, with psychotherapy continued during the latter. He improved slightly and left the hospital on a trial visit but was unable to adjust. He made few attempts to find a job. After two hours' work he left the only job he did attempt

He returned to the hospital and was given another course in insulin shock therapy concurrently with individual psychotherapy. He showed little or no improvement, and the prognosis for a satisfactory adjustment appeared poor. W. M. H.

P. React. Depr.	F:22:S:14	+13	87<u>24</u>61'<u>39</u>–X	1:17:13
Schizoid				

The illness of this patient had been insidious in onset but had been present at least eighteen months. The young woman had gradually changed from a lively, friendly, alert person to one who was morose, weepy, and increasingly nervous. After she was discharged from her job because of these symptoms, she became inactive, ate poorly, lost weight, and slept little. She was distant, detached, and ambivalent toward her fiancé. She herself felt that the problems represented an outgrowth of feelings of inferiority which had been present most of her life.

In the past medical history there were numerous minor difficulties of a general hysterical type, including palpitations and vomiting. After four years of good work in high school she listlessly spent a year at a university, withdrawing to enroll in a business course which she also failed to complete. She then worked as a file clerk but was very nervous and was not good at the job. She had always been a fairly social person, yet her ways of thinking were peculiar. In college her themes were often marked "incoherent."

In the hospital the patient said, "I'm confused." She discussed her problems slowly and with long pauses. Most of her answers were irrelevant, many completely incoherent. At some times she wept freely and seemed depressed, at others she laughed and joked freely. Much of the time she seemed queer and detached. There were no obvious hallucinatory or delusory states. She took little active interest in ward activities, preferring to stay in bed. Her appetite was poor and she talked little. Occasionally for a time she would discuss things coherently, but these periods were short-lived. She could not make decisions, nor did she obey orders well. Asserting that she did not like the hospital, she appeared eager to leave until arrangements were completed for her discharge. Then, suddenly, she reversed her attitude and desired to remain. She was discharged, however, to stay with her sisters. It was feared that a definite schizophrenic pattern might later develop.

P. React. Depr.	M:23:S:83	+1	87<u>2'4</u>631–9(61)	5:13:12
B. Psth., Path. Emot.		+75	2'3<u>61</u>–9(67)	3:9:17
Schizoid				
Mutilative				

This young man was apparently well until his enlistment in the army four and a half years before admission. He found adjustment in the service difficult and while overseas began to drink excessively. This was unusual behavior for him.

One day he "almost blew up" after a month of steady combat. He felt that his nerves were "out of his skin"; he was irritable, nervous, jittery, and afraid to sleep. The next morning, while lying in a foxhole, he shot himself in the right leg with a rifle so that he would be "out for a long time." The self-inflicted wound was treated as an accident, and he was eventually evacuated and hospitalized for more than a year. During this period he went AWOL twice for no apparent reason. The second time he was punished by three months in the guardhouse and a fine of two thirds of his pay. At this time he began to develop depression, shame, and guilt, felt confused, and was under considerable tension. These symptoms led him to resume his drinking. The difficulties continued more or less chronically after his discharge, and once he attempted suicide by taking phenobarbital. After that he isolated himself entirely from social contacts and finally sought psychiatric advice.

The patient's childhood was marked by mild irregularity. He ran away from home when he was 10 but was quickly found and returned. At 17 he went to another state to live with a relative. Refusing to attend school there, he went to work; he was not very successful, however, and was returned to school by his father. At 18 he graduated from high school. His intelligence was above average. The history continued with similar irregularities until his army experience. Always bothered by feelings of inferiority, he tried to compensate by acting superior toward other people. He was asocial, ineffectual in his adjustments, and prone to temper outbursts. In school he constantly found fault with teachers. He had some talent in art but overemphasized this. He had little interest in girls. He was impulsive and exercised poor judgment in financial matters. He harbored tremendous hostility toward his mother and sister and expressed it freely.

In the psychiatric unit he was well oriented. Although depressed and serious, he would smile at times. He was for the most part withdrawn and markedly introspective. No gross disturbances of sensorium or intellect could be found. His stay in the hospital was accompanied by little change in his condition. He was put on insulin subcoma therapy, but this was discontinued because he claimed that his "mind went black," inhibiting ideas that he thought might help him solve his problems. Electroshock therapy and state hospitalization were discussed with him, but he would not consent to either course and believed he was well enough to get along outside the hospital. He clung to this decision even though the staff members felt his recovery was insufficient to justify his optimism. He was discharged to continue in the outpatient department.

P. Hypo. P. Psychas.	M:18:S:60	+4	87261′34–9	1:10:8
P. Psychas. Schizoid	M:18:S:82	+11	78′241–39	0:8:10

This patient entered a general hospital for observation because he thought he was afflicted with lockjaw. Physical studies and thorough reassurance did not wholly alleviate his fear; and with his discharge he became restless, agitated, and uncooperative, refusing to eat, dress, or leave his room. These symptoms gradually became worse and were unmodified by reasoning with him. He was then admitted to the psychiatric unit.

As a child he had always been upset by trivial injuries. A bashful boy, he had resented being teased about girls. He was so closely attached to his mother that he had found it difficult to leave her even to go to school, but he had always been critical of his father. There was a long-standing self-condemnation for being "selfish, stubborn, impolite, and unaffectionate."

During his hospitalization he was relatively at ease. In spite of marked obsessive compulsions he could always be temporarily reassured; but as soon as he left the hospital temporarily or was away from professional contacts, his convictions returned to him. There was an admitted lack of any sustained desire to get well, which he explained by saying that he had no hope or desire to do any specific thing in the future. His family was advised that he should go to a state institution; but when the patient strenuously objected, he was finally taken home, although it seemed improbable that he would be able to adjust. He was readmitted five days later because of the return of his morbid fears and later was again discharged to go to his home.

Ps. M-D., Depr. M:49:M:13 +1 8726′341–9 (59) 2:10:9

Ps. M-D., Depr. M:50:M:11 +1 72849′63– (51) 2:5:9

The patient's first attack of depression had occurred three years before admission when he developed irritability, crying spells, inability to concentrate, a feeling of hopelessness, and the thought that all his hard work had been for nothing. He made a spontaneous recovery in six months but again became depressed and irritable, with dizzy spells added to the previous pattern. He was unable to relax and was sorry for himself. He complained that his wife had not helped him with his business problems and would not go out socially. He was disturbed because his youngest son had decided to become a minister instead of going into his business. He had a number of ideas about what he had done wrong in running his business, and he had arguments with his wife about how things should have been done.

There were a few times in the past when the patient had apparently been hypomanic for short periods. He was forced to leave school after finishing the eighth grade because his parents needed someone to help them in their business, which the patient took over after their retirement. His I.Q. was 120. He was a "sober" man, a chronic worrier, and a perfectionist. He had built the business up until it was a very good one. He was well liked in the community but had no close friends. The chief reason he gave for not having gone out much with people in recent years was that they might see something wrong with him. The patient and his wife were compatible.

On admission he was found to be obese and showed some evidence of retinal arteriosclerosis. He talked freely, saying that he felt he had got considerably better before admission. He was chiefly concerned about his depression. He also worried about his business. There was no gross defect of intellect, and he seemed to have good insight into the fact that he had a mental illness. He was restless but cooperative and friendly. He made a spontaneous and steady improvement, so that at the time of discharge he seemed to be normal. It was felt by the staff that this episode would probably be followed sooner or later by others.

Ps. Sz., Paranoid M:26:M:50 +7 87<u>2</u>6413'9–(59) 3:5:29

This patient was referred by his college instructors, who feared he was about to do something serious, possibly make homicidal attacks. He was in a state of confusion with a number of bizarre hallucinations. One of these was that people carried positive and negative charges of electricity which made for attractions and repulsions (he was studying radio at the time). "One must watch these repulsions and attractions for they are apt to draw one sexually," he said. "If you aren't careful, a woman might rob you of your sex organs." In order to check this hypothesis he dodged around the tables in a class one day to avoid touching people. Concerned with a "drawing up" of his genitals in a number of social situations, he also felt that his wife was "doing strange things" to him. Arrangements were made to get him into a veterans' hospital, and during the interim he was accepted for counseling.

Coming from a small community, the patient belonged to one of the better families there. In high school he was an outstanding leader—captain of the football team and a leading character in the junior class play. In the service he found that he was no longer the center of attraction: "The army was so big, there were too many people, and there was so much that I didn't know." Strong feelings of inferiority and finally confusion appeared. Immediately after leaving the service, he married and entered college. Again he found himself in a difficult situation and the problem was increased by his wife's pregnancy. Panic and confusion followed, ending in the delusions.

During therapy the young man was apprehensive and difficult to contact because of the delusions and because of a marked Negro dialect. In the solution of his problems he leaned heavily on the therapist. Within a week's time came a rapid, dramatic resolution. He was able to analyze his problem even to the point of explaining the hallucinations: "I think people tried to help me get better but I misunderstood and thought they were trying to make me worse. . . . I guess I worried about it too much. I twisted things in the wrong direction. . . . When you get as mixed up as I was you believe anything that seems to explain it." Following the therapy he left school and took a job in a filling station. The last report we have is that his vocational performance has been exceedingly satisfactory.

A. S.

Ps. Sz., Mixed	F:24:S:80	+1	87264'39–(66)	2:13:12
		+24	86724'913–X(59)	2:19:9
		+59	879'62 43–(45)	3:9:9

For a month before admission this young woman had been increasingly irritable and generally upset. She became reluctant to have people near, although she still tried to go out with a few close friends and with her fiancé. At her friends' urging she took a teaching position in a high school, but after one week she resigned because she felt she "wasn't capable of handling it." With increased feelings of inadequacy she then returned to the home of an aunt. God had taken all her knowledge away from her, she said. She controlled herself fairly well before others until two weeks before admission when she became extremely depressed, wept hour after hour, and repeated over and over that she wished to die.

A college graduate, she had majored in home economics. There was no history of any previous mental upset, and she was active in various organizations. Her childhood had been somewhat chaotic. She stayed with her grandparents as she grew up because they enjoyed her company so much that they persuaded her parents to let her live with them. She was conceived before the marriage of her parents and it was her own conviction that she was illegitimate. The young woman's fiancé was described as being intelligent and having a dynamic personality. He was an instructor in a small college. Although he seemed to be fond of the patient and considerate of her, she expressed the thought that he did not love her. The courtship had been "too matter-of-fact," she said. The young man was unromantic and wanted her only for a housekeeper, according to the patient.

On admission to the hospital she was well composed and apparently normal. Tests showed an I.Q. of 115. Depressed and hopeless, she admitted the possibility that she might be helped, but obviously doubted it. There was no evidence of hallucinatory or delusory experiences except for the repeated assertion that God had taken all her knowledge away from her and that she must enter grade school again. At first she made little progress and cried much of the time. After seven electroshock treatments she became more cheerful, began to make plans for the future, and forgot the idea that she had lost her learning and intellect. Just before she was to be discharged she suddenly became depressed again. After this second depression she got better but at the time of discharge still maintained that she "must go to the first grade again." It was recommended that she enter a rest home for further care.

Ps. M-D., Depr.	F:43:M:96	+5	8'7269–31(88)	0:8:5
P. Psychas.		+65	476'382–(51)	5:5:17
Suicidal				

Four months before admission the patient woke up one morning obsessed with evil thoughts against God. No amount of effort on her part could free her mind of these thoughts. She became greatly disturbed and although she had had considerable religious training, she lost interest in the church. Because she had been depressed a year before and had improved after thyroid treatment, she was given the same treatment for this episode, got better, and stayed that way for about a month. She had a normal menstrual period but then developed the fixed belief that she was pregnant. A physician reassured her on the matter but he did not convince her. She lost interest in her home, her appearance, and her friends. She frequently told her husband that her condition was hopeless and that he should send her away. Once she attempted suicide by wading into the river but did not have the nerve to drown herself. Her husband did not believe this story even after he saw the wet clothes hanging in the closet. This indifference on his part apparently led to her making a threat to harm her youngest son in order to gain her husband's cooperation in considering her ill.

Earlier in life, shortly before her marriage, she had become obsessed with "immodest and immoral thoughts" and had been in a dilemma about whether she should follow a religious life or marry. She had to stop working for several weeks but recovered from this conflict without special treatment. A year and a half before admission she had a spontaneous abortion, which she believed was caused by her misdeeds.

She was a graduate of a two-year business college course and apparently had always been a good student. Afterward she obtained a job as a bookkeeper in a store operated by her present husband. As a child she had constantly been warned against the evils of men and the sins of the world. These teachings had a profound effect upon her. She was quiet and shy, showing little self-expression, and was conscientious about her work and her family duties. She always took considerable interest in her own family and its doings, having few hobbies or interests outside of the home, although she belonged to several women's clubs. Her marital life had apparently been happy.

In the hospital, concern over the presence of the "evil thoughts" about God was uppermost in the patient's mind. She considered her condition hopeless and wondered what would become of her family. Although she still had the fixed belief that she was pregnant, this did not seem to worry her. She was intact in intellect and regarded any questioning or attempts at psychotherapy as silly and a waste of money. She was obviously depressed, preferred to be alone, and was passive in reaction to the hospital routine. Gradually she became more responsive and two electroshock treatments were given. After the second one she requested that they be stopped because "they might harm the baby," but she was more alert and responsive. She cried, began to pray, and asked to see a priest. "I feel like fighting now," she said. The idea that she was pregnant gradually faded. She believed at the time of discharge that she could get completely well if she had something to occupy her mind. Some of her thoughts about God still existed; however, she said, "They are not there all the time now, and I can put them out of my mind if I have something to think about."

P. Hys. M:24:S 87<u>26</u> <u>91</u> <u>43′</u>–X (80) 1:16:4

This young man, a private, was referred to the psychiatrist because of a bizarre episode of amnesia in which he was unable to identify himself and had no recollection of either the recent or the remote past. No history of a precipitating emotional trauma could be ascertained.

Born to Italian parents, the soldier was one of ten children. Of these, seven were the children of his parents' previous marriages. Both parents were emotionally labile and quarreled frequently. The father had been an alcoholic during his earlier life. The patient made a poor record in school, although he did complete high school. He was a truant and also was brought into juvenile court on several occasions for petty larceny. In his late teens he went "on the bum" for a period and once "rode the rails" for several consecutive days. His work history followed the same uneven pattern as his school career; he changed jobs frequently and was considered unreliable.

After about ten days in the hospital the patient's confusional state cleared. Intravenous pentothal had no significant effect on this process. Because of certain discrepancies in his behavior and the test results, dissimulation was suspected. He frankly admitted hostility toward the army. Were his mother not living, he said, he would have gone to "any lengths" to obtain his discharge. Returned to duty for further observation, he did not come to the attention of the psychiatrist again. A. T. K.

P. Mixed F:29:S:329 +3 87269'43–(55) 0:15:10

The patient was admitted to the hospital because of complaints of depression, a confused feeling, loss of confidence, and feelings of social inferiority of approximately one month's duration. She reported that during the last several months she had gradually felt more nervous and insecure at her job. Her colleagues at work and her friends, she felt, were beginning to treat her as she "had always treated them," by being sarcastic, belittling, hypercritical, and the like. As she made more and more mistakes she began to believe that she was not qualified for her job.

Always nervous as a child, she had also been negativistic and a disciplinary problem. Her resistance to her mother's authority continued through adolescence but was never a problem outside the home. Her mother, the dominant member of the household, was a cold woman. The patient felt she could never talk to her mother in spite of the fact that the woman was intelligent and made a conscientious effort to do "what was right" for her daughter. The patient did fairly well in school, obtained a B.A., and then held various secretarial jobs. Although she had a number of close friendships with girls she had little personal contact with boys or men and no sexual experience. Her father, who was described as kind, affectionate, and respected, did not play much part in her life. The patient tended to be too critical of men and felt too shy and inferior to get along with those she did like. Ambitious, she was eager to achieve success through competition.

On admission the patient was extremely polite, in a "soldierly" fashion, standing at attention until asked to sit down, and so on. She had a quick, somewhat masculine gait and wore slacks. She spoke in a sincere, relevant way, crying at times when discussing some of her problems, the rest of the time sitting tensely on the edge of her chair. She was moderately depressed and expressed ideas of reference bordering on the paranoid about people in her office. People were mocking her, she believed, and life was passing her by. She was seen frequently for psychotherapy and said she looked forward to getting well and to "readjusting" herself in a "constructive fashion." After three weeks her depression was gone and she was much less anxious; she was discharged from the hospital as improved. She returned immediately as an outpatient and was seen for 21 interviews over a ten-month period. She seemed to profit by this, taking an active interest in discussing her personal problems. At the time the case was closed, she had moved away from home, had a boy friend, and was feeling optimistic. E. B.

B. Psth., Path. Emot.	F:35:M:60	+1	872'96134–	1:12:4
		+20 mos.	9864'2137–	1:15:6

Six years before admission the patient had first shown severe fits of temper, according to her husband. Although they had originally occurred about every six months they had gradually increased in frequency until at the time of admission they were recurring without provocation every few days. After building up to an attack for a few hours she would suddenly be unable to control herself and would fly into a rage that lasted for only a few minutes; during the rage she broke anything she could lay her hands on. Although she had never struck or actually injured anybody, she had threatened to harm her husband. After one of these rages she was extremely fatigued, weak, and listless; between outbursts she was restless, irritable, and nervous. She had been subject to milder temper tantrums all her life. In recent years she had also had blinding headaches, lasting for several hours, that were so severe they "felt like the top of my head was coming off." Occasionally she vomited. In the past few weeks she had neglected her household, had seemed to lose interest in her friends, and had developed various physical complaints. At some times she was very unhappy but at others she was "on top of the world."

Before the particular symptomatic history of the present illness, she had had no obvious neurotic or psychotic difficulties, although her health had not been good and there was a possibility of several psychosomatic disorders. She had had one child out of wedlock and had eventually married the brother of the child's father. Although the child lived with the patient's mother, the little girl was unaware of her parentage. The patient had always been a shy, aloof, pessimistic, and retiring person. Given to daydreams, she was always afraid of what others thought of her and had trouble looking anyone in the eye. Her grades were very poor, and she did not graduate from high school until age 21. She attributed this poor record to a lack of concentration and a failure to study. She had practiced masturbation from the time she was a small child and even after marriage had preferred masturbation to sexual intercourse.

8731'24 96–

On her admission to the hospital considerable attention was given to physiological studies and to the neurological examination, which were all negative. The patient expressed considerable jealousy about her husband's interest in other women and said that one episode was a factor in the temper rage that had led to her hospitalization. During a drive her husband had been so attentive to another woman, who was riding in the middle of the front seat, that the patient had become angry and had got out of the car, insisting that she would not ride any farther. Once she had found him in bed with another woman, and he had told her that he had had an illegitimate child before their marriage. He was an unsuccessful farmer, and the financial insecurity of their home also bothered her. She wanted better things in life and thought that she had been repressed and held down without adequate self-expression. Her I.Q. was about 125. She recognized the hospital as a place where she could probably be fairly happy because it provided her with relief from her environment. Impulsive, selfish, domineering, and immature, she had several minor temper outbursts, but in general she was cooperative, friendly, and agreeable, except when she was expected to conform to rules. Little change was effected during her hospitalization.

Ps. M-D., Depr.   M:43:M:66   +11   8731'24 96–   9:4:23

The patient's present depression began about two months before admission when he developed an inability to concentrate, was irritable, and had severe feelings of inferiority. Shortly afterward he became obsessed with delusional material made up of events that had occurred twenty years before. He said that at that time he had once been intoxicated and had boasted before a large number of people that he was a member of a famous band of outlaws; he also said that he had committed fellatio with his brother. Lately he had become concerned about the possibility that he was a victim of neurosyphilis. In his fear that he was losing his mind, he withdrew from social contacts, had difficulty in sleeping, and developed severe headaches.

Twenty years before admission he had had syphilitic lesions which apparently had been inadequately treated. Nine years before admission he had become shy and so concerned about the possibility that he might have a general paresis that he was admitted to a state hospital, where he was given malariotherapy. The serological reaction after that was negative for syphilis.

Because he had disliked school he had discontinued his education at age 13 when he was in the sixth grade, and he had spent most of his life as a traveling salesman. While he had always made a fair living he had never been completely satisfied with his lot. He appeared to others as a self-reliant person, but he had always had a tendency to become easily depressed, and by nature he was shy and sensitive. One of his avocational interests was reading medical and psychiatric publications.

In the hospital he was apprehensive about the two boasts he had made twenty years earlier, and he was afraid that he was losing his mind. There were no obvious defects in his intellect, nor were there gross defects of sensorium, but in spite of an obvious effort to appear jovial, he was suspicious, expressed marked feelings of guilt, and appeared to be agitated and depressed. He answered questions readily and in general seemed superficially alert. There was no real improvement in the hospital; at the time of discharge the depression had increased in severity, and he was so ill at ease that he was unable to participate in ward activities. It appeared that he would probably need a long hospitalization, and he was transferred to a state hospital.

P. Psychas. F:40:M:49 +5 8732 61′49–(41) 1:15:15
+39 78′326 49–(39) 3:5:16

For a year before admission the patient, always a high-strung person, had been extremely nervous. Then about six months before hospitalization she had developed indecisiveness and obsessive erotic ideas about her son and other men and about killing her child, her husband, and others such as her husband's mother. She feared being left alone because of these ideas. Treated for some time by a psychiatrist, she did not improve and was in an almost constant state of panic. She finally came to the psychiatric unit.

A college graduate with a good scholastic record, the patient had always had high standards of accomplishment. Before she was married, she taught school. She was active socially and a leader in school and community affairs. Her regard for herself was high, and apparently she had never learned to adjust with equanimity to any of her own shortcomings or possible antisocial impulses. At all costs she avoided turmoil or unpleasantness in her relations with others. She was proud of maintaining an excellent personal appearance. Her watchword was *conformity,* and she was almost ritualistic in her pattern of living. The marital situation appeared to be fair.

On admission the patient was agitated and tearful and kept repeating, "I just can't go on another minute." There were no gross disturbances of sensorium or intellect. She continually sought reassurance and protection, and she was pessimistic and depressed during the first week or two. After electroshock therapy she was much better but almost immediately relapsed. She was given more shock treatment and improved again. At this stage she was discharged to return to her home. The prognosis was doubtfully good.

P. Mixed F:14:S:30 +3 873′42–(66) 7:6:7
P. Hys.

This girl had been admitted to the pediatric service and had spent five months there before the psychiatric unit admission. The diagnosis in the earlier admission was hysterical blindness. At first, in the pediatric ward, she was a difficult patient, extremely apprehensive and anxious. She shunned other patients, cried continuously, had several "convulsions," and demanded attention. During the second month she became more sociable and cooperative, although the depression and crying continued periodically. She was discharged to a foster home, but this did not work out because she was unable to form a parent-child relationship and she misinterpreted many minor incidents. Both the patient and the foster parents were eager to make the placement a success, but apparently the girl could not change rapidly enough to "accept" a good home. She ran away and was then brought to the psychiatric unit.

The patient was in the eighth grade at the time of the present admission. Her I.Q. was above 130. She had few friends, young or old. Before the present problems appeared she had been in good physical condition. Always a sensitive girl, she was somewhat withdrawn, ill at ease, overly careful not to hurt anyone's feelings in conversation. Her home life was complicated and unhealthy, with a mother who was an unhospitalized but definite case of schizophrenia and a stepfather who was punitive toward her. In such an atmosphere there was no opportunity for the girl to form a normal parent-child relationship.

In the unit the patient was worried about her difficulties in getting along with people and being liked by them. Concerned about her future, she wondered if she could overcome her hypersensitiveness and lead a normal life. Her fear that she might say something to hurt someone was marked. At first she was dramatic and fearful, inaccessible and asocial. As she became better acquainted with other patients and the staff she showed more stability and appeared to be happier. She took part in group activities and in general improved steadily. She was finally discharged to go to another foster home.

Ps. Sz., Hebe. F:16:S:20 +20 8742'1369 (53) 7:15:19

This girl's present illness began four years before admission when she was ordered to bed for a year because of "thyroid trouble." When she returned to school it was difficult for her to make friends, and she said it was "hard to get into circulation." She wanted to be a leader yet realized she did not have the qualities necessary to be one. She stayed away from her schoolmates, began to be afraid of visiting her relatives, and felt that she would cause trouble by "not doing things right." One day during the last year she came home saying that a boy had "looked at her in the wrong way." After that the phrase became an obsession with her and she told people that she was "looking in the wrong place." Recently she had begun to hear voices, particularly a child's voice that said, "Come in," or "Come here," and singing.

The girl's past history was not particularly contributory. She had no real trouble with her schoolwork; she worked hard and received fairly good grades. She was in the ninth grade at the time of admission. Although her friends were few in number, those she had were close and reliable. Always a sensitive girl, she was shy and reserved, somewhat more serious than others of her age. She did not, however, particularly stand out as different. She loved to read fashion magazines and often expressed the desire to be a designer. The girl's family seemed to be ordinary.

In the hospital she was troubled by her hallucinations. She was obsessed with the idea that she had been breaking one of the Ten Commandments, the one forbidding adultery. Well oriented for time, place, and person, she appeared to have normal intellect. Usually apathetic, she became agitated at times and scratched or struck at the nurses. For hours she sat and stared into space. Sometimes she demanded favors, such as the use of the telephone or a trip home. For eight days she showed almost no change, the hallucinations continued, and she kept to herself a great deal. Then she threatened to break a window, refusing to stay "in any place which does not keep the Ten Commandments." She was placed in a disturbed ward, where she remained most of the time thereafter during her hospitalization. Despite the recommendation that she be sent to the state hospital, the girl's family finally decided to take her home to see if she could be handled there.

P. Anxiety State	F:20:S:30	+3	874231'96–X (43)	6:17:12
Suicidal		+20	87'439126–(30)	4:7:17
		+169	8'71436–9 (51)	4:8:14

The patient had been emotionally upset for several months before admission. The upset consisted of depression and anxious preoccupation marked by thoughts of suicide. Later, interviews revealed that these symptoms were derived from guilt feelings about masturbation and from a conflict between her sexual impulses and her religious scruples. She had had crying spells since age 12. These were partly related to weekly beatings her mother received at the hands of her drunken father. During the past year the patient had seen physicians, chiropractors, and osteopaths for various somatic complaints that had kept her in bed a good part of the time. She regularly felt dizzy, noticed a blurring of her vision, and suffered from insomnia and nightmares.

The patient had grown up in an atmosphere pervaded by the drunk and malevolent father. She was a high school graduate with a good record, and she had been employed as a clerical worker for several different firms. For a while she had studied for missionary work. Apparently well liked, she had many friends, including several boy friends. She was easily upset and frequently complained to her mother when she got up in the morning that she felt depressed.

She was fretful and at times anguished while in the hospital. This behavior apparently stemmed from her religious and moral feelings about her sexual desires. She was open about a frequent fantasy in which she had a child of her own. Her mood shifted often from normal to somewhat depressed. She was immature and was prone to resort to attention-getting behavior. Her treatment consisted of psychotherapeutic discussions; the intention was to permit complete self-understanding and an expression of her problems. After the first week there were no more episodes of acute anxiety and she began to get some degree of insight. She appeared a little more mature. Obviously the process begun in the hospital would have to continue over a considerable time if she was to get much better.

P. Anxiety State	M:25:S	87 426'391–(78)	4:13:11
P. Psychas.			

This college student came to the office complaining of crying spells, constant worry, and inability to sleep in spite of sedatives.

He was exceedingly condescending in speaking of the poverty and lack of cultural background of his father and mother. In spite of a strong religious background, they continually bickered. The patient was attempting to work his way through college but was undecided about his goal, which vacillated between the ministry and music.

His concern about his vocational goal was predominant in his first visits but soon was replaced by a concern about his masturbatory activity. He was rigid, extraordinarily punitive, demanding, critical toward girls, and alternately supercilious and self-punitory. After four interviews he alleged improvement in his insomnia and his ability to concentrate, apparently as a result of developing better defenses against his sexual concerns. C. K. A.

B. Psth., Mixed	F:19:S:26	—63	8742'6913–(45)	2:15:6
Alcoholism		+70	87'492 16–3 (49)	1:10:10
Suicidal		—74	8742'6139–X (47)	1:21:9
		+132	78'492–3 (53)	1:8:11

The patient was admitted to the hospital with "a feeling of unworthiness" following an alcoholic orgy. The onset of the problem was insidious. She had first been referred to the outpatient department after a suicide attempt some five months before admission, when she had taken an overdose of barbiturates. There were three previous attempts at suicide, the first by drinking lysol when she was 15 years of age. Later she attempted to slash her wrists, and shortly after, she took an overdose of barbiturates. Since age 15 she had had "hysterical attacks" in which she would cry and shake. She also had insomnia, tachycardia, palpitations, headaches, pressure sensations in her chest, "sticking in the throat," and many other symptoms. These gradually gave way to a "don't care" attitude with withdrawal. She was a "lone drinker" when she was financially able and had been smoking two packages of cigarettes a day for eight years. An affair with a young man and a drinking spree left her with such profound guilt feelings and feelings of hopelessness that she came to the hospital.

876'12–4

Although she finished the eighth grade without difficulty and did fairly well, she was removed from school at the age of 13 by her parents. Unable to hold any office job longer than two months, she was relatively efficient in housework. Lacking aggressiveness and initiative, she always shrugged her shoulders at difficulties. Since the age of 7, she had been stealing small articles. Preferring slacks, she would never wear a dress. She was friendly and somewhat detached. Her father was a very stern man, a pathological drinker who was often brutal and offensive. The entire family was marked by tension, nervousness, and general marital discord.

On admission the patient showed overt concern about trivial matters such as cigarettes, which she was not allowed to have. She blocked when questioned about family and sexual matters, smiled inappropriately, and pretended disregard for her problem. She explained many of her difficulties on the grounds of "terrible" environmental influences. Her intelligence was dull normal. Although she was well oriented and apparently mentally clear, she was vague in giving details and was reluctant to mix with other patients. Seemingly she was ill at ease and shy. She was caught breaking the ward routine on a number of occasions and her two closest associates on the ward were young psychopathic patients. It was felt that during the hospitalization she developed some little insight but she was unable to organize her assets well enough to institute any definite plans. No particular approach seemed to be effective with her, and she was discharged with the recommendation that she be more adequately supervised.

P. Hys.	F:17:S:34	+6	876'12–4	1:8:6
P. Hypo.		+18	87129'634–	2:7:8
Schizoid				

The patient was apparently well until six months before admission, when she suddenly became homesick while visiting a sister. She demanded to be taken home to her mother, claiming that was all she needed. On reaching home she did appear normal for five months, then complained that her body felt numb and dead. She scratched her leg to make sure that she still had blood. When questioned she described her physical condition with an apparent lack of concern and expressed confidence that it could be cured by the doctors.

In school the patient failed the second and fourth grade, and left in the middle of the eighth grade at age 16. After that she lived at home and worked for brief periods as a domestic. Always a quiet, shut-in individual and closely attached to her family, she did not make normal social contacts and did not adjust to periods of work away from home. In each such job she was torn between her desire to quit and her fear of telling her employer she wanted to leave. Reluctant, also, to admit her feelings to her family, she solved the dilemma repeatedly by faking physical illness. Her intelligence was low normal.

On admission the patient complained that she felt numb, as if her body were dead. As she described this there was no show of emotion. She was quiet, talking little either with staff members or with other patients, but she was, in general, cooperative. As time went on the somatic complaint and the peculiar feelings disappeared and were no longer evident by the time of discharge. She returned to her home but it was felt not unlikely that she would later show a definite schizophrenic pattern of symptoms.

P. Mixed	F:23:S:25	?	876231'49–X (55)	3:19:10
Schizoid		+25	7'92368–(37)	2:3:14

This young woman's acute illness, which was marked by depression, feelings of unreality, and inability to make decisions, had begun insidiously four months before admission with a general loss of interest in activities and a difficulty in making decisions. Leaving her job, she returned to her home but was restless, depressed, and seclusive. There were frequent crying spells and she was irritable toward other members of her family. She had had one previous nervous breakdown four years earlier, which apparently had followed a similar pattern. That collapse she attributed to difficulties with a woman she had worked with. Apparently she had made a good recovery after several months.

A high school graduate, she had worked in offices and had been considered a satisfactory employee. She engaged in a fairly active social life and had many friends. A love affair had been terminated because of religious differences, but when the present illness began she returned to this man. Regarded as an easygoing, friendly person, she was conscientious and not usually moody. Her intelligence was high average. To a somewhat more than average degree, she was dependent upon her mother and her older sister.

In the hospital her sensorium and intellect were normal. She was apathetic and somewhat retarded. A defensiveness was apparent, but she tried to cooperate. With the hospitalization she improved considerably and appeared to recover from the acute illness. There was no definite evidence of bizarre mentation or other schizoid signs, but the staff felt that there were definitely pre-schizoid factors in the case. At the time of discharge she was relatively better and left the hospital to continue in the outpatient department and to take up a new job.

B. Psth., Asocial	M:19:S:9	+1	879 46'2–(45)	4:15:9

The present problems of this patient apparently dated back at least seven years to a state training school commitment by the juvenile court because of incorrigibility. He had been paroled on six different occasions but each time had broken parole or had returned to the school voluntarily. The authorities had tried various things, including farm placements and several kinds of jobs. He would return home when he was paroled, but there he would quarrel with his parents and would become so angry that he would leave for several hours. Shortly before admission to the hospital he stayed away from home longer, rooming with other boys from the reform school. Living on his own cost money and he returned to borrow from his mother. She refused to give him any money and he took his brother's radio and sold it. His parents had him picked up again by the parole agent, and he was brought to the psychiatric hospital for examination.

He finished the sixth grade at age 11, after having considerable difficulty in school. His I.Q. was in the average range. He then became a behavior problem; stealing was the main reason for his first commitment. When he was about 12 and on parole he began drinking heavily and running around with a group of "rowdies." He seemed unable to learn from his experiences and could not establish a personal relationship with anyone except other reform school boys. He was never willing to accept criticism or help. The family was free of obvious contributory factors.

The patient had a difficulty in his speech but no true stammer. He showed no hostility to the hospitalization. In fact he seemed well satisfied with it. Superficially he was extremely unrealistic. This was evident particularly in his statements about his behavior and his future. Although he became upset and angry when referring to his family, he always appeared to be on a superficial level emotionally. He fitted in fairly well with the ward routine and appeared comfortable and unconcerned. Every indication was that he lived only from day to day. After considerable study he was discharged to stay in a carefully selected foster home. There was little expectation that this would work and it was thought likely that he would again be returned to the reform school.

P. Mixed F:27:M:496 +73 '87961-(47) 4:3:18
P. Hys.
Paranoid

This young woman's difficulties began nearly a year before admission when she became infatuated with her dentist, a small, mild-mannered man whom she wanted to mother and protect. Obsessed with thoughts of him, she found endless excuses for visits to his office and finally, on the pretext of introducing him to a girl friend, invited him to dinner. At this dinner she decided he compared unfavorably with her husband and afterward she confessed the whole affair to her husband, who forbade her to see him again. She continued to think of him, however, and to make occasional visits and phone calls, even though she realized this annoyed him. He begged her to stop bothering him but she was unable to do so completely. Three nights before admission she had advised him to marry a young woman of his acquaintance. The next day she was told that he had committed suicide. Feeling that she was entirely responsible for his death, she became extremely upset. She went to see his body and wanted to read the suicide note to further assure herself on this point.

The patient described her father as a religious fanatic who was immoral in his personal life and who spoiled the lives of his wife and children. In her early memories of him he was a kind, jolly man, who became a preacher at his wife's suggestion. When the patient was 8 her father separated from his wife and thereafter the girl's picture of him changed. She lived with her mother and aunts while two younger brothers stayed with the father. The mother was a beautiful, intelligent woman. From the age of 9 to 18 the patient lived in an entirely female world. She was an unusually pretty girl and did well in school. She married when she was 18 at her mother's urging. The marriage was not a happy one and the patient had many complaints about her husband's unreasonableness, indifference, and unkindness, which made him deny her a career in music or drama. In addition he failed to provide well for their two children, and he made excessive demands for affection. At the time when the patient met the dentist she was feeling discouraged about her marriage and was generally blue because her life was drab and she was losing her attractiveness.

On admission the patient was cooperative and alert, and she related the details of her relationship to the dentist with evident satisfaction up to the point of his suicide. About that she was tearful, agitated, and self-accusatory. After 48 hours there was little further tearful display and the patient began to show hostility toward her husband. She had a flare for the dramatic and seemed poised and conscious of her attractive appearance. After fourteen days she was discharged as improved and was followed in the outpatient department by weekly psychotherapeutic interviews for more than a year.

There was no further improvement during this time. She continued to be obsessed by thoughts of the dentist, gradually transferring more and more of the infatuation to her therapist and continuing, in a repetitive, compulsive fashion, the unrealistic aspects of this attachment. When her transfer to another therapist was necessary she showed a fairly fixed delusion that the first therapist had, in nonverbal ways, caused her to fall in love with him and had implied that they might have an affair. Occasionally her veneer of "sweetness and light" dissolved and she expressed extreme hostility in a sarcastic way. The attempts to give this patient insight into her unrealistic reactions were fruitless. E. B.

B. Psth., Path. Emot. F:39:M:65 +31 87′9642– 5:9:13
Schizoid
Paranoid

For the past two years the patient had gradually changed in personality. She had become increasingly interested in Christian Science, and for the past six months she had been preoccupied, despondent, and neglectful of her home. She complained of frightening dreams. In the last three weeks she had had outbursts of screaming and had been so hyperactive that she had slept and eaten very little. Much of her talk was incoherent, but it pertained to religious and persecutory ideas.

There had been no previous upsets. The patient was an eighth-grade graduate. She had married a man whose religion was different from hers, and in consequence there had been many bitter quarrels between the patient and her husband's people. Although her husband thought that his relatives were no longer distressed about the religious difference, the patient was convinced that they persecuted her for it. A war veteran, her husband was receiving a small pension for "nerves and arthritis." The patient had always been an ineffectual person, juvenile in attitudes and behavior, and subject to temper outbursts. Self-conscious, shy, suspicious, and jealous of others, she had always thought of herself as "a coy little maiden whom everyone loved." Since her marriage, she had not let her husband out of her sight, even requiring him to be present when she bought clothes.

At the time of admission she was in a dreamy state with a perplexed, anxious expression, and she was unable to talk coherently. "I can't harm people and live. Let me punish myself for what I have done," she said. When asked what she had done, she said, "I wanted my husband to be happy. The greatest power in the world sends me messages." There was a poor affective contact with reality, but there was no evidence of hallucinations. She made many misinterpretations and double identifications, and she attached special meanings to chance remarks. She had little insight. "I know I'm not thinking right, but I'm better. I'm not out of the woods, but I'll never be right until I get home with my husband and children." There was little change while she was in the hospital, but since it was felt that she might be able to get along at home, and her family was pressing for her release, she was discharged.

Ps. M-D., Manic	F:38:M:40	+8	'89–12	3:4:9
Ps. M-D., Manic	F:42:M:45	+26	–4318976(43)	5:0:8

The patient had experienced recurrent nervous upsets since age 13. These came every two or three years. The one in which she was admitted was more severe than any previous attack. All the upsets were characterized by emotional instability, irritability, nervousness, alternating overactivity and underactivity, insomnia, weakness, suspiciousness, and withdrawal. She would build air castles, she would talk of composing music, writing books, and giving concerts, and she would make plans for extensive social events. In the last two or three attacks she had shown a hypersexuality characterized by hysterical behavior when her husband did not have intercourse with her. The upsets tended to be precipitated by disappointments like the loss of her job and were sometimes relieved by trips away from home. During her two pregnancies the family was most stable and the patient was a happy and contented person for the only periods of her married life.

She was a high school graduate and valedictorian of her graduating class. She went to college for a brief time, but the nervous upsets prevented regular attendance, and she dropped out. She then worked as an office employee for eleven years. After that she helped her husband as a bookkeeper in his business. In her normal periods she was entirely adequate. She was a good housekeeper, had many friends, and was active in community affairs. She was regarded as ethically somewhat "straight-laced." Sexually she was ordinarily "cool" and content with intercourse every three or four weeks.

In the hospital she had no demonstrable delusions or hallucinations. She was intact in sensorium and intellect. There was a mild flight of ideas. She was worried about her children and frequently appeared depressed. The most obvious symptom was that she was easily irritated and would have an emotional outburst whenever she was "crossed." She did not think she belonged on the psychiatric service. She demanded privileges and was difficult to manage when she was not granted them. She often stated that her husband needed treatment, not her. At the time of discharge she appeared to be nearly recovered. About four years later she was readmitted with a similar attack which likewise ran its course in the hospital.

P. Mixed Schizoid	F:20:S:70	0	8916'7432–	1:8:11

For the past six years the patient had suffered from attacks characterized by groaning, purposeless motions, refusal to answer questions, and seclusiveness. These at first were correlated with her menstrual periods, but gradually they became more frequent and severe. For a month preceding hospitalization she paid little attention to her surroundings and spent all her time in bed.

The medical and psychological history included no outstanding factors. An excellent student, she finished the eighth grade and left school in the middle of the first year of high school because of a lack of finances. She felt she had missed a great deal in life as a child because she had not taken part in social activities and had led a circumscribed existence. A hard-working, conscientious, introverted person, she had little personal warmth. She usually responded to family problems by emotional outbursts.

In the hospital she was disturbed by her whole background, feeling that she had been grossly neglected. Her problem, in her view, centered around emancipating herself from her family. Tests showed an I.Q. of 100 but she greatly overestimated her ability. She felt she possessed considerable musical and drawing talent, even though she was not able to produce proof and actually showed little interest in either subject. Her answers, though relevant, were vague and inadequate; she never spoke spontaneously; and one had the feeling that her thinking was chaotic. She was convinced that she was physically ill and needed medical attention, although she never specified what she thought was wrong with her. She took no interest in the examinations or in the activities of the ward and did not mix with other patients. Whenever it was suggested to her that she was ready to go home she showed a peculiar pattern. She would throw herself on her bed, groan, refuse to answer any questions, bite her lips and tongue, and let food fall from her mouth while eating. It was impossible to help her gain any insight into the functional nature of this behavior and she was finally discharged to try living with her family again. Her family was advised that she should be committed to a state hospital if she did not make an adequate adaptation.

Ps. Sz., Hebe. M:17:S:8 +1 89'4 137-6 8:6:19

The patient's mother had induced him to come to the hospital because he was irritable and demanding, slammed things around, and acted peculiarly, but the reason he gave for entering was that he wanted to see the university engineering building. The disorder had apparently begun about a year before when he unaccountably developed irritability and had outbursts of temper; when his parents asked him if anything was wrong he always said that he felt all right. He made poor marks in school, rushed from one task to another without completing any, and frequently made unreasonable demands such as insisting upon going fishing during a bad rainstorm. He also engaged in petty thievery, taking such things as candy, flashlights, a watch, and money, but he never was definite about why he had taken them.

He had never been able to concentrate his endeavor and he had always been impulsive in action and stubborn and spiteful when crossed. He was interested in sports and had been in the high school band, but he had never been accepted by other children because he was said to be peculiar. He tended to bully his companions and quarreled with them frequently. His best friends were persons he could dominate.

In the hospital he insisted almost continually on leaving. He would roll up his extra clothes, dash into the hall, and demand to be allowed to use the telephone or to take the next bus home. He would not listen to reasoning. Unpredictable in behavior, he would occasionally walk up to a table where other patients were playing checkers and would sweep all the checkers to the floor. He was frequently rough with other patients, insisting that they box with him, and if they were smaller than he was he handled them roughly. He was careless in appearance and would come into the women's section clad only in his pajama trousers. His answers to questions were irrelevant and vague, with frequent reversals of opinion. Asked if he had any enemies, he answered, "I have several. No, I have one, the devil. He tries to lead me into sin, but there isn't any devil. People just think so." His speech was abrupt and jerky. He insisted that he was all right, that his brother and sister needed a rest more than he did, and that he felt as well as he always had. There was no change during his hospital stay. It was recommended that he receive shock therapy and that if he did not improve he go to a state hospital, but his family refused permission for shock therapy and took him from the hospital to live on an uncle's farm.

B. Pri., Child. F:14:S:16 +1 894'671-(51) 4:13:10

The patient had been admitted to a detention center where she had disliked the "prison atmosphere" and had resented the fact that other girls used her clothes. During an argument with one of the other girls she became angry and chased the girl with a knife. After this offense she was depressed and remorseful, and admitted claiming a false ailment to attract attention. She talked of having the idea of throwing herself out of the window though she disclaimed really intending to do so. She was brought to the psychopathic unit for a general evaluation.

She had been an "unwanted child" but had lived with her parents until she was 7, being abused by them rather severely. She was then placed in a county home but ran away and returned to her own home. Succeeding years were marked by repeated attempts to adjust in her own and other homes. She accused her mother of spreading "false and dirty" stories about her. Made a ward of the state, she was put in the detention home. She went to school while there and was in junior high school at the time of admission. Her grades were somewhat above average though she did not like school. Her intelligence was dull normal. She was always moody and somewhat dictatorial toward other children. There were outbursts in which she would be violent and disagreeable. She complained that no one understood her.

In the hospital she was at first very suspicious but then talked freely, was cooperative, and appeared neat and normal in her activities. Her mental content was mostly concerned with her present activities. There was no bizarre behavior and she mixed well with other patients, though she was boisterous and demanding at times. She showed a distinct need to attract attention to herself and sought to do this by describing the aches and pains that she had. She had no marked temper outburst while on the ward. The staff felt that much of her behavior had been determined by the unfavorable environment in which she had developed. It was recommended that someone be found who would watch her very carefully and attempt to give her greater feelings of security.

B. Psth., Asocial M:30:S 89'<u>4</u>76–(43) 7:7:13
Mutilative
Drug Add.
Suicidal

This prisoner, a constant troublemaker, was referred to the psychopathic ward after he mutilated himself by cutting his Achilles' tendon. Two years previously he had injected sour milk beneath the skin of his left leg to cause an infection; this had incapacitated him for work during a six-week period.

Born in a small town, he lived there until the age of 21. Shortly after his family moved to a metropolitan area his father died. The man has spent most of the time since then in prison. School records indicate that he completed the sixth grade. When not in prison he works as a carpenter. Unmarried, he has lived with two women in common-law relationships. First in trouble at the age of 17 on a car theft charge, he was actually not guilty and was soon released. Two years later he was arrested on a burglary charge and this time received a two-year suspended sentence. According to his own statement, it was while he sat in jail waiting trial on this charge that he formed the drug habit. He remembers taking two or three doses at this time.

At the age of 20 he was arrested and given a federal prison sentence for the sale of narcotics. Because a crude hypodermic syringe, made from a medicine dropper, was found in his possession (he claimed he had found it in the clothes of another inmate), he got into trouble with the prison authorities. Transferred to a federal hospital, he was an inmate there for more than two years. After being out of the hospital for not more than a few weeks, he was again arrested for the sale of narcotics, and for this offense the sentence was three years. This time he got into trouble in the federal prison one day when a fellow inmate struck him with a floor mop and he in turn stabbed the other man seven times, resulting in the latter's hospitalization. One month after his release the prisoner was again arrested for the sale of narcotics and returned to the federal penitentiary for three years. Again transferred to a hospital, he broke out of solitary confinement and used a pipe to beat up another inmate whom he had had trouble with. At present he is being held for the sale of heroin.

The man says that he has several times tried to commit suicide. Once he cut his left wrist vein. He is obviously dissipated from the excessive use of heroin and states that he becomes ill when deprived of narcotics. Soon to be released from prison, he says that he has no plans for employment but will probably return to the use and sale of narcotics. R. C. K.

B. Psth., Asocial Mutilative M:28:S 896′2741–3X (47) 3:23:5

This prison inmate is said to have broken every rule in the prison. He is considered a constant troublemaker and is a self-mutilator, having cut his Achilles' tendons three times.

When the prisoner was still a baby his father died. His mother remarried and he spent part of his childhood with his mother and stepfather, part in an orphanage. After several years in school, where he progressed only as far as the third grade, he worked at odd jobs as a farm laborer. He spent two periods in C.C.C. camps. At the end of the first six months he received an honorable discharge. Re-enlisting later, he stayed two months, deserted, and was dismissed.

The man's first arrest, at the age of 16, was for burglary. The penalty was a two-year suspended sentence. Four years later he served an extended jail sentence for the theft of produce from a farm.

The prisoner's present sentence is for fifteen years, for robbery with firearms. In his first year of incarceration he was punished for laziness and refusing to work, for attempting to escape, and for possession of a knife. During the second year he was punished for mutiny. Three years later he led a mutiny and performed a self-mutilation. The following year he attempted to escape, mutilated himself twice, and destroyed state property. He is now in isolation, having been transferred there from the psychopathic ward.

This man has been in solitary confinement so much of the time that he is known by the inmates as "Solitary Red." Officials believe he "is a case for permanent lock-up," and they have concluded he "will always be a charge on society." The summary diagnosis was that the man is not capable of profiting from past experience. R. C. K.

Ps. Sz., Paranoid	M:21:S:441	+31	89'76–3 (53)	3:9:15
		+235	9'7468–13 (55)	3:7:11

This veteran dated his "period of change," as he termed it, from age 18 when he entered the navy. It was at this time that he was converted and "God claimed him as His own"; it was then that he "really became a Christian." The Bible tells that "us Christians are peculiar persons," he said, and so at the time of his conversion he became "peculiar." After entering the navy, the patient stopped masturbating and, subsequently, noticed a marked difference in himself; he felt stronger and "more like a man." Believing that he was one of the best men on board ship, he was always ready to fight, and the crew seemed to be afraid of him. Following his discharge from the service, he returned home but found no employment. He then began to masturbate again and felt that he was getting weaker. He became seclusive, spent most of his time studying the Bible, and decided to become a preacher. Even though it was midwinter he left his family to live at a lake cottage. From there he went to a city, wandered around broke and cold, and was picked up by the police. Taken to a veterans' hospital for psychiatric study, he was later committed and transferred to this hospital with a diagnosis of schizophrenia, grandiose, paranoid type.

The patient completed high school and entered the navy immediately after graduation. Records give no significant information about his early life or his adjustment in the navy except that he never went out much with girls and was always seclusive. In high school he engaged in athletics and enjoyed them.

The patient's course in the hospital was marked by frequent periods of assaultive and hyperactive behavior. He ran away frequently. After a course of electroshock therapy he showed some improvement and was released for a trial visit. For a few days his adjustment was good and then he began to threaten his parents, saying he would kill them and then himself. He was returned to the hospital a week later. Gradually he showed improvement and was eventually released for another trial visit, which was later converted to a discharge.

C. W. S.

Ps. Sz., Cat.	M:16:S:56	+23	897612'43–X	2:16:2
		+39	8971'624–X	2:17:8
		+50	'17 8296–4	1:5:8
Ps. Sz., Cat.	M:18:S:99			

The patient was well until two years before admission when he showed lassitude and a general restriction of interests. He recovered promptly from the initial episode. Four months before admission, following an upper respiratory infection, he had another spell. He was recovering from this when he was in a minor automobile accident; afterward he sat about the house with a vacant look on his face, occasionally complaining of a headache and dizziness. When asked questions he would say distantly, "I don't know," or "Maybe." He gradually fell into a stupor characterized by emotional apathy and marked psychomotor retardation.

Weak and sickly as a child, he spent all his time on his parents' farm. He graduated from the eighth grade at age 14 and then spent half a year in high school. Never interested in anything, he participated in activities only as a spectator. He had neither enemies nor friends; he was a shut-in, introverted person.

In the hospital his speech was bizarre. "I am going to freeze completely pretty soon because I don't talk enough," he commented. He spent most of his time lying motionless in bed and could hardly be induced to move about, even to go to meals or to the bathroom. For a while he showed a waxy flexibility. Although he gradually became better, apparently his usual self was withdrawn, self-conscious, and insecure. He was discharged considerably improved. About a year later he was readmitted with a similar attack. This attack again followed a physical illness. In the hospital this time he made several overt homosexual advances toward his physician and was unpredictably assaultive. He was transferred to a state hospital.

B. Psth., Asocial M:25:S 89762'413–X(60) 1:25:4
Ps. Sz., Simple
Mutilative

This inmate of the prison mutilated himself five times over a ten-year period by cutting his Achilles' tendons. On the first occasion when he cut the right tendon he was committed to isolation; the day he was released he mutilated himself again, cutting the tendon of his left leg this time. Isolation was again used for punishment. Thirty days later he mutilated himself a third time by cutting the tendon he had originally severed. During his third and fourth years in prison, he again cut the Achilles' tendons of both his right and left heels. He also made trouble by cursing the guards, "using profanity and being impudent," and refusing to work.

The prisoner was reared by his father and stepmother. He never saw his own mother nor did he know her whereabouts. On standardized tests he made a grade placement of 7.5. Probation authorities reported that the youth had "always" been a runaway problem and had frequently been "taken in" or warned for staying out late at night on the street. The only job outside of the prison that the prisoner ever held was for six weeks as a laborer on a truck.

Before he was 20 the youth had spent time in six detention homes, for running away from home, delinquencies, and the like. He served two terms in one prison for breaking and entering, one term in the prison of another state for forgery by alteration. In both prisons his conduct was consistently poor. He escaped from one of the prisons and was at large for a few days. He made other attempts to escape and was punished for them and for possessing a knife, mutiny, and fighting. In addition he was stabbed by another inmate because the latter "did not like the gang" the prisoner "ran around with." The prisoner was a regular member of a gang known as the R gang. The young man is at present serving ten years on two counts of theft and two of burglary.

9′–128

Placed in the psychopathic ward for observation, the inmate was found to be "legally sane, knows right from wrong, and is responsible for his acts." He was further adjudged "an agitator and a source of annoyance" and a "disturber of other mental patients in the hospital ward." The recommendation was made that he be discharged from the hospital, placed in the permanent lock-up, and "treated as other disciplinary cases of criminal psychopaths." R. C. K.

B. Pri., Child.	M:14:S:19	+1	9′–12378 (49)	3:5:6

This boy, with a companion, pilfered several automobiles in the three-month period before the present admission. In the company of the same friend, he set fire to three buildings, causing considerable damage. He was referred to the psychiatric unit by the juvenile court under an arson charge.

For several years the patient had had trouble with his side, presumably because of dilation of the colon. In addition to this difficulty he had been injured in a number of accidents; none of these injuries, however, had apparently left any enduring effects. At the time of admission he was in the eighth grade and had made a good although not outstanding record in school. Socially, he was retiring and seclusive. At times he became so irritable and angry that his face would break out in a rash. His chief interest was in building model airplanes and he was very particular in this work. He was jealous of a younger brother, and he felt that he was not wanted by his mother.

In the hospital the boy was shy but cooperative. With patients in his own age group he was somewhat boisterous. He related himself well with the staff and seemed able to discuss his problems. The whole situation appeared to be centered in his conflict with his parents, particularly his mother. It was recommended that he live away from home for a while, possibly at a military academy, although it was also recommended that his ties with his home be continued in an intermittent fashion.

Ps. M-D., Manic	M:43:M:13	+4	9′–128 (65)	4:1:16
		+10	′9–4123 (73)	4:3:16
		+11	′9–1 (78)	3:2:17

About a week before admission the patient's wife noticed that he had become restless, irritable, and highly keyed up. He was unreasonable with those about him and insisted upon working long hours at various activities.

In the past there had been two similar episodes. The first was about eight years before admission when he had had, he said, "the strength of ten men"; he had recovered in about two weeks. The second episode occurred about six years before admission; he was treated with electroshock therapy and recovered fairly quickly, although he was irritable and hard to get along with for several months.

During the years of his marriage many minor disturbances had appeared episodically. He felt that he had a "sixty-day cycle," with thirty days of hypomania and thirty days of mild depression.

The patient had left home at the age of 12 and since then had been self-supporting. He received a degree from a law school, and ultimately he became the head of a firm. Between episodes he was cheerful, got along well with others, and was active in civic and other affairs. On the other hand, when he was ill, he was moody and irritable, insisting that others did not understand him and could not do things as well as he. He described his wife as being his opposite and above him. He had felt insecure since his marriage to her and had been continually under pressure to make good. He believed that this was part of his problem.

In the hospital he was friendly and cooperative. There were no apparent abnormalities in his stream of thought. At times, especially during the first three days, he acted like a typical hypomanic. His chief concern was to be discharged so that he could get back to his neglected work. He admitted that he had thought of suicide during his depressive periods but claimed that he had never really taken the idea seriously. At first he was uncooperative, irritable, and demanding. Later, however, he improved in attitude. He was given two shock treatments in the first few days but refused to take more. At the time of discharge he was better and probably was almost recovered from the present attack.

Ps. Sz., Paranoid F:53:M:64 +18 '9–128<u>37</u>(72) 5:3:9

Following an operation on the womb at the age of 47, the patient complained of pains and she gradually developed delusional beliefs and hallucinations. She also became suspicious of her neighbors and accused them of many things. She entered the hospital as a voluntary patient.

She was the oldest of three children. Her mother was a "lady," her father a drunkard, and her family life extremely unhappy. She had been bright at school and a good musician. On leaving school at 14, she took up clerical work. She had always been an obstinate and touchy person, lacking the ability to show affection. She married at 23. When her first husband died, she remarried. She was excessively proud of her house and had no outside interests.

She was diagnosed as having paraphrenia and she underwent a course of electric convulsion therapy. She left the hospital "relieved," but with a "doubtful prognosis." M. V.

B. Psth., Path. Sexuality M:39:S:26 +3 '9–13(92) 5:2:14

From early childhood this man had accompanied masturbation with fantasies centering around men. Later he noticed that he was sexually stimulated by men dressed in tights. At age 29 he was seduced by an aggressive male homosexual and thereafter he continued to engage in homosexual activities. He claimed not to have led others into the practice and said that his drive for a homosexual relationship was not particularly strong. He was sent to the psychiatric unit for study as the result of a complaint by a young man who had been picked up by the police for some other offense. This young man was known to the police as a homosexual, and no criminal charge was filed against the patient.

The patient had maintained a very satisfactory work record and had been employed by the same concern for a long time. He had gone through high school and had taken a year of business school. He had always been a sensitive person, strongly attached to his mother and interested in art and music. He was very highly regarded by his friends and respected by those who worked with him.

In the hospital the physical and neurological examinations were noncontributory. The patient willingly discussed his homosexual activities and aside from these no abnormalities in his mentation or behavior were discovered. He was courteous and well adjusted on the ward and expressed a desire to control his sexual impulses. He felt that his many hobbies afforded him a way of compensating for his sexual impulses, and at the time of discharge the staff felt that the prognosis for good behavior was very satisfactory.

Ps. Sz., Cat.	F:45:S:25	+8	'9–1843 (53)	5:1:10
		+46	'49– (66)	7:6:18

Four days before admission the patient suddenly became irrational, overactive, and assaultive, with delusions of guilt and persecution. The first symptom was a severe headache that forced her to leave the school where she taught, and although a vacation period was only two days away, she decided to go to her parents' home in another city right away. The next day a physician advised bed rest for her, but she became hyperactive and irrational, stared blankly into space, and was oblivious of everyone. There was such bizarre behavior as creeping around on her hands and knees, stretching out her arms, and exclaiming "a child is born." She cried and whined as she wandered about the house. She thought someone was coming to get her for having stolen school funds, and she was assaultive toward her mother and the doctor. Until her hospital admission she continued to show strange actions and to express delusions.

She had attended a teachers' college, and although she had had some difficulty with her studies and had been told she would never be a good teacher, she had subsequently held a number of positions as a grade school teacher. She had been discharged from some of them. Occupationally and socially she presented a picture that observers referred to as an "old-maid schoolteacher." There was no history of any previous nervous breakdown. During her childhood she had been pampered and had shown temper tantrums. She had had at least two major operations, the last one being a hysterectomy eight years before admission. Her ability to plan for the future was poor, and her entire interest centered on her work. An overly conscientious person, she had a tendency to feel sorry for herself and to think that she worked harder than others. Emotionally she was nervous and moody. She had never been active in social affairs, and although she had had offers of marriage she had refused them because of her dissatisfaction with the men.

In the hospital the neurological and physical examinations were negative. Cheerful and cooperative on the ward, she was nevertheless anxious and concerned about her job. She had delusions of guilt and persecution about funds belonging to the school, but she was obviously over the peak of the present episode. Her sensorium was clear, but she was disoriented. She considered her illness to be a nervous breakdown. She was given shock treatment and on her fourth hospital day became oriented. Her improvement was steady, and she was discharged to return to work with the prognosis for the present episode obviously good, but the possibility of future ones appeared great.

B. Pri., Child. M:17:S:17 +7 '9–26147(49) 1:6:10
B. Psth., Asocial

The patient was admitted to the hospital upon the request of the juvenile court where he had been arraigned on a charge of burglary. The burglaries had all been concentrated in the preceding month. He had finally been caught by the police while attempting to rob a filling station. After his arrest, it was found that he had previously carried out thirteen burglaries and had accumulated a considerable amount of loot from them; the victim of one of them claimed to have lost $103, although the boy said he had stolen only $26 from the man. The patient was behind in his room rent, board, and laundry, besides being out of a job at the time he was arrested.

The boy's general health had been good. There were no previous psychotic upsets or known misbehavior of any type. The boy finished the eleventh grade and then stopped school. He had had no difficulties in obtaining better than average grades. He was well liked and people were impressed with his good manners, his appearance, and his general bearing. He was friendly and liked to meet people, was open in his attitude about himself and toward others. He said that money never seemed to last long with him. Much of his time he spent in reading books, but other things he did by fits and starts. He would take a job and stay at it only a little while, then leave it to "find a better one."

In the hospital he was well mannered, quiet, interested, and clean-cut. He had no abnormal ideas or trends. Although he smiled and talked readily, he claimed to have been inwardly depressed over the events of the past few weeks. He caused no trouble and was entirely a good patient. No good explanation could be made diagnostically that would explain the series of burglaries. He had always been free with money and had been noted for transient fits of interest in various activities, but there seemed to be no adequate basis for his misbehavior. He was discharged to be placed on parole and carefully followed for a time in the outpatient psychiatric clinic.

P. Anxiety State M:26:S:49 +13 '9–6<u>27</u>(57) 8:0:17
P. Hys.

This patient had developed symptoms suggesting an anxiety neurosis. He complained that his heart sometimes stopped beating, that he was afraid of impending death, and the like. He was certified, following an acute hysterical episode aggravated by alcohol, and was admitted to the hospital.

The youngest of seven children, he had always been nervous. He was sociable but did not play games as a child. On leaving school he had a succession of jobs (apprentice baker, shop assistant, and storeman), keeping none of them for more than fourteen months. He joined the army at 18 and was invalided out with psychoneurosis after four years' service.

He had previously been diagnosed as having an anxiety neurosis; the cause of his present admission was the hysterical episode, which cleared up in a day or two. M. V.

Ps. Senile F:50:S:81 +38 9'–<u>871</u>43(59) 5:2:8
Ps. Invol. Melan.
Suicidal
Deteriorated

Three months before admission the patient made a blood donation and had several teeth extracted on the same day. She became weak and began to complain of nervousness, restlessness, insomnia, weakness, and anorexia. She lost interest in her work. A physician prescribed a "nerve" medicine and sleeping tablets. Later she was taken to a general hospital and subsequently to three other hospitals and to "specialists." She had to take sleeping pills all the time, being unable to sleep without them. She complained of being bothered by strangers. On the day of this admission, her brother found the patient at home unconscious with the gas turned on. She had also taken innumerable sleeping tablets.

The patient developed what was called a "thin face" when she was 10 and was thereafter very sensitive about it. When she was 13 she suffered an inflammation of the hip that left her with a slight limp. She was an eighth-grade graduate and had no trouble in school. After school she worked at various jobs and later kept house for her brother and his daughter after his divorce. She ran her brother's home efficiently and had a garden that was the envy of the neighborhood. She read many books in her leisure time. Jolly and well liked, she was considered a stable person. She became very lonesome, however, after her niece left home to be married. When her sister got a defense job, the patient became jealous and also applied for a job; she was accepted on the condition that she have her teeth repaired.

In the hospital she showed mild depression but a more obvious nervousness and agitation. There was much fluctuation from day to day. Her sensorium was clear but there were psychometric evidences of organic brain deterioration, which was assumed to be the result of arteriosclerotic changes. She felt certain that she was going to lose her mind. This was the only obvious symptom after she recovered from the effects of the gas poisoning and the sleeping pills. She complained of nervousness and misery, and there were periods when she was greatly agitated. Many times she would cry out that she could not stand the pain in her head and that nobody understood her. The diagnostic picture was unclear. The menopause preceded the illness by about five years. The arteriosclerotic changes were felt to be significant. Although she was never unmanageable, she was transferred to the state hospital, chiefly because of the recurrent agitation.

Ps. Invol. Melan. F:55:M:41 —1 ′912–46(74) 7:4:13
Deteriorated

The patient's complaints were periodic headaches, accompanied by pain in one eye, and "nervousness," both of which began about two years before admission. A physician whom the patient had initially gone to because of the burning sensation in her eye had been unable to find a cause, and the pain had frequently recurred. About a year before admission the pain had caused the patient to "lose consciousness" for several hours, but she had suffered no other effects. She had had other attacks when she had experienced nausea, vomiting, and numbness "as though a thousand needles were sticking her."

There was nothing contributory in the past history. She had completed only three grades in school, stopping when she was 12. Her I.Q. was about 90. She got along well with people and had many friends, but she was shy and somewhat reserved in meeting new people. A meticulous, frugal person, she kept her affairs to herself. She was quick to react to disappointments and criticism.

The neurological examination in the hospital was not clearly normal; in fact, there were occasional and transient signs that indicated a possible organic disorder, although none was found. The patient was concerned about her headaches and nervousness, and she was more worried about finances than the circumstances seemed to warrant, but she was free of obvious mental disturbances. On many occasions she was observed crying, but she always tried to conceal her tears, and she was friendly and helpful on the ward. She answered questions adequately and showed no extreme volubility or flight of ideas, but there was a blocking of thought before she responded. When she spoke, she uttered her words quickly, noticeably accenting the sentences. During her stay the dpression improved, and the prognosis was hopeful, although the factor of organic involvement could not be adequately evaluated.

P. Mixed F:20:S:20 +8 9′1286437–(57) 5:5:10
Schizoid

This young woman's initial complaint, for which she sought medical help, was a dull pain in the left upper quadrant. This pain had been present for three years. A persistent pain in the left lower quadrant, of one year's duration, had followed treatment by a chiropractor. The pains were aggravated by work, by standing, and by riding in a car, and the intensity was reduced only by resting. She was unhappy and able to do little work. After a thorough physical study no diagnosis was arrived at and she was transferred to the psychiatric hospital.

The patient described her father as domineering, restrictive, unreasonable, a heavy drinker, and brutal to his wife and children. The mother was described as pleasant and easygoing, but not close to the patient. The patient worked in her father's store, a difficult job because he was exacting and quick to punish her. She learned to hide her anger because it was the only way to get along with him. Always nervous, she had no interest in boys or marriage because of the unhappiness in her home.

When admitted the patient claimed she had been railroaded into the hospital, and she was suspicious and hostile but otherwise flat emotionally. On mental tests her thinking appeared to be confused and it was difficult for her to formulate an answer to a question without getting far afield or forgetting the question entirely. She had little spontaneity and the only information she offered of her own accord was a long, defensive account of the mistreatment she had suffered, not only from her father, but from the rest of her family. They "tormented" her, she said, and so also did teachers and doctors. The physical examination was essentially negative, but the possibility of a herniated disc could not be ruled out. Her initial suspiciousness of the hospital subsided a little and she appeared to enjoy herself and did not complain of pain. Psychotherapy was aimed only at establishing a friendly, permissive relationship. After her first weekend visit home she reported how tense she felt there and said that this accentuated her pain. Later she refused to go home, which caused her parents to appear on the scene, demanding her discharge. "What's the use, they always do it their way sooner or later," the patient said, and she left with her parents even though against medical advice. Her condition might have responded to psychotherapy, but a more malignant picture could be expected in the future unless some change occurred in her situation at home. E. B.

Ps. Toxic M:45:D:46 +30 9′132–678 (47) 1:2:6
B. Psth., Asocial
Drug Add.

Three years before admission the patient developed severe diarrhea and after investigation he was told that he had lead poisoning. Following that he was in and out of hospitals repeatedly. He lost weight until he had gone down from 215 to 127 pounds. He took considerable amounts of barbiturates. Two and a half weeks before admission he arrived unexpectedly at the home of his brother. At that time, his brother said, the patient "looked terrible and acted like a stranger." He collapsed several times, talked irregularly, skipped over words and phrases, and was apparently hallucinatory. The brother thought that this was brought on by seconal capsules, which always made him "wild." He finally became so irrational that his brother was forced to call the police and have him taken to a hospital.

Until the present illness the patient had always been healthy, strong, and active. He was educated in a parochial school and was described as "backward," never having been able to grasp fundamentals. He failed several grades and left school because of his lack of interest. He became a machinist and married at age 21. Sometime thereafter he served ninety days in the workhouse for failure to support his wife and children. There was a possibility that he had been guilty of bigamy, and his second wife had divorced him about nine months before admission. He was described as having always been friendly and forward; he liked a good time. He was aggressive, doing what he wanted to do with little regard for others, was never sincere, and did not accept responsibility. He had always depended on his parents for financial aid and for important decisions in spite of the fact that he had been a skilled worker, able to make very good wages on his own. Though it was vigorously denied by the patient, there were a number of indications that he had forged checks and had got into other financial difficulties. During his hospitalization the police of another state attempted to get control of him for some illegal act.

In the hospital he was underweight, dyspneic, drowsy, and hallucinatory. His sensorium was clouded; his mental content was irregular and could not be studied because his discourse was irregular and unsatisfactory. He appeared indifferent to his surroundings. After several days he became rational, cheerful, and cooperative. Some physical complaints remained up to the time of discharge but in other ways he steadily improved. The prognosis for the acute episode was good but for the general behavior pattern underlying the episode it was considered to be very poor.

F:45:S '91327-6(41) 4:2:9

This woman was a supervisor of packers and wrappers in a large department store. A college graduate with fifteen years of experience in the store, she came to the center for testing in the course of an executive evaluation program initiated by the store. Her management considered her loyal and conscientious but difficult to work with. She had persistent trouble with the union.

She had a long period of military service during the war. After her return to the store she had several operations for carcinoma. There were clinical evidences of considerable anxiety and unrest which extended back to a period before the surgery for cancer. In the interview she showed active interest in the results of the ability and interest tests but did not wish to discuss the personality material. In the interview with our physician she did not admit that she knew the seriousness of her medical diagnosis. She was eager to discuss her job, particularly the pressure and difficulties involved and the fact that it took two people to do the work while she was in service. She had a complaint toward the management for not sending her better people to supervise and not realizing the magnitude of her job.

Somewhat nostalgically she reviewed in the interview her early training in a fashionable eastern college and her interest in drama and literature. The interviewer received the impression that she was a bitter woman who felt that her present job was somewhat beneath her but that it was attended by difficulties seldom understood by other people. The interviewer felt that a more suitable job placement and access to employee counseling or psychiatric help would have been constructive if it had been offered some years ago. At this time the prognosis for improving her job adjustment was poor. D. F. C.

P. Mixed M:58:M:21 +6 91'823–6 6:11:14
Mental Deficiency

Two months before admission the patient had been attacked by the inmates of a mental hospital where he was an attendant, and although there was no serious physical injury he had suffered a scalp laceration and numerous body bruises. After this attack he had shown emotional instability and had had periods of confusion. Several times he had left home without notifying his family; on one occasion after an absence of two days he had been discovered in another state, where he had traveled by freight train.

He had never been particularly robust and was said to have had a heart lesion as a child. A sixth-grade graduate and a poor student, he had an I.Q. of 71. He had worked at irregular jobs until his marriage, and then he had begun to work as a hospital attendant. His wife treated him with very little consideration and was said to have been unfaithful to him. A weak person and easily led by others, he was selfish and stubborn, but he met strangers readily and had established at least a few warm friendships.

In the hospital the physical and neurological studies were negative. The patient showed a marked concern about his financial difficulties and about his inability to work. The fact that the state had given him only two thirds of his pay while he was "recovering from his injury" disturbed him. Data of this kind indicated that a compensation neurosis was possible. He repeatedly said that he might have suffered permanent brain injury. He adjusted well to ward life and was an excellent patient. He gradually came to be reassured about his injuries, and he became impatient with idleness. At the time of discharge he was eager to go back to work, and he was relatively free of the symptoms.

P. Hypo. F:41:M:18 +8 918634'72– 9:8:19
Paranoid
Schizoid

The patient had a long list of somatic complaints which numerous physicians had been unable to find a cause for. The complaints had markedly increased following her marriage, and during the last ten months irritability had been added. She insisted that the other members of her family wash their hands carefully to avoid bringing germs into the house. On one occasion when she was thinking about something else her husband asked her to pass the salt, and she so objected to this interruption of her reverie that she threw the shaker at him.

Despite her many complaints there was no history of any severe illness other than an appendectomy and the removal of both ovaries, presumably because of a cystic condition. She was an eighth-grade graduate and apparently had been an average student. After leaving school she worked as a hotel maid and in addition wrote for the local newspaper. A stubborn, self-centered person, she craved sympathy and attention, and when she did not get her way she was irritable and difficult to live with. She met strangers easily and was socially normal. She was very religious, spending considerable time in prayer, and the fact that her husband was a heavy drinker disturbed her. Because her husband had not taken her ailments seriously the patient felt even more neglected. Although the two were unhappy, neither of them wanted a divorce.

In the hospital the patient was very eager to discuss her physical complaints —and every portion of her body was the seat of some difficulty. There were no gross disturbances of intellect or sensorium, but there was a certain vagueness and volubility about her conversation which verged on circumstantiality. Contented in the hospital, she was cooperative and entered into ward activities fairly well, but psychotherapeutic progress was difficult, and when she was discharged there had been little change. The prognosis was poor.

Ps. Sz., Paranoid M:35:M:26 +6 91'87342-(47) 7:5:16
Alcoholism

This veteran was admitted to the hospital on the recommendation of a mental hygiene clinic where he had sought assistance. His first emotional disturbance had occurred while he was overseas with the army; at that time he had been involved in a fight with other members of his unit and immediately following this had become psychotic. He was diagnosed as having dementia praecox and was considered homicidal. He showed improvement after shock treatment and was discharged to duty. A month later he entered another army hospital complaining of headaches, crying spells, and a fear of crowds. He was diagnosed as having severe psychoneurosis, mixed type.

Shortly after his discharge from the army the man became "jumpy and nervous," refused to leave his house, and believed that someone was after him and was going to kill him. He was subsequently admitted to a veterans' hospital, where he was overactive, surly, morose, irritable, and excitable, and displayed paranoid features. The diagnosis was undifferentiated psychosis with schizophrenic and alcoholic factors. Three years elapsed between that hospitalization and the present admission, although the patient felt that his symptoms (fear, auditory hallucinations, and paranoid ideas of influence) had been getting worse for the last two years.

'92178364–

The patient, a Negro, grew up in a southeastern city and attended grammar school there. Little was known of his early life but his family history consisted of marital difficulties, excessive drinking, and assaultive and irresponsible behavior.

In this hospital the patient was quiet, pleasant, cooperative, and agreeable. He gave the impression of being intellectually somewhat above average. He was well oriented and the only abnormal trends shown were mild and vague ideas of influence, which were associated with superstition. During his brief stay in the hospital he had five psychotherapy contacts in which he gained some insight. He was discharged after an excellent hospital adjustment. C. W. S.

P. Mixed F:18:S:21 +1 '92178364–(59) 1:8:7

The patient was admitted to the hospital because of "dizzy" spells, dysuria, irregular menstruation, and pain in her side. These symptoms had appeared, for the most part, in the last eight months. There was also said to be a change in her personality. The patient said she knew nothing about her spells except what others told her. A sister witnessed the first one, in which the patient "looked as if she were going to faint, stood with a blank look on her face, and said over and over, 'Where am I?,' 'Yes, yes,' and 'No, no.'" Apparently she was not unconscious and she did not fall. She spent some time in the hospital but did not improve. The dysuria was fairly constant and the pain tended to be present in the morning and evening. The patient was afraid she was developing epilepsy.

This patient was born blind but had otherwise been a fairly healthy girl. At the time of admission she was in her eleventh year at school but was still in the eighth grade. Her intelligence was about average. She read Braille and could print it; the MMPI was administered in Braille. She had also stuttered all her life. She felt that her family should take a greater interest in her and during the last year she thought that they were talking about her. She was lively in school and something of a behavior problem. In general she got along well with other girls and seemed to be a relatively normal person.

In the hospital she appeared as a somewhat obese girl; otherwise she was neurologically and physically free of symptoms. An electroencephalographic study did not indicate any epileptic tendency. She was well oriented and cheerful; her stream of thought was logical. She was cooperative though somewhat apprehensive, adjusted well to the hospital routine, and was pleasant and friendly. She received considerable sympathy and attention; apparently she was not used to this and enjoyed it very much. Her stay on the ward was uneventful except that she claimed to have had one spell; it was not observed by anyone else. The diagnostic summary expressed considerable confusion about her condition. It was obvious that she was dissatisfied with her home life and that she was experiencing extensive fantasy, part of which she admitted to be sexual in content. At times she also showed mild defensive and paranoid trends. Since several of her ten brothers and sisters were mentally defective or epileptic, there was the additional possibility of some organic cerebral defect.

Ps. Toxic M:60:M:20 +16 9'246378– 6:7:18
Alcoholism
Deteriorated

Until fifteen years before admission the patient had been a reasonably adequate person. At that time he had suffered a nervous breakdown following a prison sentence for bootlegging, and simultaneously marked personality changes had occurred. He began drinking much more heavily, became completely uncompromising and stubborn on certain subjects, and developed peculiar ideas. The next years were marked by peculiar behavior and frequent attempts to stop drinking by taking "cures." For one period he became fanatically religious, at other times he expressed pathological ideas of reference and had manic spells. At the time of the present admission there were definite evidences of a nervous system involvement as well as mental confusion and clouding of consciousness.

Early in the patient's life he had shown a talent for and an interest in the medical profession. He had learned readily and had displayed considerable mechanical skill. His energy output had always been unusually great, but he had never been able to apply it in any constant fashion. Known as cheerful, he was at ease with others and exhibited interest in group activities. He had a definite tendency to do things that would increase his prestige in the community.

In the hospital the neurological examination showed scattered but definite findings indicating some general deterioration. Despite the patient's assurance of his well-being and composure, the staff sensed a state of tension and anxiety underneath. Almost everything he said centered around four general subjects: his wife (toward whom he had ambivalent feelings), religion, gardening, and his own personal prestige. On these subjects his conversation was saturated with inconsistencies, and there were numerous instances of fabrication. The patient, entirely oblivious to these symptoms, could gain no insight into them. He answered questions directly and with seeming reasonableness. He was extremely voluble and he could not be kept on any one subject long. A portion of the patient's symptoms disappeared during his three-week stay. The blurred vision persisted, however, and the religious fanaticism and the bizarre ideas continued. He was discharged to a state hospital.

Ps. M-D., Manic F:30:M:42 +2 '927–6(43) 2:2:14

The illness of this patient began insidiously several months before admission with signs of "nervousness." She began to isolate herself from her friends and her normal activities. Not apparently depressed, she was instead "lackadaisical." She herself said that she was more irritable than usual and also that she was stimulated by many things that would not ordinarily have affected her. This general problem became progressively worse until three days before admission when she became "acutely upset." She felt faint and was panicky. The succeeding day she had another spell when she felt paralyzed and experienced a "close tightness in my chest." Again she improved but the next day had another panic spell and thought "I was going to blow my top." This feeling led to her request for admission to the psychiatric unit.

She had had one previous nervous breakdown about nine years before admission, when she apparently went through a depression. The attack lasted nearly two years; part of this time she spent in a state hospital. She finished the third year of high school, then left and went to work. A year or two later she married and from that time on worked only in her home. She was an introverted, egocentric person and was said to have a "strong inferiority complex." She was retiring but friendly and was well liked by the small group she was associated with, though she tended to spend most of her time alone. She was narcissistic and spent long hours fixing her hair and dressing. She had almost no other interests, did nothing in the way of physical exercise or sports, and had no hobbies. There was considerable friction between her and her mother-in-law, which she blamed for her first episode of illness. Her husband had a number of nervous habits which she had tried to change, with little success, and she complained that there had recently been no "thrill" to her marriage. She was also unhappy because she had no children.

In the hospital she was neat and appeared composed and coherent. She frequently made flighty responses to questions, however, though these occurred without any signs of emotional disturbance. The staff felt that the patient was trying too hard to appear well and normal. She never adjusted well to the hospital routine, frequently breaking rules in minor ways, asking for special privileges, and the like. Her behavior was childish and unreasonable. There was a recurring cycle during which she first claimed that she was ready to go home and then subsequently appeared depressed and nervous. She was very difficult to work with. Her husband finally took her home against advice.

Ps. Toxic M:53:M:22 +1 '9287143–(71) 4:5:14
Alcoholism
Drug Add.
Deteriorated

The patient had been a chronic drinker for ten years, recently drinking about a quart of whiskey a day. At one time he had been a member of Alcoholics Anonymous and had managed to stop drinking for several periods, the most recent lasting nine months. He tried taking seconal to relieve the aftereffects of intoxication and when he stopped drinking he increased his doses of seconal. He underwent several hospitalizations in the attempt to break these habits and he entered the hospital on a voluntary admission to try again to free himself of drinking.

His physical health had always been good. He was an eighth-grade graduate, and after leaving school he traveled about the country for a time as an itinerant worker. He finally settled down and held several minor executive positions. With the increase in his drinking, however, he lost job after job and his employment level declined. He was an active, outgoing person with a great deal of energy, and he liked to impress other people. When drunk he was cheerful and congenial, but without alcohol he was often irritable and difficult.

In the hospital there was a generalized tremor and other scattered neurological indications of intoxication. He seemed to have a real desire to break his habits but was always reluctant to follow procedures that were difficult for him. There was psychometric evidence indicating brain damage. On his third day in the hospital he had a peculiar convulsive seizure which was followed by confusion. After that he had a number of other periods of confusion, during which he would be noisy and uncontrollable. He improved and appeared normal at the time of discharge. The prognosis was considered poor, however, and it was feared that the brain damage might progress.

Ps. Paranoid	F:33:M:35	+3	9'31–2786 (45)	3:1:13
Ps. Sz., Paranoid		+8	9'31–728 (47)	3:1:14
Ps. Paranoid	F:34:M:56	+18	984'6–2 (57)	8:13:17

This woman's pattern of difficulties, consisting of delusions, abnormal behavior, and somatic complaints, had been present for three weeks. The onset had followed the failure of a club sale which she was in charge of. In a sudden fit of temper she told other club officers that they were doing their jobs badly. Immediately after this scene she began to complain constantly of symptoms which were connected with diabetes, cancer, syphilis, and tuberculosis, all of which she thought she was suffering from. Abandoning outside activities and housework, she went to bed. About this time she developed the delusion that her parents were not actually her own, and that her husband was really her father. Also, she accused her husband of having affairs with other women and of having fathered thousands of children. The delusions gradually subsided and she apparently was almost well; then she became depressed and felt she was near death. At one time she started downtown to buy furs and clothes, telling her husband that they were about to inherit a legacy. Later an abnormal sexual desire appeared. Just before admission she urged her husband to use his power to "clean up" the town.

The past history showed no previous physical or psychological upsets that were pertinent. A top student in both high school and normal school, she taught school until her marriage at age 22. A well-liked, gregarious person, she was happy, active, and successful socially and in community enterprises. She was, in fact, an outstanding woman in her community and church. She was reserved, tidy, and never extravagant. Her married life had been happy, and there were three children.

In the hospital the physical and neurological examinations were negative. The most obvious factor in her illness was her concern about the true identity of her parents. One of the most important things that could be done while she was in the hospital, she felt, was the identification of her true parents. She completely lacked insight into her psychiatric disorder, and she vigorously insisted that she was in the hospital solely for the treatment of her somatic complaints. Immediately put on insulin shock treatment, she received seventeen treatments, with definite improvement. The somatic symptoms disappeared promptly, and the emotion behind the paranoid delusions disappeared in large part. Not friendly with other patients, she spent much time alone. Just before her discharge, when asked how the treatment had helped her, she stated decisively that it had relieved her of pain but that her trouble had never been mental. The prognosis was felt to be good, and she was discharged to her husband.

One year later she was back in the hospital with the same pattern of symptoms. The pattern had reappeared about a month before admission. This time she was given both insulin and electroshock treatment. In the hospital she had periods of uncontrollable elation with hostility and suspicion. Again she improved somewhat symptomatically and was discharged to her husband.

Ps. Paranoid F:29:M:64 +3 '93184-2(43) 0:3:9

The patient was brought to the hospital by her husband, who said that following their marriage eight years before he had noticed that his wife was at times intolerant and suspicious about minor incidents. Rather than go out evenings she had preferred to sit at home, and while he had not been concerned about this, he had become irritated by some of her attitudes. Later she had been unduly depressed over his absence on a business trip but had recovered when he returned. She had had another depression while he was with the army in Japan, and a psychiatrist diagnosed her ailment as "mood depression." She sat staring and worrying about her husband for hours, and she came to the conclusion that he was dead and that others were writing his letters for him. On his return she quickly recovered. At various times she had had other exacerbations of paranoid ideas. After the birth of her second child she had thought that people were jealous of her, that her father and a lawyer were attempting to dope her, and that neighbors were taking small articles from her home. More recently she had suffered a miscarriage; then she had accused her husband of doping her with coffee and of scratching her at night on the shoulders and ankles. She said she found the doping instrument and that when she scratched herself with it she immediately went into a deep sleep.

In the past medical history there was a "female"operation at 16. She had also had hay fever for many years. She had graduated from high school with honors and had attended a business college for a year. She had then worked successfully as a sales girl until her marriage and had been able to handle several part-time jobs later. Her high school social life had been restricted by her mother, who did not let the girl go out. The patient was an excellent housewife and handled the affairs of her home and her children very well. Except for a weekly card club she had few hobbies. She had always "talked down" the neighbors and her husband's friends and avoided meeting them if possible, but when she did meet them she was very pleasant. She had few personal friends.

In the hospital she showed definite paranoid trends, with delusions of reference and persecution. She said emphatically that her husband had scratched her with the wire she had found, and she told exactly how it was done. She admitted that she had periods of depression and moodiness, but she did not consider them unusual in view of her home problem. She insisted that she was not ill. There was no gross disturbance and she was well oriented. Her I.Q. was 119. She showed an excellent attitude and manner, but there was an air of martyrdom in her demeanor. She was very active in ward activities and showed considerable leadership. She would have seemed entirely normal if it had not been for the delusions of persecution and reference. Since a coma could not be brought on by insulin therapy, electroshocks were given. After three treatments she changed somewhat and became adolescent in attitude, giggling and joking frequently. She was discharged to her husband's care and it was arranged for her to continue at the outpatient clinic.

P. Hypo. F:55:D:29 +1 9'324–(55) 9:4:15

Four years before admission the patient noticed vague painful and constrictive sensations about her neck and upper chest. These lasted a very short time; they came on with exertion and were accompanied by perspiration and breathlessness. Gradually, persisting pains in her head developed and these began to interfere with her sleep. Another source of worry and disturbance to her was a callus on her heel.

Sixteen years earlier the patient had been diagnosed as a diabetic; that condition had since been fairly well controlled. She also had been operated on for a goiter and had had, among other medical procedures, three pelvic repairs, nine dilations with curettements, uteran suspension, tube ligation, and two operations for glaucoma.

Following high school she took an eighteen-month nurses' training course. Before her marriage she led an average social life with girls but associated little with boys. Of a pleasant disposition, she was above average in intelligence and appeared to have been happy, well adjusted, and emotionally stable. However, she admitted to a "lot of troubles that I cannot talk about." Somewhat seclusive and reserved, she selected her friends with care. The patient had married a man who had proved to be an irresponsible drunkard, and he had finally deserted her, leaving her with one son. When the latter grew up he married and moved away, assuming no responsibility for his mother. For the last ten years she had lived alone.

In the hospital the patient was clearly oriented but preoccupied with her somatic complaints. Her problems, she believed, must be due to a recurrence of the former thyroid trouble. She was friendly and cooperative. While she had a partial insight into her condition, she was defensive and avoided discussion of personal matters. It was difficult also to bring her to realize that many of the symptoms were unrelated to physical findings. Concerned about being on relief,

9'34 168–

she was eager to get a job. The callus on her heal she feared might be cancerous and she was convinced that if she could just have another operation, this time to remove the callus, she would be completely well. It appeared that she had almost consciously developed an attitude of well-being and complete and active adjustment to the world. Because of this defense mechanism she changed little in the hospital, and at her discharge the prognosis was guarded.

Ps. M-D., Manic Paranoid   F:41:D:21   +1   9'34 168–(39)   4:6:14

Two months before her admission the patient began to develop paranoid ideas about her work. She thought that her employer would not raise her wages because he was angry with her and that people in the office were talking about her. She also had delusional ideas about marrying a person she referred to as "George." In a letter to her employer she resigned her position, giving marriage to George as her reason for leaving. George talked to her over the radio, she said, and he played for her the music she heard. She insisted that doors be kept open for him, and she frequently telephoned gasoline stations to ask for him. When she came to the hospital she thought she was coming to be married.

Several years before admission the patient had divorced her husband so that she could marry a man named George, whom she had been fond of. They had talked of having sexual relations, but something had always thwarted their plans. When she was free, George denied having had any intention of marrying her. As a result she became so obnoxious in her insistence on marriage that her father was asked to come to the town where she worked and take her home. Her recovery was rapid, but a year later she developed a delusional system centering around George. She again recovered in three months.

As a child the patient had been quiet, sensitive, and very well behaved. She graduated from an agricultural college and taught for four years, but she changed positions frequently because of dissatisfaction with her salary. She had been a good student, and her family had always been proud of her. She was an outgoing, cheerful, and friendly person. Her marriage had been adequate and satisfying; it was possible that the divorce resulted from her illness rather than from maladjustment. There was evidence that she had been frustrated by not having children of her own. The patient was the oldest of six children, four of whom had been feeble-minded, and she and her husband had not wanted to risk having feeble-minded children.

During the patient's stay in the hospital she was elated and euphoric, refusing to sleep at night and roaming through the halls causing a disturbance. She expressed her delusional ideas about George very freely and seemed to immerse herself in them. After ten subshock doses of insulin there was rapid improvement, and all the symptoms practically disappeared. She began to plan for the future and asked how to prevent a recurrence of the illness.

B. Psth., Asocial M:36:M:16 —44 '9346–(71) 6:4:18
Ps. Toxic —86 4'2937 86–(59) 7:2:23
Alcoholism

The complaint of this patient on admission was a "terrific hangover." He had begun to drink at the age of 16. After a girl he had been intimate with became pregnant, he had continued to attend high school, drinking, he said, "to cover up my embarrassment." Later he had married the girl, but he had never lived with her and they were divorced when he was 20. At 22 he had married a woman who was three years older than he and whose education was superior to his. At age 26 he had begun to go on drinking sprees that lasted for seven days at least once a month. After serving in the navy for two months, he had been discharged for drunkenness. He had joined Alcoholics Anonymous under pressure and had remained sober for three months. Since then he had been in practically every hospital and sanitarium in the metropolitan region he lived in, but only to recover from the sprees. A bout of drinking finally resulted in the present admission to the psychiatric unit, although he had been seen as an outpatient for some time.

At the time of admission he was managing a soft-drink stand, and with the help of his wife, was doing fairly well. He had had many jobs, mostly as a salesman or in other work involving social contacts. Although he was a friendly person, he maintained a superior attitude and showed indifference to most activities and to his friends and his family. An only child, he had been spoiled and pampered by his parents.

In the hospital he said this was the first time he had ever wanted to stop drinking, but he resented the idea of staying in the hospital for more than a few days since it would hurt his business. He felt guilty about all the trouble he had caused his family and was convinced that he would be able to stay sober if he came regularly to the outpatient department. He had an I.Q. of 126. The psychological tests and other procedures showed him to have considerable hostility toward his wife and his mother in particular. Polite and friendly toward everyone, he made a halfhearted attempt to engage in games and other ward activities, but he acted as though he were superior to the other patients, and he was guilty of slight infractions of the rules. He was discharged after recovering from his acute state, but prognostically there was little likelihood that he would change his behavior.

Ps. Sz., Paranoid M:30:S:1460 +790 9'348–(51) 9:2:24

This veteran was first admitted as a transfer from an army hospital with a diagnosis of dementia praecox, paranoid type; this was later changed to dementia praecox, hebephrenic type. He left the hospital against medical advice and a second admission (the present admission) was effected two years later. The commitment papers indicated that he entertained delusions of grandeur about himself—he thought that he heard his name mentioned over the radio, that he had certain friendships among the Axis powers, and that he could stop the war at any time. His principal line of conversation concerned his "great ability."

Just before admission he became violent in his home, pulling telephone wires from the wall and slapping his sister, and it was necessary for the police to take him to a hospital.

The patient graduated from high school at age 18 and later attended another high school to take a course in accounting. Before his illness, he was cheerful, easygoing, and had many friends. He did not use alcohol, smoked a little, and enjoyed outdoor sports. At the time of his induction into the army he was engaged. Records indicated that his military adjustment was satisfactory. His illness had first become manifest when he wrote a letter to his commanding general and sent a telegram to the president proposing that he be discharged so that he could take over important governmental duties in Washington.

On admission, the patient was relevant, coherent, and oriented; he seemed to be under tension. Somewhat euphoric, he was overtalkative and showed ideas of grandeur. He ran away from the hospital and was returned four months later. During these months he had been at home, where he refused to work and got into trouble with neighbors. He was given a course of electroshock therapy without apparent improvement. He continued to be grandiose, euphoric, and hyperactive, many times getting into difficulties with other patients and with nurses. C. W. S.

Ps. M-D., Depr. F:34:M:9 +5 '93862417–(49) 5:4:15
Suicidal

Five months before admission the patient's husband had broken his arm, and about the same time he had failed to get a promotion. He became irritable and began to drink and to wander off for days at a time. He was at the time engaged in business activities that were supposed to be kept secret and he refused to discuss them with his wife; she began to "hound and nag" him and finally had him admitted to a psychiatric service. While the husband was in the hospital the wife became sullen and depressed and he asked to be discharged so that he could go home and take care of her. She began to have a "give up" feeling, felt there was no use in trying any more, and, as she put it, came to feel that a person she had thought to be perfect was not perfect. She could not sleep and on one occasion took four sleeping pills. One day she asked her husband to get a gun so that she could end it all. While waiting for hospital admission she thought she was going to have a heart attack and after admission she thought she had died.

She had had three previous attacks of depression at ages 14, 24, and 32. These were precipitated by disappointments in love affairs. She had attended college for a year but dropped out because she had difficulty getting from one class to another. Then she worked in her father's bank for a number of years. She was a friendly person and appeared well above average in intelligence. All her life she had been overprotected and "fondled." She had had poliomyelitis and had come out of it with a leg deformity that had encouraged more parental overprotection. Until the present difficulty her marriage had been a happy one and she had one son she was very fond of.

In the hospital she was concerned about her illness, was confused and disoriented, and had feelings of unreality and death. She was obviously depressed but attempted to cover it up. Her answers to questions were adequate but her speech was slow and she appeared to have difficulty in thinking. Shortly after entering the hospital she made a remarkable improvement. Her feelings of unreality and death disappeared, and the depression was not as severe as when she was admitted. She began to look forward to leading a normal, happy life with her husband and child.

Two months later she was readmitted after an attempted suicide. At the time of her first discharge her husband and father were supposed to call for her. Her father came but her husband failed to appear. He called and said he would be home early that evening. She went home and when her husband did not come, she began to worry and to feel "let down." She could not sleep and the next morning took an overdose of sedative. Her husband returned home, found the note she had left for him, and immediately called an ambulance. She was taken to a general hospital and eventually transferred to the psychiatric unit again. On this admission she appeared tired, drawn, disheveled, and concerned about her recurrent depression, and she again attempted suicide. She had hope of getting well but believed it would be a struggle. She improved during her stay and was open and friendly around the hospital, enjoying the routine. She was again discharged, apparently recovered from this attack.

Ps. Sz., Paranoid   M:23:S:168   +101   '94–213(51)   3:2:16
Ps. M-D., Manic

This patient was admitted with a diagnosis of manic-depressive reaction, manic. For a period of several weeks before hospitalization he had been extremely restless and excitable. He paced up and down and emphasized his remarks by slapping his fist into his hand or against objects. His conversation revealed ideas of grandeur. He spoke of himself in the third person and talked of political aspirations and F.B.I. connections. In addition he annoyed the police department by seeking protection because he believed a man intended to kill him.

The patient completed high school at the age of 18. His school record indicated that he had "high and low moods" at school and was inclined to be boisterous and a "show-off." After high school he enlisted in the navy and was discharged on points after three years. While in the service he had some trouble because of drinking and fighting. After his discharge he began to show restlessness and tension and worried considerably about having contracted a venereal disease while in the service. His mother had suffered a "nervous breakdown" after the birth of an older child.

After the patient was given electroshock therapy he showed improvement. The MMPI was administered two months after the completion of the electroshock therapy. At the time of the examination, he was responding well in group psychotherapy and was selected for individual psychotherapy. During psychotherapeutic contacts over a period of two months he began to show some insight and his restlessness gradually diminished. In early sessions he paced the floor while talking, but as time went on he became calmer and in a number of ways showed better emotional control. During therapy he showed much concern about matters relating to sex and childbirth. He had learned as an adolescent that his mother had been in a mental hospital after the birth of his older sister, who was a cripple. This had been a shock to him and he worried about the inheritance of mental disease. At the time of discharge from the hospital the prognosis appeared favorable. C. W. S.

Ps. M-D., Manic F:20:S:47 +8 9'4–26(59) 4:2:15

One month before admission this young woman donned the fatigue uniform of a friend in military service and turned in a false fire alarm. When the police and fire departments arrived the patient was overactive and talking foolishly. When she insisted that she wanted to ride in the fire engine to the station house, she was taken to the precinct police station where her behavior became increasingly bizarre. Insisting that she was undergoing some sort of test, she wanted to telephone family friends. Taken to a hospital, she continued to show marked hyperactivity and a flight of ideas for a few days. After a short remission of these symptoms they returned again and she was brought to the psychiatric hospital.

Following three years in one university, the young woman was arranging, at the time of the illness, to transfer to another university to finish her course. Always an adequate person, she was interested in sports and in social affairs and led an active life. Among the children in her family, she was regarded as the most stable. The family was congenial and there were no other factors that appeared contributory to the present illness.

In the hospital she showed such an extreme flight of ideas that determination of their content was difficult. She made many references to her family and friends and a good many oversexual comments about babies. The patient was flirtatious and aggressive. Elated and without any insight, she demanded that she be allowed to go home. Although markedly overactive, she was cooperative and permitted an examination. At times she appeared afraid to be left alone. She continually misidentified members of the staff and nurses, confusing them with her friends and relatives. She had occasional paranoid ideas. During the hospitalization she gradually returned to nearly normal behavior and moods. The paranoid ideas slowly disappeared and she came to recognize that she had been ill. She was discharged after plans had been made for her to increase her independence from her family and to follow a course of action that would relieve her of psychological stresses.

B. Psth., Asocial F:20:D 9'4–26(70) 6:5:17
Ps. Psth.
Suicidal

Uncontrollable crying and inability to tell the truth brought this university student to the mental hygiene clinic. She came voluntarily and asked for help. Earlier the girl had been hospitalized for several weeks for what may have been a schizophrenic psychosis, although information about this episode was incomplete. The event precipitating the present hospitalization was an abortive suicide attempt.

Little could be elicited about the girl's background because of her pathologic lying. She complained of her early home situation, but facts were not available to corroborate her stories. She said she had been married briefly and for some years had engaged in hitchhiking and other unconventional activities.

The girl was an obese, unattractive person. She blamed much of her difficulty on her home situation. Treatment consisted of three interview sessions over a two-month period, with no perceptible change in her lying, although her crying rapidly subsided. C. K. A.

Ps. Paranoid F:37:M:27 +26 9'4–63(45) 2:3:15

The patient had been married about eighteen months before admission and about a month before, she had completed a normal pregnancy and had delivered her first child. On the fifth postpartum day she had developed a severe paranoid psychosis, characterized by ideas that the nurses were mistreating her baby and that her food was poisoned. She also had ideas of reference and hallucinations of a bizarre type. This psychotic period had disappeared suddenly after a few days, but about three weeks after her discharge from the hospital she had returned complaining of many somatic pains. No good basis for them was discovered in the physical examination. From that time on she showed increased irritability, sensitiveness, insomnia, and inability to relax. She was then admitted to the psychiatric unit.

She had apparently been healthy until the onset of the present illness. Although she had been somewhat overprotected by her mother, she had seemingly been a normal child, and she had done well in school. After finishing high school she worked for her father, but although she enjoyed the work very much, she left home at age 25 to escape the overprotectiveness of her mother. After graduating from a business college she took a job in another city as a secretary, but when her family moved to the same city she again had to live with them. Even after her marriage she had continued to live with them. She was a somewhat immature person, but no other facts about her character seemed contributory.

In the hospital she talked freely even about the intimate details of her life. She expressed a multitude of somatic complaints, worried about inconsequential things, cried very easily, was extremely sensitive, and had ideas of reference that made her conscious of everything she did and its possible interpretation by others. Superficially she made every effort to appear at ease and in a good light, but she had a haggard, intense expression and would frequently burst forth with such statements as this: "If only I could relax. Sometimes I'm all right for an hour or two, then I get tired and my legs and arms begin to ache all over again and then I begin to cry." She mixed freely with other patients, but only because it was part of the hospital routine. Her smiles and speech, while appearing normal, were forced. About a week after admission she was given electroshock treatments and after the fourth treatment changed definitely for the better. At the time of discharge she felt she was entirely well again.

Ps. Sz., Mixed	M:20:S:108	+30	9'4–672 (45)	3:7:13
Alcoholism				

This veteran's first hospitalization for a mental disorder occurred at 19 while he was in the navy. Given electroshock therapy, he was discharged from the service with a disability compensation for schizophrenia in remission. On his return home his behavior was considered bizarre and entirely different from his pre-service personality. His employer reported that he lied continually and was disliked by the other employees. At home he got up in the middle of the night, played phonograph records, slammed doors, and walked around laughing and making vulgar remarks. His parents were alarmed one night when they awoke to find him standing over their bed looking at them "in a very strange way." At this time he was also drinking heavily. Four months after his discharge from the service he was committed to this hospital following an arrest for burglary.

The patient was a high school graduate. Little information was available about his social and personality adjustment before he entered the service, but it was said that he had been an average student at school and had presented no problems at home. For his two years in the navy there was also no record of his adjustment other than the hospitalization and the discharge for schizophrenia.

At the hospital the patient made a marginal adjustment. He attempted to escape once but otherwise appeared indifferent to his surroundings and his difficulties. At the psychotherapy clinic he was judged to be a poor candidate for intensive therapy because of his indifferent attitude. He was considered immature and definitely lacking in emotional stability and insight. No specific treatment was given and he was finally discharged. C. W. S.

Ps. M-D., Manic	F:35:M:50	+1	9'4–<u>72</u>31 (53)	4:4:12
		+5	4'98–6 (51)	3:6:17

Six months before admission and four months after the birth of her third child the patient began to show an obviously abnormal increase in psychomotor activity. She slept only two or three hours a night, neglected her home and children, began to spend money foolishly, and engaged in a multitude of outside activities.

These symptoms gradually increased until she became unmanageable and was hospitalized for study and treatment.

The woman's past history was clear of contributory factors except for a six-month period six years earlier when she had had a similar attack. A trained nurse, she had been active athletically, socially, and professionally. Her self-assurance was abundant and she was regarded as extroverted. With people she was usually cheerful and social. The patient's husband, a lawyer, was tense and overly conscientious. Both the husband and the patient used sedatives and alcohol in moderate excess. There was some sexual maladjustment, the patient having never been able to obtain an orgasm without masturbation. There were three children.

In the hospital there were no obvious disturbances of mentation or orientation. She said, "Two months ago I suddenly saw what life was all about and everything was clear to me." She planned to write a book and let the world "know the truth." She rationalized her excessive activity and said that it was "natural in a person with three children and a country home." She felt she had been tricked into coming to the hospital. There were marked emotional swings from euphoria to anger and tears. She totally lacked insight into her condition as a mental illness. She was alert, overly active, agitated, and suspicious. After twelve electroshock treatments she gradually improved; the overactivity decreased, she began to eat and sleep normally, and she adjusted well to ward activities. She gained some insight and seemed to have benefited enormously from the hospitalization. When she returned to her home she was given a strict warning to decrease her use of alcohol and sedatives.

Ps. M-D., Manic F:59:S:20 +4 941'3687-(39) 3:11:10

The present episode began two weeks before admission. The patient gradually increased her activities and talked aimlessly for hours. Another day she spent hours running from one place to another and engaging in flighty conversation without any reason. She had the delusion that someone was taking movies of her. She called a brother who was more than a thousand miles away to talk of things well known to both of them and of no consequence. Just before admission while driving with some friends she stopped the car, got out, talked to herself, and was apparently very agitated. Since there was a river nearby, her friends were afraid that she would become suicidal and took her to a physician. For two or three days she was hilarious, could not carry on an intelligent conversation, and did not recognize her brother. By the time of admission to the hospital she had shown considerable improvement.

In the past history there was a period during which she had suffered from hypothyroidism. This condition was treated successfully. About seven years before admission she had a maniacal attack and was treated with electroshock therapy. One year before admission she felt a compulsive desire to get away, and she apparently avoided an attack of hypomanic activity by traveling to another state. A college graduate with a master's degree in the social sciences, she was successful at promotional work and had held positions of considerable responsibility. Her social life was almost entirely dependent on her work. A domineering, self-made, and exacting woman, she was somewhat egotistical and extremely self-confident. Because she had felt a responsibility to her father, who was divorced, she had never married.

In the hospital, she said the episode was the result of the "many burdens" on her. She showed some flight of ideas but was otherwise fairly close to her normal behavior. She became rapidly even more normal and after she had made plans for retiring from her position and in other ways reducing the strain on her she was discharged. The prognosis was thought to be good.

Ps. Paranoid F:34:M:43 +5 9′41683– 4:8:19

This woman was admitted to the hospital as a voluntary patient; she had ideas about her husband's infidelity and a manifest hatred of him. Her first accusation of his unfaithfulness had occurred three years before when, at a party, she noticed him walking down the basement stairs with another woman guest. From that time on she objected to his taking part in any activity which included other women. She frequently misinterpreted his behavior; for example, car horns she interpreted as "signals from chippies." She believed her husband was an habitué of a house of ill fame in the neighborhood. Most of these accusations were indefinite and the persons involved were referred to as "they." Gradually she neglected her home and children. During one period she pulled down the shades and turned on the lights in the daytime. Strange behavior such as smiling vacantly and signaling to strangers was noted. The event precipitating admission to the hospital occurred when, in a rage, she picked up a butcher knife and ordered her husband from the house. At various times she had reported seeing strange women in the house, but when questioned by a physician about them she was evasive and said that "perhaps they were only shadows."

The past history showed no apparently contributory factors. She had attended a university for two years but had failed in several subjects and had withdrawn. Until her marriage she taught in a parochial school. She had managed her home and children well although she resented interference. Admired for her independence and clear thinking, she was able to dominate a situation, and, in fact, her husband had always looked to her for guidance. The patient was, however, selfish and egocentric, wanting the best of everything regardless of cost. During the present illness she had become extravagant and careless in money matters and had also lost many of the friends she had earlier made.

In the hospital she appeared well, poised, and conventional. Denying the need of psychiatric attention, she nevertheless did accept the hospitalization reasonably. She avoided discussion of family or personal affairs because she felt "they are unalterable and of no importance in my case." She said, "I needed just this kind of a rest and I'm going to make the best of it." Smilingly she evaded all attempts at psychotherapy. "I wouldn't have come to the decisions I have if I didn't have adequate proof. It's a long and gruesome story," she commented. With a longer stay in the hospital she became somewhat less inaccessible and aloof but no genuine change occurred by the time of discharge.

M:23:S:50 +18 9'428 673–(53) 3:12:3

This young man had a history of repeated indecent exposure, for which he was charged by the police. He got headaches and had to masturbate at the sight of girls. He had been involved in several accidents and had sustained a fractured skull. He was admitted to the hospital for observation as a voluntary patient.

He was the second of three children. After receiving an elementary education he worked in a factory as a lorry driver until he joined the ground staff of the Royal Air Force.

His symptoms were regarded as post-traumatic character changes, but no definite diagnosis was made. M. V.

M:32:? '943–1X (57) 11:3:16

This man, an industrial engineer, was referred by his employer because he was not performing satisfactorily on his job. He did not finish enough work in a day, seemed to have few ideas to contribute, and was not happy in the job location. The employer wished to know if a change in his assignment or supervisor or other adjustments would improve his effectiveness.

He himself had no direct complaints about his job but was critical of the management, disliked the town, and did not feel he was being given suitable work experience. He had a concept of himself playing a professional role in a community where he could be a leader, and the present setup did not fulfill his ambitions.

Tests of his ability indicated that he could not compete successfully with the other engineers in his group and that he was not suited for on-the-job training of the type he was receiving. While coming in for counseling interviews, he was dismissed from his job, which complicated the situation but permitted him to survey all possibilities for his next move. Influenced largely by the kind of social belongingness he believed he would feel in another kind of work, he chose to make a radical change in his vocation. The security and the local prestige offered by public school jobs in relatively small communities were attractive to him, and he decided to consider high school teaching rather than industrial work, even though it meant acquiring more training in education. D. F. C.

Alcoholism **M:50:M:45** **+3** **'943–6(51)** **8:4:22**
Drug Add.
Paranoid

Although it was an overdose of barbiturates which finally brought this man to the hospital, he had been "jittery" for the past six months and had used drugs and alcohol excessively much of his life. For almost twenty years there had been episodes of heavy drinking. These bouts had lasted from a few months to several years. Between the bouts he stopped drinking voluntarily or sought hospital help. In the "dry" spells he led a normal and responsible life. Some months before admission he joined Alcoholics Anonymous and after that did not take alcohol in the usual form but substituted a mixture of terpin hydrate with codein and also began to take excessive amounts of phenobarbital and seconal. These intoxicated him to the point where he sometimes smashed furniture. A month before admission he tried a private rest home but left because of "hospital jitters." After eight or nine sleepless nights he took a box of phenobarbital pills and was found in a groggy, resentful condition. Brought immediately to the hospital, he was given a gastric lavage.

In World War I the patient began to drink in moderation soon after he joined the army. A graduate of a two-year business college, he was first a successful salesman, later a general manager. Between drinking episodes he was cheerful and hard working. His interests were wide and he got along well with people. On the other hand, during the periods of drinking he lied, showed irritability, and at times threatened that "someone is going to get hurt." During these periods he lost interest in things and was unable to sleep.

In the hospital the patient was incensed at being locked up, believed he had done nothing wrong or unusual, minimized his illness, and was untruthful about his drug addiction. His mentality appeared intact; he was well oriented and in general normal, except for the remnants of the symptoms from the sedation. Harboring a steady resentment against the staff, he was irritable and short with interviewers and insisted that he had been taught a lesson. Uncooperative and resentful, he refused to fit into the hospital routine. He was demanding of the nurses and abused them for going about their duties. As time went on he began to select certain staff members toward whom he became more friendly. In general, however, he never really relaxed his hostilities. Neither did he develop any degree of insight into the severity of his problems, insisting at all times that he "understood what was wrong" with him and had learned "what to do about it."

B. Pri., Child. M:17:S:3 +2 9'43–6712 2:4:8

This boy was admitted to the hospital because of misbehavior consisting chiefly of truancy, and, in addition, restlessness, inability to concentrate, and generally unconventional behavior. For many years he had had difficulty in getting along with his father. Never a success in high school, he had recently been cutting classes and had shown such poor cooperation that he was finally expelled.

The boy had an I.Q. of 130. He was an affable lad who usually got along with adults as well as youngsters of his own age. He was six feet four inches tall and weighed 160 pounds. Only a few details about his actual misbehavior were available, but apparently it had not been severely asocial.

In the hospital he was at ease, casual, and almost overly friendly. He regarded his admission to the hospital lightly; he did sober down a little when the reasons for it were explained to him, but he soon brushed the whole matter off and entered into ward activities with considerable interest and absorption. He had no thinking disorder that could be elicited. He spoke of no worries and there was nothing unusual about his appearance or manner. Unduly friendly with one or two of the women patients and flip with the nurses, the lad was somewhat of a nuisance on the ward, and it was clear that if he remained in the hospital for any length of time he would surely be in considerable trouble. It was recommended that he be placed in a strict boarding school away from home, and that an attempt be made to get him interested in a difficult curriculum of studies.

Ps. M-D., Manic	F:44:D:66	+1	94'3-7 (47)	5:4:14
Paranoid		+56	'94-21786 (49)	4:2:13
Ps. M-D., Manic	F:46:D:37	+2	914'23687- (51)	2:9:10
Ps. M-D., Manic	F:48:D:37	+2	9'4183-67 (55)	8:6:12

The patient was first brought to the hospital because of intermittent periods of nervous agitation, various somatic complaints, and apparently unfounded suspicions. This pattern had been going on for about five years; during this time she suffered from repeated attacks of "nervous exhaustion" in which she was sleepless and irritable. Each attack was preceded by a period of overactivity. She had been hospitalized on numerous occasions, occasionally in the state hospital. Associated with the attacks were jaundice, cholecystitis, severe headaches, and frequent colds, all of which she seemed frequently to exaggerate. Lately the patient had developed suspicions involving her relatives, whom she accused of tampering with her mail and of taking her alimony payments. She had consequently become engrossed in legal procedures, making herself a considerable nuisance to all those concerned with her.

The patient's past health had been fairly good. She had had a number of difficulties that seemed possibly psychosomatic in character. About five years before admission she had undergone a hysterectomy, which marked the onset of the present pattern of symptoms. The medical indications determining this operation were unknown.

She had been trained as a chemical technician and after graduation had worked until her marriage. She had had to assume the support of her family at various times during her marriage and she had had to work steadily after her divorce, which had occurred three years before admission. She was a pleasant person and a diligent and conscientious worker; she was described as cheerful, kind, and thoughtful almost to excess. She had had a happy early life and thought highly of her parents. The first twelve years of her marriage had also been happy but her husband then had begun to drink excessively and to associate with other women. This change in his behavior ultimately led to the divorce. The patient was very sensitive about the unhappy outcome of her marriage and it was felt that she still loved her former husband.

The physical examination on admission was essentially noncontributory except that she was obese. The neurological findings were also negative. She was concerned with her health, her legal affairs, and her ill-defined suspicions of her relatives. Her sensorium and intellect were unaffected; her emotional tone varied between elation and slight depression and irritability. She felt that there was nothing wrong with her mentally and that her problem was wholly somatic. She was voluble and circumstantial, and at times she showed a moderate flight of ideas. She was pleasing in appearance and accessible to the interviewers, apparently trying hard to be cooperative. She gradually got somewhat better and, though she was obviously not completely recovered, returned to her home.

About eighteen months later she was readmitted with a similar pattern of complaints. This time she was given shock therapy and again her hyperactivity decreased until she could return home. Three years later she was again admitted. The admission and the pattern were similar but this time there were, in addition, bizarre somatic complaints, and the psychotic elements were judged to be more severe. She was discharged for admission to a state hospital.

Ps. Sz., Paranoid	M:28:S:23	+7	9'43–71 28 (37)	3:4:12
Ps. Sz., Paranoid Mutilative	M:28:S:93	+13	9'84–13 (26)	3:4:11
Ps. Sz., Paranoid	M:28:S:179	+23	9'43–78 (32)	3:4:10

This man was first hospitalized for a mental illness while in the army and was discharged from the service with a diagnosis of paranoid state in partial remission. Two years after his discharge he was hospitalized in a veterans' hospital and received electroshock therapy. Immediately following this he entered a private hospital where he received insulin therapy. From there he came to this hospital for his first admission. He was disoriented, confused, and showed paranoid delusions. In a few days there was a total spontaneous remission and he was discharged.

The patient returned home and resumed work but in a short time had an acute exacerbation of the psychosis, with numerous paranoid delusions. Believing he was back in the army and was being followed by his former commanding officer, he went to a police station for protection. While waiting there he thrust his hands through a window, cutting his wrists. Returned to the hospital, he again made a spontaneous remission and was discharged after a period of good adjustment. A few weeks later he turned up at another veterans' hospital after breaking windows and creating a disturbance while drinking. After treatment he showed improvement and was discharged but soon returned under similar circumstances, was subsequently committed, and was transferred to this hospital.

The patient completed high school with average grades. Sociable and popular with students and teachers, he participated in sports, particularly football and swimming. The first sign of a personality difficulty appeared during his adolescence when he showed a great deal of hostility toward his father. This culminated in a fight in which he severely beat his father. Soon after this, following his graduation from high school, the patient entered the army, where he served for five years. Shortly before his hospitalization in the army he had an altercation with another soldier, who resembled his father in physical structure and countenance. After his return home from the service his parents noticed a great change in him. Many nights he was troubled with severe nightmares which disturbed the whole household; often he dreamed of an airplane crash in which a friend had been killed. The patient worked at a number of different jobs, leaving most of these impulsively because he felt that other workers were watching him.

During the veteran's several hospitalizations his symptoms followed similar patterns. He had periods of confusion and extreme paranoid delusions, followed by complete remissions. He showed much hostility toward his parents, particularly his father. While under the influence of alcohol the patient had visual hallucinations, usually the face of his father and the face of the soldier who resembled his father. It was seeing these faces in windowpanes that caused him to break windows a number of times. During the hospitalization just preceding the last exacerbation he received insulin and electroshock therapy and intensive psychotherapy. During the latter he showed considerable insight. At the last admission the patient was in a partial remission and showed some superficial insight, bland affect, and defensiveness. C. W. S.

Ps. M-D., Manic F:23:M:45 +1 9'4678321-X 12:5:21

The present problems of this girl could be understood only in the light of her history. A student in a home economics course at a university two years before admission, she slept and studied irregularly, worked only for "a good time," failed to make credits, and was dismissed after two quarters of work. She told romantic tales to classmates about her family's wealth and bragged about her powers with men. After being dropped from the university, she attempted to find a job but apparently made a poor impression. She then began to forge checks and to charge clothes, using her father's name. One day she made a down payment on a new automobile with a bad check and ran away with a 19-year-old student. She lived with him until they were found by her parents. Not only did she show no remorse over this but in fact was very gay.

Later, during a visit to a small town, she went out with a young man, who, she claimed, forced her to have sexual intercourse with him. Fearing pregnancy, she insisted that he marry her within a week. The couple lived together for two months in continual strife, then she returned to her parents' home. On various occasions she stealthily returned to her husband, sometimes stealing money to pay the fare. Away from her husband she tended to be depressed and withdrawn, and she frequently phoned him and wrote letters to him. Following her last visit she said she was "through with him"; he was "no good" and was the cause of her nervousness. He had told her he had gonorrhea. At this time her mother brought the patient to the hospital for advice.

The earlier years of the patient's life were relatively uneventful. She finished high school, was considered an average pupil, and in general appeared to have been normally social and friendly. She made friends quickly but tired of them soon. Described as always gay, she was energetic and interested in sports. She felt a much closer attachment to one of her sisters than to either of her parents.

On admission the patient voiced the belief that she was in the hospital "because my husband wants to get rid of me." "He doesn't want me around because he is going to inherit some money," she said. Her husband had mistreated her, had said malicious things about her, and had gone out with other women, according to her claims, which were probably founded on fact. There was no evidence of delusional or hallucinatory experiences. She was well oriented and, in general, intact in sensorium and intellect. There was a mild elation with pressure of thought and hyperactivity. She laughed continually, frequently reiterating, "Nothing is the matter." Gradually her mood improved to the point her parents considered to be normal for her. She remained gay and voluble, always ready to dance and enter into any activity. There was evidence of poor judgment, such as too open criticism of other patients. She gained some insight, and she recognized that she had had a mood disturbance for a year. "I can't imagine why I did all those things, and I know I made my parents suffer," she said. However, she showed no real feeling as she made this statement. At discharge she was apparently fairly well recovered from the acute episode.

Ps. Sz., Simple F:37:S:49 +1 946 87′23–(43) 1:8:11
Paranoid

The present illness of this patient dated back roughly ten years to a disappointing love affair. The patient, deciding her fiancé was not to be trusted, broke her engagement. Two years later the company for which she worked moved out of the city, and she was left without a job. Her mother noticed that she became irritable at this time. For a few months she held another job, then suddenly refused to go to work and stayed home in bed. For hours she talked about the past and demanded that her mother sit and listen. Persuaded to make a visit in another city, she went but did not get better and was placed in a rest hospital for a time. Next she took a job as a receptionist for a doctor but was so careless of her dress that she was a disgrace to the office. Moreover, she lost several hundred dollars by confusing the accounts. Another period in a rest hospital followed and then she worked at odd jobs. Most of the time, she helped around the house, took walks, and played bridge. Such poor relations existed between the patient and her mother that many days they did not speak to each other except when necessary. The mother described the patient as changeable, unreliable, and full of paranoid delusions. Just before admission the patient was depressed and talked of suicide.

All through school she earned good grades but had to work hard for them. After high school graduation she attended a business school for eight months, and then, after working a few months, she began to attend a nursing school. When she found that she disliked the work in the wards she withdrew. Described as a happy-go-lucky, friendly, sensitive, self-conscious person, she was also stubborn. Outdoor sports such as skiing and skating interested her. She was known as a fast worker.

In the hospital there was no evidence of hallucinatory experiences, but she had delusions of persecution and believed that her mother discussed her frequently with the rest of the family. She showed marked indecisiveness. Her sensorium and intellect in other ways seemed normal. Although she was somewhat depressed, she had a fairly appropriate emotional tone. Because she was confused and depressed she recognized that "there was something wrong," but she blamed everything on her surroundings. It was difficult to get a coherent story from her or, for that matter, any concerted effort of any type. On the ward she adjusted fairly well but was eager to leave. However, she made no plans at all for leaving and showed no appreciation of the problems she would meet if she returned to the environment she felt had caused all her troubles. Aloof and unfriendly most of the time, she did not get along well with other patients. Eventually she was transferred to a state hospital.

Ps. Sz., Simple M:27:S:33 +28 9'478–3X(55) 10:2:20

This veteran first entered a general hospital on the advice of his employer, who believed that the man needed a rest because he was "nervous" and overactive on the job. The patient gave no complaints and did not agree that he should be hospitalized. Although he realized that he had been hyperactive at work, he explained, "I've always worked that way—I don't like to be idle." He admitted having had dizzy spells at work but said he had never lost consciousness. After a brief hospitalization he was discharged and returned to his job in a garage.

Within two months he was returned to the hospital. His employer reported that the man's actions were still peculiar. The patient several times jumped into a car and drove at a breakneck speed around the parking lot until he had everyone running for cover. An examination at this time showed no physical defects but a definite blunting of affect. The patient showed poor judgment and a great deal of autistic thinking. He was diagnosed as having schizophrenia, simple type, and was transferred to this hospital.

When the patient was a child his parents acted in a theatrical troupe. When the company traveled, which happened frequently, the patient was left with his grandparents. When the patient was 15 his parents were divorced. He attended school until the ninth grade and apparently made a satisfactory adjustment there. It was said he had always played well with other children. During three and a half years in the army he saw considerable action and received a number of citations. After his return home he destroyed all his citations, except one which his mother hid, and refused to discuss his war experiences.

At this hospital the patient exhibited definite emotional leveling. He was apparently indifferent toward the hospitalization; nevertheless he could not understand why it was judged necessary. At a staff conference the diagnosis of schizophrenia, simple type, was suggested. However, the majority of the staff felt that more information was required and he was classified "undiagnosticated" pending further study. Shortly thereafter, he was taken from the hospital, against medical advice, by his mother and stepfather. C. W. S.

B. Pri., Child. F:16:S 94'7863–(59) 2:4:11

This girl was brought to the clinic by her parents after she had been expelled from a private school for bringing liquor into the dormitory. Her parents were afraid that she might not finish high school and also wondered about vocational possibilities for her. They were interested in learning how they could help her to get along better.

The second of three children, the girl had presented no particular problems until her entry into junior high school. There she began to skip school, was impudent to her teachers, and did poor work. This resulted in her transfer to the private school. The difficulties were most marked in the months just before the visit to the clinic; she was belligerent toward everyone at times and accused her parents of not loving her. Her parents said the client hated her older sister, who was a good student, "like poison" and was jealous of her. Since the age of 14 she had received medication for a thyroid deficiency. This had been recently stopped because she smoked heavily and the physician thought her heart was being overstimulated. The girl smoked forty cigarettes a day, and when forbidden to smoke at home she left the house early in the morning in order to smoke before school began. It was said that she was willing to give up anything for cigarettes. Her parents stated that she was full of promises which she never kept but added that she was a good helper at home and seemed fond of her baby sister.

In two interviews at the clinic, the client appeared bland and pleasant and offered no active objection to any of the procedures. However, she gave the impression of exerting herself little and caring not at all about what she did. She expressed no feeling about her expulsion and no concern about her future. It was not until after repeated and direct questioning that she admitted she knew why she had been brought to the clinic. She said that she had no idea of what she wished to do vocationally, but added that she would "get a job." On the Otis test she obtained an I.Q. of 107, and her interests, according to several inventories, seemed to be mechanical and scientific. She was referred to a psychiatrist for treatment. M. V. B.

Ps. M-D., Mixed	M:17:S:23	+1	9′48–2$\underline{37}$	2:8:17
Ps. M-D., Mixed	M:17:S:37	+3	94′$\underline{86}$–7213	0:14:9
		+9	49′68–2$\underline{71}$3	0:15:11

This patient was first brought to the hospital (first set of admission data) five months before the present admission when he developed marked irritability and increased psychomotor activity. On being discharged from the hospital after this first admission he got along fairly well for two months. Then as he gradually became hyperactive again, he gave impromptu singing and whistling concerts in public places, conducted himself pretty much as he pleased, and was irritable when requested to comply with any rules or regulations at home or at school. At the time of admission he planned to go to New York to sing and whistle for radio programs. On one occasion he hitchhiked from one city to another and back in the same day without any apparent purpose.

His past history and home status were noncontributory. Described as having always been a normal boy, he was possibly somewhat more social and active than the average, but he had not been outstanding in any way.

In his opinion he had been railroaded into the hospital, having been given a choice between coming to the psychiatric unit or going to a state hospital. He explained that he was good at "singing, whistling, imitating famous people," and he intended to appear on radio shows, but he felt that a certain amount of practice was necessary. This he tended to do on the ward. He talked at great length about a girl he said he was engaged to. Aside from these ideas and activities, he was free from gross symptoms. He felt he was in excellent condition both mentally and physically. He was well oriented and intellectually intact. He regarded examinations as very silly. He would play ping-pong, dance a jig, smoke a cigarette, and whistle, all at as nearly the same time as possible. When his activities increased, it was decided to give him a period of narcotherapy, but there was no beneficial effect, and he was transferred to a state hospital.

Ps. M-D., Manic	F:26:S:63	+108	9′48–7	2:2:14

Following an attack of influenza about a year before admission the patient began to complain of fatigue and lost some weight, but in spite of the fact that her strength was not up to par she enrolled for a course at a university. Later she was especially depressed when she learned that a close male friend of hers was engaged to be married, and four days before admission she became acutely disturbed, running out into the street in the nude. She was transferred to the psychiatric unit from a private sanitarium.

The patient had finished high school and had taken training in nursing. She had worked as a public health nurse for a year and a half, changing then to a job as a dormitory nurse and dietician at a small college. Ambitious and a hard worker, she learned readily, did well in all her schoolwork, and was regarded as an unusually self-reliant person. There were no other factors in the past history that were particularly contributory.

In the hospital she was incoherent, uttering such statements as these: "Hit, please." "Thanks, kid." "Oh thanks, Mabel." She was suspicious of the examiners and frequently appeared to be responding to auditory and visual hallucinations. At times, when she mentioned the name of the young man who had married another girl, she became momentarily tearful. Disoriented for time, place, and person, she displayed a marked lability of emotion, although her predominant mood was euphoric, with a marked motor excitation. In spite of episodes of overactivity and irritability, she gradually became more comfortable, but even at the time of discharge she was not well and still found it difficult to apply herself seriously or effectively to relatively simple tasks. However, she had acquired enough insight into the fact that she had been ill and had become sufficiently cooperative to enable her to return home.

Ps. M-D., Manic	M:45:S:40	+3	9′48–7 (55)	4:4:16

Seven or eight months before admission the patient's brothers, with whom he worked, noticed that he was becoming progressively more gregarious and voluble, hyperactive, irritable, and expansive in business ideas and policy. They observed that he paid increased attention to women, drank more alcohol, and showed other symptoms of overactivity. Placed under a doctor's care, he was hospitalized but in a few days returned home. At home he became so overactive and irritable that he was taken to jail and from there was brought to the psychiatric unit.

A university graduate, he had always done well in school and had been successful in business. A friendly and forward person, he was a hard worker and previously had always been, as far as anyone could tell, entirely normal.

In the hospital he thought only of returning home. His reasons were that he felt good and liked it better at home. He was normal in intellect and well oriented. Most of the time his emotional tone was stable. His only insight was the idea that he was "possibly nervous from overwork." At first, despite his desire to return home, he showed some interest and appreciation in the hospitalization, but later he became morose and critical. In conversations with other patients he advised them about their troubles, spoke with sarcasm of his treatment, and talked about everyone. His overbearing manner lost him the friends he had made at the beginning of his stay. A course of subshock insulin treatments was tried but with no resultant change in his behavior except that he became a little less active. When it finally appeared that he had quieted down to an extent that would permit a trial at home, he was discharged to the care of his brothers.

Ps. M-D., Manic	M:20:S:120	+3	9′481–6	3:10:10
Schizoid		+83	9′4–$\underline{312}$78	4:2:13

A month before admission this young man suffered a spontaneous epistaxis, and was treated for it. The attending physician noticed that the patient seemed outstandingly happy and energetic. About this time the patient's friends observed that whereas he had previously been witty but restrained he now behaved in a silly and unrestrained fashion. At home he became seclusive and resented correction, especially from his father. During this month the patient drank a great deal and smoked an unusual number of cigarettes. On the day before admission, each time his father spoke to him he replied, "For God's sake, lay off me." On this same day the patient pulled the bed clothes from the bed in his room and the slip from the pillow, before lying down. Alarmed, his parents arranged that he be admitted for study.

The patient had never been robust. In addition to the usual childhood diseases, he had had tuberculosis peritonitis at age 11 and from that time on had had repeated attacks of diarrhea, nausea, and vomiting. For the past five years he had suffered from sinusitis and an intermittent swelling of the face that appeared to be a subauricular lyphangitis. He had no previous psychotic upsets.

An honor graduate of high school, he was at the time of this illness in the second year of a university premedical course, maintaining a B average. Described as a stubborn, sensitive individual, he had always suffered from marked mood swings, his feelings were easily hurt, and he brooded over small slights. Receiving the admiration of his group seemed highly important to him, and it was difficult for him to accept the success of friends or relatives. His family was an unhappy one, the mother was lenient, the father exceedingly strict.

In the hospital the neurological and physical examinations were not contributory. The patient showed a flight of ideas, emotional instability, and a general elation. He appeared clear in sensorium. He threw bedding about, spit on the walls and doors, and was markedly overactive. He showed an impulsive assaultiveness which made it difficult to work with him. Within a couple of weeks he was much improved, although there still was increased ideation and circumstantiality. He then became worse and presented almost the same picture as he had at the time of admission. Again he improved, and a new symptom, stereotypy, appeared. He posturized and began to act in much more bizarre ways. He did not recognize his parents, although he talked with them fairly rationally. In the next few weeks he again became better and was so well that he discussed problems logically and asked permission to leave the hospital for a few hours at a time. This was granted. The third time he showed markedly increased activity, sold all his textbooks for a ridiculously low amount, talked foolishly to sales girls, and exhibited other bizarre behavior. A few days later he was describing himself as the greatest genius who had ever lived. He also misidentified other patients, claimed that some were important persons and others criminals. His seclusion in a disturbed section became necessary and eventually he was transferred to a state hospital.

B. Psth., Path. Sexuality M:24:M:13 +2 9′483–1(47) 3:4:16

Within three weeks before this patient's admission to the hospital there were two instances of abnormal behavior, both having the same pattern. He followed a woman, grabbed her shoe, ran into a dark alley, and masturbated while holding the shoe. On the second occasion he was apprehended by the police and subsequently was brought to the hospital.

This veteran was a high school graduate of apparently average or better intelligence. There seemed to be nothing significant in the family history or in the patient's developmental history; however, during his four months in the army he was hospitalized for "headaches, dizziness, sweating, and nail-biting." His wife considered him to be a good-natured person and easy to get along with. She said he enjoyed "kidding" and teasing, was a fairly calm person, but "lost his temper easily." The wife believed overwork and his consequent tiredness were responsible for his behavior. She hinted that he might be "oversexed" but would not elaborate on this point.

At the hospital the patient's mental content appeared normal; he had no paranoid trends or unusual sexual trends. He did, however, appear to have much misinformation about sex, and he showed considerable conflict about masturbation, worrying about its relationship to insanity. He was concerned about being oversexed, and both he and his wife were apprehensive about a second pregnancy. Their one child was 10 months old. The patient gained no insight into his condition and could not understand his behavior. He adjusted well in the hospital, was cooperative, and took part in all ward activities. Psychotherapy was recommended but at the insistence of the patient and his wife he was discharged against medical advice. C. W. S.

B. Psth., Mixed M:28:S:4 +1 9'483–21 (41) 4:16:5
Ps. M-D., Manic
Paranoid

The patient said his extreme nervousness was the result of a skull fracture experienced seven years before admission, but his family and friends could not assign a specific time for the appearance of the present problems. He had been a problem child and his behavior had merely become more accentuated during the last seven years. His relatives finally complained of his behavior and requested that he undergo a personality evaluation.

He had been born two months prematurely. His mother was mentally dull, and his father divorced her to marry a younger woman. The boy went to live with his father. After the skull injury the patient had been "unconscious" for four days and "out of his head" for six months, but information from relatives indicated that his behavior had been "queer" before the accident. He had been transferred from one school to another because he got into trouble and did not study. After he left school he did odd jobs but was quickly discharged. He could not stand monotony, and he was proud of the fact that he had lived the life of a tramp. Rejected by the army because of "violence," he was later discharged from the merchant marine after being AWOL several times. He regarded everyone as dishonest and out to "get you." He went from one extreme to another.

For example, he drank heavily for a while and then stopped entirely. He slept in a bathtub full of water whenever he could. Although he was independent in his actions and thoughts, he was without confidence in his own abilities. He was fatalistic and stubborn. He had had many heterosexual experiences and a few homosexual ones.

In the hospital he reiterated his idea that most people are dishonest, especially "cops, who are a bunch of parasites." In test situations he was average in intelligence, normal in general demeanor and behavior. He attributed his troubles, those he admitted, to the accident. He had a tendency to ramble. He felt that his being in the hospital was a huge joke, but he appeared mildly depressed. He was independent and arrogant toward others. After testing and study he was discharged to be returned home.

Ps. Paranoid M:36:M:37 +10 9′483–6 (49) 3:6:9

Committed by the court and brought to the hospital by the sheriff, this veteran was spontaneously assaultive and difficult to manage. On admission the patient insisted that he was not mentally ill and claimed that his trouble began when he was given barbiturates by his physician because he had been nervous, restless, and unable to sleep. He became very angry with the examiner and repeatedly stated that there was something "fishy" about his being hospitalized. He talked a great deal about hypnotism and about people trying to influence him.

This patient had been a superior student in school but it had been necessary for him to go to work after completing the eighth grade. Before his military service he had worked on a number of jobs and eventually had become a solicitor and agency manager for a metropolitan newspaper. After his discharge from the army he returned to this work, spending much of his time traveling. The patient said that his was a high-pressure job, and it kept him under some tension. His first mental illness occurred in the service while he was on a train en route home for a furlough. He became restless and fearful lest other passengers kill him. Taken to an army hospital, he was very suspicious and manic in behavior and talked a great deal about other people trying to influence him, saying that he masturbated and the like. He was transferred to this hospital with a diagnosis of acute paranoid reaction. Here his ideas of reference and influence gradually disappeared and he made a remission without specific treatment. Apparently he made a satisfactory adjustment during the four years intervening until the present hospitalization.

During his present hospitalization the patient was presented at the psychotherapy clinic and at this time he showed considerable blocking and a great deal of evasion. It was the opinion of the group that he should be given individual psychotherapy and the areas of particular importance were listed as these: "1. The reason for reoccurrence of acute symptoms with each of his wife's pregnancies. 2. His unwillingness and blocking in discussion of the family situation. 3. The reasons back of his tremendous drive for achievement on the job. Here his efforts far exceed the expectations of the employers." However, since the patient experienced a spontaneous remission of the symptoms and made a good hospital adjustment, and because he insisted on his release, he was discharged without receiving psychotherapy. C. W. S.

B. Psth., Asocial M:19:S:30 +33 9'486–13 (47) 3:10:5
Ps. M-D., Manic
Alcoholism

This veteran was first admitted to this hospital at the age of 18, a few weeks after his discharge from the navy. He had been arrested for disorderly conduct (fighting), and his symptoms were nervousness, restlessness, and sleeplessness. Hospitalized for 86 days, he was diagnosed as having a psychopathic personality, with asocial trends. One year later he was again brought to the hospital in the present admission after spending several days in jail because of drinking and fighting.

The patient had completed the tenth grade. Frequently a truant, he was once expelled for truancy. His early home life was poor; the father was a heavy drinker and at times beat his wife. Before the mother's death, which occurred when the patient was 7, his parents were separated. He had little supervision, began to get involved in delinquencies, and at age 13 was sent to a state training school for stealing. At 17 he enlisted in the navy. Nothing was learned of his adjustment in the service. After his first hospitalization he again enlisted in the navy but was soon discharged, presumably for psychiatric reasons since he had been hospitalized for "nervousness" immediately before his discharge.

At the hospital the patient showed a great deal of psychomotor activity, approaching a flight of ideas. He was grandiose, euphoric, and emotionally labile. He admitted excessive drinking and gave as his reason the fact that his fiancée was killed in a car accident while he was driving and that this preyed on his mind. The diagnosis on admission was psychosis, unclassified. His symptoms gradually disappeared; he made a good hospital adjustment and was discharged with a diagnosis of psychopathic personality, asocial trends, unimproved. C. W. S.

B. Psth., Asocial F:17:S:42 +4 94'86–213 (55) 3:4:14
Suicidal

This girl, who was admitted on a court order for delinquent behavior, first came to the attention of the courts when she attempted to commit suicide by taking lysol and suffered severe facial burns. This attempt had followed an argument with her boy friend. He had been her "steady" until he joined the merchant marine. After he left the city she began to go out with other men, one an older, married man with whom she "fell in love." When her boy friend returned home on leave and learned of this affair he told her he was through with her. After a two-day period of brooding over this, she took the lysol.

The girl was average in intelligence, had a pleasant disposition, and got along well with people. So secretive was she that little was known about her activities. She considered herself stubborn, sensitive, and shy, but other persons thought of her as cheerful and fairly attractive. She "just didn't like" schoolwork and never earned good grades. It had always been her ambition, she said, to marry and have two children. She had held only two jobs. The first she had left after an argument with the supervisor. The second, a job with a photo company, she still held at the time of admission. The home background was not extremely unfavorable, but there was a sister who had contracted lues while working as a prostitute.

In the hospital the girl showed no obvious abnormal behavior. Apparently completely relieved of her worries when she learned that she was to be put on parole after she left the hospital, she showed no interest in the rules of parole and little regard for those of the ward. Although not openly uncooperative, she caused a good deal of trouble and had no appreciation at all of the reason she was considered a subject for psychiatric study. About her past experiences she was secretive and untruthful. No obvious neurotic or psychotic symptoms could be discovered. She could not form a good personal relationship with any of the examiners and the psychotherapeutic approaches were relatively ineffectual.

P. Anxiety State M:46:M:13 +1 9′486–321 (43) 2:6:14

This man's illness began three months before admission when he experienced low back pain and pain radiating down his legs. In a week the pains became so severe that he went to a hospital, where a diagnosis of myelonephritis was made and the infection was successfully treated. To relieve the pain the patient was given a succession of heat treatments and was tightly taped across the back. These procedures accentuated rather than reduced the pain because the skin on his back and buttocks was extremely sensitive. This skin had been hypersensitive since he had suffered a burn as a child. The patient and his physician vigorously argued over the therapeutic procedures used. Before his discharge from the hospital the man was told that his kidneys were now all right but that the trouble was in his back, and he was also informed that he would never work again. These facts upset him seriously. He became nervous and tense. Later he went to a medical outpatient department, where no cause for the continuing pain could be established and, finally, he was referred to the psychiatric unit.

Eleven years before admission the patient "strained his back" while sawing wood. At that time he suffered for several hours low back discomfort with pain radiating to the legs. One month later the pain recurred and continued until chiropractic manipulation relieved it. After that he had frequent bouts of the same type of pain until the time of the present illness.

An eighth-grade graduate, he had been a moderately good student. He lived on his parents' farm until he was 20 and then worked as a farm hand and painter. Known as a stable person, he was not hypochondriacal or nervous. He had been married eleven years and had two children. The family appeared to be compatible. The patient's interests had always been restricted almost entirely to his family and to his workshop.

In the hospital he was anxious and restless. Although he had some insight into the reasons for his restlessness, he did not agree that he needed psychiatric care. In conversation he was adequate and well oriented. When discussing his illness he became angry and spoke derogatively of the medical treatment he had received. There was little objective evidence of any change during his stay in the hospital. He said he was less tense and had practically no back pain. The main psychotherapeutic approach was an attempt to reassure him, but in general he was not accessible because of his complete rejection of the idea that he had psychiatric difficulty.

Ps. M-D., Manic   F:25:M:81   +67   9'4867–21(51)   3:6:11
Paranoid
Schizoid

Fifteen days before admission the patient, while still in the hospital after childbirth, was told that her baby son was defective and that his life expectancy was ten or twelve years. The knowledge troubled her deeply, and she developed insomnia and began to experience nightmares about childbirth. This condition became even more distressing after she was discharged from the hospital. Then she began to have delusions of persecution and at the same time she became overactive. Three days before admission to this hospital she became violent, and bit and scratched her husband. She was transferred to the psychiatric unit from a general hospital. There were no previous psychotic or obviously neurotic disturbances.

The patient was a high school graduate. After one year in college she attended business college for a year. She then worked in an office for four years. She belonged to numerous clubs and took part in many sports programs. Although she was known to be a little stubborn and to have a violent temper, she made friends easily. She was a spendthrift but a good planner. The patient was well adjusted with her husband and had apparently wanted the child. The pregnancy was a normal one, except for the fact that the child had a spina bifida.

In the hospital the patient was at first inaccessible, uncooperative, and violent. Her discourse was incoherent, and she expressed many delusions. For a number of weeks she alternated between depression and hyperactivity. Seventeen electroshock treatments and twenty-four subinsulin shock treatments were effective in relieving the gross psychosis, but she developed little insight. During most of her convalescence she remained unreasonable and difficult. At the time of discharge she was clearly disturbed. She went home to her family against the advice of the staff, who recommended that she go to a state hospital for a while.

Ps. M-D., Manic Schizoid F:21:S:8 +3 9486′7–3(51) 0:6:7

Three years before admission, boredom with her job as a typist made the patient so nervous and irritable that she took a trip to "get away from home," but she returned and took another job within two weeks. Her nervousness persisted, even though she changed from job to job, and in an attempt to escape the problem she again left for another state. At this time, according to the story she told later, she was "seduced and raped" by a policeman, but she told none of her close friends of the incident. Three days later she attempted suicide by drinking lysol. After a week's hospitalization she returned home, and although she found employment she was unable to hold a job for more than a week or two. Two months before admission she was hospitalized for a gonococcal infection. Two days before admission there was a dramatic change in her mood and behavior, and she "told off" her best friends, refused to go home at night, and became "snooty" to her relatives. Her attitude was described as a "don't give a darn" one.

A high school graduate, she had not cared for school although she had been an honor student. She had always been a poor planner, but she had attempted to save money. Although she had apparently been at ease with people until her present illness, since its onset she had even been afraid of her friends. She had always been self-reliant, truthful, and devoutly religious.

In the hospital the patient was uncooperative, her attitude and manner changeable. She apparently liked attention from men. When asked to do something she did not want to do she became very sarcastic. She was destructive of bedding and clothes and assaultive toward nurses and orderlies, but she was oriented and apparently intact in general mentation. There was little evidence of inappropriate affect, but the staff felt that a schizoid factor in her behavior was almost certainly present. Her family took her out of the hospital against the advice of the staff.

M:20:S ′<u>96</u>–14(65) 3:0:13

This student came for help in overcoming his stammering because it represented a bar to his admission to a school of pharmacy. He had begun to stammer when he was about 6 years old.

An attractive boy, he seemed to be well liked by his associates. His father and mother had separated when he was about 5 years old and his father had died five or six years ago. Before coming to this university he had had a series of failures in premedical and predental courses even though he was a potentially able student.

He was treated over a nine-month period with a combination of interviews and hypnoanalytic and narcosynthesis treatments. This analysis brought into the open strongly repressed feelings of hostility toward his father and some indications of repressed affection for his mother. Some connections between these feelings and his previous academic failure were found. Although during this period his academic achievement improved considerably, there was only a slight reduction in the severity of his stammering. The treatments were interrupted by the end of the school year and no follow-up information was available. E. S. B.

Alcoholism M:39:D:29 +7 9′6–3(51) 3:6:2

This patient was admitted to the hospital from the jail in his home town where he had been locked up for drunkenness. On admission he stated, "My present situation is due to drinking. Since I got out of the army [three months earlier], I was not working steadily—only a couple days a week. I had lots of time on my hands and lots of friends and it would be just one drink after another. I came here to stop drinking."

After completing high school the patient spent two years in a junior college. Married at 28 he was divorced by his wife five years later because of his drinking. His wife remarried and continued to live in the same town. The patient brooded over this situation and used it as an excuse for further drinking.

At the hospital the veteran showed no overt symptoms of psychosis. In psychotherapy interviews it was brought out that he had many feelings of inadequacy and showed considerable dependence on his father, who had always found jobs for him and helped him out when he got into difficulties. He was regarded as a fundamentally unstable individual who used alcohol to excess as compensation. He made a very good hospital adjustment and when he left he intended to move to another town to get away from his former associates. He felt that with the help of Alcoholics Anonymous he could stop drinking.

C. W. S.

B. Psth., Asocial F:18:S:28 +6 9′64–(61) 6:7:11
Paranoid

For the past eight years, this patient's foster parents had noted in the girl progressive behavior changes toward lying, stealing, and disobedience. She had resented her foster parents and foster sister to the point of living away from home during her last year of high school. After her graduation she went to the city and there met a 25-year-old man in a hotel, went out to dinner with him, and agreed to marry him, all in the same evening. She became pregnant and, still unmarried, went from job to job. When the pregnancy became obvious she was taken to a hospital for unmarried mothers, where her baby was born about a month before the present admission. During the latter days of the pregnancy she was very unstable, causing considerable worry because of her crying and other emotional behavior. On several occasions she interpreted incidents as threats to her and her baby and she had mild ideas of reference. Shortly before admission, she fled to the father of the baby, but she fought with him and his landlady until police matrons and welfare workers arrived. She was apprehended in the process of smothering the baby and was brought to the psychiatric unit on a court order.

Her past health was not particularly bad. There were no previous psychotic episodes though she had been a behavior problem since age 10. She herself was an illegitimate child of a 13-year-old schoolgirl and a 38-year-old man who was married and had two other children. She had lived in a good foster home and had apparently been happy as a young girl. While away from home as a senior in high school, she worked for a professional man for about a year and did very satisfactory work. She was a good student in school but was secretive, egotistical, and mendacious. Toward others her own age she assumed an air of superiority that antagonized them. Much of her time was spent in the company of men. She considered law and order to be made for others than herself.

When she was first admitted to the hospital, she was obnoxious toward the other patients and the nurses, even attempting to slap one of the nurses for no apparent reason. She used vile language and would not cooperate in group activities. She spent much of her time with the men patients. When an effort was made to discuss her problems with her all she would say was that she wanted to get out. She changed little while in the hospital. There were indications of an early psychosis. Chief among these signs were her bizarre paranoid ideas and her willingness to sacrifice her baby rather than let anyone else have it. She was transferred to a state hospital.

Ps. M-D., Manic	F:36:M:73	+7	9′6478–21	2:10:7
		+41	946′8327–	4:6:14

The patient was admitted because of extreme overactivity. This had first appeared about a month before admission when she became unusually gay and expansive in her thinking. Shortly afterward she began to be overactive physically, spending most of her time writing and talking, and she was irritable and demanding.

The woman had taken a nurses' training course at a state hospital and had worked as a nurse until her marriage a few years later. Her fifth child was born eight days before the present illness began. Always a normal and apparently adequate person, the woman had few interests outside of her home, but she was known to have good common sense and to be able to handle her affairs very well.

Her conversation in the hospital was expansive and circumstantial, with a moderate flight of ideas and play upon words. She emphatically disliked her husband's mother, whom she accused of interfering with her domestic affairs. Although she was well oriented and appeared intact in mental faculties, she had no insight into her illness, accounting for her presence in the hospital by saying that her doctor wanted her to have a vacation. She wrote poetry on any scrap of paper within reach. A few weeks after admission she began to improve, and then elation gave way to a depression that was manifest mostly by crying spells.

She became friendly and as she recovered, entered into all the routine activities of the ward. In discussing her illness after her symptoms had improved, she showed fair insight into the fact that she had been mentally ill, but she could not account for the illness except with reference to the strain of her recent pregnancy and the influence of her mother-in-law. She was fairly well at the time of discharge.

B. Psth., Asocial M:36:M:26 +7 '967 382–(61) 3:5:11

Under a court order the patient was admitted to the hospital for investigation. He had committed 41 offenses of petty pilfering. He showed mild anxiety, but there were no symptoms for diagnosis. He scored an I.Q. of 108 on the Stanford-Binet test. There was reason to believe that he had a full understanding of the situation. He told the psychiatrist that he had a "compulsive urge" to enter homes through windows and steal.

He was one of eight children, and his childhood was spent in extremely poor conditions. He and his siblings never ceased to be bitter about this. He had an elementary education and worked as a laborer thereafter. He was discharged from the army after three months; the reason for the discharge was unknown. He was married and had three boys. He treated one of his sons as a girl, idolizing him and ignoring the others. His wife was unhappy and described the patient as difficult, contradictory, and touchy. He was mean in money matters and never gave his wife enough to keep the household going.

He was diagnosed as having a psychopathic personality. The investigation having been completed, he left the hospital without further treatment. M. V.

Ps. Sz., Paranoid M:24:S:161 9'678–231 (65) 3:8:14

This patient had apparently made a good adjustment until just before admission when he began to complain to his mother about their poor environment and about his lack of instruction in sexual matters. A few days before he entered the hospital he demanded that he be baptized, and this was done. After his baptism the patient began to talk about being God and being in hell. He felt that his brother was trying to hypnotize him and that neighbors were "casting an evil eye" upon him.

As a child the patient had been quiet and reserved. He preferred to stay at home, and he never had any close friends before his entrance into the service. In school he went as far as the eighth grade and always got along well with teachers and pupils. His parents were of different religions and some of the children were baptized, while others were not. At age 20 the patient entered the army and served two years. In the army he adjusted satisfactorily and was a sergeant at the time of his discharge. Upon his return home the family was impressed by the way he had matured since they had last seen him. He began to go out more, attending movies and sporting events and swimming, for example. Occasionally he went out with a girl friend. He attended a trade school and was making a good adjustment there. Shortly before the onset of his present illness it was noticed by the family that the patient seemed considerably upset about the current international situation and he expressed some concern about being drafted again.

On admission the patient was grossly psychotic. He was extremely delusional, believing he was God or the second Adam, and talking a great deal about sex and hypnotism. On one occasion he alternately wept and "preached" in a loud voice, believing that he was God and was holding the world up by his eyelids. He was given a course of electroshock therapy with only moderate improvement, and shortly thereafter he had an acute exacerbation of psychotic symptoms. After another course of electroshock therapy he showed marked improvement, with a total remission of the psychosis. C. W. S.

Ps. M-D., Manic F:36:M:17 +10 9′68–2(57) 2:10:13
Schizoid
Paranoid

Two weeks before admission the patient underwent the surgical removal of a goiter. Shortly after this she began to show a gross behavior disturbance. Before the operation the thyroid enlargement had produced a mechanical difficulty in breathing, bending, and stretching, and the relief of these symptoms seemed to be the basis for an extreme elation. She developed overactivity, extreme irritability, and anorexia. She had delusions that she was being given "dope." On several occasions she had "fainting spells" that seemed feigned.

The patient's past health had not been good. In addition to the goiter, which her physician attributed to an attack of measles at age 10, dysmenorrhea had required her to stay in bed from three to four days each month, and she had taken a "sleep tonic" for insomnia over the past five years. She also suffered from marked myopia. There had been no definite neurotic or psychotic episodes, however.

In school she earned excellent grades and finished high school. She had always had a cyclothymic disposition. Her business ability was sound, and she was active and well informed about things in general. A social, cheerful person, she was well liked. Her marriage had not been happy, according to the patient's sister, but the husband denied this and claimed that they were reasonably well adjusted. There were three children. The older daughter constantly quarreled with the patient.

In the hospital the patient showed increased psychomotor activity. Her mental content revolved around ideas of influence. "The doctor puts thoughts in my mind," she said. The "thoughts" involved syphilis, flowers, sin, and religion. She believed at times that she was sent to the hospital to study psychiatry. Marked circumstantiality and a flight of ideas made it difficult to examine her sensorium but she appeared oriented and had a good memory. She struck nurses on several occasions, but always apologized later. Her insight varied but was usually poor. She presented an unkempt, disheveled appearance. Electroshock treatment was given but she did not change. Gradually, however, she did improve until at the time of discharge she was thought to be able to continue convalescence at home. In view of some of the schizoid features present, the prognosis was thought to be unfavorable.

Ps. Sz., Paranoid M:23:M:96 +24 9′68–271X (43) 3:13:7

Shortly after this patient's marriage a few months before admission he began to undergo a personality change. Periods of confusion were noted first and at times he would speak incoherently; then periods of extreme depression appeared when he would become tremulous and would alternately cry profusely and laugh hysterically. Considerable friction developed in his relationship with his wife's parents. The patient had difficulty adjusting in his work as a sales clerk. He became unable to make out sales slips correctly and regarded Christmas decorations in the store as having some special significance for him.

The patient's school adjustment had been satisfactory. At 18 he completed high school. He was always somewhat shy and reserved and preferred to keep himself occupied with hobbies such as model airplane building and radios, rather than engage in group activities. He was very dependent upon his mother and his family was overprotective toward him. In personal habits and dress he was fastidious. The patient first noticed some degree of stress after his induction into the army. At times he became homesick to the extent that he was not able to eat and he frequently made long-distance phone calls to his parents. After his discharge from the army he made a good initial adjustment, got along well with his supervisor and fellow employees, and was considered above average in his job.

In the hospital the patient manifested many paranoid delusions and was evasive and extremely suspicious. Emotionally he was very labile. At times he became hyperactive and several times attempted to run away. He received electroshock therapy and "simmered down," but it was felt that he should be given a course of insulin shock. At the insistence of relatives, however, he was released for a trial visit and was later discharged. C. W. S.

Ps. M-D., Manic M:19:S:46 +33 9′68 34–21 0:8:10

In apparently good health until three years before admission, the patient then suddenly went to a general hospital complaining of abdominal discomfort. An examination revealed no outstanding disorder, but later that year his family noticed that he was nervous, disobedient, and somewhat inactive. He began to have difficulty with his schoolwork and was playful and restless. Two years later he was readmitted to the hospital and this time a diagnosis of acute nephritis was made. After he left the hospital he spent some time visiting a sister and felt much better until he returned to school. There his work was so poor that he was finally taken out of school. After an argument with his parents he started to hitchhike across the country, ran out of money, stole a car, and was put in jail for five weeks. At home again, he was exceptionally active, was "on the go" at all times, either to movies or to dances, until he finally entered the psychiatric unit in the present admission.

The youth was 17 when he left school; he lacked only a few credits for graduation. He had done very well earlier and had been even-tempered, active, and normal. There was no particular event in the past medical or psychological history that seemed to shed any light on his personality change.

In the hospital the physical and neurological examinations were negative. He said he had failed in school because he was "too interested in radio announcing work," which he wanted to follow as a vocation. Studying was difficult because he could not concentrate, he said. He did not want to go back to school because he felt sick and weak, but at the same time he wanted to take singing lessons and to organize a band for radio appearances. He was happy and exuberant, with marked circumstantiality and a flight of ideas. On the ward he was restless and overactive and inclined to be too familiar with others. There were no gross defects of sensorium or intellect. The psychological examinations indicated a paranoid-schizoid component along with the cyclothymic traits. In the hospital the youth gradually became more amenable to suggestions about his behavior and he developed some insight. He expressed a desire to return to school and later to go to another state for a while. At the time of discharge it seemed that he was well on the way to recovery from the present episode.

P. Anxiety State M:23:M:13 +2 9′7–21(45) 3:7:8

This veteran had reported as an outpatient for a physical examination because of foot trouble that had begun with trench foot while he was in the service. The medical examiner advised hospitalization and further study because of the possibility of Buerger's disease. The patient subsequently entered the hospital and was placed in the infirmary ward. Finding himself in a locked ward in a "mental hospital," he became very tense, anxious, and apprehensive. The second night of his hospitalization he had a spell of vomiting and complained of a "nervous stomach." He reported that he had experienced a similar stomach upset the day of his marriage.

The patient completed high school at 18 and entered the army immediately thereafter. He served two and a half years, was in combat about a hundred days as a member of the infantry glider troops, and was honorably discharged. For two or three months while overseas, he was troubled with enuresis about twice weekly. After his discharge he worked steadily as a spray painter in a factory. Married just two weeks before admission to this hospital he entered the day he returned from his honeymoon. He admitted becoming very tense during periods of excitement and he spoke of frequent dreams, mostly centering around accidents involving himself. According to the patient, he had always been "nervous and high-strung."

The patient was discharged as improved after thirteen days. Buerger's disease was not found. He was given advice about the proper care of his feet. The c 'nical findings did not clearly indicate a diagnosis of a chronically borderline manic-depressive who overreacted to stress. C. W. S.

Ps. Sz., Cat. F:25:S:137 0 9′728–1 (43) 4:4:13
Ps. M-D., Mixed +136 9′8734–(49) 3:4:14

About eight months before admission the patient began to complain of low back pain, which a psychiatrist diagnosed as psychogenic. An internist and an orthopedist, however, diagnosed her ailment as a protruded intervertebral disc. They fitted her with a brace and she returned to work. Suddenly, five days before admission, she began to act strangely, felt that the home in which she was a guest was strange and unreal, became incoherent in speech, and showed a flight of ideas. Preoccupied with sex, she accused two women friends of being Lesbians, and she spoke of the great love she had for her employer. She felt that everything had suddenly become quite clear to her, and she discussed mysticism and the occult. At times she seemed hysterical. She had delusions that she was married to her employer and was the mother of a 5-year-old son. Another time she said she was the Virgin Mary. She ate little, would not sleep, was mute, and posturized. Later she began to talk incoherently.

Always a masculine girl, she had a tall and slender stature, which she regarded as a social handicap. She finished high school and then went to a private college for two years, finally receiving a degree in French with honors from a large university. A strong desire to be independent caused her to leave home and she became a junior partner in a business. She was described by her family as friendly, able to meet people easily, somewhat emotional, and appreciative of fine clothes, good music, literature, and art. Until three years before her present illness she had had little interest in men but then had shown a marked attachment for her employer, a man of 50.

In the hospital she expressed many delusions, was apparently hallucinatory, and constantly misidentified personnel on the ward. She had no insight into her illness. She was careless of her dress and labile emotionally. Twenty electroshock treatments decreased her belief in her delusions, and she began to express guilt feelings about the affair she had been having with her employer. Then she relapsed and was given more shock therapy, including insulin shock. Her sensorium was clouded for a while but she again improved and became irritable, antagonistic, unreasonable, and unappreciative. Finally, during the three weeks before her discharge, she seemed fairly well and apparently had recovered from the present attack.

B. Psth., Asocial M:41:S:109 +45 9'742-(57) 6:4:12
Alcoholism
Deteriorated

From the age of 17 this patient was troubled by chronic and severe alcoholism. Before the war he would become grandiose and happy when he drank, but after his return from the service it was noted that he was irritable and cried continually during his drinking sprees. He brooded a great deal about his war experiences and turned to alcohol in "trying to forget." Drinking, however, only made him more emotionally upset. One of the things he worried about, especially when drinking, was a German he had killed during the war; he had later learned that this man had children. The alcoholism became gradually more severe and finally other members of his family convinced him that he needed hospitalization. They used the pretext that he should have treatment for a rheumatic complaint.

The patient did not attend school beyond the eighth grade. Throughout his school life he had difficulty and repeated several grades. The history showed more than one arrest for drunkenness. Never staying long at one job, he worked usually just enough to earn money for a "spree" and then quit.

At the hospital no psychosis was found. The man showed marked anxiety and tension. The neurological findings indicated some organic brain damage due to chronic alcoholism. C. W. S.

Ps. Paranoid M:37:M:41 +1 9'7826-31(47) 5:4:9

Apparently the first behavior changes in this patient had been noted two years before admission when he began to argue with his friends and relatives over trivial matters and developed an antagonistic manner. He treated his wife badly, occasionally striking her; he would not eat her cooking; and he would have nothing to do with their baby. They had had no sexual intercourse since the birth of their last child, although at times he had asked his wife to perform fellatio. He showed a definite antagonism toward the baby but he got along well with his 7-year-old daughter. He began reading the dictionary in order to improve his conversational ability. Becoming antagonistic toward his boss, he was for the first time negligent in his work.

He required five years to complete high school, but there was no apparent explanation for the extra year it took him to graduate. After stopping school he worked seven years at one job and then took another one which he still held at the time of admission. Apparently well adjusted and easy to get along with, he was somewhat preoccupied with improving himself. There was no history of peculiar behavior.

In the hospital he refused to talk about his present illness, simply blocking when anything personal was suggested. He said he was not sick and he constantly tried to leave the hospital. There were some evidences of a memory disturbance; otherwise, his sensorium and intellect were intact. When personal subjects were not touched on, he was cooperative and talkative. At no time in his hospital stay did he show the slightest evidence of insight into his difficulties except when under amytal. Then he talked about trouble at home and admitted that there was no basis for his delusions of infidelity about his wife, but he still refused to say that she was faithful to him. He said he had been forced into marriage by her and felt that she had been overly demanding sexually. Five electroshock treatments brought no special change. He was discharged unimproved for a try in the home community, with the recommendation that he be committed to a state hospital if he continued to have the same threatening manner.

Ps. M-D., Mixed	F:28:M:114	+1	9'783–2(61)	1:3:19
		+25	'936–2(63)	2:3:16

This young woman, a nurse, was admitted because of depression, fear of insanity, mental unrest, and recurrent diarrhea. The present illness dated from her last pregnancy, which had terminated three months before admission. For the first few weeks she had no trouble, but then she began to have discomfort when she nursed the baby. Her schedule was strenuous and the patient felt nervous. At this time, during a quarrel with a roomer, she became very angry. Following this incident she developed diarrhea and anxiety, but she rejected the symptoms and considered them "all foolishness." There was some bleeding from hemorrhoids and she was afraid of a malignancy. As the unrest and anxieties continued she began to fear that she was losing her mind.

Throughout her schooling in private schools, the patient did better than average work and took part in extracurricular activities. She finished nurses' training at age 21. She became a head nurse, but after a year she left to be married. A leader in any group, she was self-reliant and outgoing. She had always been hypochondriacal, and as a child she had been overly sympathetic and had cried easily.

In the hospital she was worried and anxious and continually talked about "giving in to this." She felt there was little that could be done for her in the hospital. Agitation and depression were the dominating signs of her illness. Despite her obvious search for sympathy, she could not admit this desire. Intact in orientation, sensorium, and intellect, she was relatively cheerful and cooperative during the first few days in the hospital; later she began to experience crying spells. After a series of episodes in which she first seemed to be better and then depressed electroshock treatments were tried. These seemed to help markedly and she was discharged upon the return of her husband from the army. It was felt that she would quickly recover from the present illness, although it seemed likely that others would follow.

Ps. M-D., Manic M:37:D 978′46–3 (59) 1:15:13
Paranoid
Alcoholism

The present admission to the hospital was the fifth commitment for this veteran. While in the service he had been diagnosed as having a manic-depressive psychosis. He had been hospitalized for a time and since his discharge from the army, he had gone back and forth to mental hospitals because of his inability to adjust and the recurrence of the psychosis. Before the last admission he had been picked up by the police because of some difficulty involving homosexual acts with three persons, including a 12-year-old boy. The court charges were dropped when the man was hospitalized. In the past he had also drunk excessively.

Little was known of the patient's early life except that he lived with both parents as he grew up. His general physical health had been good. Although he finished only the eighth grade, his scores on standardized tests showed him to be at the high school level in general school achievement. On intelligence tests, he was in the superior range. At the time of examination he showed increased motor activity, was overtalkative, facetious, and amorous toward fellow patients. The other patients objected to his presence. Although euphoric and grandiose, he was oriented in all spheres and denied having hallucinations or delusions. He showed little insight and poor judgment. At times he was belligerent because of his paranoid ideas toward the hospital.

Electroshock therapy was given during his hospitalization but was discontinued after only two grand mal convulsions because he objected strenuously and feared the treatments. He did show some clinical improvement after the two shocks. At present, the patient is on an open ward making an adequate adjustment. He is superficially quiet, subdued, and cooperative, but he does create some disturbance among other patients. He is receiving supportive psychotherapy, in which he shows little insight and has a tendency to rationalize his problems. W. M. H.

Ps. M-D., Manic F:15:S:126 +85 9′8–2 (51) 7:6:18

Since beginning school two weeks before admission, the patient had become progressively more voluble, hyperactive, and unmanageable. She was obsessed with the idea of being a cheerleader. Despite her poor record in school recently, she requested permission to take additional subjects. She attempted to organize and put on a party in spite of attempts to convince her that it was too big an undertaking, and she used her parents' charge accounts to get supplies for the party. A week before admission she went to a football game in the company of two older men who had been asked to look after her. She returned home late and refused to go to bed. Early the next morning her mother awoke to find the girl washing and dying some of her clothes in the kitchen. She had ruined several garments. When her mother attempted to whip her with a belt the patient "threw a fit" and shouted at her mother. A physician was called and gave her sedatives. The acute episode subsided, but she remained disturbed and agitated until the time of admission.

The past history contained nothing of particular note. There were no previous episodes of nervous breakdown. She had done fairly well in school, had been active in group activities, and had appeared normal in every way before the present episode. A nervous, high-strung person, she had always had a great deal of energy and ambition, but she was known for her tendency not to carry things through to completion. She was very attached to her mother and was especially fond and proud of her brother.

In the hospital the patient was hyperactive and excessively voluble. Although she gave the impression of being happy there seemed to be an underlying depression. She was upset by difficulties between her parents and apparently felt insecure in the family situation. She had no definite hallucinations or delusions. She was intact in sensorium and intellect. She was aware that she was hyperactive, but she did not consider herself ill or abnormal in any way. Her I.Q. was 90. After seven electroshock treatments she got better and worse by spells, gradually becoming in general somewhat better. At the time of discharge she apparently was on her way out of the present episode, but the possibility of a recurrence was considered high.

Ps. Sz., Simple Alcoholism	M:22:S:71	+7	9′8–26 (37)	5:5:15

This veteran was arrested for passing worthless checks. Because of a history of hospitalizations for a neuropsychiatric disorder, he was placed on probation and committed to this hospital.

The patient completed the ninth grade. He did not like school and frequently played truant. Inducted into the army at 18, he served two years. His first admission to a mental hospital, while he was overseas, followed an AWOL of one month. There he was retained for observation but was not treated and was returned to his unit. Since his discharge from the army two years before admission the patient had been irresponsible, had worked sporadically, and had been arrested several times for drunkenness and for passing bad checks.

At the hospital the patient showed no psychotic behavior. He was mildly hostile and negativistic. His affect was somewhat inappropriate; he showed no concern about his difficulties with the law. His hospital course was uneventful except that he left once without permission, returning the same evening intoxicated, belligerent, antagonistic, and quarrelsome. The hospital staff felt that the patient could not be helped to any great extent as far as his alcoholism or other antisocial behavior was concerned, and he was, therefore, discharged.

C. W. S.

B. Psth., Asocial	F:17:S:88	+6	9'8–7	3:7:11
Suicidal		+42	94'86–21	6:4:20

This patient was sent to the psychiatric unit from a girls' reform school for an evaluation of her suicidal trends. On one of the two occasions on which she had injured herself she had thrown herself down a flight of stairs in the hope of incapacitating herself and being confined to the hospital where she could attempt an escape. A more obviously suicidal attempt had occurred when she had broken her glasses and had slashed the veins of her wrist with the fragments. She had called for help and after being taken to the hospital, had been assaultive and destructive for three days.

The girl had gone part way through the eleventh grade in school, and with her I.Q. of more than 130 there was no question of her scholastic ability. She was a nice-looking girl. The family background was poor. Numerous members of her family had been in trouble with the law, and the patient's mother was a former inmate of the same reform school in which the patient was imprisoned. At the age of 14 the patient had "fallen in with bad company" and had run away from home with another girl about the same age. She had taken up prostitution as her main means of livelihood although she had also worked as a waitress and a clerk. The patient had lived with two Chinese until they were arrested for white slavery, and after a brief sojourn in her home state, the girl had once again run away, taking up this time with some Filipinos, from whom she contracted gonorrhea. She claimed to have married one of them under an assumed name. Following this she was sent to a reform school; she later escaped but was finally returned to the school. While she was free she attempted suicide by taking veronal and would have succeeded if a chance passer-by had not seen her.

In the hospital the patient's uppermost thoughts were concerned with ways and means of avoiding her return to the reform school. She said that she would do anything in her power to escape from the school, and it was difficult to determine whether she was really suicidal or whether her threats represented a means of escape from the reform school routine. She scoffed at personal appeals, which she called "the old pep talk." She had no sense of guilt over her behavior and disclaimed feeling any warmth in her sexual experiences. The girl had a fatalistic attitude toward the future: "There's nothing you can do. Why bother?" Her interests were masculine in many ways, but her stated ambition was in the literary field. She complied with the hospital rules but she dramatized her situation to other patients and regaled them with lurid stories of her life. Perverse, moody, and uncooperative at first, she gradually improved, but even at the last, she refused without apparent reason to do certain small tasks. Evidently with her cooperation, plans were made for her to begin university training, but on the day she was supposed to begin at the university she disappeared, and when she was next heard from she was working as a barmaid in another city. At a still later date she was the manager of a successful night club.

P. Hypo. F:52:M:24 +7 9′8<u>13</u>4–2 6:14:11
Ps. Invol. Melan.

The patient, who had been ill for about seven years, was admitted to the hospital because of depression, weakness, insomnia, anorexia, and multiple somatic complaints. At the onset of her illness, she had been hospitalized for a number of weeks and had later lived with a sister, who had given her very good care. She had gradually improved until she was able to care for herself and her son, but she had never completely recovered. For a while she had spent a great deal of her time in bed and had worried about her inability to give her son proper care.

The patient's difficulties had begun about ten years before when she had received deep X-ray therapy, resulting in an artificial menopause. Before the onset of her difficulty she had been an active, energetic woman who had lived intensely, and she had been a very capable manager. Her husband had died about eleven years before, leaving her to support a young son.

In the hospital the patient complained of weakness, difficulty in sleeping, and somatic symptoms which she described in detail. Her sensorium was clear and there were no defects of intellect, but she was something of a nursing problem because she insisted on staying in bed. Only with difficulty could she be induced to get up. She was emotionally depressed, wept, and complained bitterly of her physical suffering. She was gradually induced to take a more active interest in her surroundings, and she began to take part in games and activities. She complained less, and the complaints were less specific. The depression gradually lifted so that she felt able to cope with her life situation. She was discharged to live with her brother for a while, and it was hoped she would make a more complete recovery.

Ps. M-D., Manic M:18:S:18 +10 98′1463–(55) 3:14:10

One year before this admission the patient had been taken to a psychiatrist on the advice of the family physician because of the youth's increased tendency to depression. The depression gradually lessened during the next six months and he was thought well enough to return to school. Every consideration was given him in order to prevent a recurrence of the depression. Some months later his habits began to change gradually as he underwent the stress of training for the track team and preparing for his spring examinations. He became overactive, sleepless, and argumentative, and developed ideas of reference and persecution. The symptoms were most obvious during the week preceding hospitalization, when he began to break windows and furniture and developed grandiose ideas about his mental and physical abilities. He became so active that it was necessary to take him to jail to restrain him.

When he was 3 years old he had experienced a severe concussion and had been unconscious for two days. He had gradually recovered, but the family felt that thereafter he had always been "more nervous and excitable." He had also had severe headaches and occasional cyanosis with vomiting. These attacks continued until about two years before the present illness. It was also noted when he was young that his left arm would "twitch" when he slept, but this symptom also gradually disappeared. In school he was always a leader, took part in numerous activities, and got along well with his classmates and teachers. His progress was apparently normal until the depression began.

In the hospital the boy showed grandiose delusions, particularly about his financial and business acumen. The neurological examination was negative and his sensorium and intellect were clear. Tests revealed average intelligence. He was talkative, his answers were often facetious. The reason for his presence in the hospital puzzled him. He was overactive and showed a flight of ideas. These general symptoms continued until he was given shock treatment. The shocks were unusual since each was followed by severe excitement, then headache, nausea, and vomiting. He did not improve, remained belligerent and demanding, and continually broke ward rules. When he finally refused further treatment, his family decided to take him to a private hospital for further shock therapy.

Ps. Paranoid M:31:M:22 +2 9'84–21 6:8:16
Alcoholism

The patient was induced to come to the hospital by his wife on the pretext that he could show the doctors his "powers of divine healing." His wife said that the patient had developed ideas of reference after a period of alcoholism about a year before admission. His mood had been one of depression, and he thought people jeered at him because he drank. Later he developed an inordinate interest in religion, spending hours and days in prayer. Except for one occasion there had been no drunken spells after the onset of the illness. About two months before admission he began to develop ideas of having unusual power. He thought the highway department was using his ideas, that he was to be the next governor, and that God was working through him. He applied for a job on the Supreme Court, giving as a reference the author of a book on theology he had read. He spent money foolishly, became suspicious of his wife, and felt that she was not fit to care for their children.

Before the present illness he had been in relatively good health. A sporadic drinker for ten years, he had had periods of remorse and abstinence, and at one time he had gone to a hospital for a "liquor cure," but in that admission there was no evidence of psychosis. He had had two years of college work, and in his jobs he had been a very good workman, but because of his poor judgment his finances were always muddled. At the time of admission his family was on relief. He was described as an easygoing person, always optimistic and overly confident. His great initial interest in new projects was always poorly sustained. When others attempted to get him to be more steady, or to show more effective judgment, he became argumentative and irritable, especially when he had been drinking.

In the hospital the physical and neurological examinations were noncontributory. The patient was eager to express his unusual powers. He felt that he had been reborn. "I've been called from above. I'm here to explain my calling so that I can go ahead with my federal work," he said. There were many other vague and generalized ideas of reference, and generally paranoid delusions, but there were no gross aberrations of intellect or sensorium and no evidence of hallucinatory experiences. Occasionally he became irritable because of his confinement and restrictions. Evasive and slightly on the defensive, he insisted, "My mind is clearer than ever." When confronted with the possibility that he was mentally ill he disagreed and, adopting a superior attitude, said he was misunderstood because the staff had not heard the same "still small voice" he had. He was discharged to be transferred to a state hospital.

Ps. Sz., Mixed M:22:S:48 +18 9'84–631 (34) 3:9:14
Alcoholism

The patient was arrested and brought to the hospital because he had threatened his employer with a gun. The man's history revealed that he had a number of times threatened various members of his family, at one time holding a loaded revolver at his brother's head.

At 16 the patient completed the tenth grade and left school. His general health was always good. Periodically he drank excessively. He considered himself "quick-tempered" and complained of having frequent periods of depression since his service in the navy, but he blamed the depression on "boredom." He always felt the need of excitement; while in the service he preferred being in action and would become depressed "when things got dull." After his discharge two years before admission he stayed at home, working only occasionally. His employment history was a record of trying one job after the next, becoming restless in each. Never able to settle down, he avoided responsibility and thought at times of "going to the Orient" or some other spot where there was guerrilla warfare.

When examined in the hospital he was oriented, in good contact, cooperative, and agreeable; he discussed his problems freely but without any apparent concern or evidence of affect—even when telling about his homicidal threats. He frankly admitted having no feelings of love or affection for his family or for anyone else. The Rorschach test revealed some schizoid characteristics and showed a preoccupation with "blood" and "gunfire." He made a fairly good hospital adjustment but showed no insight. Because he was regarded as potentially dangerous, an attempt was made to have him committed to a state institution. This was unsuccessful and against medical advice the patient was discharged at the insistence of his parents. C. W. S.

P. Hys. F:25:M:6 +3 984′13–X 6:19:19
Schizoid

The patient, a little more than eight months pregnant, had had an uneventful pregnancy until about three days before admission when she developed crampy, abdominal pains which she interpreted as labor pains. On the third day she became restless, tried to get out of bed, and asked about her baby as though it had already been born. When the attack, which lasted about a half hour, was over, she said that she had been blind and that although she had heard people talking she had been unable to understand what they said or to answer them. (The experience was not hallucinatory since she was referring to what actual people had said.) After three other attacks during which she talked "foolishly" the patient was admitted to the hospital.

The patient had been in good health before this episode. She had graduated from the eighth grade. Married about two years at the time of admission, she had worked as a waitress until her pregnancy was well advanced. She was happily adjusted to her husband, and they were completely satisfied with their narrow, simple interests. At one time the patient had decided to become a nun and had spent three months in a convent.

In the hospital the physical and neurological examinations were negative. The pregnancy was entirely normal, but the patient, who was eager to have the child, was worried because a previous pregnancy had terminated in a spontaneous abortion. There were no evidences of a disturbance in her sensorium or intellect. The patient was somewhat labile emotionally, crying and becoming upset on small provocation. She felt that the attacks had been caused by nervousness, which she attributed to a lack of sleep and to a fear that she would abort. She adapted well to hospital life and was active in it. The psychological and other examinations failed to indicate a reason for the attacks, and after a complete examination she was discharged. It was felt that the medical reassurance would probably carry her through the pregnancy.

P. Mixed F:20:S:49 +49 98′4367–(61) 4:4:19
P Hys. +13 mos. 86734′219–(74) 2:12:9
Ps. M-D., Mixed

The patient had experienced her first menstruation at about age 14. After this first period, which apparently was normal, she had an amenorrhea for a year until hormone therapy established a menstrual cycle. She thereafter experienced pain requiring bed rest on the first one or two days of each period. Later, a two-week cycle with a generalized collicky pain began and she developed anorexia with weight loss. No medical approaches seemed to help her. Shortly before admission she was brought to the city by her sister, who left her at a boardinghouse. The patient was lonely and frightened, refused to eat, became depressed, cried frequently, and slept only a few hours each night. She was finally admitted to the hospital as an emergency because she had a "convulsive seizure" at the boardinghouse. She was described as having "threshed about, and rolled her head from side to side."

The only pertinent incident in the patient's past medical history in addition to her pre-admission menstrual trouble was an accident when she was 14. She fell on an icy street and experienced a brief period of unconsciousness; she was hospitalized and during her fourteen days in the hospital had to be put in a disturbed section because of her agitated behavior.

She had been raised in an orphan asylum and at the age of 14 had moved to a boarding home where, she said, "everything was wonderful." She completed high school at age 17, having made an average record, and she was essentially self-supporting thereafter. At one time she charged an elderly carnival worker with attempted rape. The patient frequently expressed ambivalent feelings of love and hate toward her father, chiefly because there was a story that he had had incestuous relations with the patient's sister, a delinquent later committed to a reform school.

On admission the general physical examination and other studies were essentially negative. The patient showed great concern about her menstrual difficulties and the associated symptomatology. She talked spontaneously about her family problems, expressing the desire to kill her father. She had little insight into the possible psychological background for her somatic complaints. She was usually courteous and thoughtful in a superficial way and sought favor with the nurses and doctors by frequent expressions of gratitude for the treatment she received. She varied from apparent depression to hypomania, finally saying in a somewhat euphoric way that she now understood herself perfectly and would have no further trouble.

Ps. Sz., Mixed M:20:D:264 +14 9′84<u>63</u>–X(47) 13:4:17
Ps. M-D., Manic

This veteran's present illness apparently began during his military service. When he returned home following his discharge he appeared restless and was almost constantly talking about girls and sexual matters. He told many conflicting stories. On one occasion he became boisterous at a public meeting. He could not concentrate on his work. Within the week before admission he was involved in four automobile accidents and was arrested for careless driving. He was committed and hospitalized at the request of his parents.

The patient completed high school at the age of 18. During his senior year he worried considerably about his studies and a physician advised him to drop some courses and not to study so hard. His parents were considered rigid, and they disapproved of dancing and other frivolous activities usually engaged in by young people. While in the service the patient was married at age 19 to a Japanese girl. This marriage ended in divorce after only eight months because of sexual inadequacy on his part and the promiscuity of his wife. During his military service he was AWOL several times and had two courts-martial. The present illness came on while he was stationed on an island in the Pacific. Given leave for 24 hours to visit his wife, he ran around the country for six days instead, attended dances, and was sexually promiscuous. Picked up by the military police, he was hospitalized for gonorrhea and subsequently transferred to a neuropsychiatric service because of grandiose and bizarre ideas. There he was overtalkative and got into minor difficulties but received no specific treatment. He was given a medical discharge for schizophrenic reaction, unclassified.

Less than a month after his discharge from the service the patient was admitted to this hospital. He was verbose and grandiose and talked a great deal about an "invention" of his. The diagnosis on admission was manic-depressive, manic. He was given a course of electroshock therapy and responded well to treatment. After making an excellent adjustment on the privileged ward, he was released for a trial visit to his home. A social service report four months later indicated that the patient was making a satisfactory adjustment. C. W. S.

Ps. M-D., Manic	M:18:S:29	+7	98′467–2	4:13:11
		+60	9′4–3	3:8:7

The patient was admitted to the hospital because of restlessness, agitation, insomnia, and loss of weight. He had been in good health until about a month before admission when he had had an influenza attack marked by weakness and high fever. Although he had recovered in about six days, he had then become unusually active, working all day and spending many hours organizing a 4-H club. He ate and slept poorly, began to lose weight, and was unable to concentrate for long on any one thing. He was almost incessantly developing ideas, many of them bizarre. A few days before admission he was markedly depressed over the death of a friend.

Before the present illness he had been an apparently normal boy with many friends. A fair student, he had always been active and interested in many things. At the time he developed his illness he was in a university. His parents said that he had been gradually increasing his activities even before the acute illness.

In the hospital he showed marked circumstantiality, a flight of ideas, and volubility in his discourse. He told how he had tried to direct the activities of his friends. Certain persecutory ideas about members of the community developed. He said that he had always been depressed when people did not agree with him but that he now felt fine and was very happy. "I feel so good I could jump out the window," he commented. Although he appeared elated and was very restless, there was no evidence of hallucinations or a gross sensorium defect. He slept little. It was difficult to handle him because of his high activity, and gradually this condition became worse as he grew more demanding and less reasonable. Toward the end of his hospitalization he had brief depressed periods when he sobbed quietly. Delusions of reference and persecution appeared sporadically. At the time of discharge he was belligerent and potentially assaultive, and he was transferred to a state hospital.

B. Psth., Asocial	M:17:S:25	+1	984′67–312 (32)	2:14:5
		+19	98′476–13 (43)	4:14:6

The patient had been a behavior problem nearly all his life. He had first appeared in juvenile court five years before admission because of incorrigibility, truancy, and the like. He had tried to run away from home ever since age 3. At the time of his first court appearance he was placed in a foster home. His behavior improved somewhat but he developed many somatic complaints. He was finally returned to his own home and a year later again appeared in juvenile court. This time he was sent to a reform school. He was put on parole but after stealing a revolver and some shells he was sent back to the school. At this time he claimed to be bothered by dreams of a sexual nature. These dreams were so realistic that he could scarcely believe they did not occur, and he seemed unable to distinguish between real and dream facts. On this basis he explained his fantastic tales about his life.

He was of dull normal intelligence and had finished the eighth grade with great difficulty. As far back as five years before admission, when interviewed by a child psychiatrist, he had told fantastic stories of planned holdups, sexual relationships, and the like. He had always been irritable and quick-tempered and had been very conscious of feelings of inferiority, which he attempted to compensate for by antisocial behavior. His mother was a rigid person who had dominated her husband and had completely rejected the child from the time of his birth.

In the hospital the boy was very verbose, talking almost continually about his girl friend, about sexual intercourse, and about the fights he had had. He appeared morbidly preoccupied with these subjects and made no discrimination between fact and fantasy. He told long tales of army life, although he had never been in the service. When reminded that these stories were obviously not true, he would become moody and uncooperative. He was insecure and seemed unable to form a psychotherapeutically useful relationship with anyone. He was sent back to the reform school unimproved and with a poor prognosis. Relatively few positive suggestions for his management could be made.

P. Hys. M:17:S:38 +7 9846'712- 3:13:3
Ps. Sz., Mixed +27 89472'63- 0:15:7

The patient had been in good health until about a month before admission when he became ill with laryngitis and acute appendicitis. The appendectomy was deferred for a time because of the respiratory infection. His postoperative course when the operation was performed was uneventful and he seemed well until he had a recurrence of the laryngitis, together with an attack of mumps. During this illness he had a high fever and was confused for 24 hours. While convalescing he became irritable and overtalkative and showed marked resentment against parental supervision. On one occasion he borrowed his father's car and drove it without permission 400 miles to a distant city. There he had an extended long-distance telephone conversation with his girl friend. On coming back to his home town, he was met by his brother and father, and when he saw them he became belligerent, putting up a fight until he suddenly sank to the ground unconscious. Although he remained unresponsive until the next morning, he returned to school the following day, and aside from depression and irritability there was no further difficulty until one evening about a week later when he started out to see his girl friend against the wishes of his parents. They went after him and he ran out into the back yard with a rifle, threatening to shoot if his brother came any closer; after one shot into the air he shot himself in the thigh. He was then admitted to the hospital.

A senior in high school at the time of admission, the patient had been a convivial boy with many friends and had got along well in school before his illness. During the year before admission he had developed a resentful attitude toward his parents because they did not allow him to stay out late at night, but aside from their strictness in discipline the home was a fairly good one.

In the hospital the physical examination showed two superficial bullet wounds in the left hip, but X-rays indicated that the bullet had caused no severe damage. The neurological examination was noncontributory. Usually noncommunicative and evasive, the patient spoke of being discouraged and depressed because his doctors had been unable to help him, but he did not give any explanation for shooting himself, and he disclaimed any suicidal impulses or bids for sympathy. His explanation of the automobile trip was that he must have lost his mind. He gave vivid descriptions of the two times he fainted, once after the fight with his father and his brother, and once after he shot himself. On the whole a submissive, unhappy individual, he had frequent crying spells. He repeatedly stated, "There's nothing wrong with me. I'd be all right if my mother and father would leave me alone." With longer hospitalization he admitted that he had been irritable and resentful.

A severe reaction to tetnus antitoxin injections may have acted as a kind of shock therapy. His crying spells, which had been frequent at first, occurred less often. He became less critical of the way in which his parents treated him, and he began to express the desire to return home and to go back to school. Throughout his stay in the hospital he remained a retiring, noncommittal patient who could not be adequately approached psychotherapeutically. Although it was felt that toxic exhaustive factors contributed to the development of the original symptoms they could not be precisely evaluated.

Ps. Toxic Alcoholism **M:43:M:9** **+1** **98'4672–31(47)** **1:11:5**

The patient was admitted with a severe tremor, auditory and visual hallucinations, and cramping abdominal pain. In addition there was a psychological pattern including extreme and long-standing jealousy of his wife, which was especially pronounced when his wife talked to patrons in his beer parlor. He believed she had illicit affairs with other men, and about four months before admission he began to worry more than usual about it. A moderate drinker for twenty years, he began drinking as much as a pint and a half of whiskey a day, in addition to several bottles of beer, to "calm himself down." He tolerated this fairly well for a while, but then he began skipping meals. Three days before admission he woke up to find himself shaking severely. He also began to experience hallucinations, seeing and hearing his wife and friends when they were not present. He saw impossible things, such as water and vomitus floating on the floor, and he lay in bed in this condition with no food for several days before his admission to the hospital.

At 15 he had left home because he could not tolerate his mother's religious views. He had contracted what he believed to be gonorrhea when he was 16. He had been forced into marriage because of the girl's pregnancy. Working at odd jobs until he finally bought a tavern, he had always been able to support his family fairly well, and he was regarded as an able person. He kept things to himself but made friends easily and had good judgment and the ability to handle money.

In the hospital the neurological examination showed evidence of an alcoholic neuritis. When admitted he was obviously experiencing hallucinations and he claimed to be thinking chiefly about his wife. Although he was friendly and oriented, intact in sensorium and intellect, he was restless and unable to concentrate. There was no psychometric evidence of alcoholic brain damage. With extra vitamin dosage and attention to his diet he became much better within a few days, and the tremor began to disappear. He left the hospital against advice. Since hygienic measures represented the only progress made with his problem, it was felt that his continued jealousy of his wife would in all probability lead to another alcoholic psychosis.

Ps. M-D., Manic M:28:M:75 +48 9'867–43 0:9:6

The patient had exhibited an unusual interest in politics approximately two months before admission. When this was followed by the development of acute anxiety, delusions of persecution, and restlessness, he was taken to a general hospital, where he was overtalkative and restless to such a degree that he required sedation and restraint. At that time he was fed by tube, and he was so active that he nearly collapsed from exhaustion. There was some decrease in the severity of the symptoms, and by the time he was admitted to the psychiatric unit he had improved to the extent that he was eating some meals voluntarily.

There had been no previous psychotic upset, and the past history contained nothing particularly contributory. A cheerful individual, the patient had not been inclined to worry and had not been subject to mood swings. He was devoted to his family and he had made many sacrifices for them. He was apparently very happily mated. A laboratory chemist, he was efficient in his work.

In the hospital, when the attending physician introduced himself, the patient asked, "Are you an M.D.? Do you know what an M.D. means? No, I mean in Latin. *Medicinae doctor.* Do you know any chemical German? What does hex mean? It means a witch. That nurse that just came in looks like a witch." Many of his remarks had a religious coloring, and he frequently used medical and chemical terms. He knew where he was, but he was so distractible that it was difficult to determine the extent of his orientation. Although most of the time he was elated, he was often irritable, sarcastic, and antagonistic, particularly when his stream of thought was interrupted, and he made no effort to cooperate in the examinations. There was a marked motor restlessness, and he required spoon and tube feedings because he would not feed himself. He showed no concern about himself or his family. At times he was vulgar, and much of his conversation related to drinking. As he gradually improved he required less sedation. When his condition was such that he could be allowed to come to the quiet section for short periods, he insisted on being discharged, because, he said, "There is nothing the matter with me, and there isn't any reason why I should be kept here against my will." Later he became reconciled to the necessity of staying in the hospital "until I get well." His improvement continued until the time of discharge, when he had apparently recovered to almost his normal self. The prognosis was fairly good in view of his response to treatment, the presence of many personality assets, and the fact that his wife, a capable individual, could probably help the man combat any future upsets.

Ps. M-D., Manic F:47:M:27 +2 986′721–(45) 2:11:7

Three weeks before admission this patient had a crying spell while talking to her husband over the phone. When he got home he found her irritable, depressed, and emotionally unstable. For the next two weeks she slept poorly and cried frequently. She worried about her children, about the coming of summer, and about other things. She did not want people around. She gave up her housework and spent most of her time in bed. Two days before admission she became euphoric, restless, and hyperactive. She made repeated lists of things she wanted to do and was very flighty. Her husband thought the present illness might be due to anxiety engendered by home responsibilities and worry about her daughter, who was in a hospital for a nervous disorder.

There were two previous episodes, one twenty years before when she was hospitalized for six weeks, and the other approximately ten years later, after her father's death, when she was in a hospital for four weeks. A college graduate, she had made very good grades and had been active in sports and in social affairs. Married early, she had been a housewife thereafter. She was social, cheerful, buoyant, vivacious, and a good planner. She tended to be somewhat meticulous.

In the hospital she was extremely excited, irritable, loquacious, and emotionally labile. She was also rambling and circumstantial and made frequent gestures and bizarre grimaces. She had a tendency to disrobe. She was often evasive and negativistic, and she thought that being in a locked ward was detrimental to her recovery. She was often playful, however. Under routine hospitalization she showed progressive improvement. On discharge she was well out of the severe attack but was still talkative and active. The prognosis for the present episode seemed obviously good, though there was an equally obvious probability that she would have other attacks.

B. Psth., Asocial M:19:M 9′8726–X (57) 5:23:5
Mutilative

This prisoner was one of a group of four self-mutilators. All severed their Achilles' tendons. The youth used a dirk knife and later refused to have his wound attended to by the prison physicians. He is now in isolation.

When the boy was 3 years of age his father died, leaving the mother with three children and no resources. It was not until the boy graduated from high school that he began to get into trouble. His first offenses consisted of petty thievery. At 18 he married a girl four years his senior, but the marriage failed, and his wife left him to return to her home to have a baby.

Before the burglary leading to his present sentence, the prisoner was arrested four times. His record included car pilfering, malicious mischief, and drunkenness. For these he was given, respectively, probation, a suspended sentence, a no-bill by the grand jury, and a fine. Although his present conviction is for eight burglaries he admits to only three and claims that his co-defendant was involved in the eight, he in not more than three. The loot from these burglaries consisted of cigarettes, cigars, chewing gum, candy, perfume, and hams. The youth was finally arrested one night while inside a department store, which he had entered by breaking the lock. On this charge his sentence is for two years.

The prisoner, a youth of low intelligence, is lacking in maturity and given to self-pity. He is also a malingerer. It has been noted that he has been used by a group of inmates who are more intelligent and more malicious than he is. Further observation suggests that he is off to a very poor start and needs therapy which is not available in this prison. R. C. K.

P. Psychas. F:26:S +25 987′4316–(49) 4:5:17

This young woman came to the clinic complaining of a fear of blushing, a condition which had existed for an indefinite period of time but had become worse in the past six months. It manifested itself particularly when it was necessary for the client to converse with her superiors at work, but it made her uncomfortable and self-conscious in many other situations as well. She also described herself as being troubled by a feeling that her contemporaries had greater "inner content and poise" than she.

The client was the fifth in a family of seven children. Her father was a self-educated Irish-Canadian "inventor," who was sixteen years older than his convent-trained Irish wife. Until the client was 9, her father's inventions brought the family a comfortable income, but after that he had no success and refused to find other work, leaving the responsibility for supporting and rearing the children to his wife. The girl resented her father's laziness and often lost her temper with him. During the period when she was coming to the clinic she began to keep out of such quarrels since, she said, they only upset her, left her with guilt feelings, and changed his attitude not at all.

The client, a secretary for a big firm, was a high school graduate and took college work at night school for two years. She had an average number of dates and her ambition was to be married, although formerly she had wanted a "fling" before settling down and had rejected a suitor who, she later decided, would have made an ideal husband. Marriage to her meant responsibility and children, rather than companionship. Her scores on the Bell Adjustment Inventory showed unsatisfactory in the home and emotional sections. Her interests as measured by several inventories appeared somewhat weak; her highest score was a B rating for housewife on the Strong Interest Inventory, and on the Kuder Preference Record she was only at the eighteenth percentile for clerical workers. Another of her desires was to be a singer, and she said she did well in vocal lessons. Her extreme self-consciousness, however, made an appearance before even a small group impossible.

Five therapeutic interviews at intervals of several weeks were held after the two preliminary testing sessions. The client seemed eager to do something about her problem, but her concern was so centered on her fear of blushing that it was necessary for the therapist to initiate all other topics of discussion. The client brought out her feelings of self-consciousness and her lack of ambition and "nerve," and she described her underlying depressed feeling that life was rushing by too quickly and her consequent concern about the problem of death. The only time she was not afraid of death was when she sat in church. She wanted to be married but at the moment had no prospects. Life seemed lacking in purpose. Later the client obtained relief, although the blushing continued. The prospect of an overseas job with the government, she felt, offered the possibility of adventure and would alleviate the emptiness of her existence. It seemed that in the absence of a greater drive to explore and deal with her inner problems, and in view of some crystallization of her interests, this might substitute for interview therapy. It was thought also that if an opportunity for marriage appeared this might even better dispel her vague dissatisfaction with life.

M. V. B.

Ps. Sz., Paranoid	M:23:S:64	0	9'87 462-(59)	2:7:12
		+9	9'67824-3(61)	2:7:12

The present illness of this patient had an abrupt onset about a month before admission when he came home from a Saturday night in town fearful, agitated, and weeping. He told the story that "they" had put something in his pop that had knocked him over and that they had already shot his brother and if he disclosed their identity they would kill him. In another episode a week later he felt he was being watched while having his hair cut. He said that the last month had seemed unreal and like a nightmare to him and that he had frequently felt confused, even forgetting the familiar routine in his farm work. The farm animals had "inspired" him and he had felt "uplifted" when around them because they were so kind and never harmed anyone. He had tried to overcome his illness by working harder than ever before.

The past medical history was relatively negative except for persistent constipation and hemorrhoids. He had always lived on a farm. He was a shy person, and his conduct had always been good, almost too good. His brother said that the patient enjoyed talking to older men and had never adequately related himself to his own age group. He had hated to see others hurt or to hear them talked about in a derogatory fashion. Criticism hurt him and he could not tease or be teased by anyone. At a school picnic he had observed some of his friends drinking and necking and he told them that he thought their behavior was wrong. After that he was ostracized by his fellow students; this so bothered him that he went to school in another town. He had never had a girl friend but said that he had friends among his own sex.

In the hospital the patient was apathetic. His thought content centered mainly around his condition and he showed mild self-depreciatory and hypochondriacal trends. His stream of thought was characterized by vagueness, rambling, irrelevancy, and occasional metonymic distortions. A great deal of blocking was noted. He frequently stopped in the middle of sentences for a long time, occasionally taking up unrelated subjects after such pauses. There was a striking flatness of affect. He adjusted well to the hospital routine, although during the last of his stay he became irritable and less cooperative. Insulin shock treatment seemed to help some, at least with reference to the paranoid ideas and delusional content. On discharge he was well oriented and spontaneous in speech; probably he was back to his usual state.

B. Psth., Asocial Deteriorated M:39:M:145 +15 9'876–213 (67) 3:9:12

On the recommendation of a judge this veteran was brought to the hospital following his arrest and a hearing on the charge of nonsupport. It was the opinion of the court that since the veteran had had some difficulties in the army, and in adjusting since his discharge, he should be studied at a psychiatric hospital.

The patient, part Indian, had grown up on a reservation. He attended several schools, and although he possessed average intelligence, he did not complete high school until age 21. He served 34 months overseas and saw considerable action. After being hospitalized several times for wounds (once for a head injury, when he lost consciousness and hemorrhaged from the mouth, nose, and ears) and for combat fatigue, he was discharged with a diagnosis of a moderately severe anxiety state, chronic, manifested by increasing tension and hysterical tendencies. There was a history of several arrests for drunkenness and for assault and battery before his induction, and while in the army there were several courts-martial for AWOL and insubordination. In the three years between his discharge and his hospitalization he had no steady employment and wandered around the country doing farm work and odd jobs.

The patient was admitted with a tentative diagnosis of psychopathic personality. While at the hospital he developed convulsive seizures. Subsequent neurological studies led to a diagnosis of cerebral trauma, resulting from concussion, with a delayed appearance of the convulsions. The staff summary said: "It would be difficult to state how much of his personality abnormalities are due to, or associated with, his cerebral pathology. It appears that he has had a lifelong pattern of psychopathic behavior and it is probable that no great personality changes have occurred from his head injuries, though his behavior may have been less well controlled following the concussion." C. W. S.

INDEXES

High-Point Index

This index shows all codes represented in the *Atlas*. The codes appearing as single entries refer to a summary in the *Atlas* under that code. Where entries have an indented code below the main entry, the indented code is the master code under which the former code may be found either as a second MMPI or as a variant of the master code or of a secondary code (see Examples A and B on page xviii). In all *Atlas* summaries one code is called a "master" since it locates the summary in relation to other summaries. This index shows, then, all master codes and all cross-reference codes, giving for the latter the master code to locate the summary.

1327'869– M
132'76984–
132'8–4 M
132'8–94 F
'2183 479–
132'847–9 M
1328476'–9 F
3128476'–9
132'864–9X F
123'864–9X
132'8749–6 M
1328'7496– M
213'867–
13'2876–9 M
31'2876–9
132'87649– M
1'32978– M
1342786'– M
1234'678–9
134'287–9 F
13'428 76–9 M
'13469– M
'1347928– F
413872'69–
13'49287– F
13'628 79– M
31'628 79–
13'6472–9 M
31'6472–9
136'82497– F
163'2894–
1'37246– F
13'724869– F
13728'4– F
'376842–1
1'378– F
13'79268– F
'1382–9X F
1'382–96 F
138 24 79'– F
13'82 4967– F
13824'976– F
13'8274– F
13'829– F
13'829– M
'13 84–X F
'31 84–X
13'847– F
'138 49–6 M
'183 49–6
1389'2764– F
1938'742–X
13'92–4 F
31'92–4
139'26–4 M
132'4–6
1'39428– M
139'74628– F
319'74628–
'14236–8 M
'21346–8
'1426– F
'2146–
'1427386– F
72'8631–
1'42836–9 M
418'236 79–X
'14369– M
'13469–
'1437928– F
413872'69–
14'38 267– M
14 382'67–9 M
14'78 23–6 F
4'817326–9
'1482– M
1482'36–9 M
14'82739– M
148372'69– M
14 9386'27–X F
'162394–7 F
'163–97 M
163'2894– F
16'83792– F
61'83792–
'17–98436 M
2173'6489–
'1723486– F
72'8631–
'172 386–9 M
'127 386–9
1723'864– M
12'639–84
1723'896– M
17263'48–X F
'1728–4 F
'7128–4
172834'69– M
2173'6489–
172836'49– M
2137'68–9
'1729843– M
87213469'–
17328'4– F
'376842–1
'1743928– F
413872'69–
'17 8296–4 M
897612'43–X
17829'634–X M
178'3942– M
718'3942–
18236'74– M
'182 374–9 F
182736'4– M
182736'4–9X M
18273'946– M
12873'946–
'1832–9X F
'1382–9X
183 24 79'– F
138 24 79'–
18327'6– F
278'3194–
'183 49–6 M
'18 673–9X M
'3–6X
18 7324'69– M
148372'69–
187326'49– M
189'6327– F
819'6327–
'192374– M
123'497–
'193–7 F
19'34 28–7 M
193'74628– F
319'74628–
1938'742–X F
19'823–6 M
91'823–6
'2–138749 M
'2–39 M
'2–47 F
'2–63 M
'2–6789 M
'2–694 F
'2–861739 F
21'3–98 M
2'134– M
21'3 487–6
'21346–8 M
2'13468– M
2'134687–9 M
12'38467–9
2134'6879– F
624'3819–
213'476– F
123'476–
213'479– F
21'348–9 M
21'3 487–6 M
213 4876'–9 F
8123 764'–
213 6'4897– F
87231'469–
21'368–94 F
2'137– M
27'36 184–
21'37–4689 F
1'32–4968
213'7–9 F
321'47–9
213'76–9 M
231'76–9
2137'64– F
2671'4398–
21376'48–9 M
821347'69–
21376'8– F
31'92–4
213'768– F
2137'68–9 M
21376'8–9 M
21376'84–9 M
132'76984–
213'78– F
213'78–9 F
312'78–9
213'784– M
213'784–9 F
312'784–9
213784'6–9 F
31276'84–X
2137'86– F
21'3786– M
12'3786–
21378'6–9 M
213'8–94 F
'2183 479–
2138'467– F
213'86–9 M
213'867– M
213'867–9X F
21'387–9 F
213'87–94 M
21387'4–9 F
2138'746–X M
2318'746–X
213876'4–9 F
2'1437– F
214'379– M
124'379–
'2146– F
216'379– F
63 12'794–
21637'98– F
2'17346–9 F
217'348–6 F
'2173486– F
72'8631–
2173'6489– M
2'17368–9 M
2'71368–9
217'3684–9 F
26'7 13 48–9
217'38–9 M
21'7384–9 F
21738'4–9 M
217'3846– M
21 738'469–X M
74812 36'9–
217386'– M
217'386– F
21738'649– M
21738'96– M
27381'46–
2'174– F
'2176–98 43 M
217'638–9 M
2'17 64 938– F
'2178–4 F
'7128–4
'2178–94 M
'2718–94
2'1783–9 M

HIGH-POINT INDEX

'21 783–9 F
'12 783–9
2'17834–9 M
827631'4–
'217836–9 F
217843'69– M
2'1786– M
21786'34– M
2178'639– M
8279'641–
'2179843– M
87213469'–
'2183 479– F
21837'4– F
'2183 479–
218 47'369– M
218'63–79 M
2'1873–9 F
21873'694– F
28731'694–
'23–6 F
2'31– M
'231–98 46 F
13'2748–6
2'314– M
21'3 487–6
'23146–8 M
'21346–8
2'314687–9 M
12'38467–9
231476'89– F
231'478–9 M
2'31478–96 M
23'1 487–6 M
21'3 487–6
231 4876'–9 F
8123 764'–
231'64789– F
231 6'4897– F
87231'469–
231'674– F
23'17–94 F
2317'46–9 M
3217'46–9
23'17 468– F
2731 48'6–
231746'89– F
231'748– F
43'2167–9
2317'486– M
13'2–9
2317'486–9 F
231'76–9 M
2317'64– F
2671'4398–
23 1764'8–9 F
32 1764'8–9
231'76498– F
2'31768–9 M
2'71368–9
2317'68–9 M
217386'–

231768'–94 F
23 1786'–9
23'178– F
231'78–9 F
312'78–9
'23178–9X F
231'784–9 F
312'784–9
2'31784–9 M
827631'4–
23178'4–9 M
27836941'–
2317846'–9 F
23178'46–9 F
231'674–
231784'6–9 F
31276'84–X
23 1786'–9 F
23 1786'4– F
32 1786'4–
23178'64–9 F
231'8–94 F
'2183 479–
2318'467– F
2138'467–
2318'746–X M
231876'4–9 F
213876'4–9
'234–7168 M
'234–9 F
23417'86–9X F
7284136'–9
23'46871– M
'2347–9 F
2783'416–9
2'3471–9 M
23471'68–9 F
23'47168–9 F
3'427 816–
'234 71986–X F
'243 71986–X
2'3478– M
2'31478–96
'23478 16– M
2'378146–
23'47816–9 F
23478'6– F
26'4378–
23'47 861–9 F
2348'671–9 F
2'3487–9 F
2483'7–
23'487–9 M
23'46871–
'2349– F
69'487–X
'2349–7 M
2'361–9 M
872'4631–9
'23679– F
'238749–6

2'3 697–8 F
3'2 697–8
2'37– M
'237–9X F
237'1– F
2371'864–9
'2371486– F
72'8631–
237148'6–9 F
23'71486–9 F
237'1648– F
23716'48–9 F
23716'84– F
237'18–49 F
273'8614–
237'184– F
37128'46–
2371'86– M
2'37186–49 F
6'31284–
2371'86–9 M
2731'86–9
2371'864–9 F
2371'864–9 F
23'7416– F
'238749–6
23741'86–9 M
'237 619 84– F
7291'836–
'23768– M
'32768–
2'37681– F
2'73681–
2'378146– M
237816'–9 F
23 1786'–9
237816'4– F
278316'4–
2378461'– F
23'789461– F
'2379–4 F
2'38–1 M
2381'476–9 F
819'6327–
'2381 479– F
'2183 479–
2381'76– F
2831'76–
23817'694– M
2318'746–X
2384176'9– F
2'3849– M
2'8349–
238'7146– F
23871'694– F
28731'694–
'238749–6 F
'239418– F
'329418–
'24–698 F
27'438 19–6

'2413– F
'4213–
'24136–8 M
'21346–8
2'413687–9 M
12'38467–9
'2416– F
'2146–
2416'3789– F
2'417– F
2'174–
24 186'73–9 F
42 186'73–9
'243–69 F
'423–69
'243–7168 M
'234–7168
'243–9 M
24'317– M
23741'86–9
2431'78–9 M
728134'96–
'24367– F
'42367–
'2437–9 F
2783'416–9
2'4371–9 M
2'3471–9
'243 71986–X F
24'3768– M
42'67 389–
2'4378– M
2'31478–96
'24378 16– M
2'378146–
2438'1679– F
243817'69– F
2'4387–9 F
2483'7–
'2439– F
69'487–X
'2439–7 M
'2349–7
2467'3819– M
'24 6783– F
2467'831– F
62487'3–
2468'7–1 F
4268'7–1
'246879– F
'247– F
'247–8 F
27'438 19–6
'2471386– F
72'8631–
2471836'– M
821347'69–
2471'9638– M
24738'6– F
26'4378–
'24783– M
728436'19–

247'8361-9 M
427'8361-9
247836'91- F
472836'91-
2478'63- F
278'46-
247981 36'-X M
274981 36'-X
'248367-9 M
2483'7- F
248371'6- M
2483716'-9 F
2843716'-9
'24839- M
'28349-
24'87-9 M
24'876193- F
24'8763- M
24'879- M
'249 13- M
4'8193-
249'7836-X M
'26-483 M
2'613487-9 M
12'38467-9
26'13748-9 F
2613'7489- F
2'61738-9 M
2'71368-9
'264-913 M
'624-913
264'1783-9 F
26'4378- F
264781'3- F
2648'7-1 F
4268'7-1
2'64871-X F
61'83792-
'264879- F
'246879-
2'67-1 M
2'67-91 M
72864'319-
26'7 13 48-9 F
267'138- F
271'4836-
2671'4398- F
2'673-9 F
27834'61-9
2'673-94 M
27'831-9
2'67381- F
2'73681-
2'6743- F
'267438-9 F
27834'61-9
2674'8139- F
267'81349- M
182736'4-
26'783-9 F
2'687-9
26794'183- F

'268 14 37-9X F
2683'7194- F
2'687-9 F
26871'34- F
268'7314- F
628'7314-
'26874- F
'28674-
26'8749- M
2'6973- M
2'6983- F
472836'91-
'27-3 F
2'7-9 M
'27-9 F
27'1-4 M
2'71346-9 F
2'17346-9
2'713468-9 M
12'38467-9
271'348-6 F
217'348-6
'2713486- F
72'8631-
271348'6-9 M
23741'86-9
271348'69- M
2'71368-9 M
27136'84- F
271'3684-9 F
26'7 13 48-9
27138'- F
1'32-4968
2713'84-9 M
27138'4-9 M
2'713846- F
27138'46-X M
27138'46-9 M
271384'6-9 F
31276'84-X
271'3864-9 F
2713'896- F
2137'86-
2'714- F
2'174-
271'4836- F
27148'36-9 M
27'31846-X
271486'3- M
2'71638-9 M
217'38-9
2'71 64 938- F
2'17 64 938-
'2718-4 F
'7128-4
'2718-94 M
2'7183-9 M
2'1783-9
2'71834-9 M
827631'4-
2718346'-9 M
2718364'-9

27183'64- F
2718364'-9 M
271836'4-9 F
271843'69- M
728134'96-
2718'639- M
8279'641-
'2719843- M
87213469'-
273'1- F
2371'864-9
2731 48'6- F
27314'86-9 M
273'18-49 F
273'8614-
27318'4-9 M
2731'86-9
27 318'46- F
72 318'46-
27'31846-X M
2731'846-9 M
2731'86-9 M
27318'64-9 F
2731 48'6-
2731'864-9 F
2371'864-9
2'7341-9 M
2'3471-9
2734'16- M
2734'681-9 F
23716'48-9
2734'681-9 F
27'463891-
2734'816- M
2'73486- M
27'36 184- M
'273 619 84- F
7291'836-
2'73648-1 M
27'36481-9 F
2'73681- F
273'6849- F
27381'4- F
27381'46- M
27'38146- M
273'8146-9 M
27381'64- F
2738'1694- F
273'8614- F
274'136-9 M
27'43- M
27431'86-9 M
27436'18-9 M
27436'189- M
'27438 16- M
2'378146-
274'3819- M
27'438 19-6 F
27438'6- F
26'4378-
27'4618 39- M
72168'934-

2746'1983- M
27'463891- F
'2748- M
78213649'-
274836'91- F
472836'91-
274'86- M
27486'31- F
274981 36'-X M
2'76-1 M
2'67-1
'276-9 M
2'76-91 M
72864'319-
27'6 13 48-9 F
26'7 13 48-9
276'138-9 F
2'763-9 F
27834'61-9
27'63148-9 F
276'138-9
27'63489-1 M
2'7643- F
2'6743-
'276438-9 F
27834'61-9
2764'8139- F
2674'8139-
276'81349- M
182736'4-
2'7683-9X M
'27684- F
'28674-
278134'6-X F
278134'69-
2781346'-9 M
2871346'-
278134'69- F
278'13496- F
278134'69-
2781'364-9 M
2781364'-9 M
2871346'-
2'78139- M
2'87139-
278'14396- F
2781463'9- F
278134'69-
27'831-9 M
27831'46- F
32 1764'8-9
2783'146- F
28713'6-9
278316'- F
28713'6-9
278316'4- F
27831'69- M
72831'69-
2783'169- M
27'831-9
27831'694- F
28731'694-

278'3194– F
2783'416– F
436'28–7X
278'3416–9 F
2783'416–9 F
27834'61–9 F
278361'4– F
273'8614–
278'3641–9 M
27'831–9
278 3641'9– F
287 3641'9–
27836941'– M
278'436– M
278'436–9 F
2784'3916– M
7284'3916–
278'46– F
27 84631'9– F
8721436'9–
27 846'319– F
72 846'319–
27861'3–9X M
278 61'34– M
728 61'34–
2786'134–9 M
27'8631– F
72'8631–
2786'314–9 M
278631'49–X M
27836941'–
278634'9– M
2786'41–9 F
27864'13– M
72864'319–
2786413'9– F
2876413'9–
278643'–9 F
278'3416–9
2786'4931– F
7286'4931–
27'8916– M
278'964 31– M
72864'319–
27'91384– F
72'91384–
2791'8346– F
'2794–1X F
27'94 836–1 M
27'98631– F
2'813467–9 M
12'38467–9
2813'467–9 F
819'6327–
281347'69– M
821347'69–
'2813 479– F
'2183 479–
2813746'9– F
281376'4–9 F
213876'4–9

281 47'369– M
218 47'369–
2'81734–9 M
827631'4–
28173496'– F
138 24 79'–
281736'4– F
281763'4–X F
281736'4–
2831'476–9 F
819'6327–
28316'74– F
2831'76– F
28317'694– M
2318'746–X
'28349– M
2'83674– F
28 371'46–9 F
28371'469– F
28713'6–9
283716'4–9 F
2837416'9– F
28647319'–X
28'3764–9 F
283764'1–9 F
312784'6–9
'28437 16– M
2'378146–
2843716'–9 F
2846'7–1 F
4268'7–1
28467'3–X M
82467'3–X
2846731'9– M
28471369'– F
28647319'–X
2847'1639– M
28473'6– F
26'4378–
'286 14 37–9X F
'268 14 37–9X
286'3471–9 F
286417'93– M
28647319'–X F
28671'34– F
26871'34–
2867'1493– F
2674'8139–
286'731–9 M
286'7314– F
628'7314–
286'7341– F
'28674– F
2871346'– M
287'13496– F
278134'69–
28713'6–9 F
2'87139– M
287139'46– F
278'14396–
28713'946–X F
278'3194–

287'1463–9 M
287164'39– M
28731'46– F
32 1764'8–9
2873'1469– F
2873146'9– F
2378461'–
287316'– F
28713'6–9
287316'4– F
278316'4–
287316'49– F
28731'694– F
2'87361– F
2'73681–
287'361– M
27'831–9
287361'4– F
273'8614–
2873614'9– M
287 3641'9– F
'2874–69 M
287'436–9 F
278'436–9
287 61'34– M
728 61'34–
287'61349– F
28763'149– F
287631'49–X M
27836941'–
2876'341– M
2876413'9– F
287'9136– M
28947'613– M
'29–316 M
2371'86–
'29–41 M
'293418– F
'329418–
'294–6 F
'294 13– M
4'8193–
'2946– M
294'7836–X M
249'7836–X
2'9673– M
2'6973–
2'9683– F
472836'91–
'2974–1X F
'2794–1X
'3–2 F
'3–29 F
314'892–
'3–6X M
'31–468 F
'31–47 F
'31–6742 F
'1327–89
'31–87962 F
'31–94 M
2137'68–9

'31–987 M
3'12– M
'312–97 M
1482'36–9
'3124–678 F
312'48769–
'31246–8 M
'21346–8
31'246–9 F
3'1247–6 F
31'2478– F
3'427 816–
312'478–9 M
312'4786–9 F
132'4786–9
31'24867– F
13'24867–
31248'7– F
3'12487– F
312'48769– F
31248769'– F
312'49–6 F
31'24 968– F
31'26–9 F
3'126–98 F
31'2648– F
312 6'4897– F
87231'469–
31'26784–X F
31267'894–
3126'789–4X F
1326'789–4X
31267'894– F
31'2684–9 F
3'12687–9X F
31'26874– F
31268'79– F
31286'79–
'3127–89 F
'1327–89
31'2748–6 F
13'2748–6
'3127486– F
72'8631–
312748'6–9 F
31'27 48 69– F
'3127 64–9 F
312'7648–9 F
312784'6–9
31'27684–X F
31'27684–X F
31267'894–
31276'84–X F
312'78–9 F
312'784–9 F
312'7846–X F
132'6784–9
312784'6–9 F
312'7849– F
312784'96– F
3721 486'–

HIGH-POINT INDEX

'4327-9 F
2783'416-9
'4327186- F
72'8631-
'43278 16- M
2'378146-
43278'6- F
26'4378-
43281'796- F
42381'796-
'43 286-9 M
'34 286-9
432'8967- F
423'8967-
'4329- F
69'487-X
4'3297 86- M
'9346-
'43 619 278-X F
'34 619 278-X
'436 218- F
'7243-
4'36271-9 F
3'46271-9
436'28-7X F
4367281'9- F
2378461'-
436'821-79 F
436 8912'7- F
463 8912'7-
'43 69-2 F
'34 69-2
4'3726-9 F
'43728-9 M
4'379- F
4'38- F
4'83-
'438-9 F
'43816- M
'4-19
43'829 761- M
'4386- F
2483'7-
'4386-1 F
2483'7-
4387126'9- F
4387'219- F
8437'219-
4'389 16 27- M
31'4782-
'439- F
'243 71986-X
'439- F
81934'726-
'43962-718 M
462378'91-
'4398672- F
'3948672-
4398'7126- F
4'6-132 F
46'-79 F
'46-9 M

'46-9213 M
'64-9213
46183'792- F
416'9378-
461'9378- F
416'9378-
462378'91- M
4'627381-9 F
4'276381-9
462738'19- F
4'62793-1 M
4'72693-1
'4628-97 F
'4268-97
4'6287- M
4628'7-1 F
4268'7-1
'462879- F
'246879-
'4629-X M
'462987-3 M
4'63- F
'463-2 F
4'6318- F
'463 218- F
'7243-
4'6328- F
4'6372-9 F
4'3726-9
'4638- F
46381 27'9- F
46'3819- F
463'821-79 F
436'821-79
4'638 2179- F
463 8912'7- F
46'3897- F
46'829 37-
46391 28'7- F
64'97-1
'46392-718 M
462378'91-
'46398- M
7289'6-
'467- F
76'284-
4673'2189- F
467'839- M
'4679-1 F
2'6743-
468'21 93- F
468'23- M
46'829 37- F
4'683271-9 F
46'83721- M
4'68379- F
2416'3789-
4'68379-1 F
46872'319- M
46879'31- F
86479'31-

46'89237- F
436'28-7X
46'89317- F
468'972-1 F
486'972-1
'469328- F
4'6938-7 F
'469 728-1 F
24'876193-
46'98-13 M
'4698237-1 M
'64-1
4'69 83- M
4'96 83-
4698'3-2 M
2'73486-
4698'713- F
'4712486- F
72'8631-
'472-1 F
76'284-
47213'98-X M
42713'98-X
'47238 16- M
2'378146-
472'3819- M
728436'19-
47238'6- F
26'4378-
'47239- M
8716243'9-X
47'239- M
4'726381-9 F
4'276381-9
'472 6389- M
'427 6389-
4'72693-1 M
472836'91- F
4'7293 86- M
'9346-
4'7298-1 M
4'72693-1
4'7326-9 F
4'3726-9
'47398-2 M
47 6'2381- F
4763'2189- F
4673'2189-
476'382- F
8'7269-31
476'82193- M
47682'93- F
476'839- M
467'839-
'4769-1 F
2'6743-
'478-13 M
4782'6913- M
2'73486-
478'296- F
72 846'319-

'4783- M
728436'19-
4'789-6 F
'478 96-1 F
86479'31-
'479-1 M
'497-1
'479238-6 M
4'79 286-1 M
'479 38- M
'48-2 F
'84-2
4'8-263 M
4'8-69 F
'48-7 F
'48 12- M
'4812-7 M
782134'6-9
481'236 79-X M
418'236 79-X
'48 13 2679-X M
48139'672- F
'4816- F
'4186-
4'817326-9 F
4'8193- M
4'82- F
6'98341-7
'482 136- F
'428 136-
48231'796- F
42381'796-
'48237 16- M
2'378146-
4823716'-9 F
2843716'-9
48'23917- F
423871'96-
'4826-97 F
'4268-97
4826'7-1 F
4268'7-1
48 267'3-9 M
4'8273-9 M
48273'6- F
26'4378-
'4827 63-X M
48276'31- F
4827'6913- M
2'73486-
4827'963- M
48'291 367- M
'48296-13 M
'42896-13
48'2973- M
4'83- F
'483-269 M
'4-19
'4836- F
2483'7-
4836'712- F
26871'34-

4837'219– F
8437'219–
4837926'1– F
4'839– F
4'83–
'4839672– F
'3948672–
'486– M
'486–9 M
4'8617– M
4862'7931– F
4'863271–9 F
4'683271–9
'48 67–13 M
'84 67–13
48679'31– F
86479'31–
4869'1372– M
486'972–1 F
'487–13 M
'478–13
'487–6 F
487'2136– M
48 72 13'69– F
84 72 13'69–
487'236–9 M
4872361'9–X F
48'726– M
48'72936– F
'4873– M
728436'19–
48'7391– F
48 761'923–X F
48'7623– M
487'6932– M
'4879–6 F
'487 96–1 F
86479'31–
'489– F
'489– M
'489–273 M
'849–273
4891'367– M
'4892– F
4'8923– M
48'9263– F
86 1'23479–X
489'263 17– F
4'893 16 27– M
31'4782–
4'8937– M
4'8937– F
489376'21– F
4'896– F
4'896–2 F
4896'271–X F
'489 73–2 M
'498 73–2
48976'2–1 M
'49– F
'9–1843
'49–1267 M
4'9–26 M
'49–2817 M
4'9–6378 12 M
49'–673 M
'491–673 M
4'9–6378 12
4'9138– M
492'3671– M
4'9237– M
4'9237 86– M
'9346–
'492 38– M
'429 38–
4'9278–1 M
4'72693–1
492'7836–X M
249'7836–X
4'92 867– F
4'29 867–
'493–6 M
'943–6
'49318– M
49'326–1 M
'4936– M
'49362–718 M
462378'91–
49'3816– F
'4938672– F
'3948672–
4938'7126– F
4398'7126–
4'96–71 M
'496 728–1 F
24'876193–
4'9678–132 F
49'68–2713 M
9'48–237
49'68–72 M
'4968237–1 M
'64–1
4'96 83– M
4'96837– F
496'87– F
489'263 17–
'497–1 M
'497–6X M
'49 7231–6 F
4'97 286–1 M
4'79 286–1
'497 38– M
'479 38–
497823'61– F
6247'389–
'498– F
'489–
'498– M
'489–
49'8–6 F
4'98–6 F
9'4–7231
4981'367– M
4891'367–
'4982– F
'4892–
'4983– M
4'983 16 27– M
31'4782–
4'9837– M
4'8937–
49'86–213 F
94'86–213
49'87–1 M
49'8716–3 M
49'872–3X F
'498 73–2 M
'49876–21 M
49876'2–1 M
48976'2–1
498'763– F
'6–29 M
'6–39184 F
27'463891–
'6–7149X F
'6–7893 F
61273'94– F
231'674–
'613–97 M
'163–97
'6149–73 F
61'83792–
61'83792– F
6189'473– F
6819'473–
6'19 834– M
871'236 49–
'62–483 M
'26–483
'6238– F
'624–913 M
624'3819– F
6243'8719– F
6423'8719–
6247'389– F
6247'8319– M
7284'3916–
6248'7–1 F
4268'7–1
62487'3– F
'624879– F
'246879–
6'2748–1 M
6274'8139– F
2674'8139–
627'8139– M
62'783–9 F
2'687–9
'62784– F
'28674–
'6279– M
72168'934–
'628 14 37–9X F
'268 14 37–9X
628'7314– F
6287'4319–X M
'63–7184 M
'36–7184
63 12'794– F
6'31284– F
'6327 841–X F
'6328– F
'6238–
634'12– F
'634 218– F
'7243–
6342'7891– F
6432'7891–
6'34 78–91 F
4'6328–
6'34819– M
6'48319–
'637814– F
'637842–1 F
'376842–1
'639– M
'63972– F
'69372–
'64–1 M
'64–9 M
'46–9
'64–9213 M
'6419–73 F
61'83792–
642'3819– F
624'3819–
6423'8719– F
6427'389– F
6247'389–
6428'7–1 F
4268'7–1
'642879– F
'246879–
64287'93– M
'6429–X M
'4629–X
'643 218– F
'7243–
6432'7891– F
6'43 78–91 F
4'6328–
64'3819– F
46'3819–
6'43879– F
'6479–1 F
2'6743–
648'23– M
468'23–
648273'19– F
64'8297–1X F
'6483–92 F
'648317– F
31876'249–
6'48319– M
6'4832–79 F
6'8432–79
648'7923– F

64879'31– F
86479'31–
64'89237– F
436'28–7X
64'89317– F
46'89317–
6489'721– F
86497'1–
64897'3–X F
'3482697–
64'97–1 F
'6498237–1 M
'64–1
6498'7–3 F
46'89317–
'67–3 F
'7243–
'67–91 F
826743'1–9X
6724'389– F
6247'389–
6724'8139– F
2674'8139–
'67284– F
'28674–
'6729– M
72168'934–
6'729–4 M
'673814– F
'637814–
'673842–1 F
'376842–1
'6749–1 F
2'6743–
6749'2813– M
72168'934–
678'12–4 F
876'12–4
6'791234– M
6'971234–
'67932– F
'69372–
68 1'23479–X F
86 1'23479–X
6812473'9– F
8612473'9–
6819'473– F
68213 794'–X F
'682 14 37–9X F
'268 14 37–9X
'6823– F
'6238–
68 231'47– F
86 231'47–
6'8243–9 F
682'7314– F
628'7314–
6827 413'9– M
683'127–9 F
2'1873–9
68 347129'– F
462738'19–

6842'3791– F
6842'7–1 F
4268'7–1
'6843–92 F
'6483–92
6'84319– M
6'48319–
6'8432–79 F
6'847–1 M
68472'31– F
6847'239– F
6847291'3– M
68479'31– F
86479'31–
68497'3–X F
'3482697–
6'87–319 F
687'12–4 F
876'12–4
6'87214 39– F
687234'19– F
68'724– F
'68724– F
'28674–
687'249–1X F
6874'23 91–X F
6879'43–2 M
'689– M
6'89–271X M
9'68–271X
6'89–3127 F
68'9147– M
689'47–X F
'689713– F
6897'2341–X F
6897'421– F
'69–14 M
'96–14
'6914–73 F
61'83792–
6'91 834– M
871'236 49–
'69372– F
'694–873 M
2'6973–
69'438271– F
27'98631–
69'48 123– F
'6948237–1 M
'64–1
69'487–X F
6'971234– M
'6973– M
'698– M
'689–
'698–2 M
6'98–271X M
9'68–271X
6'98341–7 F
'698713– F
'689713–

6987'2341–X F
6897'2341–X
'69874–2 F
'7–63 F
'7123486– F
72'8631–
'712389– F
278316'4–
'7128–4 F
'7129843– M
87213469'–
713'26849– M
'71 8296–4 M
897612'43–X
'7183–9X M
'71832469– M
'78312469–
'718342– F
687234'19–
718'3942– M
71'863 29– M
7'2–148 M
'72–3 F
'27–3
'7213486– F
72'8631–
72138'– F
1'32–4968
'721389– F
278316'4–
7'21638–94 F
'7128–4
72168'934– M
'7218–4 F
'7128–4
721843'69– M
728134'96–
'7219843– M
87213469'–
7'23148–69 F
27'438 19–6
72 318'46– F
7231'846–9 M
2731'846–9
723'18694– F
28763'149–
7'23418 69– M
'723 619 84– F
7291'836–
723'6849– F
273'6849–
7238'491– F
23'71486–9
'7243– F
72'43– M
27'43–
'72438 16– M
2'378146–
72'438 19–6 F
27'438 19–6
72438'6– F
26'4378–

724836'91– F
472836'91–
72486'3–1 M
6'2748–1
7'248631–9 F
4'638 2179–
72'63489–1 M
27'63489–1
7264'8139– F
2674'8139–
7'26814 39– M
72'684– F
76'284–
7'2689–4 M
72813'46– F
728134'6–X F
278134'69–
7281346'–9 M
2871346'–
728134'96– M
728'3–96 M
728314'69– M
872361'49–
'72831469– M
'78312469–
72831'69– M
72831'96– M
72'836–49 F
72'8361–9 F
7283'614– F
728361'4– F
273'8614–
728'3614–9 F
72'84–1 M
728'4136–9 F
7286'4931–
7284136'–9 F
72841 36'9– M
728413'69– F
27'438 19–6
728436'1–9 M
78234'169–
728436'19– M
7284'3916– M
'728 46–9 F
'782 46–9
72 84631'9– F
8721436'9–
72 846'319– F
728'4963– F
72849'63– M
8726'341–9
728 61'34– M
72'8631– F
72863'14– F
2138'467–
728'63419– M
'72864– F
'28674–
7286'43– M
728643'19– M
72864'319– M

HIGH-POINT INDEX

HIGH-POINT INDEX

82471369'– F
28647319'–X
8247163'– F
8274631'–
82473'6– F
26'4378–
824761'3–9 M
821347'69–
82476139'– F
28647319'–X
8247639'1– M
8427639'1–
8'26137–9 F
'826 14 37–9X F
'268 14 37–9X
8261'7349– F
82617'439– F
86217'439–
826'3471–9 F
286'3471–9
826'3714– F
82647139'– F
86471239'–
82647319'–X F
28647319'–X
82671'93–X M
86721'93–X
826'7314– F
628'7314–
'82674– F
'28674–
826743'1–9X F
8269'7143– F
82713'694– M
827139'46– F
278'14396–
82714369'–X F
82716'349– M
182736'4–9X
827164'39– M
287164'39–
8273146'9– F
2378461'–
827316'94– F
28713'6–9
827361'4– F
273'8614–
8273641'– F
827'4– M
'8274–69 M
'2874–69
8274631'– F
82746'3 19– M
827 61'34– M
728 61'34–
827'61349– F
287'61349–
827631'4– M
8276'341–9 M
8726'341–9
8276413'9– M
8726413'9–

82769413'–X F
278'3194–
827'9613– F
28713'6–9
8279'641– M
8'2971634– F
628'7314–
8297631'4–X M
'4–19
'8312–9X F
'1382–9X
'831247– M
8312 764'– F
8123 764'–
8316724'9– F
3816724'9–
83217'694– M
2318'746–X
83247'6– F
26'4378–
832 61'749– F
6821̲3 794'–X
8341'7926– M
12873'946–
'83427 16– M
2'378146–
8347'219– F
8437'219–
8'367924– F
3'867924–
'837– F
28'3764–9
837164'2–X M
8'372164–X F
83726'419– F
86947231'–X
83 74126'9– F
2378461'–
837'42– F
873'42–
'839–6 F
3'867924–
'83 91–X M
'8394672– F
'3948672–
'84–2 F
'84 12– M
'48 12–
84'1239– F
'182 374–9
'84 13 2679–X M
'48 13 2679–X
841'39267– M
31'628 79–
8'4172– M
'8417369–X F
'8147369–X
842 173'96– M
824 173'96–
8423716'–9 F
2843716'–9

'84237 16– M
2'378146–
84'23917– F
423871'96–
8426'7–1 F
4268'7–1
84 267'3–9 M
48 267'3–9
8426793'– F
4872361'9–X
84273'6– F
26'4378–
8427639'1– M
8427'936–X M
84'2973– M
48'2973–
8431'7926– M
12873'946–
8437'219– F
'8439672– F
'3948672–
84639'712– M
'84 67–13 M
84671239'– F
86471239'–
'84672– F
'8467 23– M
846792'31–X M
84679'31– F
86479'31–
'84697–13 M
'86947–13
84 72 13'69– F
847'2639– F
8473 216'9– F
84 761'923–X F
48 761'923–X
84'769–13X M
'8479–2 M
'84793–2 M
'847 96–1 F
86479'31–
'849–273 M
84'9 137–6 M
89'4 137–6
'86–3 F
86 1'23479–X F
8'612 394–7 M
8612473'9– F
8613'472– F
'86143–7 M
861792'34– F
86213 794'–X F
68213 794'–X
'862 14 37–9X F
'268 14 37–9X
8621'7349– F
8261'7349–
86217'439– F
86 231'47– F
86239 14'7–X F

86271'349– M
182736'4–9X
862'7314– F
628'7314–
'86274– F
'28674–
862743'1–9X F
826743'1–9X
86279413'–X F
278'3194–
863'127–9 F
2'1873–9
86 347129'– F
462738'19–
8642'7–1 F
4268'7–1
86439'712– M
84639'712–
86471239'– F
'86472– F
'84672–
8647'239– F
6847'239–
8647291'3– M
6847291'3–
864792'31–X M
846792'31–X
86479'31– F
86497'1– F
867'12–4 F
876'12–4
'8671423– M
8'672–3 M
86721'93–X M
86'724– F
68'724–
86724'913–X F
87264'39–
86729'431– F
86732'41– F
86734'219– F
98'4367–
867 423'19– M
867 49'321– M
'86791– F
'87961–
8679241'3–X M
867942'13–X M
86794'23–1X M
8679'43–2 M
6879'43–2
'869– M
'689–
8'69–271X M
9'68–271X
'86947–13 M
869'472– F
86947231'–X F
86'97234– M
869'724–3X M
8712346'9– M
871'236 49– M

HIGH-POINT INDEX

HIGH-POINT INDEX

93'1428-6 F
39'1428-6
931'74628- F
319'74628-
'93184-2 F
9'324- F
'932418- F
'329418-
934- M
2'71368-9
9'34-67 M
'698-2
9'34 168- F
'9346- M
9'348- M
'9348672- F
'3948672-
'936-2 F
9'783-2
'9376- F
728'4963-
'93862417- F
'94-1267 M
'49-1267
'94-213 M
'94-21786 F
94'3-7
9'4-26 F
9'4-26 F
9'4-3 M
98'467-2
9'4-31278 M
9'481-6
9'4-63 F
9'4-672 M
94'-673 M
49'-673
9'4-7231 F
941'23687- F
94'3-7
9'4128637- F
9'1286437-
941'3687- F
9'41683- F
9'4183-67 F
94'3-7
94'187 26- M
274981 36'-X
9'426378- M
9'246378-
942'7836-X M
249'7836-X
9'428 673- M
'9428713- M
'9287143-
'943- M
2'71368-9
'943-1X M
'943-6 M
9'43-67 M
'698-2
9'43-6712 M
94'3-7 F

9'43-71 28 M
9'43-78 M
9'43-71 28
9'43 168- F
9'34 168-
94'326-1 M
49'326-1
'9436- M
'9346-
'9438672- F
'3948672-
9'46-31 F
'69874-2
9'4678321-X F
'9468237-1 M
'64-1
946'8327- F
9'6478-21
946 87'23- F
'94 7231-6 F
'49 7231-6
9'476-1 M
49'87-1
9'478-3X M
947823'61- F
6247'389-
94'7863- F
9'48- M
1327'498-
9'48-13 M
9'43-71 28
9'48-237 M
94'8-6 F
49'8-6
9'48-7 F
9'48-7 M
9'481-6 M
9'483-1 M
9'483-21 M
9'483-6 M
9'486-13 M
948'6-2 F
9'31-2786
94'86-21 F
9'8-7
94'86-213 F
9'486-321 M
94'86-7213 M
9'48-237
9'4867-21 F
9486'7-3 F
94'867-31 F
4'9678-132
94'87-1 M
49'87-1
94'8716-3 M
49'8716-3
'96-14 M
9'6-3 M
9'6128437- F
9'1286437-
9'624378- M
9'246378- M

'9634- M
'9346-
9'64- F
9'64-31 F
'69874-2
'964-873 M
2'6973-
9'64183- F
9'41683-
9'6478-21 F
'9648237-1 M
'64-1
96'487-X F
69'487-X
9'6487-21 F
9'4867-21
964 87'23- F
946 87'23-
'9673- F
728'4963-
'967 382- M
9'678-231 M
9'67824-3 M
9'87 462-
'968- M
'689-
9'68-2 F
9'68-271X M
9'68 34-21 M
9'7-21 M
'972-6 F
'927-6
9'728-1 F
'9728143- M
'9287143-
'9736- F
728'4963-
9'742- M
9'746-1 M
49'87-1
9'7468-13 M
89'76-3
9'7486-21 F
9'4867-21
'976 382- M
'967 382-
9'7826-31 M
9'783-2 F
'9783-2 M
'7893-2
'978 32- F
'789 32-
978'4316- F
987'4316-
978'46-3 M
9'78 462- M
9'87 462-
9'8-2 F
9'8-231 F
2438'1679-
9'8-26 M
9'8-7 F

9'8126437- F
9'1286437-
9'8134-2 F
98'1463- M
'9827143- M
'9287143-
'98314-2 F
'93184-2
'9834672- F
'3948672-
9'84-13 M
9'43-71 28
9'84-21 M
9'84-631 M
984'13-X F
9'84163- F
9'41683-
9'8417-6 F
498'763-
9'843-6 M
9'483-6
98'4367- F
9'846-13 M
9'486-13
984'6-2 F
9'31-2786
9'846-321 M
9'486-321
9'8463-X M
98'467-2 M
9'8467-21 F
9'4867-21
984'67-312 M
9846'712- M
98'4672-31 M
98'476-13 M
984'67-312
984763'21- F
14 9386'27-X
'986- M
'689-
9'86-271X M
9'68-271X
9'86274-3 M
-34
9'86 34-21 M
9'68 34-21
9864'2137- F
872'96134-
9'867-43 M
986'721- F
9'8726-X M
'9873-2 M
'7893-2
'987 32- F
'789 32-
9'8734- F
9'728-1
987'4316- F
987'46-3 M
978'46-3
9'87 462- M
9'876-213 M

Low-Point Index

This index shows the low-point scales of all the codes represented in the *Atlas*. Codes are given with the low-point scales printed first. A semicolon indicates the division between the low and high points of the code. The master code under which the summary for each entry may be found is given in normal order (the high-point code printed first) indented below the main entry.

LOW-POINT INDEX

-2;'69874 F
'69874-2
-2;'7893 M
'7893-2
-2;'84 F
'84-2
-2;'8479 M
'8479-2
-2;'84793 M
'84793-2
-2;89'764X M
2'31478-96
-2;'93184 F
'93184-2
-2;'936 F
9'783-2
-2;9'68 F
9'68-2
-2;9'783 F
9'783-2
-2;9'8 F
9'8-2
-2;9'8134 F
9'8134-2
-2;984'6 F
9'31-2786
-2;98'467 M
98'467-2
-21;'49876 M
'49876-21
-21;'89 F
'89-12
-21;9'483 M
9'483-21
-21;94'86 F
9'8-7
-21;9'4867 F
9'4867-21
-21;9'6478 F
9'6478-21
-21;9'68 34 M
9'68 34-21
-21;9'7 M
9'7-21
-21;9'84 M
9'84-21
-213;'94 M
'94-213
-213;94'86 F
94'86-213
-213;9'876 M
9'876-213
-21378;9' M
9'-12378
-21 43768;'9 F
'243 71986-X
-21786;'94 F
94'3-7
-218;9' M
9'-128
-231;9'678 M
9'678-231

-231;9'8 F
2438'1679-
-2317;6'89 F
6'89-3127
-23178;9'4 M
9'481-6
-237;9'48 M
9'48-237
-2416;'93 M
12386'7-
-26;4'9 M
4'9-26
-26;9'4 F
9'4-26
-26;9'4 F
9'4-26
-26;9'8 M
9'8-26
-26147;'9 M
'9-26147
-263;4'8 M
4'8-263
-269;'483 M
'4-19
-27;'36 F
'36-27
-27;'9 F
46'829 37-
-271;9'68X M
9'68-271X
-2713;49'68 M
9'48-237
-273;'849 M
'849-273
-2731;9'4 F
9'4-7231
-2786;9'31 F
9'31-2786
-'279;'34 F
'34-279
-2817;'49 M
'49-2817
-29;'3 F
314'892-
-29;'6 M
'6-29
-2913;'64 M
'64-9213
-3;'27 F
'27-3
-3;'462987 M
'462987-3
-3;49'8716 M
49'8716-3
-3;49'872X F
49'872-3X
-3;6498'7 F
46'89317-
-3;'67 F
'7243-
-3;7'8426 F
78 2694'31-

-3;78'492 F
8742'6913-
-3;'86 F
'86-3
-3;8'672 M
8'672-3
-3;869'724X M
869'724-3X
-3;87'492 16 F
8742'6913-
-3;896'2741X M
896'2741-3X
-3;89'76 M
89'76-3
-3;9'4 M
98'467-2
-3;9'478X M
9'478-3X
-3;9486'7 F
9486'7-3
-3;9'6 M
9'6-3
-3;9'67824 M
9'87 462-
-3;978'46 M
978'46-3
-3;9'86274 M
-34
-31;46'98 M
46'98-13
-31;'478 M
'478-13
-31;8'7269 F
8'7269-31
-31;94'867 F
4'9678-132
-31;9'64 F
'69874-2
-31;9'7826 M
9'7826-31
-31;9'84 M
9'43-71 28
-31;98'4672 M
98'4672-31
-31;98'476 M
984'67-312
-312;4'6 F
4'6-132
-312;984'67 M
984'67-312
-3127;6'89 F
6'89-3127
-31278;9'4 M
9'481-6
-316;'29 M
2371'86-
-318749;'2 M
'2-138749
-319;6'87 F
6'87-319
-31984;'6 F
27'463891-

-321;9'486 M
9'486-321
-321;9'8 F
2438'1679-
-34 M
-34
-346;'879 F
'746-139
-36;'7 F
'7-63
-361;'29 M
2371'86-
-361;9'84 M
9'84-631
-3716;'92 M
68'9147-
-3721;9'4 F
9'4-7231
-39;'2 M
'2-39
-39;78'241 M
87261'34-9
-4;126'378 F
126'378-4
-4;1326'789X F
1326'789-4X
-4;132'8 M
132'8-4
-4;139'26 M
132'4-6
-4;'17 8296 M
897612'43-X
-4;'2379 F
'2379-4
-4;27'1 M
27'1-4
-4;312'9786X F
1326'789-4X
-4;31'92 F
31'92-4
-4;31'96728 F
31'96728-4
-4;3'21 796 F
3127'9486-
-4;6'729 M
6'729-4
-4;'7128 F
'7128-4
-4;7'2689 M
7'2689-4
-4;7'8 M
78'2693-4
-4;78'2693 M
78'2693-4
-4;82'1637 M
82'1637-4
-4;876'12 F
876'12-4
-41;'92 M
'29-41
-4123;'9 M
9'-128

LOW-POINT INDEX

–4126;'93 M
12386'7–
–418;7'2 M
7'2–148
–4183;'9 F
'9–1843
–4189 F
–4189
–4281739 M
869'724–3X
–43;9'867 M
9'867–43
–4318976 F
'89–12
–46;132'78 F
31'26–9
–46;'38 M
'38–46
–46;'912 F
'912–46
–463;'879 F
'746–139
–467;'9 F
'2–47
–467823 F
–467823
–468;'31 F
'31–468
–4689;21'37 F
1'32–4968
–47;'2 F
'2–47
–47;'31 F
'31–47
–47 13 M
–47 13
–4718;'36 M
'36–7184
–47869;'13 F
'31–87962
–483;'26 M
'26–483
–49;123'7 M
123'7–94
–49;21'368 F
21'368–94
–49;23'17 F
23'17–94
–49;237'18 F
273'8614–
–49;2'37186 F
6'31284–
–49;72'836 F
72'836–49
–4968;1'32 F
1'32–4968
–6;1'234 F
312'49–6
–6;132'4 M
132'4–6
–6;13'2748 F
13'2748–6

–6;132'8749 M
132'8749–6
–6;'183 49 M
'183 49–6
–6;21'3 487 M
21'3 487–6
–6;217'348 F
217'348–6
–6;'23 F
'23–6
–6;'238749 F
'238749–6
–6;27'438 19 F
27'438 19–6
–6;'294 F
'294–6
–6X;'3 M
'3–6X
–6;3'1247 F
3'1247–6
–6;312'49 F
312'49–6
–6;'31428 F
'31428–6
–6;3'79148 F
31'297–
–6;'389 F
3'867924–
–6;39'1428 F
39'1428–6
–6;41'78 23 F
4'817326–9
–6;4'2X M
4'2–6X
–6;'421378 M
'421378–6
–6;4'29 M
4'29–6
–6;4'789 F
4'789–6
–6;'479238 M
'479238–6
–6;'487 F
'487–6
–6;'4879 F
'4879–6
–6;'497X M
'497–6X
–6;'49 7231 F
'49 7231–6
–6;49'8 F
49'8–6
–6;4'98 F
9'4–7231
–6;89'4 137 M
89'4 137–6
–6;'91327 F
'91327–6
–6;91'823 M
91'823–6
–6;'927 F
'927–6

–6;'943 M
'943–6
–6;9'481 M
9'481–6
–6;9'483 M
9'483–6
–6;9'8417 F
498'763–
–627;'9 M
'9–627
–63;'2 M
'2–63
–63;'7 F
'7–63
–63;9'4 F
9'4–63
–631;9'84 M
9'84–631
–6378 12;4'9 M
4'9–6378 12
–64;'38 M
'38–46
–64;'912 F
'912–46
–6412;'93 M
12386'7–
–643;'879 F
'746–139
–647;'9 F
'2–47
–647823 F
–467823
–648;'31 F
'31–468
–6489;21'37 F
1'32–4968
–67;9'4183 F
94'3–7
–67;9'43 M
'698–2
–6712;9'43 M
9'43–6712
–672;9'4 M
9'4–672
–6723;'9 F
'294–6
–673;'419 M
4'9–6378 12
–673;49' M
49'–673
–6742;'31 F
'1327–89
–678;'3124 F
312'48769–
–678;9'132 M
9'132–678
–6789;'2 M
'2–6789
–681739;'2 F
'2–861739
–69;1'2 M
1'2–96

–69;13'2478 M
13'2478–69
–69;2'31478 M
2'31478–96
–69;'2874 M
'2874–69
–69;'423 F
'423–69
–69;4'8 F
4'8–69
–69;7'23148 F
27'438 19–6
–69;7'41238 M
7'41238–96
–69;'74238 F
27'438 19–6
–694;'2 F
'2–694
–698;'24 F
27'438 19–6
–7;13'249 F
13'249–7
–7;'162394 F
'162394–7
–7;'193 F
'193–7
–7;19'34 28 M
19'34 28–7
–7;'2349 M
'2349–7
–7;3'94681 F
3'94681–7
–7;'4182 M
782134'6–9
–7;436'28X F
436'28–7X
–7;4'6938 F
4'6938–7
–7;'48 F
'48–7
–7;6'98341 F
6'98341–7
–7;8'612 394 M
8'612 394–7
–7;'86143 M
'86143–7
–7;94'3 F
94'3–7
–7;9'48 M
9'48–7
–7;9'48 F
9'48–7
–7;9'8 F
9'8–7
–71;4'96 M
4'96–71
–71 28;9'43 M
9'43–71 28
–714 M
278'436–
–7149;'6X F
'6–7149X

LOW-POINT INDEX

–7168;'234 M
'234–7168

–718;'43962 M
462378'91–

–7184;'36 M
'36–7184

–72 F
–72

–72;'36 F
'36–27

–72;49'68 M
49'68–72

–7213;94'86 M
9'48–237

–72186;'94 F
94'3–7

–7231;9'4 F
9'4–7231

–728;9'31 F
9'31–2786

–73;'6149 F
61'83792–

–7312;6'89 F
6'89–3127

–741 M
278'436–

–74 13 M
–47 13

–76;9'43 M
'698–2

–768;'3124 F
312'48769–

–768;9'132 M
9'132–678

–78;9'43 M
9'43–71 28

–78143;9' F
9'–87143

–7893;'6 F
'6–7893

–78962;'31 F
'31–87962

–79;218'63 M
218'63–79

–79;436'821 F
436'821–79

–79;46' F
46'–79

–79;6'8432 F
6'8432–79

–792;'4X F
'4–792X

–796 F
–796

–8;'21346 M
'21346–8

–8;'247 F
27'438 19–6

–8;31'29 46 F
31'29 46–8

–8;324'619 M
342'619–8

–8;3'2 697 F
3'2 697–8

–814;7'2 M
7'2–148

–8143;'9 F
'9–1843

–82176;'94 F
94'3–7

–84;12'639 M
12'639–84

–846;'31 F
'31–468

–8469;21'37 F
1'32–4968

–861739;'2 F
'2–861739

–871;'43962 M
462378'91–

–8714;'36 M
'36–7184

–87143;9' F
9'–87143

–873;'964 M
2'6973–

–8793;'6 F
'6–7893

–87962;'31 F
'31–87962

–89;12'3467 F
12'3467–98

–89;'1327 F
'1327–89

–89 43;'2176 M
'2176–98 43

–89 46;'231 F
13'2748–6

–9;1234'678 M
1234'678–9

–9;1234876' M
1234876'–9

–9;123'6874 F
123'6874–9

–9;12'37 F
1'32–4968

–9;12'38467 M
12'38467–9

–9;123'864X F
123'864–9X

–9;1'238674 F
1'238674–9

–9;'127 386 M
'127 386–9

–9;'12 783 F
'12 783–9

–9;13'2 M
13'2–9

–9;132'4 M
132'4–9

–9;132'478 M
132'478–9

–9;132'4786 F
132'4786–9

–9;'13248 M
'13248–9

–9;13'248 M
13'248–9

–9;132'6784 F
132'6784–9

–9;132'847 M
132'847–9

–9;134'287 F
134'287–9

9;13'428 76 M
13'428 76–9

–9;'1382X F
'1382–9X

–9;1'42836 M
418'236 79–X

–9;14 382'67 M
14 382'67–9

–9;1482'36 M
1482'36–9

–9;'182 374 F
'182 374–9

–9;182736'4X M
182736'4–9X

–9;'18 673X M
'3–6X

–9;2'134687 M
12'38467–

–9;21'348 M
21'348–9

–9;213'7 F
321'47–9

–9;21376'48 M
821347'69–

–9;2137'68 M
2137'68–9

–9;21376'8 M
21376'8–9

–9;21376'84 M
132'76984–

–9;213784'6– F
31276'84–X

–9;21378'6 M
21378'6–9

–9;213'86 M
213'86–9

–9;213'867X F
213'867–9X

–9;21'387 F
21'387–9

–9;21387'4 F
21387'4–9

–9;213876'4 F
213876'4–9

–9;2'17346 F
2'17346–9

–9;217'38 M
217'38–9

–9;21'7384 F
21'7384–9

–9;21738'4 M
21738'4–9

–9;217'638 M
217'638–9

–9;2'1783 M
2'1783–9

–9;2'17834 M
827631'4

–9;'217836 F
'217836–9

–9;2'1873 F
2'1873–9

–9;231'478 M
231'478–9

–9;231 4876'
8123 764'–

–9;2317'486 F
2317'486–9

–9;231'76 M
231'76–9

–9;2317'68 M
217386'–

–9;'23178X F
'23178–9X

–9;23178'4 M
27836941'–

–9;2317846' F
2317846'–9

–9;23 1786' F
23 1786'–9

–9;23178'64 F
23178'64–9

–9;'234 F
'234–9

–9;23417'86X F
7284136'–9

–9;2'3471 M
2'3471–9

–9;23'47168 F
3'427 816–

–9;23471'68 F
23471'68–9

–9;23'47816 F
23'47816–9

–9;23'47 861 F
23'47 861–9

–9;2348'671 F
2348'671–9

–9;23'487 M
23'46871–

–9;2'3487 F
2483'7–

–9;2'361 M
872'4631–9

–9;'237X F
'237–9X

–9;237148'6 F
237148'6–9

–9;23'71486 F
23'71486–9

–9;23716'48 F
23716'48–9

–9;2371'864 F
2371'864–9

-9;2371'864 F
2371'864–9
-9;23741'86 M
23741'86–9
-9;237816' F
23 1786'–9
-9;2381'476 F
819'6327–
-9;'243 M
'243–9
-9;2431'78 M
728134'96–
-9;'2437 F
2783'416–9
-9;'248367 M
'248367–9 ·
-9;24'87 M
24'87–9
-9;26'13748 F
26'13478–9
-9;264'1783 F
264'1783–9
-9;26'7 13 48 F
26'7 13 48–9
-9;2'673 F
27834'61–9
-9;26'783 F
2'687–9
-9;'268 14 37X F
'268 14 37–9X
-9;2'687 F
2'687–9
-9;'27 F
'27–9
-9;2'7 M
2'7–9
-9;271348'6 M
23741'86–9
-9;2'71368 M
2'71368–9
-9;271'3684 F
26'7 13 48–9
-9;27138'4 M
27138'4–9
-9;27'1384 M
27'1384–9
-9;27138'46 M
27138'46–9
-9;271'3864 F
271'3864–9
-9;27148'36 M
27'31846–X
-9;2'71638 M
217'38–9
-9;2718346' M
2718364'–9
-9;2718364' M
2718364'–9
-9;271836'4 F
271836'4–9
-9;27314'86 M
27314'86–9

-9;27318'4 M
2731'86–9
-9;2731'846 M
2731'846–9
-9;2731'86 M
2731'86–9
-9;27318'64 F
2731 48'6–
-9;2734'681 F
27'463891–
-9;2734'681 F
23716'48–9
-9;27'36481 F
27'36481–9
-9;273'8146 M
273'8146–9
-9;274'136 M
274'136–9
-9;27431'86 M
27431'86–9
-9;27436'18 M
27436'18–9
-9;'276 M
'276–9
-9;276'138 F
276'138–9
-9;27'63148 F
276'138–9
-9;'276438 F
27834'61–9
-9;2'7683X M
2'7683–9X
-9;2781346' M
2871346'–
-9;2781364' M
2871346'–
-9;2781'364 M
2781'364–9
-9;27'831 M
27'831–9
-9;278'3416 F
278'3416–9
-9;2783'416 F
2783'416–9
-9;27834'61 F
27834'61–9
-9;278'3641 M
27'831–9
-9;278'436 F
278'436–9
-9;27861'3X M
27861'3–9X
-9;2786'134 M
2786'134–9
-9;2786'314 M
2786'314–9
-9;2786'41 F
2786'41–9
-9;278643' F
278'3416–9
-9;2813'467 F
819'6327–

-9;28 371'46 F
28 371'46–9
-9;283716'4 F
283716'4–9
-9;28'3764 F
28'3764–9
-9;283764'1 F
312784'6–9
-9;2843716' F
2843716'–9
-9;286'3471– F
286'3471–9
-9;286'731 M
286'731–9
-9;28713'6 F
28713'6–9
-9;287'1463 M
287'1463–9
-9;31'246 F
31'246–9
-9;312'478 M
312'478–9
-9;31'26 F
31'26–9
-9;31'2684 F
31'2684–9
-9;3'12687X F
3'12687–9X
-9;312748'6 F
312748'6–9
-9;'3127 64 F
'3127 64–9
-9;312'78–9 F
312'78–9
-9;312'784 F
312'784–9
-9;312784'6 F
312784'6–9
-9;312786'4 F
312786'4–9
-9;3128476' F
3128476'–9
-9;31'2876 M
31'2876–9
-9;31'6472 M
31'6472–9
-9;3'214 F
3'12487–
-9;321'47 F
321'47–9
-9;3'21478 F
3'21478–9
-9;3217'46 M
3217'46–9
-9;321'7648 F
312784'6–9
-9;32 1764'8 F
32 1764'8–9
-9;32178'46 F
231'674–
-9;324'176 M
324'176–9

-9;'3246 M
'3246–9
-9;3271'864 F
3271'864–9
-9;3'412768 M
3'412768–9
-9;'34 286 M
'34 286–9
-9;3'46271 F
3'46271–9
-9;371'2468 F
'3127 64–9
-9;3721864' F
1326'78–X
-9;3'81624X M
3'81624–9X
-9;'413 F
'413–9
-9;'42 F
'7–63
-9;4217'83 M
4217'83–9
-9;42 186'73 F
42 186'73–9
-9;42'3678 M
42'3678–9
-9;4'23781 F
4'23781–9
-9;4'276381 F
4'276381–9
-9;427'8361 M
427'8361–9
-9;43'2167 F
43'2167–9
-9;4'3726 F
4'3726–9
-9;'43728 M
'43728–9
-9;'438 F
'438–9
-9;'46 M
'46–9
-9;4'683271 F
4'683271–9
-9;4'817326 F
4'817326–9
-9;48 267'3 M
48 267'3–9
-9;4'8273 M
4'8273–9
-9;'486 M
'486–9
-9;487'236 M
487'236–9
-9;6'8243 F
6'8243–9
-9;683'127 F
2'1873–9
-9;'7183X M
'7183–9X
-9;7'248631 F
4'638 2179–

LOW-POINT INDEX

–9;72'8361 F
72'8361–9

–9;728'3614 F
728'3614–9

–9;7284136' F
7284136'–9

–9;728'4136 F
7286'4931–

–9;728436'1 M
78234'169–

–9;7'4231 M
728134'96–

–9;'7684 23 M
728 61'34–

–9;781236'4 M
781236'4–9

–9;7813'62 M
7813'62–9

–9;78213'46 M
78213'46–9

–9;782134'6 M
782134'6–9

–9;'782 46 F
'782 46–9

–9;782'463 F
782'463–9

–9;824761'3 M
821347'69–

–9;8'26137 F
8'26137–9

–9;826743'1X F
826743'1–9X

–9;8'71436 F
874231'96–X

–9;872'4631 M
872'4631–9

–9;87261'34 M
87261'34–9

–9;8726'341 M
8726'341–9

–91;2'76 M
72864'319–

–91;6'4378 F
4'6328–

–91;'67 F
826743'1–9X

–913;'624 M
'624–913

–91384;'6 F
27'463891–

–9164387 M
–9164387

–92;'3 F
314'892–

–92;'6483 F
'6483–92

–9213;'64 M
'64–9213

–93;'2 M
'2–39

–94;123'7 M
123'7–94

–94;123'8 F
'2183 479–

–94;21'368 F
21'368–94

–94;213'87 M
213'87–94

–94;23'17 F
23'17–94

–94;231768' F
23 1786'–9

–94;237'18 F
273'8614–

–94;2'673 M
27'831–9

–94;'2718 M
'2718–94

–94;'31 M
2137'68–9

–94;7'21638 F
'7128–4

–9468;21'37 F
1'32–4968

–96;1'2 F
'162394–7

–96;1'2 M
1'2–96

–96;1'382 F
1'382–96

–96;2'31478 M
2'31478–96

–96;'2874 M
'2874–69

–96;'4 M
'4–96

–96;'4 M
'4–96

–96;728'3 M
728'3–96

–96;7'41238 M
7'41238–96

–964;'2 F
'2–694

–9647;32'1 F
32'1–9647

–97X F
–97X

–97;'163 M
'163–97

–97;'321 M
1482'36–9

–97;'4268 F
'4268–97

–97;436'821 F
436'821–79

–97;46' F
46'–79

–97;6'8432 F
6'8432–79

–972;'4X F
'4–792X

–98;12'3467 F
12'3467–98

–98;'1327 F
'1327–89

–98;21'3 M
21'3–98

–98;3'126 F
3'126–98

–98;'4 M
'4–98

–98 43;'2176 M
'2176–98 43

–98436;17 M
2173'6489–

–98 46;'231 F
13'2748–6

–987;'31 M
'31–987

–9873;'6 F
'6–7893

–98762;'31 F
'31–87962

Contributors' Index

This index shows the master codes of the summaries contributed to the *Atlas* from clinical sources other than the Psychiatric Unit. Each of these contributors is indicated by initials that follow the case summary where it occurs in the *Atlas*.

CONTRIBUTORS' INDEX

2731'846–9
'276–9
2'7683–9X
278'436–9
27861'3–9X
2'83674–
'462987–3
6287'4319–X
6'48319–
687'249–1X
72831'96–
72'84–1
728643'19–
78 26'4319–
'83 91–X
869'472–
'9–12837
'9–627
9'428 673–
'967 382–

Diagnosis Index

This index shows the codes related to the diagnostic and descriptive terms used with the summaries. Generally, the only code given is the master code that will locate the given summary. However, when the patient had two admissions and there was a different diagnosis for the second admission, the code for the second admission is listed but is followed, as in earlier indexes, by the master code.

Where the given diagnostic or descriptive term is listed in the first position on the summary, indicating that it is the main diagnostic term for the case, the code is here preceded by an asterisk. All other codes are cases where the diagnostic term was added as a secondary description.

For notes on the meanings of the terms as used in the *Atlas*, see pages xi–xiv preceding the case histories.

DIAGNOSIS INDEX

*4'83– F
*4862'7931– F
'487–6 F
*48'726– M
48 761'923–X F
*48'7623– M
*4891'367– M
*'4892– F
*4'8923– M
*489'263 17– F
4'8937– F
*48976'2–1 M
*'49–1267 M
*4'9–26 M
*49'–673 M
*4'9138– M
*492'3671– M
*4'9237– M
*49'326–1 M
*4'96–71 M
*4'96 83– M
*4'96837– F
*'497–1 M
*'498 73–2 M
*'49876–21 M
*'624–913 M
*62487'3– F
*'639– M
*71'863 29– M
*7286'43– M
*'8124 63– M
84639'712– M
*'84 67–13 M
*847'2639– F
*86479'31– F
*8'672–3 M
*867942'13–X M
*86794'23–1X M
*8714263'9–X M
*879 46'2– M
*89'476– M
*896'2741–3X M
*89762'413–X M
'9–26147 M
9'132–678 M
*'9346– M
*9'4–26 F
*9'486–13 M
*94'86–213 F
*9'64– F
*'967 382– M
*9'742– M
*9'8–7 F
*984'67–312 M
*9'8726–X M
*9'876–213 M

B. Psth., Mixed

*1326'78–X F
*13824'976– F
13'847– F
*'1482– M
*17829'634–X M
*2317'486–9 F
*'248367–9 M
*24'876193– F
*'268 14 37–9X F
274'136–9 M
*278'3416–9 F
31248'7– F
31427896'– F
*319'74628– F
*3'412768–9 M
416'9378– F
*4217'83–9 M
42'739816– F
*'427 6389– M
'429 38– M
*4'29 867– F
4'31867– M
*46'–79 F
46183'792– F
416'9378–
*'462987–3 M
*4'63– F
*463 8912'7– F
*4673'2189– F
467'839– M
46'83721– M
*4698'713– F
*4'8–263 M
*48139'672– F
*'4827 63–X M
4837926'1– F
*48'7391– F
*'6973– M
*824 173'96– M
*82713'694– M
*8279'641– M
*86471239'– F
*8742'6913– F
*9'483–21 M

B. Psth., Path. Emot.

*132'478–9 M
*1'32978– M
*13'829– M
14 9386'27–X F
*'183 49–6 M
*217'348–6 F
2'378146– M
*2734'816– M
*2'73486– M
*2746'1983– M
28947'613– M
*3'12487– F
*3'214–9 F
3'12487–
'329418– F
'34–279 F
*39'1428–6 F
'4–96 M
*423'8967– F
4'2798–1 M
4'72693–1
'428 136– F
*431276'8– M
*4'379– F
*46'3819– F
*46'98–13 M
*4827'963– M
4869'1372– M
*4'896–2 F
*'4936– M
*'6–7149X F
*6'2748–1 M
*6423'8719– F
64287'93– M
*6847'239– F
*817296'34–X F
*'84–2 F
*8427'936–X M
*'84672– F
8473 216'9– F
*8612473'9– F
*86732'41– F
872'4631–9 M
*872'96134– F
*87'9642– F

B. Psth., Path. Sexuality

*14 382'67–9 M
*'21346–8 M
*31'6472–9 M
*46'83721– M
*'48 12– M
*4'817326–9 F
*48'291 367– M
*'486– M
*4'8617– M
*487'2136– M
*487'236–9 M
*'489– M
*4'8937– M
*'497–6X M
*6847291'3– M
*7'26814 39– M
*'84793–2 M
86479'31– F
*871'236 49– M
*'9–13 M
*9'483–1 M

B. Simple Adult Maladj.

*'13–47869 F
'31–87962
*182736'4– M
*2348'671–9 F
*264'1783–9 F
*2'73648–1 M
*27436'189– M
*'31–87962 F
*31'29 46–8 F
*324'176–9 M
*3'867924– F
*'423–69 F
*'46–9 M
*46872'319– M
*47682'93– F
*4'896– F
*627'8139– M
*'689713– F
*'69372– F
*72'8631– F

Deteriorated

13824'976– F
*'2–6789 M
'2176–98 43 M
2'1786– M
231'76–9 M
26'7 13 48–9 F
31'24 968– F
412'7386–X M
418'236 79–X M
4'263–19 M
'4268–97 F
4'2798–1 M
4'72693–1
4'72693–1 M
'4827 63–X M
64287'93– M
68'9147– M
'7893–2 M
817296'34–X F
821347'69– M
82713'694– M
8714263'9–X M
9'–87143 F
'912–46 F
9'246378– M
'9287143– M
9'742– M
9'876–213 M

Drug Add.

132'478–9 M
*13'249–7 F
1'32978– M
2'17 64 938– F
23471'68–9 F
'248367–9 M
27381'4– F
28947'613– M
'294–6 F
3'12487– F
31'27 48 69– F
'3127 64–9 F
3217'46–9 M
'3246–9 M
3'2 697–8 F
'427 6389– M
4'63– F
'4638– F
492'3671– M

4'96–71 M
'497–1 M
63 12'794– F
782149'36– M
867942'13–X M
89'476– M
9'132–678 M
'9287143– M
'943–6 M

Epilepsy

13824'976– F
2'137– M
27'36 184–
27'36 184– M
32 1786'4– F
'4892– F
72 846'319– F

Mental Deficiency

–796 F
123'864–9X F
14'38 267– M
17263'48–X F
21378'6–9 M
24'8763– M
2843716'–9 F
312'478–9 M
46'829 37– F
487'2136– M
'6–7149X F
6874'23 91–X F
72 318'46– F
78146 32'9– M
'7893–2 M
84'1239– F
'182 374–9
8'612 394–7 M
8612473'9– F
861792'34– F
86 231'47– F
86794'23–1X M
91'823–6 M

Mutilative

124'379– M
14 9386'27–X F
18236'74– M
19'34 28–7 M
24'8763– M
286417'93– M
28713'6–9 F
'3–2 F
39'4 287 16– M
'4267– M
'42896–13 M
43'829 761– M
47'239– M
4891'367– M
492'3671– M
4'9237– M
49'326–1 M

4'96–71 M
'497–1 M
6247'389– F
'639– M
7'2893– F
84'769–13X M
86794'23–1X M
872'4631–9 M
89'476– M
896'2741–3X M
89762'413–X M
9'84–13 M
9'43–71 28
9'8726–X M

P. Anxiety State

*'13248–9 M
*132694'78– M
1327'498– M
*1'378– F
*187326'49– M
*213'7–9 F
321'47–9
*'217836–9 F
*2471'9638– M
*2'7683–9X M
*28'3764–9 F
*312'86749– F
*'3246–9 M
*3712'4986– F
*423871'96– F
*476'82193– M
*6'43879– F
*687234'19– F
*687'249–1X F
*6'971234– M
*713'26849– M
*7'23418 69– M
*7291'836– F
*781236'4–9 M
*7821346'9– M
*782149'36– M
837164'2–X M
*874231'96–X F
*87 426'391– M
*'9–627 M
*9'486–321 M
*9'7–21 M

P. Hypo.

*12'3467–98 F
1234'678–9 M
*1234876'–9 M
123'497– M
*123'7–94 M
*12'3786– M
*12'38467–9 M
*123'847– M
*12386'7– M
*1'238674–9 F
*126'378–4 F
*12'639–84 M

*1'32–4968 F
*13'2478–69 M
*132'4786–9 F
'13248–9 M
*13'248–9 M
132'6784–9 F
*13'2689– F
31286'79–
*132'847–9 M
*132'8749–6 M
*13'49287– F
*1'37246– F
*13'79268– F
*1'382–96 F
*13'82 4967– F
*13'8274– F
*13'829– F
13'829– M
*13'847– F
*2'13468– M
*213'479– F
*21'37–4689 F
1'32–4968
*2137'64– F
2671'4398–
*213'768– F
*2137'68–9 M
*21376'8–9 M
*213'784– M
2137'86– F
*213'867– M
*213'867–9X F
*21'387–9 F
*21637'98– F
*2'17346–9 F
*217'38–9 M
*21'7384–9 F
*21738'4–9 M
*217386'– M
21738'649– M
*217'638–9 M
*2'1783–9 M
*23 1786'–9 F
*23471'68–9 F
23741'86–9 M
*2384176'9– F
264'1783–9 F
*267'138– F
271'4836–
*2671'4398– F
27486'31– F
278'14396– M
*278634'9– M
*283716'4–9 F
*2'87139– M
2876413'9– F
*31'246–9 F
31248769'– F
312'48769– F
*31'24 968– F
31'26–9 F
*31'2648– F

*31267'894– F
*3'12687–9X F
*31'26874– F
*31'27684–X F
*312784'6–9 F
*312786'4–9 F
*3128476'–9 F
*31286'79– F
*31'2876–9 M
*31'297– F
*31'42789– F
*31427896'– F
*'31428–6 F
*31'4782– M
314'892– F
*321'47–9 F
*'376842–1 F
*3816724'9– F
*'413–9 F
*42 186'73–9 F
*42381'796– F
62487'3– F
627'8139– M
*7812364'9– M
*78146 32'9– M
*7842'1936– M
*'7893–2 M
*8123 764'– F
8279'641– M
*86 231'47– F
*87261'34–9 M
876'12–4 F
*9172 48'36– F
278'14396–
*918634'72– F
*9'324– F
*9'8134–2 F

P. Hys.

*–4189 F
–467823 F
*–72 F
*–796 F
*12378'46– M
*132'4–6 M
*132'4–9 M
*13'24867– F
*132'6784–9 F
*'1327–89 F
*1327'498– M
*134'287–9 F
13'829– F
*1938'742–X F
*'2–39 M
*2'137– M
27'36 184–
*213'78– F
*2137'86– F
213'867– M
*'2146– F
*231 6'4897– F
87231'469–

DIAGNOSIS INDEX

*23'17–94 F
23 1786'–9 F
*'2379–4 F
*238'7146– F
26871'34– F
*'2718–94 M
*2731'846–9 M
*27'36 184– M
*2'73681– F
283716'4–9 F
28763'149– F
'294–6 F
'31–468 F
*'31–47 F
*'31–987 M
*3'12– M
31248'7– F
*31248769'– F
31'24 968– F
31267'894– F
*31'26874– F
*312'784–9 F
312784'6–9 F
*3127'9486– F
*312'8674– M
3'142679– F
31'42789– F
*314'892– F
*31'48976– F
*31'7982– F
31876'249– F
*31'96728–4 F
*'321–97 M
1482'36–9
*3'21478–9 F
3'4216 78– F
'34 286–9 M
*'38–46 M
3'867924– F
*'4–792X F
*413872'69– F
*47 6'2381– F
4'817326–9 F
4837926'1– F
*498'763– F
628'7314– F
*6432'7891– F
*6874'23 91–X F
*72831'96– M
*7813'62–9 M
8279'641– M
*'831247– M
*'83 91–X M
*8427639'1– M
*'86947–13 M
872'19346– F
*87231'469– F
*8726 91 43'–X M
873'42– F
*876'12–4 F
'87961– F
'9–627 M

*984'13–X F
98'4367– F
*9846'712– M

P. Mixed

*1'234–6 F
312'49–6
*123'476– F
*123'864–9X F
*'127 386–9 M
*'12 783–9 F
*12873'946– M
*132'478– M
*132'478– M
*1326'789–4X F
*13'2748–6 F
*132'78– F
*132'8–4 M
*132'87649– M
*13'428 76–9 M
*139'26–4 M
132'4–6
*1482'36–9 M
*14 9386'27–X F
*17263'48–X F
*'182 374–9 F
182736'4– M
*21'3–98 M
*21'3 487–6 M
21'368–94 F
*213784'6–9 F
31276'84–X
*21378'6–9 M
*2138'467– F
*217'3846– M
*2'17 64 938– F
*217843'69– M
*21786'34– M
*'2183 479– F
231476'89– F
*231'64789– F
*231'76498– F
*23'178– F
*2317846'–9 F
*237148'6–9 F
*23'71486–9 F
*2371'86– M
*23741'86–9 M
2378461'– F
*24738'6– F
26'4378–
*2613'7489– F
*26'8749– M
*2'713846– F
*2718364'–9 M
*271836'4–9 F
*27'38146– M
*273'8146–9 M
*2783'146– F
28713'6–9
*27831'46– F
32 1764'8–9

*278316'– F
28713'6–9
*278'3194– F
*27'98631– F
*2813746'9– F
*28371'469– F
28713'6–9
*283764'1–9 F
312784'6–9
*2843716'–9 F
*'28674– F
*2871346'– M
*28713'6–9 F
*287'1463–9 M
*287164'39– M
*3'1247–6 F
*312'478–9 M
*31'2478– F
3'427 816–
*312'48769– F
*312'49–6 F
*31'26–9 F
*31'2684–9 F
*312748'6–9 F
*31'27 48 69– F
*'3127 64–9 F
*31276'84–X F
*312'7849– F
*31'82476– F
*31'92–4 F
*32'1–9647 F
*3217'46–9 M
*32 1764'8–9 F
*32 1786'4– F
*3'27 1684– M
*3'27169– F
*3271'864–9 F
3'427 816– F
*3781269'4– F
312'86749–
*416'9378– F
*'4213– F
4'2367819– F
*427'3819– M
728436'19–
*42'739816– F
*4'276381–9 F
431276'8– M
*4398'7126– F
*46183'792– F
416'9378–
*462378'91– M
*462738'19– F
*4'8193– M
*48'72936– F
*48 761'923–X F
*'489– F
*628'7314– F
*63 12'794– F
*'64–1 M
*6'729–4 M
*'7128–4 F

*718'3942– M
*7'21638–94 F
'7128–4
*'7243– F
*72 846'319– F
*78132'496– F
78'964231– F
86947231'–X
82713'694– M
*82714369'–X F
*827316'94– F
28713'6–9
*8274631'– F
*82769413'–X F
278'3194–
*827'9613– F
28713'6–9
*84'1239– F
'182 374–9
8427639'1– M
86947231'–X F
*872'19346– F
*872361'49– M
*87269'43– F
*873'42– F
*8743261'– F
87231'469–
*876231'49–X F
*'87961– F
*8916'7432– F
*9'1286437– F
*91'823–6 M
*'92178364– F
*98'4367– F

P. Psychas.

*–467823 F
*1723'896– M
*'2–694 F
21387'4–9 F
2173'6489– M
217843'69– M
*21786'34– M
2'1873–9 F
*231'478–9 M
231 6'4897– F
87231'469–
*23417'86–9X F
7284136'–9
23'46871– M
237'1– F
2371'864–9
23'71486–9 F
*23716'84– F
2371'864–9 F
2'6973– M
*2'7–9 M
2718364'–9 M
27314'86–9 M
27381'64– F
2738'1694– F
*273'8614– F

274'136–9 M
27431'86–9 M
27436'189– M
*274'86– M
*278134'69– F
*27'831–9 M
2783'146– F
28713'6–9
27834'61–9 F
*278'3641–9 M
27'831–9
278'436– M
2786'134–9 M
278634'9– M
27'8916– M
*287'361– M
27'831–9
*28763'149– F
312748'6–9 F
31'6472–9 M
32'1–9647 F
*'32768– M
3'867924– F
*4'638 2179– F
472836'91– F
*6842'3791– F
687234'19– F
'6973– M
71'863 29– M
*7'2–148 M
7'23148–69 F
27'438 19–6
*72 318'46– F
7'26814 39– M
72813'46– F
*728'3–96 M
*72831'69– M
72'836–49 F
*7283'614– F
*7284136'–9 F
72841 36'9– M
728413'69– F
27'438 19–6
72'8631– F
7286'43– M
728643'19– M
72864'319– M
*7'2893– F
*732816'4– M
2'7–9
*7328416'– F
*'738 69– F
7812364'9– M
7821346'9– M
*78234'169– M
*78'241–39 M
87261'34–9
782'463–9 F
78 26'4319– F
7842'1936– M
*78'964231– F
86947231'–X

'8147369–X F
*837164'2–X M
*8437'219– F
*'8467 23– M
*86947231'–X F
8716243'9–X M
872'19346– F
87231'469– F
872361'49– M
87261'34–9 F
8'7269–31 F
*8732 61'49– F
87 426'391– M
*987'4316– F

P. React. Depr.

*13'2–9 M
*138 24 79'– F
*163'2894– F
*'193–7 F
*'2–861739 F
2137'86– F
217386'– M
*2'174– F
*'2176–98 43 M
'23–6 F
231'478–9 M
*231'674– F
*'234–9 F
23'47816–9 F
*'2349–7 M
*'237–9X F
*237'1– F
2371'864–9
237'1648– F
*23716'48–9 F
*2371'864–9 F
*23'7416– F
'238749–6
23741'86–9 M
*2'38–1 M
*'238749–6 F
*2416'3789– F
*'24 6783– F
*'247– F
*26'4378– F
*2674'8139– F
*2'6973– M
*27'1–4 M
271348'6–9 M
23741'86–9
*271348'69– M
*27136'84– F
*27138'4–9 M
*27138'46–9 M
*271486'3– M
2731 48'6– F
*2734'16– M
2'73648–1 M
27'36481–9 F
*27381'46– M
2738'1694– F

*27'43– M
27436'189– M
*27'438 19–6 F
*27486'31– F
*27'63489–1 M
27'831–9 M
*27834'61–9 F
*278'436– M
*278'46– F
278634'9– M
*2791'8346– F
*'2794–1X F
*286'3471–9 F
*2867'1493– F
2674'8139–
*28731'694– F
2873614'9– M
287 3641'9– F
*287'61349– F
*28947'613– M
3'12– M
31'24 968– F
*3'126–98 F
*312'78–9 F
312784'6–9 F
31'297– F
*31'42679– F
*31876'249– F
*32178'46–9 F
231'674–
*'34–279 F
*3'4216 78– F
*3'42178– F
3'4216 78–
*'34 286–9 M
*'34 619 278–X F
*37128'46– F
*'3948672– F
*42'3678–9 M
*4268'7–1 F
*43'2167–9 F
*436'821–79 F
'4638– F
472836'91– F
*'49 7231–6 F
*61'83792– F
*624'3819– F
6847'239– F
*6'87214 39– F
*7'23148–69 F
27'438 19–6
'7243– F
72813'46– F
728'3–96 M
*72'8361–9 F
*728'63419– M
*72864'319– M
*72'91384– F
*7'41238–96 M
*74812 36'9– M
*78213649'– M
*782 46–9 F

*'782496– M
*78 2694'31– F
*82'1637–4 M
*8473 216'9– F
*86217'439– F
*869'472– F
*872461'39–X F
*872'4631–9 M
9172 48'36– F
278'14396–

Paranoid

–47 13 M
1'2–96 M
1326'789–4X F
132'87649– M
13'428 76–9 M
1'39428– M
'2–138749 M
21'348–9 M
213'867–9X F
21637'98– F
2'174– F
2'31478–96 M
2317'486–9 F
'234–7168 M
'234–9 F
2'37– M
2371'864–9 F
'238749–6 F
2438'1679– F
'248367–9 M
'26–483 M
26'13748–9 F
264'1783–9 F
26794'183– F
'268 14 37–9X F
'27–9 F
2'71368–9 M
271'3864–9 F
27'463891– F
28647319'–X F
28763'149– F
3128476'–9 F
31'29 46–8 F
3'46271–9 F
3'94681–7 F
'4–19 M
'42367– F
426'78139– M
'427 6389– M
427'8361–9 M
436'28–7X F
4'379– F
4387126'9– F
4'6328– F
46381 27'9– F
4698'713– F
4'8–69 F
48'2973– M
'486– M
'486–9 M

DIAGNOSIS INDEX

489376'21– F
49'68–72 M
'6–29 M
'6327 841–X F
'64–1 M
6423'8719– F
64'97–1 F
68'724– F
'689713– F
'69874–2 F
'7243– F
7284'3916– M
'8124 63– M
8231'4679– F
82467'3–X M
'84 67–13 M
861792'34– F
87126'493– M
'87961– F
87'9642– F
918634'72– F
9'34 168– F
'943–6 F
94'3–7 M
946 87'23– F
9'483–21 M
9'4867–21 F
9'64– F
9'68–2 F
978'46–3 M

Ps. Invol. Melan.

*–47 13 M
*123'497– M
*123'8–94 F
'2183 479–
*'2–47 F
*21837'4– F
'2183 479–
*231476'89– F
*2'37– M
*237'1648– F
*2438'1679– F
*26'13748–9 F
*2'67–1 M
*26'7 13 48–9 F
*'27–9 F
*27'1384–9 M
*27183'64– F
*2731'86–9 M
*2734'681–9 F
27'463891–
*27'36481–9 F
*2738'1694– F
*27'463891– F
*28316'74– F
*28471369'– F
28647319'–X
*2847'1639– M
*28647319'–X F
*286'731–9 M
*'31–468 F
*3'46271–9 F
*'42367– F
*4'2367819– F
*4'6328– F
*46381 27'9– F
'48–7 F
*69'487–X F
*'7–63 F
*72841 36'9– M
*821347'69– M
*8231'4679– F
824761'3–9 M
821347'69–
*8261'7349– F
*826'3714– F
9'–87143 F
*'912–46 F
9'8134–2 F

Ps. M-D., Depr.

*12378'496–X M
*132'76984– M
*1327'869– M
132'76984–
163'2894– F
*'2–138749 M
'2–47 F
*2'1437– F
*2173'6489– M
*217'386– F
*21738'649– M
*2'1873–9 F
*2'31478–96 M
*2'3478– M
2'31478–96
*23'47816–9 F
*23'47 861–9 F
*2371'864–9 F
*23'789461– F
*243817'69– F
*'26–483 M
*2'6743– F
*26794'183– F
*2'687–9 F
*2'71368–9 M
*271'3864–9 F
*271'4836– F
*2731 48'6– F
*27314'86–9 M
*27318'64–9 F
2731 48'6–
*273'6849– F
*27381'64– F
*274'136–9 M
*27431'86–9 M
*27436'18–9 M
*274'3819– M
*276'138–9 F
2'7683–9X M
*2781'364–9 M
*278'14396– F
*278316'4– F
*2783'416–9 F
*278'436–9 F
*2786'314–9 M
*2786'41–9 F
*27'94 836–1 M
*281736'4– F
286'7341– F
*287'61349– F
*2876'341– M
*2876413'9– F
3'142679– F
*'34 1287– F
*'4679–1 F
2'6743–
*489376'21– F
*49'8–6 F
61'83792– F
6'87214 39– F
*68'724– F
*'7183–9X M
'7243– F
*72813'46– F
*72'836–49 F
*728'3614–9 F
728413'69– F
27'438 19–6
*728436'19– M
*7284'3916– M
*72849'63– M
8726'341–9
*7'29618– M
7824136'9–X F
278'14396
'782496– M
*7842136'9– F
49'8–6
*8'26137–9 F
*826743'1–9X F
86217'439– F
*86729'431– F
*87213469'– M
*8726'341–9 M
*8'7269–31 F
*8731'24 96– M
*'93862417– F

Ps. M-D., Manic

–4318976 F
'89–12
*123'4687–X F
*'234–7168 M
*'28349– M
31427896'– F
*'34 69–2 F
*38419'276–X F
*3'94681–7 F
'423– M
*4698'3–2 M
2'73486–
4'82– F
6'98341–7
*'487–6 F
49'3816– F
*49'68–72 M
*6819'473– F
*68'9147– M
*689'47–X F
*6897'2341–X F
*'89–12 F
*9'–128 M
*914'23687– F
94'3–7
*'927–6 F
*9'34 168– F
'94–213 M
*9'4–26 F
*9'4–7231 F
*941'3687– F
*9'4183–67 F
94'3–7
*94'3–7 F
*9'4678321–X F
*9'48–7 F
*9'48–7 M
*9'481–6 M
9'483–21 M
9'486–13 M
*9'4867–21 F
*9486'7–3 F
*9'6478–21 F
*9'68–2 F
*9'68 34–21 M
*978'46–3 M
*9'8–2 F
*98'1463– M
9'8463–X M
*98'467–2 M
*9'867–43 M
*986'721– F

Ps. M-D., Mixed

21376'8–9 M
*231746'89– F
*23178'64–9 F
*2483'7– F
2783'416– F
436'28–7X
*2873'1469– F
*287316'49– F
*31'628 79– M
*'31 84–X F
31'92–4 F
*32'16 7948– F
*412'7386–X M
*4'3726–9 F
*'4386–1 F
2483'7–
*4837926'1– F
*49'87–1 M
*7289'6– M
*76'284– F
*8273641'– F
*841'39267– M
31'628 79–

DIAGNOSIS INDEX

*86239 14'7-X F
87'261439- F
27'98631-
*9'4-672 M
*9'48-237 M
*94'86-7213 M
9'48-237
9'728-1 F
*9'783-2 F
98'4367- F

Ps. Paranoid

-34 M
*-97X F
*1234'678-9 M
*12738'469- M
*'13469- M
*'162394-7 F
*21'368-94 F
*2'31- M
*23178'4-9 M
27836941'-
*2'378146- M
*'243-9 M
'243 71986-X F
*'246879- F
*264781'3- F
*2683'7194- F
*28 371'46-9 F
*'3-2 F
*'36-7184 M
*'4186- F
*42713'98-X M
*'43728-9 M
*'438-9 F
*'439- F
'243 71986-X
*4'6318- F
*468'21 93- F
*4'683271-9 F
*'48-7 F
*'6-7893 F
*648273'19- F
*6'8243-9 F
*6827 413'9- M
*6'8432-79 F
*6'847-1 M
*6897'421- F
*728'4136-9 F
7286'4931-
*7286'4931- F
*'78312469- M
*'789 32- F
*'8671423- M
*8712316'9- M
*9'31-2786 F
*'93184-2 F
*9'4-63 F
*9'41683- F
*9'483-6 M
*9'7826-31 M
*9'84-21 M
*984'6-2 F
9'31-2786

Ps. Postpartum

*'243 71986-X F
2786'41-9 F
286'3471-9 F
6'87214 39- F
6897'421- F
*78 26'4319- F

Ps. Psth.

*-34 M
*1'2-96 M
*1'39428- M
*26871'34- F
*426'78139- M
*4387126'9- F
*497823'61- F
6247'389-
*6247'389- F
*'6327 841-X F
*64'97-1 F
*8721436'9- F
9'4-26 F

Ps. Senile

*2'1786- M
*231'76-9 M
*418'236 79-X M
*9'-87143 F

Ps. Sz., Cat.

*21387'4-9 F
*23'46871- M
274'86- M
*287 3641'9- F
*'3482697- F
*'463-2 F
*48'2973- M
*6'87-319 F
*'69874-2 F
*7'2689-4 M
*728134'96- M
*72'84-1 M
*7'4231-9 M
728134'96-
*8269'7143- M
*82746'3 19- M
*8'372164-X F
*'86143-7 M
*897612'43-X M
*'9-1843 F
*9'728-1 F

Ps. Sz., Hebe.

*148372'69- M
*213'86-9 M
*3'81624-9X M
'467- F
76'284-
*'6-29 M
*69'48 123- F
*81934'726- F
*8613'472- F
*89'4 137-6 M

Ps. Sz., Mixed

*271348'6-9 M
23741'86-9
2783'416- F
436'28-7X
*27'8916- M
34817 62'9- F
*'4-19 M
*427'8361-9 M
*'43816- M
'4-19
'48 12- M
*'486-9 M
*4872361'9-X F
*49'8716-3 M
*6'89-3127 F
*82467'3-X M
*861792'34- F
*87246'139- M
*87264'39- F
*8927631'4-X M
'4-19
*9'84-631 M
*9'8463-X M
9846'712- M

Ps. Sz., Paranoid

*-9164387 M
-97X F
*123'6874-9 F
'2-694 F
*213'87-94 M
*213876'4-9 F
23178'64-9 F
*2381'476-9 F
819'6327-
'243 71986-X F
*24'87-9 M
*27836941'- M
*2831'76- F
28 371'46-9 F
*'2874-69 M
2876413'9- F
*'29-41 M
*316 478'29- F
*4'23781-9 F
4'29 867- F
4'3178296- M
31'4782-
*4'6287- M
*468'23- M
*'469328- F
*'479 38- M
*'48 13 2679-X M
4'82- F
6'98341-7
*48 267'3-9 M
*'4983- M
*6287'4319-X M
*634'12- F
*'637814- F
*'6483-92 F
*6'48319- M
6'8432-79 F
*68472'31- F
*6879'43-2 M
*'689- M
68'9147- M
*68'9147- M
*6'98341-7 F
*728 61'34- M
*'746-139 F
*'7684 23-9 M
728 61'34-
*7842316'9- M
*'8147369-X F
*819'6327- F
826'3714- F
*827631'4- M
*8'4172- M
*84 72 13'69- F
'849-273 M
*86 1'23479-X F
8612473'9- F
*867 423'19- M
*8679241'3-X M
*86'97234- M
869'724-3X M
*8726413'9- M
*89'76-3 M
*'9-12837 F
*91'87342- M
9'31-2786 F
*9'348- M
*'94-213 M
*9'43-71 28 M
*9'43-78 M
9'43-71 28
*9'678-231 M
*9'68-271X M
*9'84-13 M
9'43-71 28
*9'87 462- M

Ps. Sz., Simple

132'4786-9 F
132'6784-9 F
*'163-97 M
*18236'74- M
*182736'4-9X M
187326'49- M
*21'348-9 M
*218 47'369- M
*2318'746-X M
23'7416- F
'238749-6
248371'6- M
2'64871- F
61'83792-

DIAGNOSIS INDEX

'268 14 37–9X F
*'27–3 F
278'14396– F
*2786'134–9 M
*2873614'9– M
312'478–9 M
*'4–96 M
*4'31867– M
*436'28–7X F
'46–9 M
*467'839– M
*486'972–1 F
*4'9678–132 F
*49'872–3X F
61'83792– F
*68213 794'–X F
*782134'6–9 M
*7824136'9–X F
278'14396–
*78'2693–4 M
*827'4– M
*84'769–13X M
*'86–3 F
*86497'1– F
*86721'93–X M
*87126'493– M
89762'413–X M
*946 87'23– F
*9'478–3X M
*9'8–26 M

Ps. Toxic

23'789461– F
*27381'4– F
*274981 36'–X M
'3–6X M
*3'12487– F
*3'2 697–8 F
412'7386–X M
*4'2–6X M
*'4629–X M
7'2689–4 M
*9'132–678 M
*9'246378– M
*'9287143– M
'9346– M
*98'4672–31 M

Schizoid

12738'469– M
12873'946– M
13'428 76–9 M
'183 49–6 M
*'2–63 M
213'867–9X F
'217836–9 F
*'23178–9X F
24'876193– F
2'687–9 F
*27138'46–X M
2718364'–9 M
271836'4–9 F
*27'31846–X M
2734'816– M
273'8146–9 M
*'276–9 M
2'7683–9X M
278'46– F
*27861'3–9X M
'28349– M
*2'83674– F
2871346'– M
287'1463–9 M
287'361– M
27'831–9
28763'149– F
*287'9136– M
31'2648– F
31'2684–9 F
31'2876–9 M
3'2 697–8 F
*'348791–2 M
38'46172– M
'4–792X F
42381'796– F
4398'7126– F
4'8–69 F
4827'963– M
48'72936– F
'489– M
489376'21– F
49'3816– F
49'8–6 F
*648'7923– F
6842'3791– F
7'23418 69– M
7284'3916– M
*728'4963– F
7286'43– M
*728643'19– M
7289'6– M
78'241–39 M
87261'34–9
78 26'4319– F
78 2694'31– F
826743'1–9X F
8274631'– F
82769413'–X F
278'3194–
8427639'1– M
'84 67–13 M
'8467 23– M
*846792'31–X M
'8671423– M
8'672–3 M
86732'41– F
867 49'321– M
872461'39–X F
872'4631–9 M
876'12–4 F
876231'49–X F
87'9642– F
8916'7432– F
9'1286437– F
918634'72– F
9'481–6 M
9'4867–21 F
9486'7–3 F
9'68–2 F
984'13–X F

Suicidal

–72 F
1234876'–9 M
124'379– M
1326'78–X F
1'32978– M
21387'4–9 F
2'1437– F
2'174– F
231'478–9 M
231746'89– F
2317846'–9 F
237148'6–9 F
23'71486–9 F
23716'48–9 F
'243 71986– X F
243817'69– F
'24 6783– F
2'6743– F
27'1–4 M
2'713846– F
271'3864–9 F
27183'64– F
27'36 184– M
273'6849– F
27381'64– F
276'138–9 F
27'831–9 M
278316'4– F
278'3194– F
27834'61–9 F
27836941'– M
278'436–9 F
2786'41–9 F
27'8916– M
2791'8346– F
28471369'– F
28647319'–X
2847'1639– M
286'3471–9 F
28647319'–X F
286'731–9 M
2873'1469– F
2876'341– M
28947'613– M
31248'7– F
31'29 46–8 F
31'42679– F
31'628 79– M
31876'249– F
'34–279 F
34817 62'9– F
37128'46– F
3721 486'– F
4'2–6X M
4217'83–9 M
423'8967– F
427'8361–9 M
436'821–79 F
'4386–1 F
2483'7–
'439– F
'243 71986–X
467'839– M
47 6'2381– F
48'2973– M
4837926'1– F
4862'7931– F
4872361'9–X F
4'9678–132 F
6247'389– F
6'2748–1 M
'689713– F
'69372– F
'7–63 F
'7243– F
728'3614–9 F
728436'19– M
728 61'34– M
72864'319– M
7'29618– M
76'284– F
'7684 23–9 M
728 61'34–
78234'169– M
7842136'9– F
49'8–6
78'964231– F
86947231'–X
817296'34–X F
81934'726– F
82'1637–4 M
824 173'96– M
826743'1–9X F
82746'3 19– M
827631'4– M
82769413'–X F
278'3194–
841'39267– M
31'628 79–
'84672– F
847'2639– F
8473 216'9– F
86947231'–X F
8714263'9–X M
8721436'9– F
8'7269–31 F
874231'96–X F
8742'6913– F
89'476– M
9'–87143 F
'93862417– F
9'4–26 F
94'86–213 F
9'8–7 F
9'8726–X F

DIAGNOSIS INDEX

Twins

14 9386'27–X F
No profile for twin

2731 48'6– F
Twin: 72'91384–X F

'486– M
No profile for twin

4896'271–X F
No profile for twin

64'8297–1X F
No profile for twin

72'91384–X F
Twin: 2731 48'6– F

8'372164–X M
No profile for twin

Mf Index

This index gives the master codes of cases that obtained deviant Mf scores. Note that the master code is given here, but the deviant Mf may have been obtained on a secondary MMPI. One must turn to the indicated summary to match the deviant Mf with its proper code. A number in parentheses after the code indicates how many deviant Mf scores occur in the MMPI profiles for that case.

40 and under

1'2–96 M
'13248–9 M
'1482– M
21637'98– F
2173'6489– M
21738'649– M
231'674– F
237148'6–9 F
2416'3789– F
2'71368–9 M
2731 48'6–(2) F
278316'4–(2) F
27834'61–9 F
278'46– F
28647319'–X (2) F
28713'6–9 (3) F
312748'6–9 F
'3246–9 M
'329418– F
3'427 816–(2) F
'348791–2 M
3'867924– F
4268'7–1 F
4'276381–9 F
436'28–7X (2) F
462738'19–(2) F
4'6328–(2) F
4'8–263 M
4'8193– M
48'72936– F
49'68–72 M
49'8–6 (2) F
62487'3– F
634'12– F
64'97–1 F
69'487–X F
72 846'319– F
728'4963–(2) F
7'29618– M
7328416'– F
8'26137–9 F
8473 216'9– F
'8479–2 M
86729'431– F
'86947–13 M
8732 61'49– F
876231'49–X F
9'34 168– F
941'3687– F
9'43–71 28 (3) M
9'8–26 M
9'84–631 M
984'67–312 M

65–69

–34 M
–467823 F
12'639–84 M
12738'469– M
'1382–9X F
14'38 267– M
'162394–7 (2) F
182736'4– M
187326'49– M
'21346–8 M
217386'– M
21786'34– M
218 47'369– M
231476'89– F
2'31478–96 M
2318'746–X M
23'46871– M
2371'86– M
23741'86–9 (2) M
2'378146– M
'247– F
2471'9638– M
'248367–9 M
2'687–9 F
26'8749– M
27'31846–X (2) M
2734'16– M
273'8146–9 M
2746'1983– M
'276–9 M
2'7683–9X M
27836941'– M
278'436– M
278634'9– M
'2794–1X F
'28349– M
28647319'–X F
286'731–9 M
287 3641'9– F
'294–6 F
'31–47 F
31'2648– F
31'628 79– M
'32768– M
'4–19 M
'423– M
42'3678–9 M
423871'96– F
4'263–19 M
'428 136– F
'46–9 M
4'6287– M
46872'319– M
4'72693–1 M
476'82193– M
'478–13 M
'48 13 2679–X M
48 267'3–9 M
4827'963– M
'487–6 F
48 761'923–X F
'6–7149X F
624'3819–(2) F
628'7314– F
6847291'3–(2) M
687234'19– F
687'249–1X F
71'863 29– M
72168'934– M
728'3–96 M
72831'96– M
728643'19– M
72864'319– M
'738 69– F
'746–139 F
781236'4–9 M
78213649'– M
782149'36– M
7842316'9– M
827631'4– M
8427'936–X M
8679241'3–X M
86794'23–1X M
872361'49– M
872'4631–9 M
87264'39– F
873'42– F
9'–128 M
'9–1843 F
'96–14 M
9'678–231 M
9'876–213 M

70–74

–72 F
13'2–9 M
'13469– M
'182 374–9 F
182736'4– M
1938'742–X F
'2–47 F
21'387–9 F
23'46871– M
2'37– M
2'378146– M
2'38–1 M
238'7146– F
27138'4–9 M
2'73486– M
274'86– M
27'831–9 M
2786'134–9 M
27'8916– M
2'83674– F
2847'1639– M
'2874–69 M

Mf INDEX

312'86749– F
31'628 79– M
32'1–9647 F
38'46172– M
39'4 287 16– M
'423–69 F
426'78139– M
4'6–132 F
487'236–9 M
'4892– F
4'8937– M
'4936– M
'4983– M
6'2748–1 M

628'7314– F
6287'4319–X M
'69874–2 F
728436'19– M
78234'169– M
'789 32– F
837164'2–X M
'84672– F
8'612 394–7 M
867 49'321– M
869'472– F
9'–128 M
'9–12837 F
'912–46 F

'9287143– M
'9346– M
9'4–26 F
98'4367– F

75 and over

'2–694 F
2318'746–X M
2'73486– M
2'73648–1 M
27'831–9 (2) M
27'94 836–1 M
431276'8– M
462378'91–(2) M

4'683271–9 F
46'83721– M
72168'934– M
78234'169– M
8712346'9–(2) M
871'236 49– M
8'7269–31 F
8726 91 43'–X M
874231'96–X F
87 426'391– M
9'–128 M
'9–13 M

L Index

This index gives the master codes of cases that obtained deviant L scores. Note that the master code is given here, but the deviant L may have been obtained on a secondary MMPI. One must turn to the indicated summary to match the deviant L with its proper code. A number in parentheses after the code indicates how many deviant L scores occur in the MMPI profiles for that case.

L 7

123'497– M
12'38467–9 M
12386'7– M
132'478–(2) M
13'24867– F
132'76984– M
132'8749–6 M
13'49287– F
1'37246– F
1'378– F
13'82 4967– F
14'82739– M
'162394–7 F
'182 374–9 F
182736'4– M
'193–7 F
'2–47 (2) F
'2–63 M
213'768– F
213'87–94 M
213876'4–9 F
21738'649– M
2'1783–9 M
'2183 479–(2) F
'2183 479– F
218'63–79 M
231'478–9 M
2'31478–96 M
231'64789– F
2317'486–9 F
23'178– F
'234–9 F
23'46871– M
2'37– M
237148'6–9 F
2371'86– M
23'789461– F
'243 71986–X F
2467'3819– M
'246879– F
248371'6– M
26'4378– F
26'7 13 48–9 F
2671'4398– F
271'4836– F
273'8614–(2) F
27486'31– F
276'138–9 (2) F
2781'364–9 M
278316'4– F
27836941'– M
28647319'–X F
2873614'9–(2) M
287'61349– F
287'9136– M
'31–47 F
'31–87962 F
3'12– M
312'478–9 M
312'48769– F
31267'894– F
3128476'–9 F
31'29 46–8 F
'31428–6 F
'34 1287– F
'34 286–9 M
3'46271–9 F
3'491 68– M
37128'46– F
'376842–1 (2) F
'38–46 M
3816724'9– F
'413–9 F
413872'69– F
'4186– F
4'2367819– F
42381'796–(2) F
43'2167–9 F
4'379– F
4387126'9– F
'463–2 F
4'638 2179– F
46'98–13 M
48139'672– F
48276'31– F
'486– M
4869'1372– M
48'726– M
49'3816– F
'498 73–2 M
'6–7893 F
63 12'794– F
634'12– F
64'97–1 F
6874'23 91–X F
'7–63 F
7'2689–4 M
7284136'–9 F
728'4963– F
72'8631– F
78146 32'9– M
782134'6–9 M
782149'36– M
'782 46–9 F
'7893–2 M
'789 32– F
82'1637–4 M
8261'7349– F
826'3714– F
8279'641– M
8473 216'9– F
861792'34– F
873'42– F
8742'1369– F
89'476– M
'9–1843 F
'912–46 F
91'87342– M
'9346– M
9'8–2 F

L 8

1'2–96 M
12'3467–98 F
1234876'–9 M
123'497– M
123'6874–9 F
132'4–6 M
13'2478–69 M
132'478–9 M
132'4786–9 F
'13248–9 M
1326'78–X F
132'78– F
'1482– M
148372'69– M
231'76–9 M
23 1786'–9 F
237148'6–9 F
2378461'– F
'2379–4 F
238'7146– F
243817'69– F
2671'4398– F
2674'8139– F
26794'183– F
27'31846–X M
2731'846–9 M
27381'64– F
274'3819– M
278'436–9 F
2786'134–9 M
2786'314–9 M
286'3471–9 F
286'7341– F
'3–2 F
'31–87962 F
31'246–9 F
3'1247–6 F
312'49–6 F
31'26874– F
312786'4–9 F
314'892– F
31'96728–4 F
321'47–9 (2) F
'34 286–9 M
37128'46– F
'4–19 (2) M
418'236 79–X M
42 186'73–9 F
'42367– F

L INDEX

F Index

This index gives the master codes of cases that obtained deviant F scores. Note that the master code is given here, but the deviant F may have been obtained on a secondary MMPI. One must turn to the indicated summary to match the deviant F with its proper code. A number in parentheses after the code indicated how many deviant F scores occur in the MMPI profiles for that case.

12–15

1234'678–9 M
1234876'–9 M
'1482– M
148372'69– M
14 9386'27–X F
17263'48–X F
'182 374–9 F
187326'49– M
217386'– M
2378461'– F
243817'69– F
2483'7– F
2674'8139–(2) F
27138'4–9 M
27138'46–X M
2718364'–9 M
273'8614– F
274981 36'–X M
278'3194– F
278'436–9 F
27'98631– F
2846731'9– M
28647319'–X F
28713'6–9 F
287164'39– M
287316'49– F
287'61349– F
28763'149– F
2876'341– M
287'9136– M
28947'613– M
31276'84–X F
314'892– F
3721 486'– F
3816724'9– F
'42896–13 M
468'21 93– F
46'89317– F
4'817326–9 F
4872361'9–X F
48'7391– F
492'3671– M
627'8139– M
68213 794'–X F
6827 413'9– M
68472'31– F
6847291'3– M
6'87–319 F
687234'19– F
6'89–3127 F
68'9147– M
6897'421– F
'69874–2 F
72 846'319– F
728643'19– M
72864'319–(2) M
781236'4–9 M
782134'6–9 M
78 26'4319– F
8123 764– F
819'6327– F
821347'69– M
8261'7349– F
8269'7143– F
8273641'– F
827631'4– M
8279'641– M
8'372164–X F
84639'712– M
8473 216'9– F
'8479–2 M
'86–3 F
8'612 394–7 M
8612473'9– F
861792'34– F
86497'1– F
86729'431– F
86732'41– F
867 423'19– M
867 49'321– M
8712346'9– M
87213469'– M
8721436'9–(2) F
87231'469– F
872361'49– M
87246'139– M
872'4631–9 M
87264'39– F
87269'43– F
872'96134–(2) F
8732 61'49– F
8742'1369– F
87 426'391– M
8742'6913– F
879 46'2– M
894'671– F
9'31–2786 F
9'428 673– M
9'48–237 (2) M
9'68–271X M
978'46–3 M
9'8134–2 F
98'1463– M
98'4367– F
98'467–2 M
984'67–312 (2) M
9846'712–(2) M

16 and above

14 9386'27–X F
17829'634–X M
182736'4–9X M
2'31478–96 M
249'7836–X M
27138'46–X M
274981 36'–X M
278134'69– F
278'14396– F
278'3194– F
27836941'– M
28647319'–X F
'3482697–(2) F
'4–19 M
4872361'9–X F
48 761'923–X F
4896'271–X F
64'8297–1X F
68213 794'–X F
687'249–1X F
6874'23 91–X F
689'47–X F
6897'2341–X F
69'487–X F
817296'34–X F
821347'69– M
82467'3–X M
826743'1–9X F
82714369'–X F
837164'2–X M
8427'936–X M
846792'31–X (2) M
84'769–13X M
86 1'23479–X F
86239 14'7–X F
86721'93–X M
8679241'3–X M
867942'13–X M
86794'23–1X M
86947231'–X F
869'724–3X M
871'236 49– M
8714263'9–X M
8716243'9–X M
872461'39–X F
87264'39– F
8726 91 43'–X M
874231'96–X F
8742'6913– F
876231'49–X F
896'2741–3X M
897612'43–X (2) M
89762'413–X M
9'483–21 M
984'13–X F
9'8726–X M

K Index

This index gives the master codes of cases that obtained deviant K scores. Note that the master code is given here, but the deviant K may have been obtained on a secondary MMPI. One must turn to the indicated summary to match the deviant K with its proper code. A number in parentheses after the code indicates how many deviant K scores occur in the MMPI profiles for that case.